Diseases
of the Skin

ELSEVIER CD-ROM LICENSE AGREEMENT

Second Edition

Diseases
of the Skin
a Color Atlas and Text

Gary M. White MD
Chief
Department of Dermatology
Kaiser Permanente Medical Group
San Diego, California, USA

Neil H. Cox BSc FRCP
Consultant Dermatologist
Cumberland Infirmary
Carlisle, UK

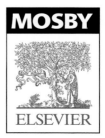

MOSBY

ELSEVIER

MOSBY
ELSEVIER

Mosby is an affiliate of Elsevier Inc

© 2000, Harcourt Publishers Limited
© 2006, Elsevier Inc. All rights reserved.

First edition 2000
Second edition 2006

ISBN 0323029973

British Library Cataloguing in Publication Data
A catalogue record for this book is available from the British Library

Library of Congress Cataloging in Publication Data
A catalog record for this book is available from the Library of Congress

Notice
Medical knowledge is constantly changing. Standard safety precautions must be followed, but as new research and clinical experience broaden our knowledge, changes in treatment and drug therapy may become necessary or appropriate. Readers are advised to check the most current product information provided by the manufacturer of each drug to be administered to verify the recommended dose, the method and duration of administration, and contraindications. It is the responsibility of the practitioner, relying on experience and knowledge of the patient, to determine dosages and the best treatment for each individual patient. Neither the Publisher nor the author assume any liability for any injury and/or damage to persons or property arising from this publication. **The Publisher**

Printed in China
Last digit is the print number: 9 8 7 6 5 4 3 2 1

Working together to grow
libraries in developing countries

www.elsevier.com | www.bookaid.org | www.sabre.org

ELSEVIER   BOOK AID International   Sabre Foundation

Commissioning Editor: *Sue Hodgson/Karen Bowler*
Project Development Manager: *Hilary Hewitt*
Project Manager: *Rory MacDonald*
Design Manager: *Jayne Jones*
Illustration Manager: *Mick Ruddy*
Illustrator: *Marion Tasker*
Marketing Managers (UK/USA): *Amy Hey/Megan Carr*

Contents

Preface

As with the first edition of this text, we have aimed to provide a comprehensive book that should have value for practitioners at many levels of dermatological knowledge; including dermatologists and their trainees, primary care or generalists and their trainees, as well as medical students. We have retained the main features of a detailed text and copious high quality illustrations. The more common disorders now benefit from a larger selection of pictures demonstrating the range of presentations and variations of any one disorder.

Each chapter opening now has a new box feature outlining the topics discussed and the sequence and hierarchy of headings. Many chapters are complete in themselves, but to avoid excessive duplication across chapters, we have used extensive cross-referencing. However, in other instances there are some topics that are briefly discussed in more than one place in order that relevant disorders can be covered within a specific chapter. The new CD-ROM that accompanies the book will also augment the ability to search for specific disorders in the text or as illustrations.

The overall layout is similar to the first edition but we have replaced about 30% of the pictures, including several new line illustrations. There are three new chapters that provide an overview of topical, systemic and physical therapies. Within each chapter we have again concentrated on diagnosis and management, but have added new information about pathogenesis to many sections. We have also specifically added major sections on differential diagnosis, with much more extensive use of bullet points and tables to explain features that favor one diagnosis over another. We have also summarized some salient diagnostic and therapeutic issues in the format of boxed 'Practice Points'; many of these highlighting common diagnostic dilemmas or therapeutic pitfalls. We hope that all of these changes will prove useful to the reader and will increase the reference value of the text.

Although most of the images are our own, as in the first edition we owe a great debt to those who have allowed us to use photographs of their patients. Individual contributors are acknowledged in the relevant figure legends, but special thanks go to Bill Paterson, Cliff Lawrence, Nick Reynolds, Mary Carr, Chris Stevenson, Tanya Foreman, Dale Collins, Raj Natarajan, Sheena Russell, Belinda Stanley, Elisabeth Higgins, Stephen Ducatman, Theodore Sebastian, Michael Murphy, Gerald Weinstein, Gary Cole, James Steger, Graham Putnam, James Rasmussen, Angelito Arias, Leo Barco, Ian Coulson and Goutam Dawn.

We would also like to thank all those at Elsevier who have been involved at various stages with this project, including Sue Hodgson, Hilary Hewitt, Charlotte Mossop, Shuet-Kei Cheung, Karen Bowler and Rory MacDonald. We would not have achieved this project without the support of our families, Gwen, Olivia and Benjamin White, and Fiona, David and Kathy Cox – they all deserve a special vote of thanks.

Gary M. White and Neil H. Cox

1 Fundamental Dermatology and Terminology

INTRODUCTION

Diagnosis of a skin disease and treatment of the patient, as with any other disorder, requires an appropriate clinical history and examination, supported where necessary by investigations. These issues are discussed in Chapter 2. However, before considering these issues, it is useful to be aware of some aspects of the basic anatomy of the skin, as this is an important factor in determining the clinical features that are observed. It is also helpful to understand the terminology that is applied to skin lesions or eruptions. An accurate description of the features using appropriate terminology is important to provide a useful clinical record, and particularly to convey a clear picture of the problem for those patients who require referral or discussion with colleagues.

BASIC STRUCTURE OF THE SKIN

The skin is a large and complex organ, which fulfills a number of important functions. In addition to the obvious physical barrier and sensory functions, it is also important as a barrier to harmful chemicals, ultraviolet (UV) radiation, and infection; is important for temperature regulation and sweating; and is required for vitamin D production. Alterations in structure and function will be described in disease-oriented chapters, the aim of this section being simply to provide a brief overview of the components of skin where these are important for understanding the physical signs of skin lesions.

The skin consists of the following.
- Epidermis—the external, cellular zone.
- Dermis—a fibrous layer that includes the blood supply to the skin.
- Subcutaneous fat—this lies deep to the skin but is often involved in pathologic processes that affect it.

These different zones and structures within them are shown in Figure 1.1 (cross-sections of the skin are conventionally illustrated in the same way that histologic sections are usually examined, with the epidermis at the top and fat at the bottom). There is a sharp interface between epidermis and dermis, which follows a pattern of downward projections known as rete pegs and is seen in cross-section as a wavy line. This interface, the dermo–epidermal junction, is the site of many important pathologic processes. Components of the different parts of skin are now discussed.

Epidermis

This, the external part of the skin, is composed mainly of keratinocytes. The basal layer of keratinocytes is an actively dividing cell population, from which the cells gradually move outward through the epidermis (upward in Fig. 1.1) while undergoing a gradual loss of nuclear material

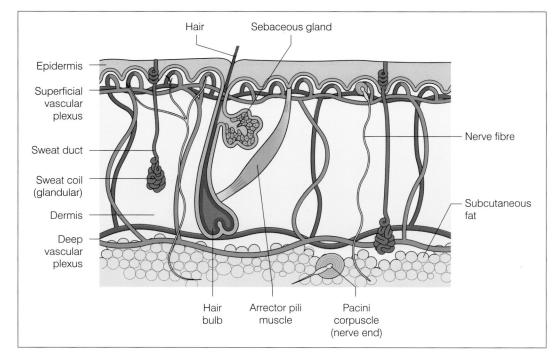

Figure 1.1 Structure of the skin. (After an original drawing by Dr. N. H. Cox.)

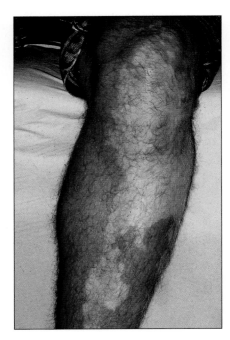

Figure 1.2 Vitiligo: a macular lesion with color change but no palpable component. (From Lawrence CM, Cox NH. Physical Signs in Dermatology, 2nd edn. London: Mosby, 2002.)

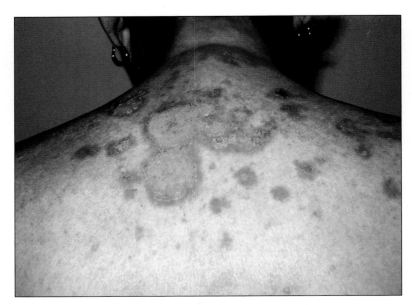

Figure 1.3 Plaques, in this case due to subacute cutaneous lupus erythematosus. These could be further described as having annular accentuation, scaling, and some central atrophy. (Courtesy of Dr. G. Dawn.)

and accumulation of keratin proteins. This maturation process creates cells with different morphology through the epidermis, from the basal cells through to the stratum corneum, as discussed here.

Basal layer

The basal layer consists of cells with rather basophilic cytoplasm and perpendicular orientation in relation to the basement membrane zone. Under normal circumstances, mitotic activity of keratinocytes is confined to this layer and produces an epidermal turnover time of about 4 weeks. In some hyperproliferative disease states, and in neoplasia, mitoses occur at other parts of the epidermis; in psoriasis, for example, the epidermal turnover is about 10-fold faster than normal, and suprabasal mitosis occurs. In neoplastic lesions, mitoses are not only increased but are often morphologically abnormal.

Situated among the basal keratinocytes are the melanocytes, which produce melanin pigment; in histologic sections of normal skin, the ratio of basal keratinocytes to melanocytes is about 10:1. Additionally, but not readily visible in routine histologic sections, the basal layer contains specialized sensory cells known as Merkel cells.

Stratum spinosum

Above the basal layer is the prickle cell layer (stratum spinosum), characterized by polyhedral cells with prominent intercellular attachments. These become more obvious in conditions of intraepidermal edema such as eczema; this causes separation of the cells, which (at least initially) remain attached to each other by their desmosal attachments, thus exaggerating the prickle or spinous appearance. Within this layer, in the suprabasal region, are specialized antigen-presenting cells involved in contact hypersensitivity, known as Langerhans cells.

Stratum granulosum

The stratum spinosum gradually merges into the granular cell layer, in which the cells lose their nuclei and acquire dense keratohyalin granules. Alterations to this layer occur in some ichthyoses, and in lichen planus it is increased in thickness.

Stratum corneum

Finally, there is an acellular layer of horizontally oriented keratin fibrils, which make up the stratum corneum, and which have an important protective barrier function. All layers of the epidermis show quite prominent body site variation, but the stratum corneum, in particular, can vary from very thin (at flexural sites) to extremely thick (on palms and soles). The outer layer of stratum corneum is constantly shed as small scales, a process that is increased dramatically in hyperproliferative

disorders and other epidermal disease states. Scaling is frequently abnormal in morphology or degree in inflammatory dermatoses.

Skin appendages

The hair follicles, apocrine glands, and sweat apparatus are specialized epidermal structures that extend down into the dermis. The larger and coarser hair follicles of the scalp and beard extend into the subcutaneous fat (an important issue in surgery of hair-bearing skin, as transecting hairs in the dermis will create areas of alopecia). The size, density, and morphology of the hair follicles vary at different body sites.

Follicular epithelium may be involved along with the interfollicular epidermis in some disease states, but hair follicles and other appendages also have their own pathology (e.g. skin appendage neoplasia), and may even be relatively spared by some epidermal disease (e.g. the intra-epidermal part of the sweat duct is relatively spared in actinic keratoses). Alterations from normal structure and function of these specialized structures will be discussed in specific disease chapters.

Basement membrane zone and dermo–epidermal junction

The basement membrane zone (BMZ), where epidermis and dermis join, is a very important site containing a number of novel proteins and structures. Immediately below the epidermal cells is an electron-lucent region known as the lamina lucida. Crossing this are anchoring filaments from the hemidesmosomes of the basal cells above, to the lamina lucida below. In turn, anchoring fibrils extend down from the lamina densa into the papillary dermis.

This zone is important, as it is a site of inflammation in several diseases, most notably in certain immunobullous disorders in which autoantibody-mediated reactions occur (e.g. bullous pemphigoid involves antibodies against the bullous pemphigoid antigen); the structural components of the BMZ are discussed in more detail in the context of this group of diseases (Ch. 16). Any of these structures may also be affected by mutations leading to congenital defects, for example the epidermolysis bullosa group of blistering disorders. The BMZ is also important in skin neoplasia, the ability to broach this region being the factor that distinguishes 'in situ' from invasive tumors, and which has prognostic significance.

Dermis

This is the fibrous part of the skin, which provides strength. It contains collagen and elastic fibers that are arranged within an amorphous ground substance, all of which are produced by spindle-shaped fibroblasts. Each of the structural components may be present in abnormal amounts in some disease states (Chs 11 and 22). The upper dermis, around the downward-

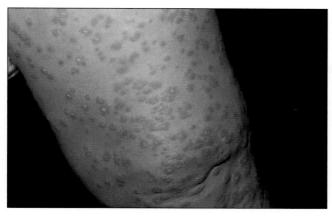

Figure 1.4 Papules, in this case due to a condition called Gianotti–Crosti syndrome. There are multiple small dome-shaped lesions with some central umbilication. (From Lawrence CM, Cox NH. Physical Signs in Dermatology, 2nd edn. London: Mosby, 2002.)

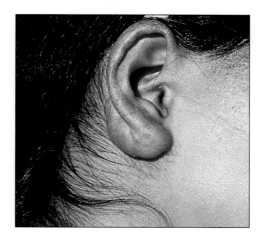

Figure 1.5 An example of a nodule, in this case a keloid on the earlobe secondary to ear piercing. (From Lawrence CM, Cox NH. Physical Signs in Dermatology, 2nd edn. London: Mosby, 2002.)

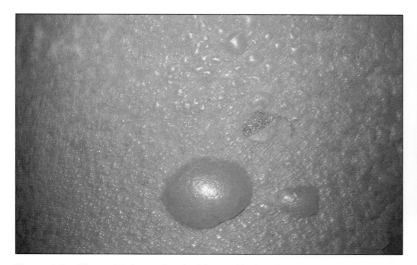

Figure 1.6 Blister: this is a unilocular blister with clear fluid content in a patient with toxic epidermal necrolysis (see also Chs 16 and 18). Intact blisters are relatively uncommon in this condition.

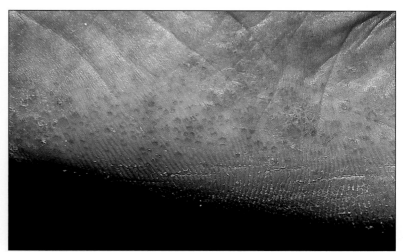

Figure 1.7 Multiple small vesicles, in this case from pompholyx.

projecting epidermal rete ridges, is known as the papillary dermis and has a looser structure than that of the deeper, reticular dermis.

The dermis has a prominent blood supply with interconnecting, horizontally oriented deep and superficial plexuses, and capillary loops projecting vertically in the papillary dermis. By contrast, the epidermis and its specialized structures acquire nutrients by diffusion, as they have no direct blood supply; thus bleeding into the skin must imply some involvement of the dermis in the pathologic process. Capillary vessels are prominent around the follicles and glandular structures. In inflammatory conditions, blood-derived lymphocytes and polymorphonuclear leukocytes enter the dermis from these vessels, and therefore often have a predominantly perivascular localization.

Also within the dermis are nerve fibers and some specialized nerve-end sensory organs.

Subcutaneous fat

This layer has importance in heat conservation and as an energy store. It is divided into lobules by fibrous septae, which contain the blood supply; the layer as a whole is relatively avascular, although some large vessels traverse it to the deep dermal plexus. This organization of vessels and septae in the fat has pathologic diagnostic significance, as some processes affect the fat throughout the lobules (such as damage by lipase in pancreatitis), whereas others affect predominantly the septal region (e.g. vasculitic processes).

TERMINOLOGY OF SKIN LESIONS

Examination of the skin is described in Chapter 2. However, to usefully record the features identified on examination, it is important to understand some of the clinicopathologic correlates of the abnormalities that may be found, and to know the terminology for the shapes and patterns of skin lesions.

Lesion morphology and surface features

This section describes the fundamental types of skin lesions (known as the primary lesions) that may occur in various disease states. Many of these can be qualified further by various descriptions of their shape, color, surface changes, and arrangement overall. For example, in a typical case of lichen planus the papules (primary lesion) could be further described as grouped, purplish, flat-topped, and slightly scaly.

Primary skin lesions
Macules and patches
These are flat, discrete areas of altered color (Fig. 1.2). In some instances, such as lentigo (increase in number of basal melanocytes), there may be fine surface scaling as a secondary phenomenon (presumably due to disturbance of the basal keratinocytes by the increased melanocyte density). Authors vary in the size cut-off between a macule (smaller) and a patch, with definitions ranging between 1- and 2-cm size limits. As such definitions are arbitrary and of no particular biological significance, it is more helpful to record the actual size.

Plaques
These are elevated lesions, predominantly flat-topped but palpable (Fig. 1.3). There is more potential for variable surface features (e.g. smooth, scaly, and crusted) than in a macule; surface features are discussed in more detail later in this chapter.

Papules and nodules
These are raised and essentially dome-shaped lesions (Figs 1.4 and 1.5). As with macules and patches, there are variable size cut-offs between papules

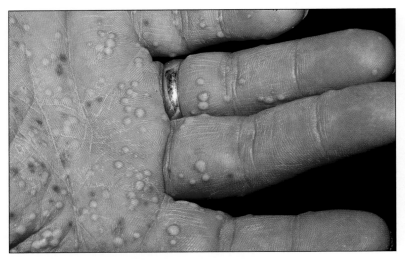

Figure 1.8   Pustules: multiple yellow pustules on the palm of the hand, in this case due to acute palmoplantar pustulosis. This should be compared with the more common chronic palmoplantar pustulosis (discussed in the context of psoriasis, Ch. 7), in which the pustules are more variable in size and in stages of evolution.

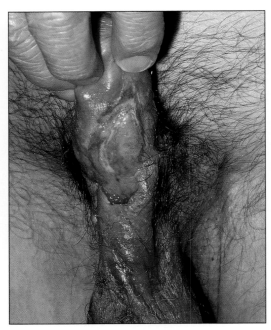

Figure 1.9   Ulcers: defects through the epidermis reveal underlying dermis or fat. This ulceration of penis was probably due to Behçet disease, although the patient did not fulfill criteria for the diagnosis, as he had no oral ulcers (see Ch. 14).

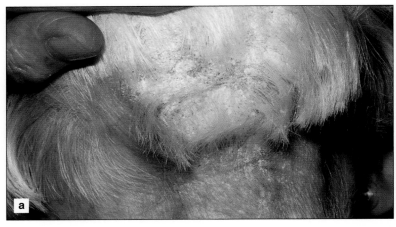

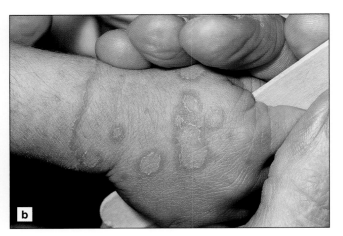

Figure 1.10   Examples of scaling. (**a**) In psoriasis, shown here on the scalp, scaling is typically well formed and has a silvery color. Compare with the different quality and pattern of the marginal scaling in (**b**) erythrokeratoderma variabilis. (Panel b from Lawrence CM, Cox NH. Physical Signs in Dermatology, 2nd edn. London: Mosby, 2002.)

(which are smaller) and nodules (which are larger). The arbitrary cut-off (either 0.5 cm or 1 cm in different publications) ignores the possibility of lesions of mixed sizes or of growth from a papule to a nodule.

The term maculopapular is applied to eruptions that have mixed features of macules and papules or plaques; although this pattern is frequent in drug eruptions and viral exanthems, it is a rather overused term that often does not accurately describe the predominant component of the eruption.

Blisters (vesicles and bullae)

Blisters can be divided into smaller (0.5- or 1-cm cut-off) vesicles and larger bullae (Figs 1.6 and 1.7). Again, this is somewhat arbitrary; in practice most vesicular eruptions (e.g. those of pompholyx eczema, Fig. 1.7) actually consist of lesions of 1–4 mm, whereas most conditions that would usually be described as bullous have at least some lesions of over 1 cm. Blisters should be documented as unilocular (e.g. in friction blister and bullous pemphigoid) or multilocular (e.g. in pompholyx eczema).

Pustules

These are similar to blisters but contain pus, which is usually yellow but may be greenish in older pustules (Fig. 1.8). Older pustules usually dry to form brownish scabs.

Telangiectasia and other vascular lesions

Vascular changes such as telangiectasia (discrete visible vessels) should be distinguished from erythema (increased redness due to increased blood flow rather than due to a fixed structural vascular abnormality) and purpura (small spots of extravasated blood), whether as components of a rash or a discrete localized lesion. Blood that is within vessels can generally be compressed out of the skin by pressure, hence causing blanching, whereas this cannot be achieved with extravasated blood. There are occasional instances where intravascular blood cannot be compressed out using simple clinical techniques (see *Diascopy*, Ch. 2).

Ulcers and other breaks in the skin

Breaks in the skin may be divided into the following.
- Ulcers—the term can be applied to any skin break but is generally taken to imply a defect extending into the dermis (Fig. 1.9).
- Erosions—these are superficial, involving the epidermis only.
- Fissures—a specific morphology of skin break resembling a small slit.
  Excoriations are a type of erosion or ulcer caused by scratching, the term describing the process by which the break has occurred rather than being used as a term for a specific primary lesion.

Weals

These are due to dermal edema. Patients often confuse weals and blisters, so a history of 'blisters' may be misleading. Gentle pressure on a blister will

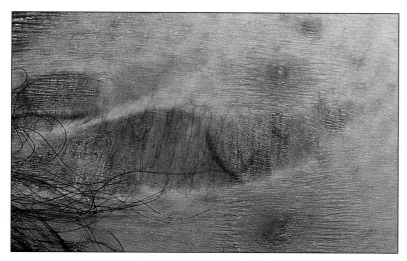

Figure 1.11 Atrophy of the skin, in this case in striae distensae. This occurs due to stretching of the skin (e.g. on abdomen or thighs in pregnancy or when the skin is damaged by excessive use of topical corticosteroids). The skin appears thinned, and dermal vasculature is readily visible in the line of the applied tension that has stretched the skin.

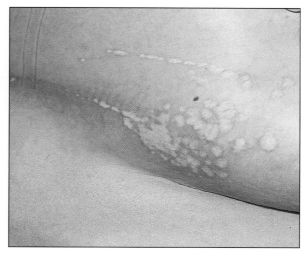

Figure 1.12 Lichen sclerosus et atrophicus. In this condition, there is epidermal atrophy together with a homogenization and edema of the upper dermal collagen. This produces a typically white color and a thinned appearance of the skin. In this patient, the two lines of lesions represent a Koebner response.

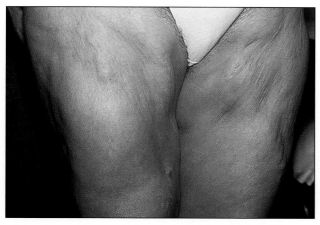

Figure 1.13 Hypertrophy. In this case, mixed fat hypertrophy and atrophy (note the normal skin color because the abnormality is deep to the skin).

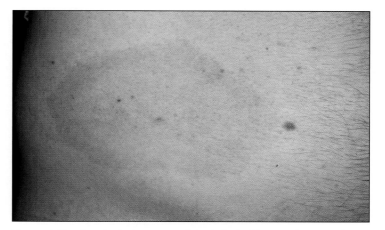

Figure 1.14 Annular lesion: a complete circle. In this case due to erythema migrans of Lyme disease. Parts of a circle are termed arcuate or arciform.

alter its shape, which generally returns to the previous shape very quickly unless the fluid content is highly proteinaceous, and firm pressure may cause the blister to spread or to break. By contrast, gentle pressure on a weal has no effect (except blanching if it is erythematous), while firm pressure may compress fluid out of it to leave an indentation that slowly refills. However, the simplest distinction is that blisters can be punctured and then leak fluid.

Surface morphology and secondary changes
It is useful to note certain surface features of papules, nodules, and plaques.

Overall shape
Papules and nodules can be further characterized as dome-shaped, flat-topped, umbilicated, etc.

Surface changes
A particularly important issue is distinction between disorders with and without an epidermal component, implied by scaling and crusting (Fig. 1.10). Thus, for example, annular lesions of ringworm (scaly) and granuloma annulare (no scaling) can readily be distinguished.
  Useful terms are as follows.
- Smooth—this may be like the normal skin surface or smoother.
- Scaly—scaling is due to flakes of keratin, which can be felt, and rubbed or scraped off the skin. It can be qualified as fine (e.g. in pityriasis versicolor) or coarse (e.g. in psoriasis), and as loose or adherent. Disorders with scaly papules and plaques are termed papulosquamous.

- Hyperkeratotic—this implies a formed mass of keratin rather than the flakiness of scaling; for example, the cutaneous horn of keratoacanthoma or the diffuse hard keratin of keratodermas.
- Crusted—crust is due to dried blood or exudate, often mixed with keratin but not due to keratin alone. Hardened surface blood is known as an eschar, or colloquially as a scab (the latter term is also applied to dried pus or proteinaceous exudates).

Texture changes (see Ch. 22)
Alterations in any skin component may cause thinning (atrophy) or thickening. Epidermal atrophy causes a fine wrinkling appearance of the skin (except over the surface of a nodule, where it may produce abnormally smooth and tight-looking skin due to the tension that is being exerted). It is often combined with dermal atrophy (Figs 1.11 and 1.12). Dermal atrophy may lead to a herniation of the underlying fat (a process termed anetoderma). Fat atrophy in the absence of dermal atrophy causes a deep indentation of the skin.

  Thickening of the skin includes epidermal thickening (e.g. lichenification due to rubbing), dermal thickening (e.g. sclerosis due to increased collagen in scleroderma, and peau d'orange appearance due to dermal mucin), and fat hypertrophy (Fig. 1.13).

  These processes, and the predominant level of the skin that is affected, can usually be identified from the physical signs, both palpable and visible (e.g. increased skin markings in lichenification, and more visible vessels due to atrophy).

Shapes and patterns, symmetry

Skin lesions produce a variety of shapes (Figs 1.14–1.16) and may have striking patterns of arrangement or grouping. Some of these lead to very limited diagnostic lists, so accurate description is critical.

Shapes of individual lesions

Examples of lesional shapes, and conditions with which they are associated, are listed in Table 1.1; some specific common examples are addressed in more detail in Tables 1.2–1.4.

Arrangements of multiple lesions

Useful terms to describe arrangements of multiple lesions include grouped (agminated), scattered or disseminated, and confluent. Other terms may be based on anatomic factors (e.g. dermatomal lesions of herpes zoster) or probable causes (e.g. photosensitivity distribution). See also Tables 1.2 and 1.3.

Blaschko lines warrant specific mention: they are developmental lines that have a swirled pattern on the trunk (more linear on the limbs), and this pattern can therefore often identify an eruption as having a congenital or genetic basis.

Koebner reaction

This specific pattern of eruption (also known as the isomorphic response) is usefully described here. A number of dermatoses have the ability to create lesions in areas of minor injury (Fig. 1.12, Table 1.4); these include frank cuts, but often the triggering insult may not overtly breach the skin. Such lesions are often linear, as scratches are a common trigger, but other shapes are seen in burns, for example. A similar process that occurs at skin puncture sites, especially if autologous blood or saline are injected, occurs in pyoderma gangrenosum and Behçet disease, and is known as pathergy.

Note that viral warts are often stated to exhibit the Koebner phenomenon, but this is incorrect: viral warts in the line of a skin injury are due to direct inoculation of virus. Sarcoidosis often occurs in scars, but affects old scars rather than new minor injuries.

Symmetry

Degree of symmetry is also a useful feature of skin eruptions. In general, markedly symmetric eruptions are endogenous in causation, although there are inevitably some exceptions (e.g. contact allergy to footwear is usually symmetric). Conversely, asymmetric eruptions often have external causes. Fungal infections of the skin are an important example, exemplified

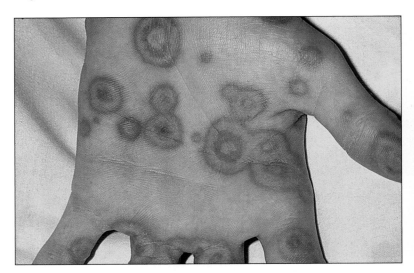

Figure 1.15   Classic target lesions, comprising multiple concentric circles, typically (as in this case) seen in erythema multiforme triggered by herpes simplex virus infection.

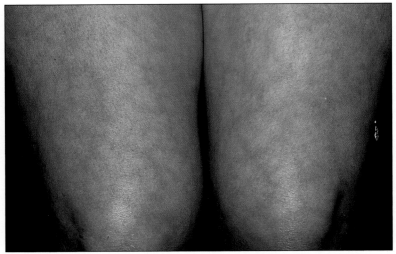

Figure 1.16   This net-like or chicken wire pattern is termed livedo (see also Ch. 14). A uniformly sized faint livedo pattern is common over fatty areas of skin, especially in babies and young women, and is a physiologic phenomenon reflecting areas of slower flow of deoxygenated blood (known as cutis marmorata).

Table 1.1	MAIN SHAPES OF SKIN LESIONS	
Shape	**Description**	**Example(s)**
Discoid (nummular)	A filled circle	Discoid eczema
Petaloid	Discoid lesions that have merged together	Seborrheic dermatitis on the trunk
Arcuate	Incomplete circles	Urticaria
Annular	Open circles with different central skin compared with the rim	Tinea corporis, granuloma annulare (see also Table 1.2)
Polycyclic	Circles that have merged together	Psoriasis
Livedo	Chicken wire criss-cross pattern	Erythema ab igne, vasculitis
Reticulate	A finer lace-like pattern	Oral lichen planus
Target	Multiple concentric rings	Erythema multiforme
Stellate	Star-shaped	Lesions of meningococcal septicemia
Digitate	Finger-shaped	Parapsoriasis
Linear	Straight line	Koebner reaction to a scratch in lichen planus (see Tables 1.3 and 1.4)
Serpiginous	Snake-like	Cutaneous larva migrans

Table 1.2 EXAMPLES OF LESIONS OR GROUPINGS OF LESIONS THAT PRODUCE ANNULAR MORPHOLOGY

Scale	Typically annular	Often include annular component
Present	Ringworm Erythema annulare centrifugum	Psoriasis Seborrheic eczema Pityriasis rosea (herald patch) Impetigo Subacute cutaneous lupus erythematosus Mycosis fungoides
Absent	Granuloma annulare Jessner lymphocytic infiltrate 'Annular erythemas' Erythema annularis telangiectoides Serum sickness	Urticaria Erythema multiforme Lichen planus Sarcoidosis

(After Lawrence CM, Cox NH. Physical Signs in Dermatology, 2nd edn. London: Mosby, 2002.)

by unilateral palmar involvement, a situation that should routinely prompt inspection of the feet for tinea pedis. Asymmetric hand eruption also occurs in cooks, hairdressers, and others who hold a tool in the dominant hand while handling wet or irritant materials with the non-dominant hand.

Color

Skin color involves contributions from several pigments, including:

- melanins (red, brown, or black; these usually provide the dominant pigment in normal skin),
- blood (red, purple, or blue),
- carotenoids (yellow; Fig. 1.17), and
- dermal fibrous tissue (white).

A wide range of skin colors occur in different physiologic and pathologic states. The subtleties of color may not be appreciated without experience. For example, patches of vitiligo (loss of melanin) and of nevus anemicus (loss of red color due to vasoconstriction) are both often termed 'depigmented' by non-specialists, but the vitiligo is white or pale pink, whereas nevus anemicus is usually a pale yellowish brown color (i.e. hypopigmented rather than depigmented). Some shades of color are quite characteristic (e.g. the yellow-orange color of xanthomas), and others are sufficiently useful that they narrow the list of likely diagnoses (e.g. purplish

Table 1.3 EXAMPLES OF LESIONS OR GROUPINGS OF LESIONS THAT PRODUCE LINEAR MORPHOLOGY

Determinant of pattern	Example(s)
Blood vessels	Thrombophlebitis, Mondor disease (linear thrombophlebitis on the trunk) Eczema related to varicose veins Temporal arteritis
Lymphatics	Lymphangitis Sporotrichosis, fish tank granulomas
Dermatome	Herpes zoster, zosteriform nevus, zosteriform Darier disease, zosteriform metastases
Nerve trunks	Leprosy (thickened cutaneous nerves)
Developmental and Blaschko lines	Pigmentary demarcation line, linea nigra Epidermal nevi, incontinentia pigmenti, hypomelanosis of Ito, linear psoriasis, linear lichen planus, lichen striatus
Skin stretching	Striae due to growth spurt (on lower back)
Infestation	Larva migrans (wavy, not straight, lines)
External injury	
Plants	Phytophotodermatitis
Allergens	Elastoplast, nail varnish (neck), necklace, waistbands, etc.
Chemical	Caustics (e.g. phenol)
Thermal	Burns
Physical	*To normal skin* Keloid scar, bruising, dermatitis artefacta, amniotic constriction bands *To abnormal skin* Purpura (cryoglobulinemia, amyloid, vasculitis) Blisters (epidermolysis bullosa, porphyrias) Inoculation Warts, molluscum contagiosum *Koebner phenomenon* Psoriasis, lichen planus, others (Table 1.4) *Other* Scar sarcoid
Other determinants	Linear scleroderma (limb, central forehead) Senear–Caro ridge (on hands in psoriasis) Dermatomyositis (linear pattern on dorsum of fingers; Gottron sign) Interstitial granulomatous dermatitis (rope sign)

(After Lawrence CM, Cox NH. Physical Signs in Dermatology, 2nd edn. London: Mosby, 2002.)

Table 1.4 DISORDERS THAT MAY SHOW THE KOEBNER REACTION[a]	
Commonly	**Less commonly**
Psoriasis	Small vessel vasculitis
Pityriasis rubra pilaris	Erythema multiforme
Lichen planus	Elastosis perforans serpiginosa
Lichen nitidus	Necrobiosis lipoidica
Vitiligo	Eruptive xanthomas
Lichen sclerosus	Scleromyxedema
	Pemphigus

[a]Viral warts are often stated to exhibit the Koebner phenomenon, but this is incorrect: viral warts in the line of a skin injury are due to direct inoculation of virus. Similarly, vasculitis in scratch marks or pressure areas may occur immediately after the insult, and is probably due to local hydrostatic pressure changes and trauma causing vascular leakage, rather than actually provoking the vasculitic process.

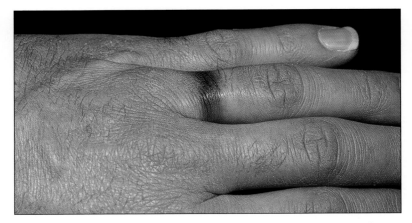

Figure 1.18 Black dermographism. Gold rings are a common cause, usually after there has been a solvent or abrasive agent under the ring. In this case, the culprit was a sunscreen containing titanium, which presumably had an abrasive effect.

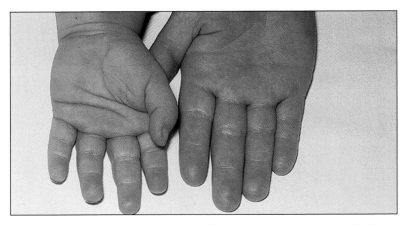

Figure 1.17 Skin color may be rather subjective, but the hand on the left in this picture is clearly more yellow than the normal control. This patient had carotenemia, which may occur as a metabolic defect or in hypothyroidism, but is commonly dietary due to excessive carotene intake.

The presence of scaling alters color by introducing air–keratin interfaces that reflect light. This can be exaggerated (notably in psoriasis) by scratching the scaly surface, and can be reduced by applying oil or water. Thus many patients will note that scaly skin lesions look redder when they take a bath or apply topical medications.

Inflammation of the skin disrupts pigmentation. Postinflammatory hyper- or hypopigmentation is a common feature of many dermatoses but causes much diagnostic confusion; hyperpigmentation in particular may take a considerable time to resolve. It is important to understand that when melanin pigment is positioned deep in the dermis, rather than at the usual epidermal level, the different refraction of light gives it a more blue color; this explains the overall grayish brown color of dermal postinflammatory hyperpigmentation, and also the purple color of lichen planus (red from inflammation plus blue-brown from disturbed pigmentation).

External pigments may also stain the skin (Fig. 1.18); on occasion, dyes leached out of new clothing may cause diagnostic confusion.

Colors that may be diagnostically useful are listed in Table 1.5.

PATHOLOGIC TERMINOLOGY IN RELATION TO THE SKIN

A detailed discussion of skin pathology is beyond the scope of this volume. However, a basic knowledge of pathologic terminology is useful to help in understanding the nature of skin diseases and the clinicopathologic correlations that lead to diagnosis (Table 1.6). It is also inevitable that many of those taking an interest in the skin will be faced with descriptive laboratory reports, for which an understanding of terminology is important. Although details of the pathology of individual disorders is generally beyond the scope of this book, brief explanation will be given in the appropriate chapters where this may be helpful.

or violaceous coloring of lichen planus or dermatomyositis). Thus an accurate description of shades of red or other color changes can be diagnostically useful (Table 1.5).

Blanching of the skin on pressure is often ascribed great diagnostic importance but is a feature of virtually all dermatoses and of normal skin: any skin with patent blood vessels will be less red when these are occluded. The converse, however, is a useful sign of extravasation of blood, as discussed earlier. The color contribution from blood in the skin is altered by the degree of blood flow, where it is occurring (from superficial or deep vessels), state of blood oxygenation, and abnormal hemoglobins (e.g. methemoglobin and carboxyhemoglobin).

Table 1.5   COLORS THAT MAY BE DIAGNOSTICALLY USEFUL

Color	Example(s)
Black	Melanin (e.g. some nevi, melanoma) Exogenous pigments (e.g. tattoos, pencil or ink) Exogenous chemicals (e.g. silver nitrate, gold salts; Fig. 1.14)
Blue-grey	Deeply situated blood (e.g. some angiomas) Deep melanin (e.g. blue nevus) Inflammatory (e.g. orf) Drugs (e.g. phenothiazines, minocycline)
Dark brown	Melanin near surface (e.g. melanocytic nevi) Exogenous pigments (e.g. dithranol staining)
Pale brown	Melanin near surface (e.g. lentigo, freckles)
Muddy brown	Melanin in superficial dermis (e.g. postinflammatory pigmentation)
Purple	Vascular lesions (e.g. angiomas) Other disorders where telangiectasia is a prominent feature (e.g. lupus pernio or chronic sarcoidosis, dermatomyositis)
Dusky blue	Reduced hemoglobin (e.g. poor arterial supply, cyanosis) Methemoglobinemia
Violaceous and lilac	Lichen planus Edge of plaques of morphea Connective tissue disorders (e.g. dermatomyositis)
Pink-red	Many exanthemata and common disorders, such as psoriasis
Red-brown	Inflammatory (e.g. seborrheic eczema, secondary syphilis) Hemosiderin (e.g. pigmented purpuric dermatoses)
Scarlet-red	Lesions with strong arterial supply (e.g. pyogenic granuloma, spider nevus) Altered hemoglobin (e.g. carbon monoxide poisoning)
Orange	Hemosiderin (e.g. lichen aureus) Inflammatory (e.g. pityriasis rubra pilaris)
Yellow-white or yellow-pink	Xanthomatous disorders
Yellow-orange	Carotenemia (ingested carotene, myxedema)
Yellow-green	Jaundice
Green	Exogenous pigment (e.g. copper salts)
White-ivory	Lichen sclerosus et atrophicus, morphea
White (or pale pink, depending on vascularity)	Albinism, piebaldism Vitiligo, halo nevus White dermographism, steal effect around vascular lesions

(After Lawrence CM, Cox NH. Physical Signs in Dermatology, 2nd edn. London: Mosby, 2002.)

Table 1.6   EXPLANATION OF SOME COMMON TERMS IN DERMATOPATHOLOGY

Term	Meaning	Comments
Acantholysis	Separation between cells of prickle cell layer	Occurs in pemphigus.
Acanthosis	Thickening of epidermal prickle cell layer	For example, in psoriasis.
Apoptosis	A form of cell death	Seen in lichenoid disorders, for example.
Atrophy	Thinning	Needs to be put into context of what is normal for the body site. Epidermal atrophy usually involves flattening of the normal rete ridge structure, rather than simply a miniaturization of all levels.
Dermo–epidermal junction	The basement membrane zone below the epidermis	Important in bullous diseases and site of inflammation in lupus erythematosus, lichen planus.
Desmoplastic	A change in collagen to cause dense bands	Occurs in various fibrous dermal lesions, uncommonly in malignant melanoma.
Ectasia (ectatic)	Dilatation of vessels	Refers to blood or lymphatic vessels.
Epidermotropism	Cells migrating from dermis into epidermis	Especially used to describe atypical lymphocytes in mycosis fungoides.
Granulomatous	Pattern of inflammation	Collections of lymphocytes and histiocytes with peripheral palisade, giant cells, often central collagen damage; seen in sarcoid, granuloma annulare, cutaneous tuberculosis, etc.
Hydropic degeneration	Necrosis of the basal keratinocytes	Occurs in lichenoid eruptions and some connective tissue diseases.
Hyper- and hypo-	Increase and decrease, respectively	For example: hypergranulosis, increased thickness of the granular layer (e.g. in lichen planus); hyperkeratosis, increased thickness of the stratum corneum (occurs in many disorders).
Interface dermatitis	Pattern of inflammation at the dermo–epidermal junction	For example, in lichen planus.
Necrobiosis	Pattern of damage and regeneration of collagen	Literally means death and life. Seen in granulomatous disorders.
Necrolysis	Cell death causing separation between cells	Occurs in drug reactions (toxic epidermal necrolysis) and in glucagonoma (necrolytic migratory erythema).
Pagetoid spread	Pattern of non-epidermal cells in the epidermis	For example, in melanoma; atypical cells migrate up through the epidermis.
Panniculitis	Inflammation of the fat	Usually divided into lobular and septal (or mixed) types.
Parakeratosis	Retention of cell nuclei into stratum corneum	Occurs in several inflammatory disorders (e.g. psoriasis).
Polarizing light	Microscopic technique	Used to identify foreign material, fragments of hair shaft in dermis, urate crystals in gout, etc.
Transepidermal elimination	Material being extruded through the epidermis	May be damaged endogenous material (e.g. collagen, elastic tissue) or foreign material (e.g. sutures).

2 Approach to the Patient

INTRODUCTION

The diagnostic importance of the physical signs described in the first chapter, and the benefits of accurate description of these, are clear. However, while close-up morphology may be diagnostic in some instances, such as in most cases of psoriasis, in others it only identifies an area of diagnosis. For example, close-up morphology that is clinically eczematous may occur in a variety of different endogenous eczemas, contact dermatitis, some drug eruptions, early bullous pemphigoid, and so on. Further diagnostic clues come from the history of the lesion or eruption, and from its overall pattern and body site distribution. This chapter discusses the factors to consider in the dermatologic history, specific aspects of the cutaneous examination, specific body site aspects (usually termed regional dermatology), and clinical investigation.

Treatments will be discussed in more detail in specific disease chapters and in Chapters 3–5.

HISTORY

The dermatologic history includes specific details of the presenting complaint, but may also require a broader discussion of family history, occupation, general medical and other disorders, and drug treatment. In some instances, notably localized benign skin lesions, an extensive history is often not required to reach a diagnosis. However, even in these cases, there may be important patient history such as previous skin neoplasia, family history of skin lesions, drug therapy that might cause bleeding or otherwise interfere with a local anesthetic procedure, etc.

In practice, many dermatologists use a 'look, talk, look again' approach; an early look at the problem may be able to focus the discussion if the morphologic diagnosis is apparent. For example, in a patient with 'hand dermatitis', a detailed occupational history is likely to be time wasted for all concerned if the initial look makes it apparent that the diagnosis is scabies. However, in less clear-cut cases, a more detailed history and re-examination of the eruption may be necessary.

The following is a list of potentially important aspects to include in the historical record; some may not be applicable to all cases, but neither is the list exhaustive for all clinical situations.

Basic demographic details (Table 2.1)

Age

Many disorders have a predilection for certain age groups, or the features may vary in different age groups (e.g. psoriasis in children is often guttate or flexural in pattern).

Sex

Some disorders are specific to men or women, some have a different frequency between the sexes (e.g. the helical and antihelix lesions of chondrodermatitis of the ear), and some may have sex-linked inheritance.

Race and country of origin

Some disorders have racial predilection, or may appear differently depending on racial origin. Examples include the high incidence of systemic lupus erythematosus in African-Caribbeans, the strong

Table 2.1 MAIN DETAILS FOR A DERMATOLOGIC PATIENT HISTORY	
Category	**Details**
Demographic	Age Sex Race and country of origin Place of residence Occupations(s)
History of the presenting complaint	Symptoms Duration, evolution, periodicity Response to treatment(s) Previous episodes Previous skin disorders
Family history	Similar disorders Other familial conditions
Medical history and medications	General health, specific system enquiry Regular medications; changes preceding skin condition
Hobbies	Especially chemical or plant exposure
Effects of the condition	Work Social, family, and relationships
Social factors	Smoking, alcohol Issues that might interfere with treatment

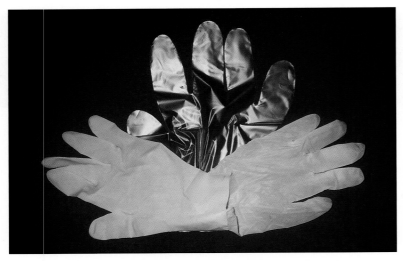

Figure 2.1 Different glove materials. Gloves used by workers are an important part of the history: whether they are used at all, whether they provide adequate protection, or whether they might cause dermatitis (e.g. rubber glove allergy, in which the rash often finishes abruptly at the wrist or mid-forearm). Latex gloves (yellowish color, on the left), for instance, are a common cause of potentially severe reactions in health workers and occasionally in their patients. Polythene (colorless) and vinyl (white) gloves are suitable alternatives.

predominance of prurigo pigmentosa in Japanese, and the skin cancer risk of red-haired individuals of Celtic origin.

Place of residence

This may be important in infectious disease outbreaks and in the practicality of some treatments (such as having to travel for phototherapy). Previous places of residence may be relevant, especially tropical countries (for the risks of skin cancer related to sun exposure and as endemic areas for infections).

Occupation(s)

This is of particular importance in regard to occupational contact dermatitis (Ch. 6), but may also have implications regarding the practicality of some treatment modalities if these are available only in normal hours of work. In some instances, a detailed account of processes and chemicals, protection methods, and previous occupations may be required. Hands are the commonly affected site in occupational dermatitis, and it is useful to record details of hand protection—gloves (Fig. 2.1), barrier creams, etc.—as well as the agents to which the patient is exposed. Some dermatoses associated with specific occupations and hobbies are listed in Table 2.2; see also Fig. 2.2.

History of the lesion or rash
Symptoms

Itch is the most common symptom, but the perceived intensity and the response to it varies considerably between individuals with objectively similar severity of eruption. Indeed, in some patients the only visible 'rash' is actually the results of the patient scratching or picking at the skin (Fig. 2.3); this can be very difficult to address, as there may be little insight into the fact that this is happening, and explaining that scratching is causing the damage may be viewed negatively. Some rashes, such as scabies (Fig. 2.4), are characteristically very itchy in most patients. However, even classically itchy rashes may vary in the response they provoke: lichen planus is also very itchy, but scratch marks are rarely seen by comparison with eczema or scabies, for example. Both for diagnostic purposes and to monitor therapeutic response, it is helpful to record the patient's view of degree of itch using a semiquantitative system such as severe, moderate, or mild.

Factors noted by the patient that aggravate or improve symptoms may provide diagnostic clues; similarly, the response, or lack of response, to previous treatments may be diagnostically useful (as discussed later).

Some disorders are typically described as painful rather than itchy, and the quality of pain may vary. Examples include the following.
- Erythema nodosum—typically produces a throbbing pain (Fig. 2.5).
- Chilblains—cause a burning or throbbing pain.
- Chondrodermatitis of the ear (Fig. 2.6)—causes a sharp, pricking pain that wakes patients when they lie on it.
- Erythropoietic protoporphyria in children—typically causes a burning sensation without a clinically apparent rash.
- Some skin nodules (such as neuromas, glomus tumors, and leio-

Table 2.2	SOME OCCUPATIONS AND HOBBIES AND THEIR DERMATOLOGIC PROBLEMS
Activity	**Examples of possible dermatologic implications**
Agricultural	Irritant dermatitis (e.g. disinfectants), contact allergy (e.g. rubber chemicals in gloves or footwear), hazards from animals (e.g. tinea, Fig. 2.2; atopy)
Gardening	Irritant or contact allergic dermatitis related to many plants, contact allergy to gloves
Building trade and do-it-yourself	Irritant dermatitis from cement (also causes chemical burns), plaster, solvents, preservatives, fiberglass; frictional palmar dermatitis from tools; vibration white finger related to use of some tools; contact allergic dermatitis (especially to chromate in cement, epoxy resin, formaldehyde resins, colophony in soldering flux)
Cars (trade or home)	Irritant dermatitis from solvents, paints, hand cleansers; contact allergic dermatitis from paints, resins, metals, rubber gloves; rubber chemicals in tire manufacture may cause dermatitis or rarely chemical leukoderma
Cooking (work or home)	Irritant dermatitis (detergents and hand washing, juices of meat, fruit, and vegetables); contact allergic dermatitis (or urticaria in some cases) from fruits, garlic, spices, meat, fish, gloves
Cleaning (work or home)	Irritant dermatitis from detergents; contact allergic dermatitis to fragrances or antimicrobials in detergents, polishes, etc., or to gloves
Healthcare work	Irritant dermatitis from cleaning agents and hand washing, latex allergy (urticaria or dermatitis), medicament allergies (dentists: also risk of allergy to balsam flavorings and to resins)
Hairdressing	Irritant dermatitis from shampoos, bleaches, etc.; contact allergic dermatitis from perfumes, dyes, bleaches, lanolin, antimicrobials; contact urticaria due to henna
Textiles (work or hobby)	Irritant dermatitis from solvents, bleaches, detergents and hand washing; contact allergic dermatitis from dyes, formaldehyde resins (finishes), mordants

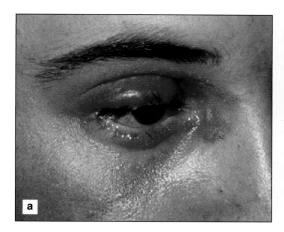

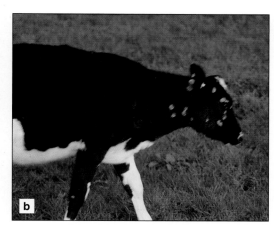

Figure 2.2 Cattle ringworm. When an unusual site is affected (**a**) the diagnosis may be unsuspected by medical staff, even though the affected farmers usually know that their stock are infected (**b**).

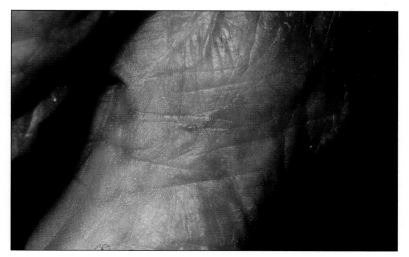

Figure 2.4 Scabies infestation. This usually causes severe itch, and careful examination of the fingers, web spaces, and wrists is important to detect the characteristic curvilinear burrows, as shown here. Scabies is discussed in more detail in Ch. 27.

Figure 2.3 Sometimes the only 'rash' is that due to the patient scratching. Complete sparing of the area on the back that cannot be reached (the butterfly sign) is diagnostically useful, as it suggests that there is a systemic rather than a cutaneous reason for itch.

important and needs to be considered in the clinical context. Some important examples include the following.

- Changes in nevi. Malignant change in nevi is virtually always a process that involves both enlargement and color changes over a few months; by contrast, a 'mole' that has gone black overnight is more likely to be a simple traumatized nevus or angioma.
- Diagnosis of urticaria. In the case of urticaria, the rash is often not present at the time of the consultation (or is a bit vague), yet the diagnosis can be made with reasonable certainty provided questions are carefully worded. Quite often, the urticaria may have been present for a prolonged period; however, the individual lesions last for less than 24 h and often migrate during this period (Fig. 2.7), this short timescale being almost unique to urticaria. Asking about the duration of the rash ('How long have you had it?') may be taken to mean the overall duration or the duration of lesions on the day in question; both are important, but it is the short duration of the individual lesions that diagnoses the eruption as urticaria. The critical question is therefore 'When the rash is there, how long do individual patches last before they fade?'
- Progression of annular lesions. Many annular lesions spread centrifugally over a period of time. The detectable rate of change varies considerably, for example progression of erythema annular centrifugum (Fig. 2.8) is usually over days, of tinea corporis over weeks, and of granuloma annulare over months.

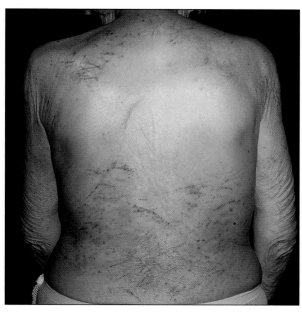

Figure 2.5 Erythema nodosum. This disorder causes deep dermal and fat inflammation, presenting as poorly defined inflammatory nodules. These are typically tender, and often require treatment with oral non-steroidal antiinflammatory drugs. This patient was unusual in having chronic lesions.

myomas)—these are characteristically tender when they are subject to pressure (including palpation by a physician!).

Duration, evolution, and periodicity

In the case of localized individual lesions, the duration and changes over time are usually straightforward. The timescale of changes is particularly

The evolution of an eruption may be characteristic, for example in pityriasis rosea, in which a solitary herald patch precedes the eruption by a couple of days, or in pyoderma gangrenosum, in which there is (usually rapidly) progressive ulceration (Fig. 2.9). The site of initial involvement in a rash can also be a useful feature, for example a generalized eczema in a patient with preceding venous eczema is likely to be a secondary autosensitization eruption (see Ch. 6). Similarly, many rashes have

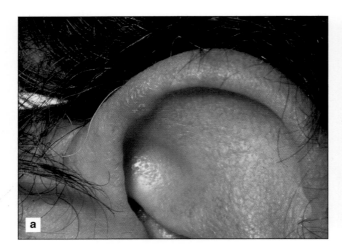

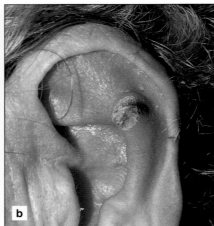

Figure 2.6 Chondrodermatitis nodularis. This lesion occurs characteristically on the helix or antihelix of the ear on the side on which the patient sleeps. It causes a sharp pain that may wake patients from sleep. Treatment is excision of the underlying cartilage. This condition varies between the sexes, helical lesions (**a**) being most common in men and antihelix lesions (**b**) in women.

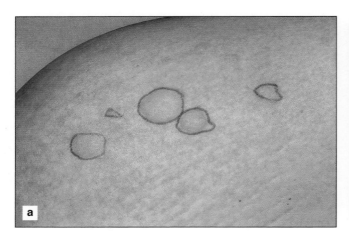

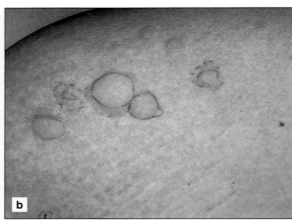

Figure 2.7 Urticaria. The margin of lesions was marked with ink (solid line) when initially examined (**a**), and again after 30 min (dotted line in **b**), showing asymmetric expansion of the lesions. Small unmarked weals at the upper part of the figure have become more prominent, being little more than erythematous patches at baseline. (From Lawrence CM, Cox NH. Physical Signs in Dermatology, 2nd edn. London: Mosby, 2002.)

Figure 2.8 Erythema annulare centrifugum. An accurate history is useful, as this annular inflammatory dermatosis slowly migrates and enlarges over a period of weeks (see also Ch. 11).

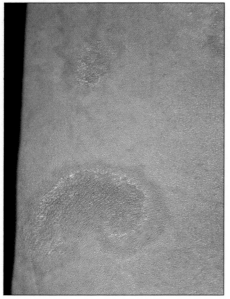

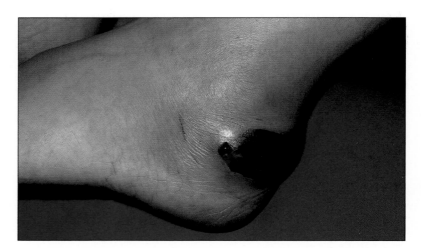

Figure 2.9 Pyoderma gangrenosum. This form of inflammatory ulceration usually has a rapid rate of progression and significant discomfort, which distinguish it from most commoner causes of ulceration of the skin (see also Ch. 14). Infections, in particular, must be excluded. Note the peripheral pustules, a feature of active disease.

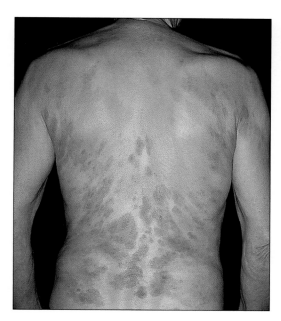

Figure 2.10 Mycosis fungoides. This starts on covered areas of the body, such as the buttocks, lower trunk, or thighs, and in most cases gradually worsens over months (see also Ch. 33).

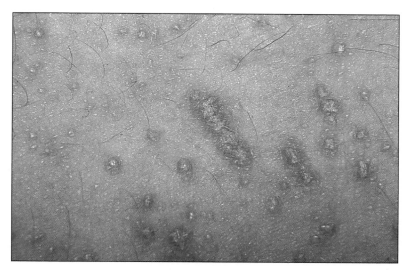

Figure 2.11 Koebner reaction in lichen planus, producing linear lesions at a site of scratching. Patients may volunteer that they have noticed lesions at sites of injury in other disorders as well, such as psoriasis (see list of disorders producing a Koebner reaction, Table 1.4).

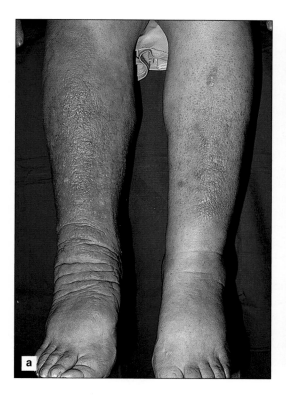

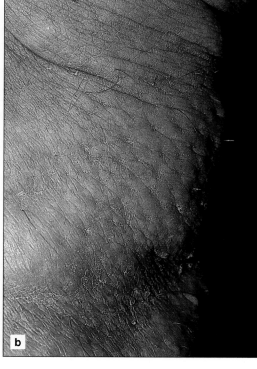

Figure 2.12 (**a**,**b**) Pretibial myxedema is a good example of a dermatologic condition that occurs in conjunction with systemic disease (see also Ch. 12). Lesions occur on the shins, and close examination reveals a peau d'orange appearance of the skin.

characteristic sites of involvement which may not all be apparent at the time of examination, but which may be appreciated from the history (Fig. 2.10).

It is always worth asking the patient about perceived triggers and provocative factors (Fig. 2.11), even if some are readily discounted. In particular, it is important to be aware that some infective and drug triggers may precede an eruption by several weeks. Provocative triggers and periodicity are of particular importance in eczematous processes. In some instances an answer is obvious, for example the recurrence of a photosensitivity rash every spring; in some cases, the explanation for a certain timing of episodes may become apparent after patch testing has identified a causative contact allergen. Improvement in a rash during holiday periods is often taken to imply that the cause is an occupational contact dermatitis; however, this assumption is not necessarily correct, as such improvement could also occur because the patient has not been in contact with a relevant household contact allergen, or it might represent improvement due to sunlight.

Response to treatment(s)

Many patients will have tried treatments bought over the counter,

prescribed for a previous problem, or borrowed from friends before they see a primary care physician. Many will also have used agents prescribed by a referring physician before they see a dermatologist. It is important to document the response (or lack of response) to these treatments, mainly because they may give clues about the diagnosis or may have altered the features of the disorder, but also because credibility is lost if the secondary care physician prescribes an agent that has been tried and failed. As examples, a supposed localized fungal infection that has failed to respond to a few weeks of antifungal therapy is almost certainly not fungal, while a true fungal infection treated for the same few weeks with a topical corticosteroid may be virtually unrecognizable. Bear in mind that previous treatments, especially herbal medicines or treatments bought over the counter, may not be volunteered unless the patient is directly questioned.

Careful questions about the original shapes and patterns of the eruption or lesion, as described in Chapter 1, may be required.

Previous episodes

In the case of localized lesions, previous similar lesions may suggest the diagnosis and lead to earlier intervention. For example, patients with three or more previous basal carcinomas have a very high risk of a further new

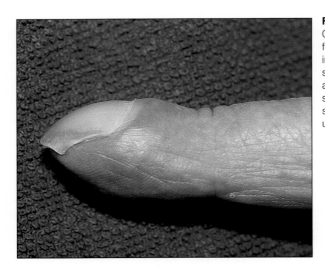

Figure 2.13 Clubbing of the fingers usually indicates a systemic disease and results in swelling of the soft tissues under the nail.

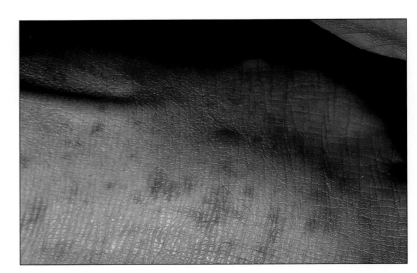

Figure 2.14 In purpuric disorders, the fact that lesions are palpable is of great importance, as it implies that the cause is a vasculitic process (i.e. that there is an inflammatory component rather than simple leakage of erythrocytes, as might occur in thrombocytopenia, extravasation secondary to vascular fragility, etc.). This photograph has used side-lighting to demonstrate this.

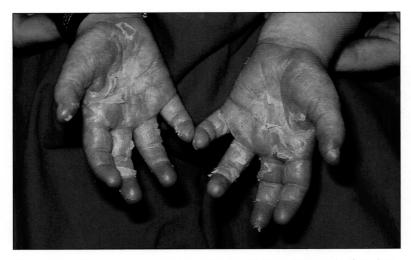

Figure 2.15 The importance of a general history of recent illnesses is often clear in patients with a viral exanthema, in whom the rash may occur several days after the malaise or sore throat has settled, especially if the main feature is desquamation, as in this case.

basal carcinoma within 5 years, and any new lesion should be treated with suspicion.

In the case of rashes, previous episodes may be useful or even critical for diagnosis of a cause. For example, recurrent poststreptococcal episodes of guttate psoriasis are not unusual, so the diagnosis can often be suspected once an earlier event has been diagnosed. In the case of occupational hand dermatitis, knowledge of previous proven hypersensitivity may be of huge value in diagnosis and avoidance.

Previous skin disorders

These may be of importance, particularly in the diagnosis of eczemas. For example, irritant hand dermatitis is not uncommon in adult patients with a history of childhood atopy, even though the patient may not recognize this as being the same process as the eczema behind their knees as a youngster. On the other hand, it is important not to be misled by a history of a previous skin problem, especially if the diagnosis is unsubstantiated; to use the same example, the fact that a patient has previous atopic dermatitis does not preclude a subsequent contact allergic dermatitis.

Family history

This is usually asked in relation to other family members who appear to have the same disorder, and may be relevant for:

- genodermatoses with a specific inheritance pattern (the most likely being uncommon pediatric conditions with blisters or ichthyosis);

- disorders with a polygenic or more complex mode of inheritance, such as psoriasis (especially with young adult onset, where the family history is often positive);
- problems in which specific inheritance is relatively uncommon but which may occasionally be inherited (such as lichen planus or basal cell carcinomas); and
- non-inherited patterns of disease, such as infestations.

In some instances, the family history may not be positive for the presenting disorder but for associated diseases, for example in the following.

- Eczemas—to identify potential atopy (the association between the atopic disorders eczema, asthma, and hay fever).
- Autoimmune diseases (e.g. associations between vitiligo, thyroid disease, and pernicious anemia).
- Some neoplasms of skin (e.g. sebaceous tumors) may be linked with a familial tendency to internal neoplasia.

Medical history and medications

A general medical history may be important in determining causes of some skin disorders, as several multiorgan diseases are first manifest in the skin (Figs 2.12–2.15); dermatology has interfaces with all other medical specialties (Chs 11–14). Recent events, which may be viewed as minor and not volunteered by patients, include sore throats (a typical trigger of guttate psoriasis) and influenza-like symptoms (which may precede a viral exanthem or urticaria).

Medications (over the counter and prescribed, topical and systemic, and including 'natural' herbal preparations) may cause skin eruptions, some patterns being linked strongly to a small number of specific agents, and the dermatologic history should document medications in the period prior to occurrence of an eruption. Questions to ask if patients are suspected of having a drug eruption are given in Ch. 18.

Knowledge of current medication may also be important to avoid interactions, particularly with increasing use of potentially toxic systemic therapy in dermatology. Previous systemic drug hypersensitivity and external contact allergies may be important when planning therapy. Aspirin is particularly relevant as a potential cause of bleeding in patients having skin surgery, but its use is often not documented or volunteered by patients. Foods may also be important, especially for episodic urticaria.

Hobbies

These are less likely to be relevant than the occupation as a cause of dermatitis, but a number of chemicals are encountered in common hobbies. These include epoxy resins (adhesives), rubber chemicals (footwear, gloves, and handles of sports equipment), and plant substances (gardening) (Table 2.2 and Ch. 6).

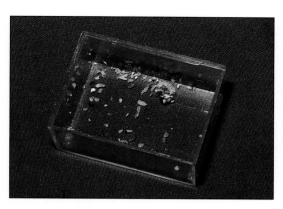

Figure 2.16 The matchbox sign. A collection of carpet fluff and small fragments of wood and skin produced by a patient with delusions of parasitosis. (From Lawrence CM, Cox NH. Physical Signs in Dermatology, 2nd edn. London: Mosby, 2002.)

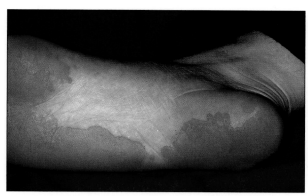

Figure 2.17 Pitted keratolysis. This condition is essentially site-specific, affecting the sole of the foot (rarely, a similar appearance may occur on the hands).

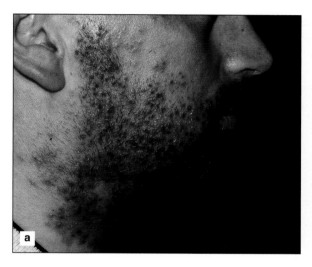

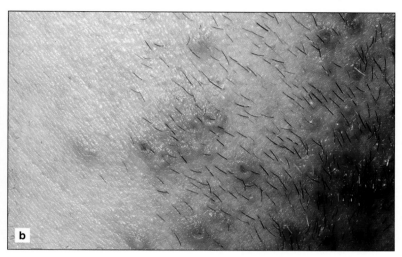

Figure 2.18 Herpes simplex folliculitis is confined to areas where there are adequate follicles. (**a**) View to show distribution in the beard area. (**b**) Close-up shows typical morphology of herpetic vesicles and follicular distribution.

Effects of the condition

There has been recent interest in the effects of skin problems on lifestyle, relationships, costs to the patient, and costs to the community from workdays lost. Various quality of life questionnaires have been developed, which are particularly applied for health economics research. In routine practice, it is helpful to know at least the patient's main concerns. These issues apply particularly to chronic skin eruptions, especially those with severe itch, with visible rash, or requiring complicated time-consuming treatments; however, many patients with discrete lesions also have concerns and in particular often want reassurance that skin malignancy is not a consideration.

Sometimes patients may be hugely affected by a problem that appears clinically trivial to the observer (in some instances, to the point of this being psychologically abnormal and requiring expert help). Such issues require careful documentation.

Social factors

Several social factors may influence treatment modalities. Work commitments may make it difficult to use messy treatments, or to attend an outpatient treatment facility if this cannot offer out-of-hours appointments. Factors such as having several young children may determine the feasibility, and alcohol intake the desirability, of hospital admission.

Excessive alcohol intake, apart from being a risk for behavioral difficulties with inpatients, appears to worsen several inflammatory skin disorders (if nothing else, it leads to poor treatment compliance), and sufficient alcohol to cause abnormal liver function may contraindicate use of systemic agents such as methotrexate.

Cigarette smoking has a close association with palmoplantar pustulosis (see Ch. 7, Fig. 7.14) and is useful support for this diagnosis. About 90% of patients are smokers at the onset of the condition; unfortunately, resolution of the pustules does not follow cessation of smoking. In patients treated with antimalarial drugs for collagen vascular disorders, smoking significantly reduces the benefit that can be achieved.

Depending on the healthcare system in which the practitioner works, financial considerations for the patient (such as extent of insurance cover), or for the healthcare system (such as agreements on cosmetic procedures), may also be an important part of the history.

EXAMINATION OF THE SKIN

Examination of the skin should be performed in an environment with appropriate privacy and with good illumination. Mobile lighting is required for close-up inspection and to side-light the skin, a useful maneuver in assessing texture and minor degrees of elevation above the skin surface. A good examination light is important for examination of the mouth, and a torch to test for transillumination. A hand lens is often useful for detailed examination, and a ruler is essential for recording lesion sizes. Other tools and techniques of value are listed below.

Ideally, the entire skin should be examined as, even if not obviously pertinent for localized lesions, there may be important incidental findings. It may also provide unexpected clues to the diagnosis of the presenting condition. Similarly, it is sometimes crucial, and often helpful, to examine the mouth and specialized skin structures such as the nails. However, performing a full skin examination in all patients routinely may not always be feasible. It can be time-consuming to prepare the patient, to perform the examination, and to explain incidental findings that may have no significance; additionally, some patients are embarrassed by the prospect of a full skin examination that they have not anticipated (e.g. if they have presented with a simple lesion on an arm). In practice, whether it is possible to routinely perform full skin examination is likely to be largely determined by the expectations and volume demands of the healthcare system in which the practitioner works. It may also be influenced by the

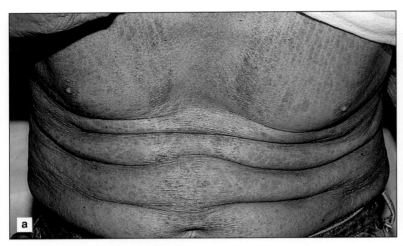

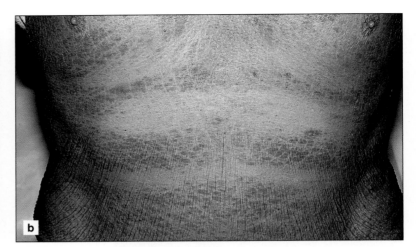

Figure 2.19 (**a**,**b**) Stretching the skin reveals features that may not initially be apparent. Close up, it reduces vascularity and enables other colors to be seen. In this case, the characteristic sparing of creases (the deckchair sign) of a disorder known as papuloerythroderma (Ofuji disease) is made apparent.

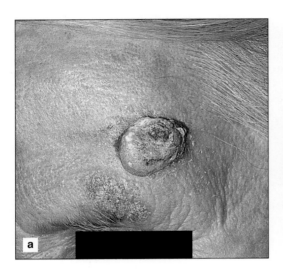

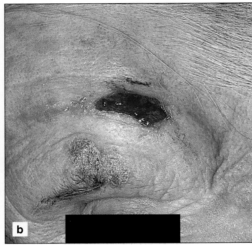

Figure 2.20 (**a**,**b**) Picking the skin is vital to evaluate some crusted conditions. In this case, an apparently large nodule was simply lifted off and demonstrated to be a large heap of infected crust overlying a small area of benign granulation tissue.

likely yield of significant lesions; for example, it is potentially more valuable in areas of high melanoma prevalence than in areas of low prevalence.

General examination

Many factors of potential diagnostic benefit may be apparent even before any formal examination. Thus arthritis, jaundice, thyroid disease, etc. may all be appreciated at a distance. The same applies to some dermatoses on the face, and general cutaneous features, such as overt solar damage, are readily visible and appreciated before a more detailed examination. Other physical signs may be presented during the consultation (Fig. 2.16). Olfactory stimuli such as alcohol, or smell from ulcers, may also be very apparent.

The extent of the general medical examination required will obviously vary depending on the diagnostic area, and will not be detailed here. The body site affected may be specifically important (Figs 2.17 and 2.18), and may affect the appearance of some eruptions, for example erythematous scaling rashes such as psoriasis occurring in the flexures have a brighter red color and may lack scale compared with their morphology at other sites. Similarly, some rashes or localized lesions have a particular predilection for specific sites (see later in this chapter).

Examination modalities and special techniques

Examination of skin lesions should determine the shape, elevation, symmetry, morphology of the border, color, vascularity, and presence of hyperkeratosis or crusting. The terminology for the shapes and patterns is described in Chapter 1. Simple visual inspection of the skin can be significantly enhanced by a variety of simple techniques, and by using other sensory modalities, such as touch. Some of these, all of which are commonly performed as part of clinical examination, are listed briefly.

Additional tests that require less routine equipment, or that have a laboratory component, are discussed separately.

Palpation

It is rare for dermatologists to diagnose a rash or localized lesion without touching it (Figs 2.14 and 2.19). Simple palpation of the skin will give information about the following.

- Surface texture and quality of scaling—texture of scaling differs between dermatoses, and the generally dry skin of atopic dermatitis is best assessed by touch.
- Deeper texture—is the lesion firm or soft?
- Site of a lesion within the skin—is it dermal, subcutaneous, etc.?
- Thickness of lesions—particularly applied to nodular lesions.
- Skin temperature—for example increased in infection and several inflammatory conditions, but typically decreased over chilblains.

There are several useful extensions of simple palpation, which include the following.

- Squeezing—for example, tethered dermal nodules such as dermatofibromas will dimple into the skin when squeezed. Some lesions may express pus or mucin when squeezed.
- Picking the crust off moist skin lesions—this is useful for visualization of the base (Fig. 2.20); a diagnosis can rarely be made when the only visible feature is crust.
- Linear pressure and rubbing—linear stroking of the skin may elicit a dermographic response in urticaria (Ch. 9), and rubbing the skin can be helpful in diagnosis of urticaria pigmentosa by producing the Darier sign (Fig. 2.21).
- Scratching a scaly rash—this may demonstrate the fine, bran-like scale of pityriasiform processes, or the striking silvery scaling of psoriasis.

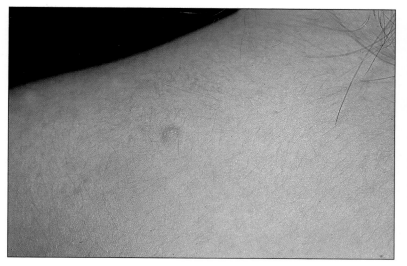

Figure 2.21 Darier sign. Rubbing the skin lesions of urticaria pigmentosa and other forms of mastocytosis causes degranulation of mast cells. The release of histamine and other inflammatory mediators produces perilesional erythema or a weal and flare reaction.

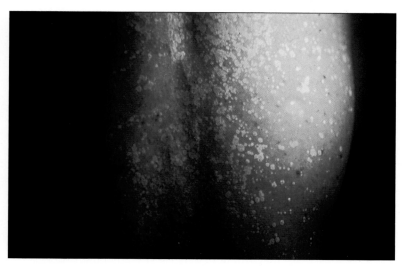

Figure 2.23 Wood's light examination. In this case demonstrating the yellow fluorescence of pityriasis versicolor, although in normal lighting the lesions would appear pale brown.

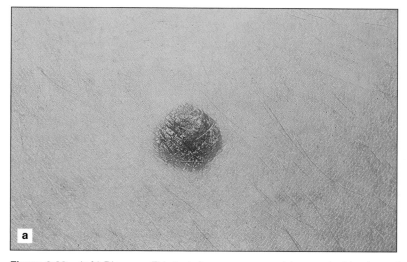

a

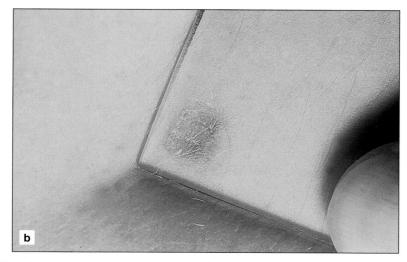

b

Figure 2.22 (**a,b**) Diascopy. This technique compresses intravascular blood out of skin lesions to demonstrate other color changes, or to demonstrate extravasated blood. It is usually performed using a glass microscope slide or, with a greater degree of safety, with a stiff strip of colorless plastic. In this case, diascopy of a Spitz nevus reveals the underlying brownish color of melanin that is otherwise largely obscured by the prominent vascular component.

Paring lesions

Some keratinized lesions have to be scalpel-pared to confirm a diagnosis. This particularly applies to the differential diagnosis between warts and corns on the sole of the foot; the former have small, dark dots due to thrombosed vessels when the surface is pared, whereas corns have a small, pearly, central nodule of compact keratin.

Diascopy

This is the use of a firm, colorless translucent strip to compress blood out of the skin and to enhance the visibility of other colors (Fig. 2.22). It is particularly valuable in diagnosis of granulomatous disorders, which have a residual yellowish brown color, and to detect melanin pigmentation in highly vascularized nevi. It will also distinguish between intravascular and extravasated blood; however, there are some pitfalls to this technique when evaluating tiny spots of possible purpura, as some small and tortuous angiomas are unable to be emptied of their blood content by the rather diffuse compression that is applied.

Skin surface microscopy

Several instruments are now available for skin microscopy (dermoscopy). Traditionally, this was used for examination of abnormal nail fold capillaries in connective tissue disorders, but more recently has been used in the diagnosis of pigmented lesions, especially in the differential diagnosis between nevi and melanoma. There are numerous specialist publications on this topic and the many diseases that it can help to diagnose; for example angiomas and basal cell carcinoma have features that are often characteristic, and scabies mites can be visualized.

Wood's light

Wood's light is a long-wavelength (around 364 nm) UV light, which is useful in several areas in dermatology (Fig. 2.23). Examples of different types of use include the following.

- Infections—it is used to demonstrate fluorescence in some infections (usually for cat and dog type of scalp ringworm, erythrasma, and pityriasis versicolor, but *Pseudomonas* spp. also fluoresce).
- Porphyria—the urine in porphyria cutanea tarda fluoresces reddish pink.
- Pigmentation—it accentuates epidermal pigmentation, and is therefore useful in the diagnosis of some pigmentary disorders. For example, the pale areas of vitiligo (loss of epidermal melanocytes) are exaggerated under Wood's light, whereas the pale skin of nevus anemicus (which is due to vasoconstriction, with normal epidermal melanization) becomes invisible.
- Natural pigments—in chromhidrosis, patients notice coloured sweat; this is due to lipofuscins in the sweat, which fluoresce green (see Ch. 23).

LABORATORY AND INTERVENTIONAL TESTS

A wide range of tests may be required in patients with cutaneous signs of systemic disease, and in monitoring therapy, but these will not be addressed here. This section discusses tests that are performed on the skin but that require some additional equipment or laboratory facilities.

Testing for contact hypersensitivity

Patch tests

Patch tests (Fig. 2.24) are a frequently performed procedure in the investigation of type 4 hypersensitivity reactions (contact dermatitis), for which the tests are usually applied for 48 h (Ch. 6). The same basic technique, but with application times of a few hours, is used in investigation of contact urticaria.

Prick tests

These tests for type 1 hypersensitivity are less commonly performed in dermatology. The more common agents that give positive results are the aeroallergens involved in atopy, but these are generally more relevant to management of asthma than of eczema. Prick tests can be useful in some food reactions and in some immediate hypersensitivity reactions (e.g. to latex). They are of limited value in urticaria, as many cases are not allergic in mechanism, but may be useful to confirm a suspected allergen in some instances. Prick testing in urticaria is also limited by the fact that pricking the skin in such patients will often cause a weal regardless of the test agent.

Radio-allergo-sorbent test (RAST)

This test and similar immunologic tests are performed on blood samples to detect type 1 hypersensitivity. They are more expensive than prick tests, and the range of substances that can be tested is smaller, but they have the advantage of safety in patients with severe hypersensitivity reactions, such as that occurring with peanuts.

Testing for fungal infection

Fungi of relevance to the skin include yeasts such as *Candida* spp., dermatophytes (ringworm fungi), and less common organisms that cause deeper infections.

Skin swabs

These are performed primarily for identification of bacterial infection, but are also appropriate if candidal infection is present. In the case of deeper infections, culture of biopsy tissue is more helpful.

Skin scrapings

These are the pertinent investigation for cutaneous dermatophyte fungal infection (ringworm) and for pityriasis versicolor (a yeast infection). They are obtained by scraping the skin surface with a blade, ideally from the edge of a lesion where scaling is most apparent. Generally, in the case of dermatophytes, the evaluation of skin scrapings will consist of both initial direct microscopy (after softening the keratin with 20% potassium hydroxide) and culture to identify the precise type of dermatophyte present. Sometimes fungi are visualized using special stains as well. Culture is not routinely performed for suspected pityriasis versicolor.

Hair and nails

Fungal infection of the scalp due to some dermatophytes, notably the infection acquired from cats and dogs, will fluoresce under a Wood's light. Hairs can also be plucked for microscopy and culture, as performed for skin scrapings. Nail clippings for identification of fungal infection are an important investigation, as treatment usually involves relatively long-term systemic therapy. In the most common types of infection, affecting the distal nail, detection rates are best if the nail is clipped back as far as possible to the proximal edge of the clinically abnormal zone.

Testing for viral infection

Direct identification of viral infection from skin samples is performed primarily for herpesvirus infection. Viral culture is infrequently used in routine practice now, due to improved immunologic techniques.

Tzank smear

This technique involves scraping the base of a viral vesicle, transferring the material on to a glass slide, staining as for a blood film, and observing cells with viral cytopathic changes by direct microscopy. It has the advantage of speed and simplicity but does not identify the virus if positive (e.g. it does not distinguish between herpes simplex and herpes zoster). It can also be used to confirm a diagnosis of molluscum contagiosum using material expressed from a lesion.

Electron microscopy

This is also a rapid technique for identification of herpesvirus infection but is not widely available. It is also useful for other large viruses, for example to confirm a diagnosis of orf.

Immunologic methods

In detection of herpesviruses, enzyme-linked immunosorbent assay (ELISA) is useful, as it does not require viable virus and can be performed on scrapings as described earlier, or even on crust from an older vesicle. More sophisticated immunologic methods, such as in situ hybridization and the polymerase chain reaction (PCR), are used to identify the presence and type of human papillomavirus in skin lesions.

Biopsy of lesions

This is not frequently required for diagnosis of viral diseases but may demonstrate characteristic histology in some instances, such as viral warts or molluscum contagiosum. Additionally, since the advent of PCR techniques, biopsy material may be used to detect infection with agents such as human papillomavirus or Epstein–Barr virus.

Obtaining samples for histology

Most histologic specimens submitted by dermatologists are those obtained during excision or other treatment of localized lesions such as skin cancers; surgical techniques are discussed in more detail in Chapter 5. However, there are also many situations where sampling part of a skin eruption is beneficial to guide or support a diagnosis. This is usually to obtain a sample for histologic examination but may be to obtain specimens for microbial culture. For diagnostic purposes, there are various types of biopsy tissue-removal procedures (discussed in this section). Most are performed with injected local anesthesia, but some do not require this (e.g. fine-needle aspiration or small superficial shave biopsies to confirm a diagnosis of basal cell carcinoma), and some may be performed with topical anesthesia.

When submitting specimens to a laboratory, it is helpful to indicate which technique has been used, and also whether the specimen is an excised lesion, a portion from within a lesion, or a biopsy into the edge of

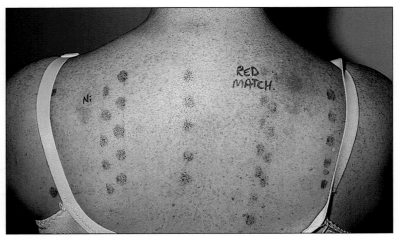

Figure 2.24 Patch testing. This patient has had test strips removed to reveal positive tests to nickel (in metal items) and phosphorus sequisulfide (in red match heads, a cause of facial eczema). The blue-black dots are ink marks adjacent to the site of test application, so that any positive reactions later can be localized and identified.

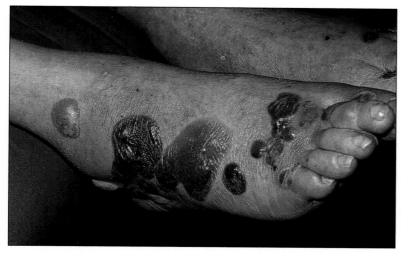

Figure 2.25   Hemorrhagic bullae in a patient with pemphigoid. In this condition, direct immunofluorescence tests show deposits of IgG and complement C3 at the dermo–epidermal junction (see Ch. 16).

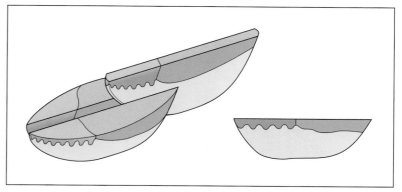

Figure 2.26   Diagram demonstrating how the laboratory will process a diagnostic ellipse into the edge of lesional skin. The aim is to have about one-third normal and two-thirds lesional skin, cut so that the histopathologist can see the interface between the two. By contrast, excision of a localized lesion will be processed perpendicular to the axis shown here (compare with Fig. 5.9). As specimens will shrink, and are generally pale after formalin fixation compared with the in vivo appearance, it is essential to tell the laboratory what technique has been used. A simple diagram is often best. (After an original drawing by Dr. N. H. Cox.)

a lesion; all these may influence the orientation of the specimen during processing and the interpretation of the results. In some instances, fresh unfixed skin may be required; this may either be frozen for immunologic stains (e.g. in blistering eruptions, Fig. 2.25, or for some lymphocyte markers), or be cultured (especially in mycobacterial or deep fungal infections). Immunofluorescence of blistering eruptions is discussed in more detail in Chapter 16.

In the laboratory, the fixed tissue is processed as thin slices and stained, usually with hematoxylin (blue) and eosin (red). However, other special stains may also be used, depending on the likely pathologic process, to identify collagen, melanin, fungi, mucopolysaccharide, etc.

The main biopsy techniques are described here.

Excision biopsy
This is applied primarily to localized lesions, for which the aim is often both therapeutic and diagnostic. See Chapter 5.

Curettage
This involves scraping a lesion from the skin surface, usually with some form of hemostasis or cautery to the base. It is most commonly performed for treatment of localized lesions such as seborrheic keratosis or small basal cell carcinomas, and is discussed in Chapter 5. It is definitely not appropriate for diagnosis of rashes, and the pathologic specimen obtained is suboptimal generally if the issue is mainly diagnostic.

Shave biopsy
This technique uses a scalpel or razor blade to obtain a superficial sample of a localized lesion. Some small lesions can be removed completely by a saucer-shaped shave biopsy. The base is treated as for a curettage. It is mainly used for treatment rather than for diagnosis but can be of diagnostic value; it is particularly useful in confirming a diagnosis of basal cell carcinoma prior to radiotherapy, as many basal cell carcinomas can be painlessly and quickly biopsied in this way without need for local anesthesia.

Incisional biopsy
Incisional biopsies may be of various types. The most frequent and easiest to interpret histologically is an ellipse-shaped biopsy through the edge of a rash or lesion, consisting of two-thirds lesion and one-third adjacent normal skin. This has the advantage of providing the pathologist with the edge of the lesion, which is often informative, and also with adjacent normal skin as a control (particularly useful if immunohistochemistry is required). Note that the laboratory workers need to be told what has been done, as they will process a diagnostic ellipse of this type by cutting along the length of the specimen (Fig. 2.26).

A more rapid technique, but one which provides smaller specimens and generally is limited to lesional skin, is use of punch biopsy.

Hair disorders
Culture for fungal infection has already been discussed. Other investigations are discussed in this section.

Hair microscopy
This may involve light and electron microscopy, and is performed for identification of hair shaft defects, especially congenital hair shaft disorders with easily broken hair.

Hair pluck analysis
The ratio between growing (anagen) and involuting (telogen) hair roots can be determined using plucked samples of 20–50 hairs, and can be diagnostically useful in some situations (Fig. 2.27).

Scalp biopsy
This can give useful information about scalp disorders with effects on hair growth. The processing of scalp biopsies for histologic examination may be either along the line of the hair root or, in some instances, transversely.

Testing for disorders of sweating
Special techniques, such as pilocarpine stimulation, can be used to quantify sweat production but are primarily research tools. Identifying discrete areas of increased or decreased sweat production can be performed in a semiquantitative manner and is important in some genodermatoses with abnormal sweating, or in neurologic disorders with damage to sympathetic nerve fibers to the skin (such as reflex sympathetic dystrophy, Frey syndrome, or some cases of carpal tunnel syndrome). The starch–iodine test is the most frequently used in these situations (Fig. 2.28).

Phototesting for photosensitivity disorders
This specialized area is discussed in Chapter 17.

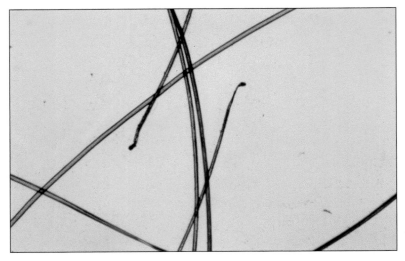

Figure 2.27   Hair microscopy.

Radiology and ultrasound

These are rarely used other than for investigation of systemic features of disease. However, radiology may be useful in detection of cutaneous calcinosis (e.g. childhood dermatomyositis) and calcification of cartilage (e.g. of the ear in recurrent cold injury), or for illustrating bony abnormalities (Fig. 2.29). Ultrasound of skin is used primarily as a research tool but may be useful in monitoring sclerodermatous processes or in the assessment of angiomas.

REGIONAL DERMATOLOGY AND SITES OF PREDILECTION

Some disorders have a sufficiently strong predilection for specific body sites that this can be diagnostically useful. In some instances, it is useful to have a list of likely diagnoses when a lesion or eruption is localized to one specific site (Tables 2.3 and 2.4, Figs 2.30 and 2.31). Most disorders listed are discussed in other chapters, but a specific list of flexural rashes and lesions has been provided in Table 2.4, as rashes at these sites often create diagnostic difficulty (see also Fig. 2.32).

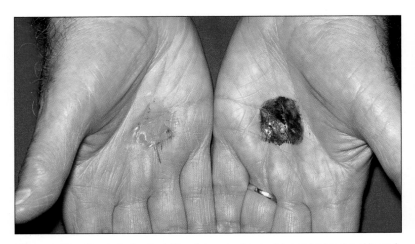

Figure 2.28   Starch–iodine test. Starch in anhydrous oil is applied to the skin and then painted with iodine in anhydrous alcohol. In the presence of water, starch and iodine form a blue-black reaction product, so active sweating can be identified as small black dots over the sweat duct orifices. In this case, the patient complained of asymmetric color, sweating, and grip; this was due to sympathetic nerve damage from previous thoracic surgery, most easily demonstrated by the asymmetry of sweating illustrated. The sweating of his 'good' hand is so marked that the black reaction product of the test has pooled.

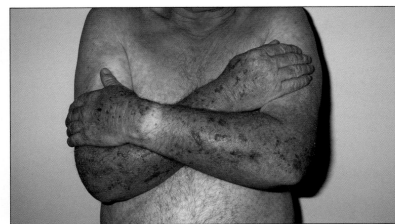

Figure 2.30   Photosensitivity affects exposed areas of skin, typically the face, V of the neck, and exposed parts of the arms. Note the sparing of the area under a watch strap.

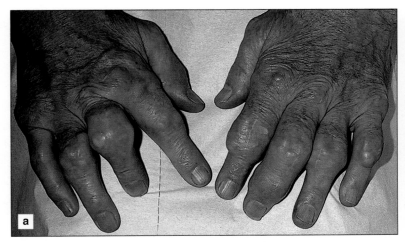

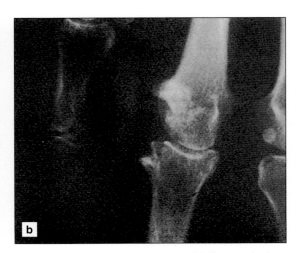

Figure 2.29   (**a**) Radiology is not used extensively in dermatology but can be helpful, as in this patient with tophi due to gout. (**b**) The punched-out erosions occurring in the phalanges of the case shown in (a).

Table 2.3   SOME DISORDERS THAT HAVE PREDILECTION FOR SPECIFIC BODY SITES

Body site	Disorders
Scalp	Hair disorders and alopecia, psoriasis, seborrheic dermatitis, lichen simplex (nape of neck), pilar cysts, organoid nevus (a hamartoma), cutaneous metastases of internal malignancy
Eyelids	Atopic dermatitis, contact allergy (cosmetics, nickel), seborrheic blepharitis, angioedema, dermatomyositis, basal cell carcinoma, xanthelasma
Face	Acne, atopic dermatitis, seborrheic dermatitis (especially eyebrows and nasolabial crease), causes of butterfly rash (rosacea, erysipelas, lupus erythematosus, lupus pernio, erythema infectiosum), photosensitivity, nevi and freckles, actinic keratoses, basal and squamous cell carcinomas, keratoacanthoma, lentigo maligna
Lips	Dermatitis (atopic, contact), cheilitis (angular, actinic), angioedema, contact urticaria, impetigo, erythema multiforme, warts, vascular lesions (venous lake, pyogenic granuloma), squamous cell carcinoma
Hands	Dermatitis (dyshidrotic, pompholyx, contact), psoriasis and palmoplantar pustulosis, keratodermas, dermatophyte infections, erythema multiforme, photosensitivity (dorsal hand), scabies (especially finger webs), collagen vascular disorders and vasculitis (especially nail fold and fingertip), viral warts, actinic keratoses, squamous cell carcinoma, granuloma annulare, nail disorders
Limbs	Psoriasis (elbows, knees), atopic dermatitis (limb flexures), discoid eczema, venous eczema and ulceration (lower leg), asteatotic eczema (lower leg), lichen simplex (lower leg), lichen planus (flexor forearms, shins), dermatitis herpetiformis (knee, elbow), granuloma annulare (elbows), erythema nodosum (legs), vasculitis (legs), papular urticaria or flea bites (lower leg), dermatofibroma, Bowen disease (lower leg)
Feet	Dermatitis (pompholyx, contact, juvenile plantar), psoriasis and palmoplantar pustulosis, dermatophyte fungal infection (skin and nails), pitted keratolysis, vasculitis and arterial disease, callosities or corns, verrucae
Axillae	See Table 2.4
Genital	Psoriasis or Reiter syndrome, lichen planus (penis), lichen sclerosus (penis, vulva), lichen simplex (scrotum, vulva), fixed drug eruption (penis), sexually transmitted diseases or genital warts, Zoon balanitis (glans penis), epidermoid cysts (scrotal), squamous cell carcinoma (penis, vulva)

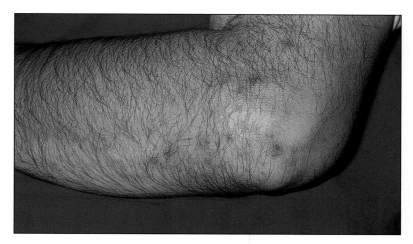

Figure 2.31 Dermatitis herpetiformis: rather minor-looking lesions, but with intense itch and with a characteristic distribution pattern including scalp, scapulae, sacrum, elbows, and knees (but beware—scabies may mimic this pattern and morphology of lesions, although it usually affects the hands as well).

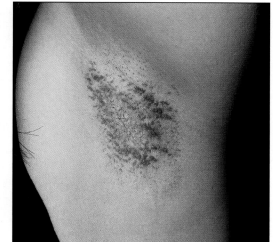

Figure 2.32 Granular parakeratosis. This flexural disorder most commonly affects axillae, and may suggest commoner diagnoses such as contact dermatitis or (because of the site and the crusting) Hailey–Hailey disease. (Courtesy of Dr. G. Dawn.)

In other cases, a particular combination of affected sites is characteristic. Some examples are as follows.

- Psoriasis—elbows, knees, scalp, low back, and nails (Ch. 7).
- Scabies—hands, wrists, elbows, waistline, genitalia (male), and periareolar (women) (Ch. 27).
- Photosensitivity—face, V of neck, dorsal hands and forearms, sparing under watch strap (Fig. 2.30 and Ch. 17).
- Atopic dermatitis—antecubital and popliteal fossae, wrists, and ankles (varies with age group; Ch. 6).
- Dermatitis herpetiformis—elbows, knees, scapulae, sacrum, and scalp (Fig. 2.31).

Certain features should prompt careful examination of distant sites, particularly in situations where the patient may not volunteer information. A few examples are as follows.

- Lichen planus. Any purple or violaceous papular rash should arouse suspicion of lichen planus. About 75% of patients have oral involvement (see Ch. 8), but this is asymptomatic in 75% of these individuals, therefore the mouth must be examined at the instigation of the doctor.
- Scabies. Genital and breast involvement is common but may not be volunteered due to embarrassment. Specific examination of these sites may be of diagnostic importance.
- Psoriasis. Nail involvement is common, especially if psoriasis affects the hands. The nail changes may be clinically diagnostic even though the skin lesions may be non-specific in some patients.

Table 2.4   SOME DISORDERS THAT HAVE PREDILECTION FOR FLEXURAL SITES

Type of disorder	Disorder	Comments[a]
Inflammatory dermatoses	Psoriasis	Common in flexures, typically red and shiny rather than the usual white scale (Ch. 7); may be termed the inverse pattern if mainly flexural distribution
	Seborrheic dermatitis	Usually with lesions elsewhere also (Ch. 6)
	Contact dermatitis	Irritant or allergic; may affect the vault of the axilla (e.g. deodorants) or axillary folds (e.g. clothing dermatitis) (Ch. 6)
	Intertrigo	Especially inframammary; may be due to simple maceration, but also secondary infection may occur (staphylococcal, streptococcal, candidal)
	Napkin rash	Many causes; the commonest are irritant and candidal (see Ch. 19)
	Lichen planus	Not often mainly flexural but may cause confusion, as flexural and genital lesions are often brown or annular, rather than the usual purplish plaques
	Hidradenitis suppurativa	Affects axillae, groin, inframammary area (Ch. 10)
	Crohn disease	Cutaneous lesions affect especially the perineum (Ch. 12)
	Atopic dermatitis	Affects elbow and knee flexures, uncommonly the major flexures, other than in infants, when the process may be generalized
Bullous diseases	Pemphigus vegetans	Rare, mainly flexural (Ch. 16)
	Hailey–Hailey disease	Inherited, variable (see Ch. 19)
Infections	Dermatophytes	Especially male groin—always look for evidence of associated tinea pedis (Ch. 26)
	Erythrasma	Brownish color, fluoresces under Wood's light (Ch. 24)
	Trichomycosis axillaris	Coated hair shafts (see Ch. 24)
	Candidiasis	Especially in napkin rash or in bed-bound elderly adults, commoner in diabetes; satellite pustules are characteristic
	Bacterial	Various types: follicular infections (furuncles), perianal abscesses, secondary infection of intertrigo, gram-negative toe web infections, etc.
	Scabies	Multiple itchy flexural nodules are highly suggestive of the relatively chronic nodular variant; penile lesions are also common in this pattern (Ch. 27)
Localized lesions	Fibroepithelial polyps (skin tags)	Common normal variant
	Neurofibromatosis	Axillary freckling is seen (Crowe sign)
	Fox–Fordyce disease	An apocrine occlusion dermatosis (see Ch. 23)
	Pseudoxanthoma elasticum	Inherited defect of elastic tissue, most apparent on the neck and axillae (Ch. 22)
Miscellaneous	Hyperhidrosis and other sweat apparatus disorders	Mainly axillae (see Ch. 23)
	Acanthosis nigricans	May be endocrine-related or paraneoplastic (see Ch. 12)
	Acrodermatitis enteropathica or zinc deficiency	Severe napkin rash and perioral rash in an infant (Ch. 19), acquired version in adults; necrolytic migratory erythema of glucagonoma syndrome may have the same pattern
	Langerhans cell histiocytosis	May present as severe napkin rash (Ch. 19)
	Granular parakeratosis	Rare; hyperkeratotic, mainly adult female axilla (Fig. 2.32)

[a]All refer to major flexures unless specified.

- Lupus erythematosus. A butterfly rash on the face can cause great anxiety for doctors, but may be due to rosacea or seborrheic dermatitis rather than to lupus erythematosus. Nail fold telangiectasia is a useful feature to confirm a connective tissue disorder but is usually asymptomatic (Fig. 2.33).

Non-cutaneous sites

The hair and nails are modified skin structures and may be abnormal in numerous dermatoses. The teeth are also ectodermal structures that may be involved in a variety of inherited disorders. Examination of the mouth and other mucosal surfaces (conjunctivae, genital) may yield useful information as part of the examination of the skin (Ch. 20).

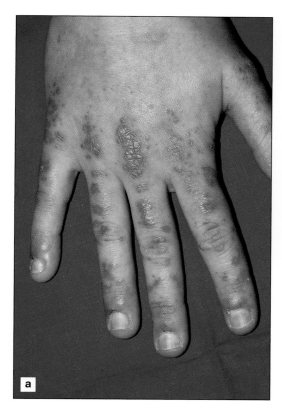

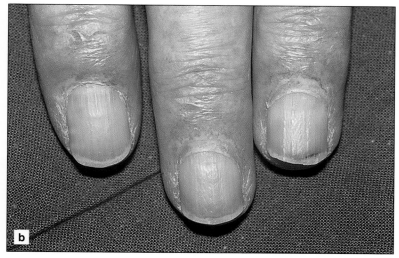

Figure 2.33 Dermatomyositis. (**a**) Streaky rash on the dorsum of the fingers. (**b**) This is a condition where examination of the nail folds is specifically useful; illustrated are the characteristic connective tissue changes of an elongated ragged cuticle and prominent capillary loops within a sclerotic dermis.

FURTHER READING

Lawrence CM, Cox NH. Physical Signs in Dermatology, 2nd edn. London: Mosby, 2002

Marks R, Dykes P, Motley R. Clinical Signs and Procedures in Dermatology. London: Dunitz, 1993

White GM. Regional Dermatology. London: Mosby-Wolfe, 1994

3 Topical Therapy

INTRODUCTION AND GENERAL PRINCIPLES

Topical therapy is the mainstay of dermatologic therapy. To be a dermatologist is to know the skin and how to improve it or cure it with topical therapy. While pills, injections, and infusions are becoming more and more important, the art and science of topical treatment is what most distinguishes dermatology from other medical disciplines. What vehicle to choose, how much to give, how often to apply it, etc. are described in this chapter. We also provide an overview of many of the more commonly used dermatologic topical therapies. Note, however, that some of these are more appropriately dealt with in disease-related chapters. For example, treatment of warts may include keratolytics, aldehydes, immuno-modulators, and cytotoxic agents; discussion of the role of each of these is more conveniently placed in Chapter 25 in the section on warts.

The following discussion of vehicle, frequency, amount, etc. applies most directly to topical steroid use, but can often be extrapolated to other therapeutic categories.

Vehicle

It may be argued that the default vehicle is the cream. Creams are relatively easy to apply and are preferred by most patients. They can, however, have a drying effect with continued use. Creams are particularly appropriate for the face, neck, and groin, and for exudative conditions. Ointments are preferred in many situations, as they provide grease that is necessary to repair the barrier function of the skin (e.g. in eczema) and to reduce the appearance of scales (e.g. in psoriasis). The ointment also provides a measure of occlusion, thus increasing the potency of the agent. However, it should be noted that it is incorrect to use an active agent in ointment form primarily to benefit from the emollient action; this is discussed further later in this chapter. Ointments also have a potential advantage in that they are often preservative-free and thus less likely to cause allergy than are creams, which are water-based and therefore usually require addition of antimicrobials.

Solutions and lotions are easily spread over large areas, as well as being well suited for the scalp and other hair-bearing areas. They may cause stinging and burning, however. A thermolabile foam preparation is quite elegant and can be used on the scalp as well. Gels are often used on the face or in body folds. Aerosol sprays (with a tube attachment for the scalp) have been used for ease of application. For example, they may ease treatment of the legs in patients with limited mobility.

Frequency of application

Most prescription topical agents are applied once or twice a day. More frequent application is usually a waste of the medication. Frequency of application is usually category-specific. Topical retinoids are applied once a day, while topical steroids and macrolactam immununomodulators (tacrolimus and pimecrolimus) are usually applied twice daily (abbreviated to b.i.d.).

Amount to dispense

The amount of cream needed to cover the average adult's entire body is 20–30 g. If one is going to treat a total body skin rash with topical therapy b.i.d. for 1 month, one would need $30 \times 2 \times 25$ g = 1500 g or twenty-five 60-g tubes! Thus one can see that a patient with a total body rash needs systemic therapy. If, however, only 10% of the body surface area (BSA) needs to be treated, then 150 g for 1 month is sufficient. One helpful rule of thumb for calculating BSA is that the surface area of one palm is about 0.5% of the total BSA over a broad range of ages (or a closed hand is 1%). Alternatively, the rule of nines, as used in burns treatment, can be applied to estimate larger areas (each arm, each lower leg or foot, each thigh, anterior trunk, posterior trunk, and head and neck each account for 9% of BSA). Neither method is accurate, however, for patients with a high body mass index.

For example, a hand dermatitis, affecting only the palms, requiring a topical steroid b.i.d. would require in a month

$$(30 \text{ days/month}) \times (2 \text{ applications/day}) \times$$
$$(1\% \text{ BSA/application}) \times (25 \text{ g/100\% BSA}) = 15 \text{ g/month.}$$

One can combine the last few terms to get

$$25 \text{ g}/100\% \text{ BSA per application} \times 0.5\% \text{ BSA/palm} = 0.125 \text{ g/palm per application}$$

or 0.125 g/palm per application × 60 applications/month (b.i.d.) means the patient will need 7.5 g/palm per month for b.i.d. application.

In practice, the amounts applied vary between individuals, vary slightly between creams and ointments even for the same individual, and are significantly altered depending on whether use is sparing, as for a topical steroid, or more liberal, as for emollients. These issues are discussed further in the following sections.

PRACTICE POINTS

- Think about alternative vehicles besides cream. Ointments are more potent, more emolliating, and less likely to cause allergy.
- One palm (not including the fingers) is 0.5% of body surface area for a lean person over a broad range of ages.
- Assuming b.i.d. application, 7.5 g/month are needed for each palm-sized area.

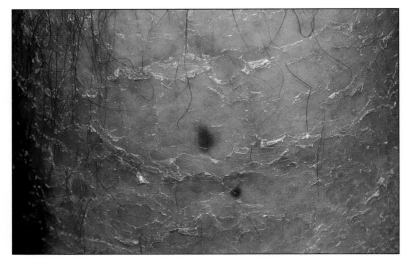

Figure 3.1 Xerosis. An emollient is necessary to reduce the scaling. A thick cream or ointment is best. Lotions contain too much water and are less effective; they can even have a drying effect.

Time of application

The best time to apply most medications is soon after washing or showering. The skin is clean, so application of a topical agent will not drive allergens and other irritants into the skin. The skin is also hydrated, increasing penetration and improving efficacy. For example, patients with eczema should apply their topical agents or emollients within a few minutes of getting out of the shower or bath. This locks in the moisture that the skin has absorbed. Waiting more than 5 min allows the water to evaporate. However, if both a topical steroid and an emollient are to be used, the steroid should be applied first, and it may be best to apply the emollient after an interval of perhaps 30 min.

PRACTICE POINTS

- In the shower or bath, the skin—like a sponge—absorbs water. The skin is 'sticky' when hydrated (increased coefficient of friction). This stickiness is lost 3–6 min after the shower or bath. Patients with atopic dermatitis should apply their medications within a 3–5 min time period.
- The active medication (e.g. steroid) should always be applied first. Some patients or their parents mistakenly apply the emollient before the steroid.
- Occlusion is an inexpensive way to augment the strength of a steroid. However, caution must be exercised, as the ultrapotent steroids may become too strong with occlusion.

Occlusion

Occluding the topical agent increases penetration and efficacy. This can be done with plastic wrap covered by a sock for the feet (gloves for the hands), vinyl suit for the body, or shower cap for the scalp. Caution must be exercised with occlusion, as it can make the ultrapotent steroids too strong.

EMOLLIENTS

The use of emollients is widespread throughout the industrialized world. Additives are common and may include botanicals (e.g. kiwifruit and apple), proteins (collagen), exfoliants (e.g. glycolic acid), sunscreens, or other potentially active agents (e.g. retinol). Ironically, however, the science of emolliating, hydrating, and exfoliating the skin is just in its infancy. What does the skin really need? Does the 30-year-old woman with no apparent skin disease need to apply a lotion to her legs? Does applying a moisturizer (without sunscreen) to the face in early adulthood prevent the development of fine lines and wrinkles later in life? (Note also that the sun

protection factor in commercial moisturizers is often too low, and applied too thinly, to really make much difference to long-term solar damage.) Further research is warranted.

What is clear is that emollients are critically important in treating certain diseases, most notably the eczemas. In eczema, the barrier function of the skin is damaged and the water content reduced. Hydrating the skin with a shower or bath followed immediately by the application of a cream or ointment (no lotions please) locks in the moisture and helps repair the barrier (Fig. 3.1). Patients feel better and the skin improves. Similarly, emollients will help to reduce scaling in numerous other dermatoses, such as psoriasis. Research is ongoing to determine the best composition of emollients to restore skin function, but at present the 'best' emollient is dictated by patient preference. This may vary according to factors such as degree of dryness, body site (e.g. face versus palms), time of day, work or social commitments, etc.—most patients therefore benefit from trying out and having available a range of agents.

What is vital, where an emollient is appropriate, is that it is used often enough and in adequate amounts to be useful. In children with eczema, for example, it is important to stress that emollients can be applied liberally and often, that they are not potentially harmful steroids, and that they will reduce itch from dry skin. Conversely, it is important that patients do not use steroid preparations for the emollient effect of their base; these should be reserved for inflamed skin. For an adult applying an emollient to all areas several times each day, at least 500 g/week is likely to be required.

In acute but non-infected exacerbations of eczema, application of emollients under damp tubular dressings (wet wraps) can be effective in some children. Particularly aimed at atopic dermatitis, in which staphylococcal infection is common, some emollients for direct application or for use in the bath are manufactured in plain versions or in versions with added antiseptic agents (e.g. benzalkonium chloride, triclosan).

PRACTICE POINTS

- The 'best' emollient is the one the patient prefers.
- The degree of dryness, body site, time of day, and work or social commitments may all influence which emollient is most suitable.
- It is vital that emollients are used often enough and in adequate amounts to be useful.
- It is important that patients do not use steroid preparations for the emollient effect of their base; these should be reserved for inflamed skin.
- Utilizing a trained dermatology nurse to explain correct use of emollients, topical steroids, and dressings is extremely valuable for patients and their parents.

TOPICAL STEROIDS

Topical corticosteroids are widely used in dermatology for their anti-inflammatory properties. They are usually applied b.i.d. initially and then can be tapered to once daily or as needed. Some are designed for once-daily use.

Potency varies greatly and is mainly a function of the steroid molecule rather than of the concentration. For example, clobetasol propionate 0.05% is ultrahigh potency, whereas hydrocortisone 1% is of low potency. The grading systems for potency vary between countries, for example a class 1 steroid in the USA is superpotent, whereas the UK system uses four grades from 'mild' to 'very potent', starting with the lower potency. Also, availability of some agents differs worldwide. To avoid confusion, we have not listed agents and potencies here but refer readers to larger or more specific texts, or to prescribing formularies pertinent to their country of work.

Vehicle influences potency as well, with ointments being 'stronger' than creams, which are in turn 'stronger' than lotions or solutions. Lotions and solutions have the problem of evaporation, which can leave inert steroid crystals that are unable to penetrate—a particular problem on scaly scalp psoriasis, for example, as discussed in the treatment section of Chapter 7. Some manufacturers make ready-diluted versions of topical steroids (typically 1:4); these are not inherently milder, although they may mean that less is used.

The choice of strength of steroid usually depends on the disease being treated and the body location (Figs 3.2–3.5). For examples, see Table 3.1.

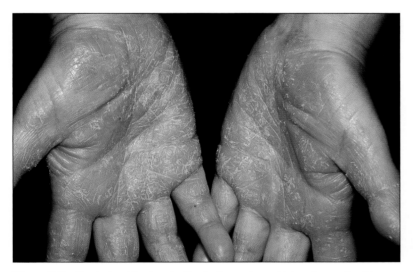

Figure 3.2 Psoriasis of the hands. Psoriasis requires a high-potency steroid, as do the palms. Together, they require a superpotent topical steroid.

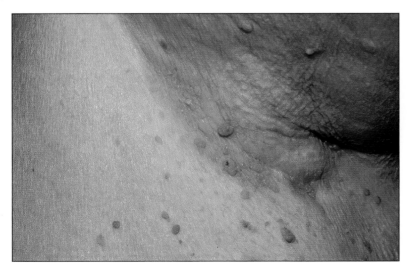

Figure 3.3 Seborrheic dermatitis of the axilla. Seborrheic dermatitis requires only a low- to medium-potency steroid. The axilla provides its own occlusion. Thus a low-potency topical steroid would be appropriate.

The general approach, which can be learned only by experience, is to choose a steroid of adequate potency to control the disease, and then to reduce potency and/or frequency. Overcautious creeping up the potency ladder means the patient has symptoms for longer (a problem in some patients or their parents who have steroid phobia), while an excessively strong agent exposes the patient to the risk of side effects if it is overused.

An appropriate amount to prescribe, for adults having b.i.d. application of a topical steroid, is discussed in some detail earlier but can be summarized as follows (bearing in mind that many topical steroids and other agents are packaged in tubes containing 30 g or 100 g, as reflected in the recommendations below).

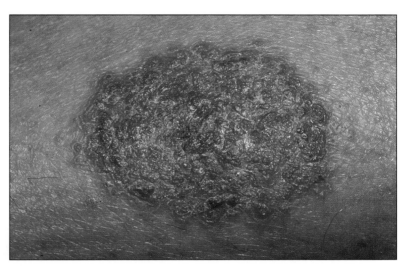

Figure 3.4 Nummular eczema. Unlike most of the other eczemas, nummular eczema requires a high-potency topical steroid.

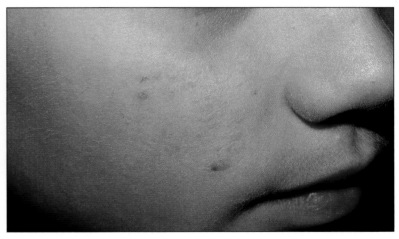

Figure 3.5 Eczema on the face of a child. A low-strength topical steroid is indicated because of the age, facial location, and eczematous process.

Table 3.1 EXAMPLES OF DISEASES AND BODY SITES THAT DETERMINE THE REQUIRED STEROID POTENCY

Steroid potency	Disease	Body site(s)
High	Psoriasis (depends on site) Nummular eczema Lichen planus (most sites)	Palms and soles Heavily lichenified skin
Medium	Atopic dermatitis (depends on site)	Trunk and legs
Low	Seborrheic dermatitis Mild eczema	Face Intertriginous areas

- Face and neck, or scalp: 15–30 g/week.
- Both hands (palm and dorsum): 15–30 g/week.
- Both arms: 30–60 g/week.
- Both legs: 100 g/week.
- Trunk, front, and back: 100 g/week.

Remember that quantities of creams or ointments required for use as an emollient are greater, as discussed earlier.

To help patients to apply the correct amount of topical steroid, a commonly used measure is the fingertip unit. Because of the uniform nozzle size of most tubes, the weight of a strip of cream or ointment squeezed from a tube and extending from the tip of the finger to the crease at the distal interphalangeal joint in an adult is 0.5 g.

Less frequently used methods for topical or local steroid use include:

- steroid-impregnated tape (e.g. for keloid scars, to confine the steroid to the application site),
- intralesional steroid injections (e.g. for keloid scars and nodular prurigo), and
- steroid mouthwash (e.g. betamethasone tablets dissolved in water for oral lichen planus).

Side effects

The use of topical steroids can lead to many side effects, including skin thinning (atrophy; Fig. 3.6), striae, purpura, folliculitis (particularly when ointments are used), steroid rosacea, and, on the face, perioral dermatitis (Table 3.2). Allergic contact dermatitis may occur as well. Systemic absorption can occur, and suppression of plasma cortisol may result in

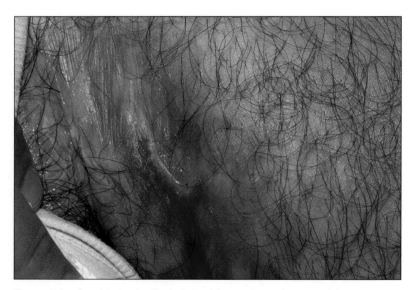

Figure 3.6 Steroid atrophy. Topical steroids over 6 months caused these changes of striae and ulceration. Stopping all steroids is indicated!

Table 3.2	CUTANEOUS SIDE EFFECTS OF TOPICAL CORTICOSTEROIDS
Type	**Side effect(s)**
Predictable	Skin thinning, striae Telangiectasia Hypertrichosis Depigmentation Tachyphylaxis and rebound effect (some disorders) Rosacea/perioral dermatitis
Idiosyncratic	Allergy to constituents
Inadvertent	Masking of non-steroid-responsive disorders (e.g. fungal infection) Worsening of secondary bacterial infection

patients using a potent steroid over a large BSA (some modern steroids are metabolized in the skin and should avoid this problem, e.g. fluticasone and mometasone).

Tachyphylaxis is not a side effect, but describes the situation in which the effectiveness of an agent decreases after several weeks of use. Its occurrence can be minimized by patients taking a periodic drug holiday.

PRACTICE POINT
- Tazarotene is the most efficacious of the topical retinoids for acne.

TOPICAL RETINOIDS

Tazarotene

Tazarotene is a topical retinoid efficacious for both acne and psoriasis. Several studies have found it to be more effective than both tretinoin and adapalene in the treatment of acne. It is usually applied once daily, but one study found it to still have significant benefit with alternate-day use. As with the other topical retinoids, its main effect is clearing the pore. For maximum benefit, it should be combined with antimicrobials that reduce *Propionibacterium acnes* counts (benzoyl peroxide, clindamycin, and erythromycin are discussed later in this chapter).

Tazarotene may also be used in psoriasis, usually with once daily application. Irritation is the most frequent side effect and can be minimized with the concomitant use of a topical steroid (e.g. applied 12 h later). An added benefit of this combination is that topical retinoids can reduce or prevent the atrophogenic effects of steroids. Finally, tazarotene 0.1% cream was found effective against photoaging, with benefit similar to that of tretinoin 0.05%.

Pregnant women are prohibited from using tazarotene.

Tretinoin

Tretinoin (all-*trans*-retinoic acid or retinoic acid) was the first widely prescribed topical retinoid. Its chemical structure is cis-retinoic acid, but it has been shown to isomerize readily to 13-*cis*-retinoic acid (isotretinoin) on the skin. It was initially used in acne for its comedolytic effect, but later it was found to decrease wrinkles and improve the signs of aging. Over the years, it has been reported beneficial anecdotally in a wide variety of dermatoses. Older formulations were quite irritating, but recent advances in vehicle formulation have minimized side effects. It is applied once daily, usually at night.

In acne, it should be given a full 12 weeks to see the maximum benefit and, as with other topical retinoids, it is usually prescribed in combination with an antimicrobial agent, for example benzoyl peroxide or an antibiotic (note, however, that benzoyl peroxide is also potentially irritant). Tretinoin helps open the pore, whereas the antimicrobial agent reduces the number of *P. acnes*.

Isotretinoin

Topical isotretinoin is used in treatment of acne; in some countries, it is also available as a combination topical product with erythromycin.

Adapalene

Adapalene is a naphthoic acid derivative that has retinoid-like activities, i.e. it mediates its effects via the retinoic acid receptors. It is both chemically and photochemically stable. It is applied once a day and is equivalent to tretinoin in terms of efficacy for acne. For many patients, irritancy is reduced compared with when using other topical retinoids. Adapalene has also been shown to reduce the signs of photodamaged skin, specifically actinic keratoses and lentigines (Fig. 3.7).

Bexarotene

Previously used orally, this has recently become available in the USA (not yet in the UK) as a topical treatment for early stages of mycosis fungoides.

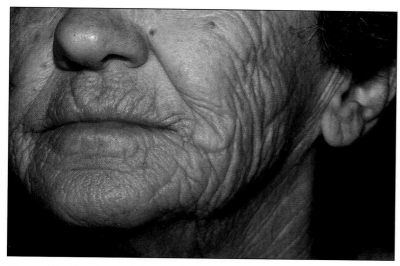

Figure 3.7 Wrinkling and photodamage. A topical retinoid as well as a sunscreen can improve the appearance over many months.

TOPICAL ANTIMICROBIAL AGENTS AND ANTIBIOTICS

Agents for acne and rosacea
Benzoyl peroxide

Benzoyl peroxide remains an excellent agent in the treatment of acne. Its ability to kill *P. acnes* is unsurpassed. Furthermore, bacterial resistance does not occur, in contrast to clindamycin and erythromycin. Washes are less effective compared with the usually recommended water-based gels. The 10% is only modestly more effective compared with the 5% and, given the higher concentration's tendency to cause excessive drying, the 5% is recommended. The patient should be warned that benzoyl peroxide can bleach carpet, sheets, and clothing. It is often best to apply at night with a topical retinoid (e.g. tazarotene 0.1% cream) in the morning.

Azelaic acid

This is only licensed for the treatment of acne in the UK, having antimicrobial and anticomedonal actions. However, it is also used more widely as a depigmenting agent in some countries, particularly for disorders such as melasma.

Topical antibiotics for acne

Both clindamycin and erythromycin are given b.i.d. to reduce the numbers of *P. acnes* in patients with acne. Unfortunately, bacterial resistance is common. Combinations of either one of these agents with benzoyl peroxide are available and should decrease the potential problem of resistance. In the UK, erythromycin is also combined with zinc for topical use in acne. Topical tetracycline is less effective.

Although some of these topical antibiotics may help in rosacea, they are often in vehicles appropriate for greasy skin and may be irritant in the typically older age group in which rosacea is more common.

Metronidazole

Topical metronidazole is used in treatment of rosacea. Several vehicles are used, and patients may need to try different options to find the one that is most acceptable.

PRACTICE POINTS
- Benzoyl peroxide is the most effective at reducing levels of the bacteria that causes acne, but be careful. It can bleach the carpets!
- Topical tetracycline fluoresces under Wood's light or UV lights as often used at discos; it is useful to confirm compliance but appreciation of the social impact of this effect is quite variable.
- If using a topical and a systemic antibiotic together, it is recommended to use the same agent.
- Use of benzoyl peroxide with a topical antibiotic in acne decreases the risk of bacterial resistance.

Agents for skin infections

Many such treatments are discussed in relation to specific disorders in Chapters 24–27, and are therefore covered only briefly here.

Bacterial infection

Several antibiotics are available topically, including the following.
- Aminoglycosides and polymyxins (e.g. neomycin). Often used for otitis and some wounds, but contact sensitivity is relatively frequent.
- Mupirocin—mainly used for staphylococcal infection, but increasingly being reserved for infections due to methicillin-resistant *Staphylococcus aureus* (MRSA).
- Silver sulfadiazine—especially used for burns.
- Fusidic acid—used for staphylococcal infection, and available in some countries as a combination product with steroids for infected eczema, but increasing bacterial resistance problems mean that use should be limited to short courses. An oral antibiotic is preferred for widespread impetigo or infected eczema.
- Metronidazole—mainly used for malodorous wounds, ulcers, or ulcerated tumors.
- Antiseptics—these have a wider spectrum of activity than that of antibiotics; many are used topically, such as povidone–iodine, chlorhexidine, etc.

Fungal infection

Agents available to treat fungal infections include the following.
- imidazoles—several are available (e.g. ketoconazole); they can treat yeasts or dermatophytes.
- allylamines (e.g. terbinafine)—they can treat yeasts or dermatophytes when used topically, and are fungicidal.
- Nystatin (a polyene)—usually reserved for the treatment of *Candida* infection.
- Amorolfine (a morpholine)—used topically for nail dermatophyte infection, but benefit is usually limited to distal infection of relatively non-thickened nails; it is useful for superficial white onychomycosis (Ch. 26) and has activity against some moulds.
- Ciclopirox olamine is available in the USA but not in the UK; it has a broad spectrum of action and is available in several formulations.
- Undecylenic acid—of notably lower potency.

Virtually all prescription topical antifungal agents are sufficient to treat simple dermatophytosis. Of the over-the-counter agents, terbinafine has the advantage of a fungicidal activity, whereas the imidazoles are fungistatic and usually less rapid in achieving benefit.

Topical imidazoles are also of value in seborrheic dermatitis (where they are sometimes used as combination products with hydrocortisone) and in treatment of pityriasis capitis and pityriasis versicolor; see also this chapter's section on shampoos.

Viral infection

Topical aciclovir and related agents such as penciclovir are available for herpes simplex infection, often by direct sale to the public and with limited efficacy.

Treatments for warts are discussed later, as they are largely not actually specifically antiviral.

INFESTATIONS

Treatments for infestations are discussed in Chapter 27.

CALCINEURIN INHIBITORS

These are topical agents primarily used for treatment of eczema (mainly atopic dermatitis), although benefit has also been recorded in several other dermatoses, such as psoriasis, vitiligo, discoid lupus erythematosus, and oral lichen planus.

Tacrolimus is a calcineurin inhibitor that is effective in treating atopic dermatitis in both adults and children. It has been shown effective in both the 0.1% and 0.03% ointments, applied b.i.d. It is particularly effective for the face and neck but, unlike with topical steroids, there is no risk of skin atrophy. Patients given it for the first time should be told to expect itching and/or burning. Significant improvement occurs within 1 week, and the majority of improvement within 4–6 weeks. Patients may apply the medication several times a week to normal skin during maintenance therapy to prevent relapse. It appears approximately equivalent in strength to betamethasone valerate. Recent studies have found tacrolimus combined with phototherapy to improve vitiligo, and personal experience supports the benefit reported anecdotally or in small studies in discoid lupus erythematosus and oral lichen planus.

Pimecrolimus is formulated as a 1% cream applied b.i.d. for atopic dermatitis. As with tacrolimus, its great advantage over steroids is its lack of atrophic side effects. It can be used on the neck and face without concern of skin thinning, in contrast to topical steroids. Clinical studies show it to be slightly less effective than tacrolimus.

Because of their safety and efficacy, some view pimecrolimus and tacrolimus as first-line agents in the treatment of atopic dermatitis. However, their cost and concerns over their possibility to promote skin malignancy in the long term (they are related to immunosuppressive agents used in prevention of organ transplant rejection) has led others to be more cautious in recommending such widespread use.

ANTINEOPLASTIC AGENTS

5-Fluorouracil

5-Fluorouracil is a topical agent that selectively kills photodamaged keratinocytes. It is effective at reducing actinic keratoses and in treatment of Bowen disease. It is applied once daily or b.i.d. for 2–4 weeks, and usually causes significant inflammation, crusting, and even erosion. It is particularly effective for actinic cheilitis of the lips. Some practitioners recommend a low-strength topical steroid for several days at the end of therapy to help return the skin to normal. Sun protection is of paramount importance both during therapy and after. Alternative regimens (e.g. b.i.d. for 2 consecutive days a week for 10–12 weeks) are recommended by many as they reduce the side effects, but such regimens involve a longer course. The most commonly used preparation is 5%, but several lower concentrations are available in the USA for a more prophylactic (secondary prevention) type of approach to actinic keratoses.

Diclofenac–hyaluronic acid

A preparation of these agents (3% and 2.5%, respectively, in a gel base) has been shown to be useful in treatment of actinic keratoses. It causes less inflammation than 5-fluorouracil does in most patients, but the benefit is less apparent.

Mustine (nitrogen mustard)

This is sometimes used topically for mycosis fungoides (Ch. 33), but it is difficult to use due to irritancy of some formulations and potential toxicity to others who may come into contact with the drug.

Imiquimod

Imiquimod is an immune modifier with antiviral and antineoplastic activities. Although initially used for treatment of genital warts, it is discussed here as it seems likely to have a role for treatment of several neoplastic lesions.

Imiquimod acts at least in part by stimulating the production of proinflammatory cytokines through Toll-like receptor 7 on the surface of dendritic cells of monocyte-macrophage lineage. This activation stimulates the patient's own immune system to attack both virally infected and tumor cells. Imiquimod is proved effective against genital warts as well as in treatment of superficial malignancies and their precursors, for example actinic keratoses, Bowen disease, superficial basal cell carcinoma, and lentigo maligna (although, at the time of writing, many of these are not yet licensed indications). It may have some benefit in the treatment of

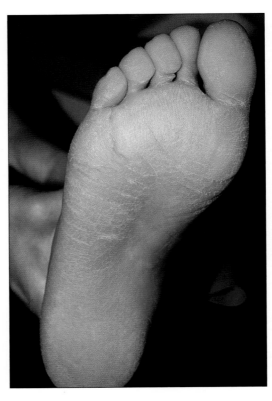

Figure 3.8
Keratoderma. Thick hyperkeratosis requires a strong keratolytic, for example urea or salicylic acid.

common warts and molluscum contagiosum. Application is three times a week for warts and up five to seven times a week for neoplasms. Severe inflammation of the skin should be expected. Some patients develop flu-like symptoms during therapy.

OTHER AGENTS AND TOPICAL INTERVENTIONS

Keratolytic agents

Some skin conditions primarily represent thickening of the horny layer of the skin. Examples include corns, calluses, some keratodermas (Fig. 3.8), and many dermatoses with a scaling or keratinizing component (such as psoriasis). For these, a keratolytic agent is needed. The following are the most commonly used.

- Salicylic acid—commonly used to help reduce scale in psoriasis, typically at 5–10% concentrations in a cream or ointment, depending on the site. Milder treatment (e.g. 2% concentration) is used for descaling in conditions such as cradle cap. Higher strengths (e.g. 15–30%) are used to treat viral warts and callosities.
- Urea—a simple organic compound composed of one carbon atom bound to two nitrogen (NH_2) groups and one oxygen (double bond). At low concentrations (e.g. 4%), urea is a hydrating agent. At high concentrations (e.g. 20–40%), it can serve as a keratolytic. When used in combination, it can enhance the penetration of the other agents.
- Others—ammonium lactate 12% and glycolic acid are also used as keratolytics. Vitamin D analogs and vitamin A analogs such as tazarotene (discussed earlier) are also helpful in scaling dermatoses.

Most keratolytics are applied b.i.d., or, in inflammatory scaling dermatoses, are applied overnight in conjunction with an antiinflammatory agent (e.g. topical steroid) during the day.

Shampoos

Shampoos are most often recommended by the dermatologist for the treatment of seborrheic dermatitis and psoriasis. The goal in seborrheic dermatitis is to reduce the number of *Pityrosporum* yeasts that seem to stimulate the immune system, causing the redness, scale, and inflammation of the skin. All the 'medicated' shampoos contain agents with antiyeast properties, for example ketaconazole, selenium sulfide, zinc pyrithione, and tar. The most common mistake patients make is to use the shampoo infrequently. Just as taking a pill once a week for hypertension is not

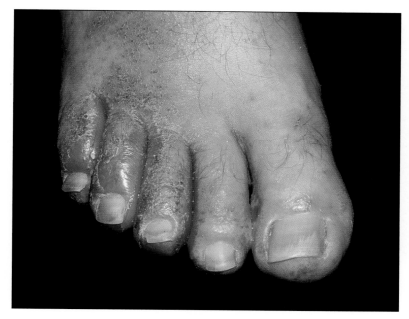

Figure 3.9 Gram-negative toe web infection. The patient must soak the feet b.i.d. to dry out the skin, reduce maceration, and remove debris and bacteria. Adding vinegar to the liquid will help reduce the gram-negative bacterial count.

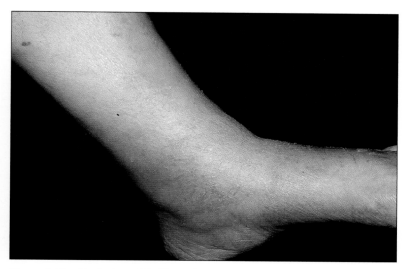

Figure 3.10 Stasis dermatitis. The patient must use support hose to reduce the swelling; this is critically important to resolve stasis dermatitis.

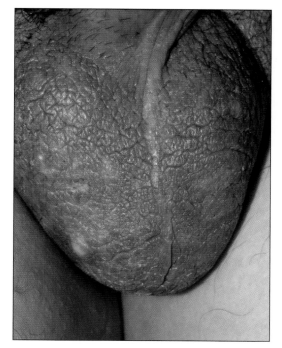

Figure 3.11 Lichen simplex chronicus. The thickened skin and more prominent skin lines indicate the patient is scratching. A brief intervention with a strong topical steroid and the simple admonition to not scratch is appropriate.

sufficient, shampooing once a week for seborrheic dermatitis is not enough. Every day or other day is needed.

Antiseptic agents such as cetrimide or povidone–iodine are available in shampoo form for use as cleansers in scalp infections.

For psoriasis, shampooing is meant to be not only antiyeast but also antiproliferative. Tar shampoos are best in this regard, as they do both. Shampoos with a keratolytic, for example salicylic acid or coconut oil, are excellent for scalp psoriasis with heavy scale.

Soaps

There are no prescription soaps in the USA or UK, although several antiseptic agents are available in formulations that can be used for skin cleansing, such as various creams or solutions containing chlorhexidine or cetrimide. Occasionally, antibacterial soaps or skin-cleansing agents (sometimes as a bath additive) are recommended for patients with chronic *S. aureus* infection of the skin. Some bath and direct application emollients are also made with an additional antiseptic component (see under *Emollients*).

Soaks and astringents

Soaks are often prescribed for exudative skin disease. The benefits are multiple and include a soothing effect on the skin, debridement, and potentially delivery of medication. Take, for example, a gram-negative toe web infection (Fig. 3.9). The patient may be told to immerse the foot in warm water with a little bit of vinegar for several minutes, remove and air dry, followed by repetition of the process—several times a day. The wetting and drying is soothing to the patient, removes excess crust and scale, and delivers vinegar to the skin, helping kill any *Pseudomonas* or other gram-negative organism that may be infecting the skin.

Potassium permanganate solution is useful as a soak for exudative pompholyx or venous eczema, having both astringent and antibacterial effects, but does stain nails and necessary utensils (e.g. a bowl for the hands) brown.

Silver nitrate 0.5% (which also causes staining) and aluminum acetate solution are also used as astringent soaks.

Eosin 2% in water is a useful astringent and antibacterial for localized areas.

Wraps

Wrapping the skin after application of topical agents can be very soothing to atopic skin. Compression bandages are critically important for healing stasis dermatitis (Fig. 3.10). Wrapping after the application of a topical steroid (i.e. occlusion) will augment the potency of the steroid.

Antipruritics and agents for pain

Most topical antipruritics are of modest benefit. The prominent exception is topical doxepin. It is so powerful that it can actually make the patient drowsy. It is best prescribed for nighttime use for treatment-resistant pruritic areas of the skin. Topical diphenhydramine should be avoided, as it can induce allergic contact dermatitis.

Menthol (1% in a cream base) has a useful cooling effect and can be helpful in situations where topical steroids for inflammation would be inappropriate (e.g. for itch due to varicella).

Topical crotamiton is also used for pruritus, as is calamine, although its benefit is limited.

Capsaicin is used to treat pain from herpes zoster but can be useful in other dermatologic conditions in which nerve pain may be implicated, such as nostalgia paresthetica and brachioradial pruritus.

Topical local anesthetics such as lidocaine–prilocaine or amethocaine are used for superficial procedures. Topical lidocaine is sometimes used for pruritus ani.

Often, the best way to reduce itching is to treat the disease. Also, when the patient is scratching due to habit, it is important to tell the patient to stop (Fig. 3.11).

Hydroquinone and related agents

Hydroquinone is a topical bleaching agent used primarily in melasma. It contains a phenol structure that inhibits tyrosinase, the key enzyme in melanogenesis. It is applied b.i.d., usually in a 2–4% preparation. At higher concentrations, it can paradoxically cause increased pigmentation in the form of exogenous ochronosis. The combination of fluocinolone acetonide 0.01%, hydroquinone 4%, and tretinoin 0.05% (Tri-Luma in the USA) is more efficacious at reducing pigmentation than any of these agents alone.

More powerful bleaching agents, such as the monobenzyl ether of hydroquinone, carry a risk of permanent depigmentation and are less widely used.

Azelaic acid (discussed earlier for acne) also has a depigmenting activity.

Antiperspirants

The most commonly used contain aluminum chloride hexahydrate. They should ideally be applied at night, when sweating is at its least. Note that antiperspirant is not synonymous with deodorant; the latter are a commercial entity that usually contain antimicrobials and fragrances as well.

Use of glycopyrronium bromide, an anticholinergic agent, for its antiperspirant effect is most commonly as an additive to enhance the effect of iontophoresis (Ch. 5), but it can also be obtained in a cream base for application to the skin. Formaldehyde also has an antiperspirant effect and is sometimes used as a treatment for plantar hyperhidrosis.

TOPICAL AGENTS DISCUSSED IN MORE DETAIL IN OTHER CHAPTERS

- Vitamin D analogs—calcipotriol, calcitriol, and tacalcitol are used mainly in the treatment of psoriasis and are discussed in Chapter 7. They can also be helpful in some ichthyoses and other keratinizing disorders. One preparation is combined with topical steroid.
- Anthralin (dithranol)—used mainly in the treatment of psoriasis (see Ch. 7). It is now most commonly used as 'short-contact' therapy, applied for about 30 min daily, so can be used in conjunction with other antipsoriatic treatments. Anthralin is an effective agent, but it can stain clothing, baths, etc.; for this reason, it is less ideal for home treatment but excellent for dermatology outpatient treatment centers. Liposomal versions may reduce the potential for staining.
- Tar preparations—tars may be derived from coal, wood (Cade oil), or fish (ichthammol and ichthyol) sources. They are antiinflammatory and antiproliferative, and are helpful in psoriasis (Ch. 7) and in some eczemas (Ch. 6). Stronger tars are messy, but attempts to make 'clean' and non-odorous tar preparations are associated with a reduction in efficacy. Ichthammol-impregnated bandages applied over a topical steroid are useful in eczema, not least as a means to reduce damage by scratching. Tar shampoos have already been discussed.
- Treatments for warts include the following.
  Salicylic acid—the mainstay of wart treatment, usually in a collodion or polyacrylamide base.
  Aldehydes—glutaraldehyde or (as a soak for mosaic warts) formaldehyde.
  Podophyllotoxin—for genital warts.
  Imiquimod (discussed earlier)—for genital warts.
- Minoxidil—used for androgenic alopecias in either sex (see Ch. 28).
- Eflornithine—used for treatment of hirsutism (see Ch. 28). It inhibits ornithine decarboxylase. Benefits vary and are not usually apparent before 1–2 months. Relapse occurs when it is discontinued.

4 Systemic Therapies

INTRODUCTION

This chapter gives an overview of the commoner systemic therapies used in dermatology, but it is not intended to be exhaustive. The emphasis is on the indications and side effects of drugs used to treat inflammatory dermatoses; some of the less commonly used agents are included if they have an important role for specific conditions, or where they have important side effects. It should be borne in mind that many such uses are unlicensed (off label). Some drugs are discussed more fully in other chapters.

ANTIBIOTICS

Antibiotics for specific infections (Fig. 4.1) will be discussed in relevant chapters. However, some antibiotics have additional antiinflammatory activity that does not appear to be related to bacterial killing. The main relevant agents include tetracyclines, erythromycin, and some sulfones and sulfonamides (discussed later).

These agents with antiinflammatory activity are useful in acne and related conditions (Fig. 4.2), in which they also have an antibacterial effect (Ch. 10), and may be an adjunct (or occasionally monotherapy) in treatment of immunobullous diseases (Ch. 16). In the latter situation, tetracyclines may be used in conjunction with nicotinamide, especially in treatment of bullous pemphigoid. Treatment is typically prolonged, as the antiinflammatory activity takes several weeks to become apparent.

Side effects from such use are generally not problematic, but candidiasis secondary to tetracyclines, and nausea due to erythromycin, are the commonest limiting factors. If used in conjunction with an oral contraceptive (as occurs quite often in women with acne), many authorities

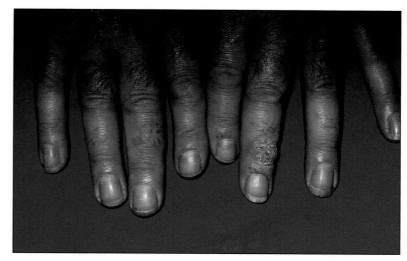

Figure 4.1 Atypical mycobacterial infection due to *Mycobacterium marinum*. Unusually, this patient had two primary inoculation sites on the fingers. Clarithromycin is usually effective.

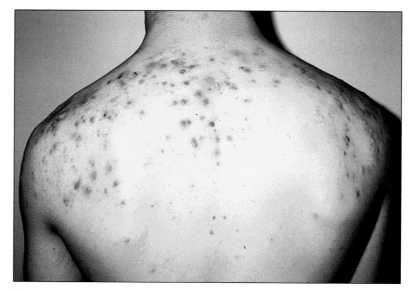

Figure 4.2 Acne: nodular lesions for which systemic tetracycline antibiotics would be a reasonable first-choice therapy, although isotretinoin may be required.

would advise use of additional barrier contraception for the first month.

Pigmentation due to long-term minocycline is uncommon, especially if treatment is for less than 2 years, but is worthy of attention (Fig. 4.3 and Ch. 18); a lupus erythematosus–like syndrome may also occur with this drug, and blood tests including antinuclear antibody every 6–9 months are prudent.

ANTIFUNGAL AGENTS

Systemic antifungal agents used in dermatology fall into several groups according to mode of action. The most commonly used for superficial mycoses interfere with ergosterol, a sterol of the fungal but not of the host cell walls. Topical agents (Ch. 26) can be used for many infections;

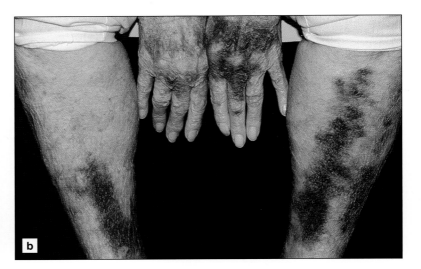

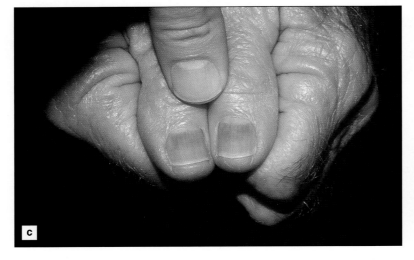

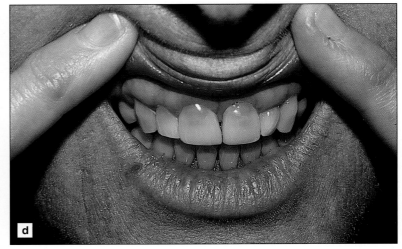

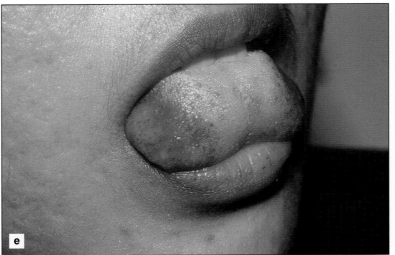

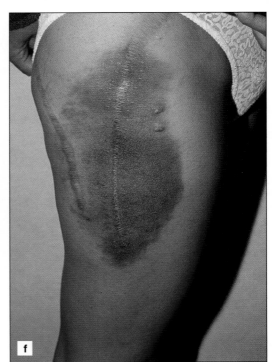

Figure 4.3 (**a–f**) Some examples of pigmentation due to minocycline. Although relatively uncommon and specifically related to long-term use of the drug, it is important to be aware of this potential side effect. The color is typically slate-gray; sites affected include the face, nails (c), teeth (d), tongue (e), and old scars (f). Note the normal nail for comparison in (c) and the old acne scars in (e). The pigmentation around the scar (f) occurred at the time of surgery and was thought to be a hematoma. It never resorbed however and this picture is 8 months post surgery. It is thought that minocycline may chelate with the iron of the blood to form a complex that the body is unable to resorb.

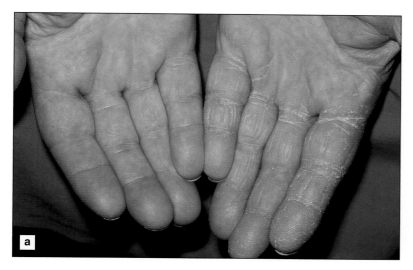

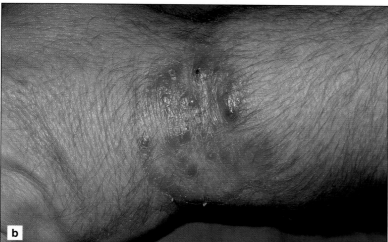

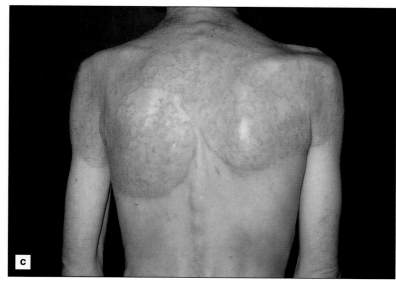

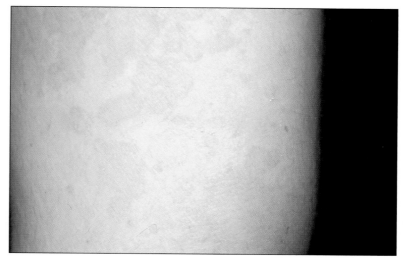

Figure 4.5 Pityriasis versicolor, a yeast infection for which itraconazole is effective.

Figure 4.4 Involvement of thick skin sites (**a**), hairy areas (**b**), and extensive skin involvement (**c**), as shown here, are indications for systemic rather than topical antifungal therapy. Note that the palm involvement in (a) is unilateral, a typical feature of fungal infection of the hands. Pustules are common at hairy sites affected by athlete's foot-type fungi, as in (b), although they are uncommon on the scalp in children affected by cat or dog ringworm. All three patients had *Trichophyton rubrum* infection, neglected in the patient shown in (c).

systemic agents are generally indicated for infection of nails, thick skin sites (Fig. 4.4a), scalp and other hairy areas (Fig. 4.4b), deeper or systemic infections, extensive disease (Fig. 4.4b), failure of topical agents, or in immunosuppressed individuals. However, it is important to make a firm diagnosis by appropriate mycologic sampling (Ch. 26) before considering systemic therapy.

The main antifungal agents are as follows.
- Azoles—these inhibit sterol demethylase to reduce ergosterol synthesis, and include imidazoles (e.g. ketoconazole) and triazoles (e.g. itraconazole).
- Allylamines (e.g. terbinafine)—inhibit squalene expoxidase to reduce ergosterol synthesis.
- Polyenes (e.g. amphotericin)—disrupt cell membranes.
- Griseofulvin—blocks microtubules.
- Flucytosine—inhibits DNA and RNA synthesis.

The commonest agents used for superficial infections are terbinafine (usually the most effective for dermatophyte infections), fluconazole (mainly used for candidal infection), and itraconazole (which has a wide spectrum of activity). Itraconazole is useful in pityriasis versicolor (Fig. 4.5), and opinion varies as to whether it should be first-line therapy or used if topical treatment fails. Griseofulvin is used rather less in developed countries, as it is fungistatic and slower to work, but it is widely used worldwide, as it is much cheaper than the newer agents. Ketoconazole is used less often systemically than in the past, as it has been associated with hepatotoxicity and therefore requires closer monitoring.

Side effects of the commonly used agents are generally few and mild, but azoles in particular have the potential for drug interactions with other medications that are metabolized by cytochrome P450. Taste disturbance is a feature with terbinafine, and provocation of discoid lupus erythematosus has been reported.

ANTIVIRAL DRUGS

Herpes simplex and varicella zoster infections are usually treated with the nucleoside analogs. These include aciclovir, its prodrug valaciclovir, or famciclovir (prodrug of penciclovir). Treatment must be started early, and at higher dose for varicella zoster (Fig. 4.6). Treatment is usually oral, but intravenous administration is used in immunosuppressed patients or those with severe infections, associated viral meningoencephalitis, chickenpox, pneumonia, etc. Patients with recurrent herpes simplex (or herpes simplex-associated erythema multiforme) may require prophylactic therapy.

Other systemic (intravenous) antiviral agents, such as foscarnet or cidofovir, may be used for herpes infections, especially in the context of HIV infection, hematologic malignancy, or other immunosuppression states; they may be useful for some other infections also. Ganciclovir is used to treat cytomegalovirus.

Antiretroviral drugs for HIV infection fall into the following groups.
- Nucleoside analogs—for example zidovudine, lamivudine, didanosine, zalcitabine, and abacavir.
- Non-nucleoside reverse transcriptase inhibitors—for example nevirapine, delavirdine, and efavirenz.

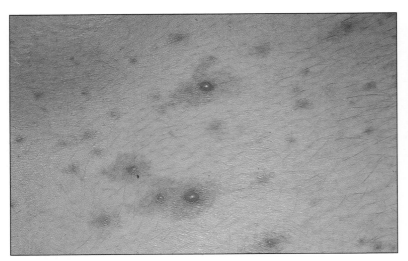

Figure 4.6 Chickenpox (varicella). Initially, there are typically small, clear blisters on an erythematous base. These subsequently become gray or pustular and then crust.

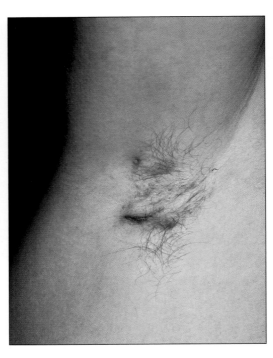

Figure 4.7 Hidradenitis suppurativa of the axilla. This condition, discussed in Chapter 10, may respond to long-term antibiotics along the same lines as their use in acne; in some patients, there is a clear hormonal influence, manifest as a tendency for premenstrual exacerbation or by a response to antiandrogen therapy.

- Protease inhibitors—for example indinavir, saquinavir, nelfinavir, and ritonavir.

Combination therapy with drugs from different groups is used; the accepted regimens vary according to factors such as viral load and are updated at intervals. Most antiretroviral drugs have significant side effects, which vary according to the class of drug as well as the specific agent; for example, several of the nucleosides may cause gastrointestinal disturbance, pancreatitis, peripheral neuropathy, or marrow suppression, while lipodystrophy is more typically seen in relation to protease inhibitors.

ANTIHISTAMINES

Oral antihistamines are widely used in dermatology. It is helpful to divide drugs with antihistamine effects into the following groups, the first two of which are marketed as antihistamines for dermatologic conditions.

- Conventional or first-generation 'sedating' antihistamines, for example chlorpheniramine (chlorphenamine), cyproheptadine, hydroxyzine, alimemazine (trimeprazine), and promethazine. (Note: patients taking these drugs should be warned about drowsiness and the potential impact on driving or operating machinery).
- Second-generation 'non-sedating' antihistamines, for example acrivastine, loratadine or desloratidine, cetirizine or levocetirizine, fexofenadine, and mizolastine.
- Other drugs that have antihistaminic or antipruritic activity, for example amitriptyline and doxepin.
- H_2 antagonists (e.g. cimetidine)—may be an adjunct in treatment of urticaria; some studies show benefit in clearing viral warts.

The importance of this division is that the second-generation agents are much more specifically antihistaminic; this is beneficial in avoidance of sedation, but it does mean that their value is limited in itch that is not primarily related to histamine (although some do have other effects, for example on eosinophils or on cytokine activity). Thus, for example, patients with eczema often derive little benefit from non-sedating antihistamines. Even in urticaria, where histamine is important, the sedative effect of an older agent at nighttime can be beneficial.

Some side effects of antihistamines are important. Most are metabolized in the liver; those that are metabolized by cytochrome P450 (especially mizolastine and terfenadine) should be avoided in conjunction with grapefruit juice or with drugs that block this enzyme (e.g. azoles and macrolides). There is a risk in such situations, or in the elderly or patients with liver or cardiac disease, of cardiac arrhythmias. Additionally, some (mainly sedating) antihistamines have anticholinergic activity and should be avoided in patients with glaucoma, hypertension, airway obstruction, or prostatism.

PRACTICE POINTS

- It can be very useful in difficult urticaria to use a non-sedating antihistamine in the daytime and a sedating agent at night.
- Non-sedating antihistamines are generally of little value in the treatment of eczema; an appropriate-potency topical corticosteroid is dramatically more helpful.
- Beware of exceeding recommended doses of non-sedating antihistamines, especially if there is a potential for drug interactions.
- Grapefruit juice interferes with the metabolism of some non-sedating antihistamines.

HORMONES AND ANTIANDROGENS

Oral contraceptive pills often have a beneficial effect on acne and related disorders, especially if premenstrual flare is apparent.

Antiandrogens have several uses in dermatology. Cyproterone acetate, used in conjunction with an oral contraceptive (either in low dose as a combined preparation, co-cyprindiol, or in higher dose by using the two separately) has a role in treatment of acne, hidradenitis suppurativa (Fig. 4.7), hirsuties, and other androgen-related disorders. It inhibits binding of testosterone to receptors and also acts as an antigonadotropin, leading to decreased testosterone production.

Finasteride is used in male alopecia; it blocks conversion of testosterone to dihydrotestosterone by inhibiting the enzyme 5-α-reductase. It is contraindicated in premenopausal women and ineffective for alopecia in postmenopausal women.

Less commonly used drugs for androgenic disorders include flutamide and spironolactone. Their lower level of popularity is because flutamide may cause hepatotoxicity, while spironolactone may cause menstrual abnormalities and electrolyte disturbances, and has been linked with a carcinogenesis risk in animal studies. There is increasing interest in use of metformin for hirsuties and androgenic disorders.

RETINOIDS

Systemic retinoids used in dermatology are discussed in more detail in relevant chapters. The main agents and indications are as follows.

- Isotretinoin—used in acne (Fig. 4.8) and less commonly in rosacea and hidradenitis suppurativa.

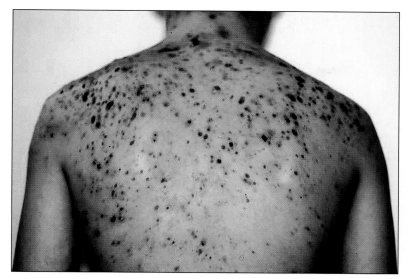

Figure 4.8 Pyogenic granuloma–like lesions are an unusual side effect of isotretinoin therapy, generally in those with severe and very inflammatory lesions initially. (Courtesy of Dr. G. Dawn.)

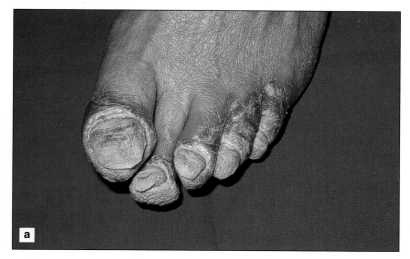

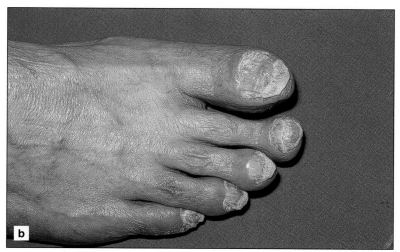

Figure 4.9 (**a**,**b**) Systemic retinoids are helpful for hyperkeratotic psoriasis of palmoplantar skin, as shown here before and after 2 months of treatment.

- Acitretin—used in psoriasis (Fig. 4.9), pityriasis rubra pilaris, some ichthyoses, and Darier disease.
- Bexarotene—a new agent, used in lymphomas.

All have, to a greater or lesser extent, effects on sebum production, keratinization, and immune function. The balance of these main effects varies between the different agents. Mucocutaneous side effects include dryness of lips and other mucocutaneous junctions. Systemic side effects may include myalgia, headache, and, of greatest importance, high teratogenic potential: pregnancy must be excluded and must not occur for at least a month after isotretinoin or 2 years after acitretin. The true frequency of depression or mood disturbance with isotretinoin is uncertain, but if it is related then it is presumably idiosyncratic.

PSORALENS

These are used with UV light and are discussed in the next chapter.

CORTICOSTEROIDS

Systemic corticosteroids are widely used in dermatology, although there are many situations where a topical corticosteroid used well is as, or even more, effective. This applies particularly to use of systemic corticosteroids for eczematous processes.

Situations in which systemic corticosteroids have a role include the following.
- Immunobullous disorders—bullous pemphigoid, pemphigus, epidermolysis bullosa acquisita, etc.
- Neutrophilic dermatoses and vasculitis—Sweet syndrome, pyoderma gangrenosum, Henoch–Schönlein purpura and other cutaneous small-vessel vasculitis (Fig. 4.10), Wegener granulomatosis, etc.
- Connective tissue diseases—systemic lupus erythematosus and dermatomyositis.
- Severe forms of common dermatoses—pompholyx, contact dermatitis, drug eruptions, erythema multiforme, and acute urticaria.
- Other inflammatory diseases—eosinophilic cellulitis or fasciitis, lichen planus (scarring, nail, or scalp), sarcoidosis, and hemangiomas (with bleeding or functional impairment).

It is important to bear in mind that milder cases, even of disorders such as the immunobullous diseases, may not need this level of therapy. It is also important to be aware that long-term oral corticosteroid use, particularly at higher dose levels, carries a variety of risks. Stopping treatment may be more difficult than never starting it in some instances (e.g. in urticaria).

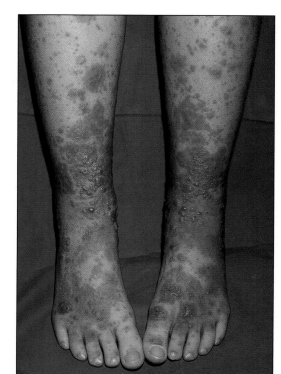

Figure 4.10 Henoch–Schönlein purpura. It is debatable whether oral corticosteroids alter the overall course of this disease, but they are undoubtedly helpful when there are large necrotic or bullous lesions, as shown here.

Corticosteroids may be combined with, or gradually substituted by, other agents such as cytotoxic drugs (discussed later) that have a steroid-sparing effect. In some cases, such as in bullous pemphigoid, corticosteroids may be used initially for their speed of action, but the dose can be reduced once a slower-acting drug such as azathioprine starts to work.

For most indications, treatment starts at higher doses (e.g. 1 mg/kg per day for bullous pemphigoid, 0.5 mg/kg per day for many inflammatory disorders) and is then reduced, ideally aiming to drop below 5 mg daily for most indications. For more severe dermatoses, such as extensive pemphigus, pulsed intravenous methylprednisolone may be used.

Side effects with long-term use include sodium and water retention, hypertension, weight gain, plethoric facies, euphoria, osteoporosis (note: give prophylaxis), suppression of hypothalamic–pituitary axis, avascular necrosis of the femoral head, myopathy, cataracts, and the cutaneous side effects of topical corticosteroids (see Ch. 3).

OTHER IMMUNOMODULATORY, IMMUNOSUPPRESSIVE, AND CYTOTOXIC THERAPIES

These agents are grouped together, as most of their use is in similar situations in dermatology, for a variety of severe inflammatory dermatoses, for vasculitis, and for immunobullous diseases. However, the range of agents to consider is wide, and some have widespread application while others are used for only a small number of indications. The main features of the more widely used of this group of agents are summarized in Table 4.1.

Malignancy risk

Many immunosuppressive drugs carry an actual or a potential risk of increased frequency of malignant disease, due to suppression of immune surveillance. This will not be discussed for all the following drugs, as the same principles apply to most of them. In general, as with immunosuppression for renal transplant purposes, the main concern is skin cancers, cervical carcinoma, and lymphomas. Of particular relevance in dermatology is the potential that previous natural sunlight or psoralen ultraviolet A (PUVA) therapy for psoriasis (Ch. 7) may increase the risk of skin cancer: there is a disproportionate increase in squamous cell carcinoma (more than the normally commoner basal cell carcinoma). Additionally, although rare as a sporadic neoplasm, long-term immunosuppressive therapy carries a very significantly increased risk (about 80-fold greater than in the general population) of Merkel cell carcinoma (Fig. 4.11).

Opportunistic infections

As with malignancy risk, all immunosuppressive agents have at least a theoretical risk of predisposing to opportunistic infection. Herpes infec-

tion, cytomegalovirus infection, candidiasis, and fungal infections should all be considered in the event of unusual or unexplained symptoms in patients on such therapies.

Pregnancy and lactation

Most of these agents are at least relatively contraindicated in these situations. Men are advised not to father children while taking methotrexate, although the evidence for this is from hematologic doses that are much larger than those used for dermatologic indications. Individual summary of product characteristics (SPC) data sheets should be consulted.

PRACTICE POINTS
- Most immunosuppressive drugs used in dermatology have several potentially important side effects; in particular, most can cause pancytopenia.
- Most are at least relatively contraindicated in pregnancy and are therefore avoided in younger female patients where possible.
- Side effects that are common to most immunosuppressive agents include a risk of infections (often unusual organisms or atypical presentation) and a long-term risk of potentially aggressive skin cancers (especially squamous cell carcinoma and the otherwise rare Merkel cell carcinoma).

Ciclosporin (cyclosporin A, cyclosporine)
This drug is used for treatment of the following conditions.
- Severe psoriasis or eczema (especially atopic type in adults)—licensed indications.
- Pyoderma gangrenosum and other neutrophilic dermatoses—can be useful as monotherapy.
- Immunobullous disorders—usually as a steroid-sparing agent.
- Severe photodermatoses such as actinic reticuloid.
- Connective tissue diseases such as scleroderma and discoid lupus erythematosus (response is varied; good responses are reported in childhood dermatomyositis).
- Chronic urticaria—especially of proven autoimmune type.
- Others—sometimes useful in lichen planus; possible benefit in alopecia areata and toxic epidermal necrolysis.

Ciclosporin has a number of side effects, some of which are potentially serious and which require careful monitoring. The most important or frequent are the following.
- Nephrotoxicity—usually increases with dose and duration of treatment; creatinine 30% above baseline should prompt dose reduction or discontinuation.
- Hypertension—also common; usually treated with nifedipine or amlodipine if it occurs (note: there are interactions with several other calcium channel blockers such as diltiazem).
- Nausea—common and may be dose limiting.
- Drug interactions—numerous, largely due to common metabolism by CYP 34A (part of the cytochrome P450 system) (Table 4.2).
- Mucocutaneous—hypertrichosis, gingival hyperplasia, and facial papules (Fig. 4.12).
- Neurologic—burning extremities, especially early in treatment, and tremor.

Mycophenolate mofetil

This is a newer agent that selectively inhibits lymphocyte proliferation. It is likely that it will share many of the therapeutic indications for ciclosporin, as listed earlier. It is mainly used as a steroid-sparing drug, but there is interest in its use in conjunction with ciclosporin. This combination has been used in psoriasis, for example, and is beneficial, as the two drugs have a different spectrum of side effects, and lower doses of each may be achievable. It is generally well tolerated, although gastrointestinal upset is relatively common. The most important dose-related side effect is bone marrow suppression.

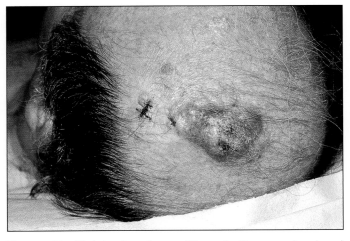

Figure 4.11 Merkel cell carcinoma of the scalp. There were lymph node metastases at presentation. There is a huge increase in the risk of this neoplasm in patients on long-term immunosuppressive therapy.

Table 4.1   THE MOST COMMONLY USED DERMATOLOGIC IMMUNOSUPPRESSIVE AGENTS: MAIN INDICATIONS AND SIDE EFFECTS[a]

Agent	Main uses	Main side effects
Corticosteroids	Immunobullous disorders, vasculitides, collagen vascular (connective tissue) diseases, severe pompholyx and other eczemas, some drug eruptions	Weight gain, hypertension, osteoporosis, avascular necrosis of femoral head, myopathy, cataract, suppression of hypothalamic–pituitary axis, striae, hirsuties (all usually related to dose and duration of treatment)
Ciclosporin	Eczemas, psoriasis, pyoderma gangrenosum, immunobullous disorders, actinic reticuloid	Nausea, anorexia, nephrotoxicity, hypertension, gingival hyperplasia, hypertrichosis, many drug interactions (Table 4.2)
Mycophenolate mofetil	Psoriasis, pyoderma gangrenosum, immunobullous disorders	Gastrointestinal upset, bone marrow suppression (especially thrombocytopenia) or infection risk, headache, hypertension, chest pain, cough, dyspnea
Azathioprine	Immunobullous disorders, lupus erythematosus, other collagen vascular disorders, systemic vasculitides, atopic dermatitis, actinic reticuloid	Bone marrow suppression (measure TPMT[b]), hypersensivity reactions, gastrointestinal upset, hepatotoxicity, drug interactions; rarely pancreatitis, pneumonitis
Methotrexate	Psoriasis, hypertrophic sarcoidosis	Nausea, bone marrow suppression, folate deficiency, hepatotoxicity (monitor transaminases, liver biopsy, PIIINP[c]), many drug interactions; rarely pulmonary toxicity
Hydroxycarbamide (hydroxyurea)	Psoriasis	Bone marrow suppression, macrocytosis; long-term use may cause lichenoid or dermatomyositis-like rash, pigmentation, or leg ulceration
Cyclophosphamide	Immunobullous disorders, systemic vasculitides	Bone marrow suppression, hepatotoxicity, bladder toxicity (cystitis or cancer)
Gold	Discoid lupus erythematosus, immunobullous disorders	Bone marrow suppression, nephritis (monitor for proteinuria), rashes and pigmentation (early rash may be urticarial, later patterns include erythroderma), diarrhea
Fumaric acid esters	Psoriasis	Gastrointestinal upset (common), bone marrow suppression
Sulfones	Dermatitis herpetiformis, other immunobullous disorders, neutrophilic dermatoses, small-vessel vasculitides, leprosy, *Pneumocystis* prophylaxis	Bone marrow suppression, hemolysis (higher risk if glucose-6-phosphate dehydrogenase-deficient), methemoglobinemia, headache, motor neuropathy, rash (rarely severe, with eosinophilia—'dapsone syndrome'), hepatitis, psychosis
Potassium iodide	Erythema nodosum, other panniculitides, sporotrichosis	Gastrointestinal upset, rash, hypothyroidism
Colchicine	Small-vessel vasculitides, Behçet disease	Gastrointestinal upset, nausea, vomiting, pain; rarely neuritis
Hydroxychloroquine and other antimalarials	Lupus erythematosus, other collagen vascular disorders, sarcoidosis, porphyria cutanea tarda, reticulate erythematosus mucinosis	Nausea, headache, rash (rarely severe patterns), retinopathy (very unlikely if ideal dose is not exceeded), pigmentation (especially mepacrine), lightening of hair color
Thalidomide	Severe aphthous ulceration, Behçet syndrome	Teratogenicity, neuropathy, sedation, mood disturbance, nausea, decreased thyroid function, rash
Monoclonal antibodies and cytokine inhibitors[d]	Severe psoriasis, lymphomas	Nausea, anaphylaxis or hypersensitivity reactions, fever, headache, blood dyscrasia, worsening of cardiac failure, infection (especially septicemia, listeriosis, varicella zoster, reactivation of tuberculosis), lupus erythematosus, demyelination disorder, uncertain risk of long-term malignancy
Intravenous immunoglobulins (IVIG)	Severe immunobullous disorders, toxic epidermal necrolysis	Anaphylaxis, hypotension, acute renal failure (exclude anti-IgA antibodies in IgA-deficient patients), headache, aseptic meningitis, urticaria or rash, nausea, flu-like symptoms
Retinoids[e]	Acne (isotretinoin), psoriasis and disorders of cornification (acitretin)	Dryness of skin and mucous membranes, hair changes, myalgia, headache (benign intracranial hypertension), hyperlipidemia, mood change, teratogenicity (high risk)
Phototherapy and photochemotherapy[e]	Psoriasis, eczemas, mycosis fungoides	Burning (UV dose-related), nausea (oral psoralen administration), carcinogenesis; see Chapter 5

[a]Some agents, such as interferons (mainly used in cutaneous oncology) and monoclonal antibodies (mainly used for lymphoma), are not included in this table, as they are mainly used in specialist settings.
[b]Thiopurine methyltransferase.
[c]Amino terminal peptide of type III procollagen
[d]Side effects vary between agents; not all listed apply to all types of monoclonal antibody and cytokine inhibitor. Side effects listed are for monoclonal antibodies used for psoriasis. See text for details of monoclonals for lymphoma.
[e]Retinoids and phototherapy (see Ch. 5 for the latter) are not primarily immunosuppressive but have some immune-modulating functions. Additionally, they are used for indications such as psoriasis, for which other drugs listed may also be used, and are mainly used in secondary care, so a summary of their use in this table is potentially useful.

Table 4.2   SOME DRUG INTERACTIONS WITH CICLOSPORIN

Type of drug	Examples	Effect
Antimicrobials	Macrolides	Increased ciclosporin levels
	Doxycycline	Increased ciclosporin levels
	Azole antifungals	Increased ciclosporin levels
	Aminoglycosides	Increased nephrotoxicity
	Quinolones	Increased nephrotoxicity
	Rifampin	Decreased ciclosporin levels
Rheumatologic	Non-steroidal antiinflammatory drugs	Increased nephrotoxicity
	Methotrexate	Increased ciclosporin and methotrexate levels
Cardiac	Some calcium channel blockers	Increased ciclosporin levels
	Statins	Increased risk of myopathy
	Digoxin	Increased digoxin toxicity
Anticonvulsants (some)	Carbamazepine	Decreased ciclosporin levels
	Phenytoin	Decreased ciclosporin levels
	Barbiturates	Decreased ciclosporin levels
Hormonal	Oral contraceptives	Increased ciclosporin levels
	Danazol	Increased ciclosporin levels
Others	Bromocriptine	Increased ciclosporin levels
	Metoclopramide	Increased ciclosporin levels
	Grapefruit juice	Increased ciclosporin levels
	Chloroquine	Increased ciclosporin levels

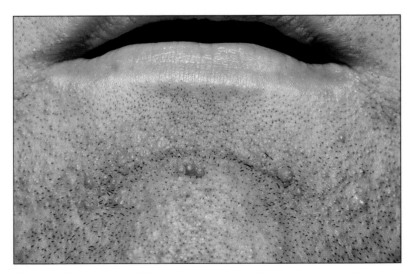

Figure 4.12 Papular facial lesions associated with immunosuppression include sebaceous hyperplasia and non-melanoma skin cancers. The flesh-colored papules illustrated appear to be specifically related to ciclosporin, and have been reported as ciclosporin-related folliculodystrophy.

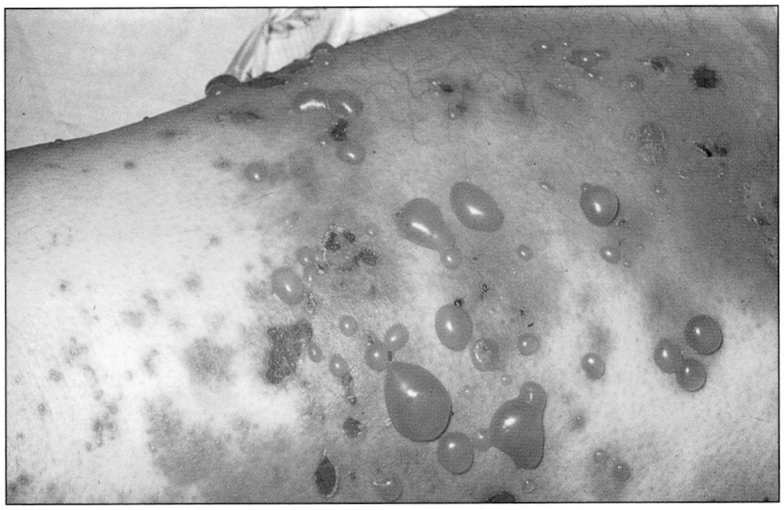

Figure 4.13 Bullous pemphigoid. Although corticosteroids are usually first-line treatment, azathioprine is often used as well for its steroid-sparing effect. (From Lawrence CM, Cox NH. Physical Signs in Dermatology, 2nd edn. London: Mosby, 2002.)

Azathioprine

This is a widely used drug in dermatology. It has a slow onset of action, and is therefore mainly used as a steroid-sparing agent rather than as initial therapy. It is used in the following conditions.

- Immunobullous diseases—bullous pemphigoid (Fig. 4.13), pemphigus, and epidermolysis bullosa acquisita.
- Connective tissue diseases—lupus erythematosus and dermatomyositis.
- Vasculitis—Wegener granulomatosis, Behçet disease, and Churg–Strauss syndrome.
- Dermatitis—atopic eczema, and chronic actinic dermatitis or actinic reticuloid.
- Other inflammatory dermatoses—pyoderma gangrenosum, sarcoidosis, and psoriasis (less commonly).

Knowledge of the metabolism of azathioprine is of some importance. It is a prodrug of 6-mercaptopurine, which in turn is metabolized by three main pathways involving the enzymes thiopurine methyltransferase (TPMT), xanthine oxidase, and hypoxanthine guanine phosphoribosyl transferase. Activity of TPMT is genetically determined; individuals with low-activity TMPT are at very high risk of azathioprine toxicity, as a greater proportion of the dose is metabolized to form toxic 6-thioguanine nucleotides. Where possible, the activity of this enzyme should be measured before starting treatment so that appropriate doses can be determined. In any event, frequent blood monitoring is required during the first month of treatment.

The main adverse effects are as follows.

- Hematologic—marrow suppression (note: this is both dose related and genetically determined as already described; it may also be increased by concurrent treatment with allopurinol, sulfasalazine, angiotensin-converting enzyme inhibitors, or other myelosuppressive drugs) and macrocytosis.

- Gastrointestinal—nausea, hepatitis (may occur as part of a hypersensitivity reaction), and pancreatitis (rare).

Methotrexate

This is an antimetabolite that interferes with folate metabolism. It is used in the following conditions.

- Psoriasis—the main indication.
- Connective tissue disease and vasculitis—especially in resistant lupus erythematosus, dermatomyositis, and various forms of vasculitis.
- Others—sarcoidosis (especially hypertrophic forms), bullous pemphigoid, and lymphomas.

Treatment is usually commenced with a small test dose to identify patients with significant side effects, and is then increased with close monitoring of blood counts and liver function. It should not be used in patients with significant renal dysfunction or in patients with known liver disease or heavy alcohol intake. Liver biopsy is normally performed in the first few months as a baseline for assessment of the potential side effect of liver fibrosis (this period allows those with other side effects or with lack of benefit to avoid this investigation). Ongoing monitoring may include routine liver function tests, further liver biopsy (after a cumulative dose of 1–3 g, depending on routine tests), and/or serial measurements of the amino terminal peptide of type III procollagen (PIIINP), a serum marker of fibrosis.

Side effects include the following.

- Nausea.
- Myelosuppression—this may relate to inadvertent drug interaction in the absence of dose increase (discussed later); treat with folinic acid rescue.
- Skin ulceration—a warning sign of methotrexate toxicity.
- Hepatotoxicity—may occur acutely, but long-term fibrosis is the important issue. (Note: it is more likely if alcohol intake is high.)
- Folate deficiency—supplementation may be required.
- Cough—a feature of pulmonary toxicity, and rare.
- Drug interactions—may increase methotrexate levels and cause toxicity; drugs include the following.
  Folate antagonists—antibiotics such as trimethoprim, sulfonamides (especially in combination as co-trimoxazole), and dapsone.
  Non-steroidal antiinflammatory drugs—usually a mild effect, but avoid intermittent use due to unpredictability.
  Others—ciclosporin, probenecid, phenytoin, phenothiazines, and tetracyclines.

Hydroxycarbamide (hydroxyurea)

The main dermatologic use of hydroxycarbamide is for psoriasis. It may cause myelosuppression, but this is usually gradual and readily reversible. The benefit seems to gradually wane in many patients over a period of years. Other side effects include macrocytosis (very common), liver or renal toxicity, gout, and flu-like symptoms. Notably, it has a number of potential dermatologic side effects, including photosensitivity, pigmentation, a dermatomyositis-like skin eruption, or, in long-term use for myeloproliferative disorders, leg ulceration.

Cyclophosphamide

This alkylating agent is not used widely in dermatology, but it is one of the first-line treatments for Wegener granulomatosis and is sometimes used in other vasculitides. It is also occasionally used in severe immunobullous diseases, such as refractory pemphigus, or in sight-threatening mucous membrane pemphigoid or linear IgA disease.

Gastrointestinal side effects, myelosuppression, and alopecia are anticipated at doses used for malignant disease; these effects are less prominent with the lower-dose oral therapy used in dermatology but may be troublesome with higher-dose pulsed intravenous treatment. The most important side effect that is novel to cyclophosphamide in this group of immunosuppressive treatments is bladder toxicity due to a metabolite called acrolein, leading to either a hemorrhagic cystitis or rarely bladder cancer. These risks are most significant with intravenous use as a cytotoxic. High fluid intake is recommended. To avoid long-term use, azathioprine is often substituted once disease control has been achieved.

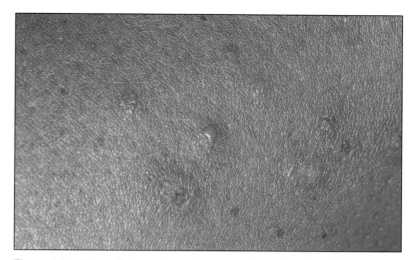

Figure 4.14 Dermatitis herpetiformis: close-up examination showing scratched papules with some tiny, intact blisters. Often these are so itchy that the blisters are destroyed by scratching. There is usually a very rapid symptomatic response to dapsone.

Gold

This is not widely used in dermatology but may be useful in resistant cases of discoid lupus erythematosus or in immunobullous diseases such as pemphigus.

Leukopenia and proteinuria may occur and must be monitored; a rash due to gold is not uncommon.

Fumaric acid esters

These agents are used in treatment of psoriasis, most commonly in continental Europe but less often in the USA or the UK. Side effects include nausea, flushing, headache, lymphopenia, and increased hepatic transaminases.

PRACTICE POINTS

- Ciclosporin has numerous drug interactions and significant long-term risks of hypertension or abnormal renal function.
- Azathioprine may cause early severe pancytopenia due to an inherited difference from the usual metabolic pathways.
- Methotrexate is given *once weekly*; it has long-term risks of liver damage, as well as dose-related hematologic side effects.

Sulfones

Dapsone is used in treatment of the following.

- Leprosy and also prophylaxis of malaria and of *Pneumocystis carinii* infection.
- Some immunobullous disorders—especially dermatitis herpetiformis (Fig. 4.14), linear IgA disease (Fig. 4.15) (and its pediatric counterpart, chronic bullous disease of childhood), and bullous pemphigoid.
- Some neutrophilic dermatoses and vasculitis—Sweet syndrome, pyoderma gangrenosum, bowel-associated dermatitis–arthritis syndrome, granuloma faciale, erythema elevatum diutinum, and cutaneous small-vessel vasculitides.
- Some other inflammatory dermatoses—examples include less common use in palmoplantar pustulosis, bullous lupus erythematosus, and relapsing polychondritis.

The main toxicity of dapsone relates to its effects on hematopoiesis. Agranulocytosis occurs rarely, but a dose-related hemolysis and methemoglobinemia occurs in all recipients; hemolysis occurs especially in patients with glucose-6-phosphate dehydrogenase deficiency, and this should be excluded in relevant populations prior to treatment. Headache is also common, probably due to methemoglobinemia. Weekly blood counts for a month, then fortnightly for a further month, monthly up to 3 months, then every 3–4 months are recommended: a reticulocyte count

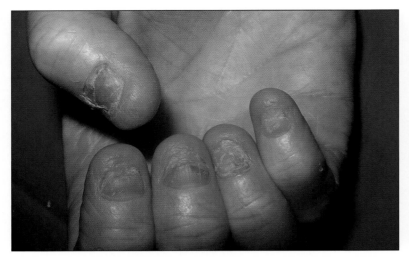

Figure 4.15 Linear IgA disease. Dapsone is the usual treatment for this condition and was initially helpful in this patient. However, over time she developed severe scarring of the conjunctivae, causing blindness (see Fig. 16.53), and of the nails (as shown here). Unsuccessful treatments to arrest her disease included corticosteroids, several immunosuppressive drugs, and intravenous immunoglobulins. Interferon-alpha proved useful but had hematologic side effects that precluded ongoing treatment.

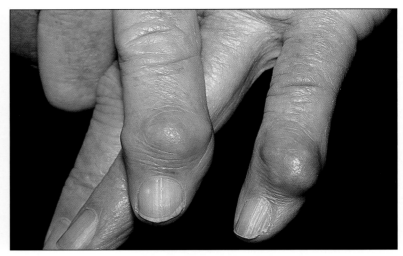

Figure 4.16 Large nodules of gout over the joints on the fingers. The deep location of these is apparent as the skin is stretched over them, with no textural changes and normal skin color. Individual tophi may be excised if required, and prophylactic treatment of the underlying metabolic disorder should be instituted with allopurinol (a rheumatologic drug that is not discussed here; it is rarely used by dermatologists but can be useful for cutaneous sarcoidosis). For painful joint exacerbations, analgesics and antiinflammatory drugs are typically used, but colchicine is often more effective.

gives a guide to the degree of hemolysis (drop in hemoglobin of 2 g/dL, and reticulocyte count up to about 5%, are usually acceptable). Vitamin E 800 IU daily may reduce hemolysis and headache; cimetidine also reduces methemoglobinemia.

Other side effects include a predominantly motor peripheral neuropathy, anorexia, and headache. Rash may occur, including toxic epidermal necrolysis; if severe rash occurs with eosinophilia (dapsone syndrome), then treatment should be stopped, as there is a risk of progression to hepatitis, psychosis, and even death.

Other sulfonamides such as sulfapyridine or sulfamethoxypyridazine are alternatives, especially for children, but are less readily available.

Potassium iodide

This is an old agent that may be useful in the following conditions.
- Infections—sporotrichosis.
- Panniculitis or vasculitis—erythema nodosum, nodular vasculitis or erythema induratum, and Wegener granulomatosis.
- Neutrophilic disorders—Sweet syndrome and pyoderma gangrenosum (but may also cause exacerbation).

Potassium iodide has an unpleasant taste, and treatment may be limited by gastrointestinal disturbance. It can cause various rashes, including iododerma, and may cause hypothyroidism.

Colchicine

Colchicine affects microtubule function and probably produces its antiinflammatory effects mainly by interfering with polymorphonuclear leukocyte function. It is mainly used in the treatment of gout (Fig. 4.16), but in dermatology it has a potential role in a number of vasculitic and neutrophilic disorders. The main use is in different forms of cutaneous small-vessel vasculitis, in urticarial vasculitis (Fig. 4.17), in Behçet disease (and other aphthous ulceration), occasionally in immunobullous diseases, and in rarities such as familial Mediterranean fever.

The main side effects when used at doses traditionally applied for gout are gastrointestinal disturbance and diarrhea, but these are unusual at the doses used for dermatoses (typically 0.5 mg two or three times daily).

Antimalarials

Chloroquine, hydroxychloroquine, and mepacrine (Atabrine) are all used in a variety of disorders, such as the following.
- Lupus erythematosus—especially discoid, subacute cutaneous (Fig. 4.18), and profundus types.

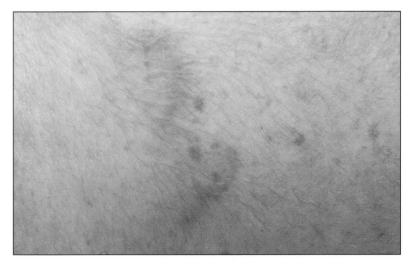

Figure 4.17 Urticarial vasculitis: purpura within lesions of urticaria, which each last several days, is typical. Colchicine may be very useful therapy.

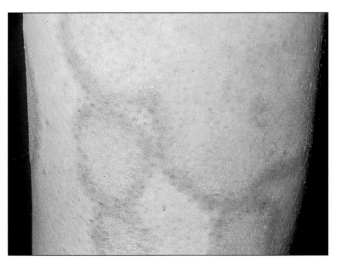

Figure 4.18 Subacute cutaneous lupus erythematosus, a disorder that often has annular morphology and photosensitivity. Many patients with this condition have an excellent response to hydroxychloroquine, a drug that generally has a good safety profile if used at appropriate doses.

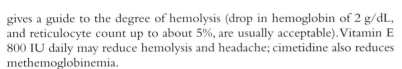

- Other disorders that may have a photosensitive component—polymorphic light eruption, Jessner lymphocytic infiltrate, reticular erythematous mucinosis, and dermatomyositis.
- Porphyria cutanea tarda.
- Sarcoidosis.

In most of these, the mechanism(s) of action are uncertain and probably multiple. Sarcoidosis is often relatively resistant by comparison with lupus erythematosus. In porphyria cutanea tarda, the drug (at lower dose than for the other inflammatory disorders listed) acts by binding porphyrins and enhancing excretion; this approach therefore does not work in patients with severe renal failure.

The main therapeutic issues with antimalarials for dermatologic indications are as follows.

- The time taken to see benefit—these agents have strong tissue binding and may take about 2 months to reach a steady state (also, the same period for their effect to disappear).
- The potential for ocular toxicity—part of the tissue binding is to the retina, and at higher doses or with prolonged treatment there is some risk of macular changes and impaired central vision; this is extremely unlikely if recommended dose limits are followed (e.g. hydroxychloroquine dose below 6.5 mg/kg lean body mass). This side effect does not occur with mepacrine.
- The marked diminution in benefit in patients with lupus erythematosus who smoke cigarettes.
- Other common side effects—nausea and headache are not uncommon. Mepacrine causes pigmentation and may cause a lichenoid drug eruption.
- Lack of benefit—if smoking has been excluded, lack of benefit can sometimes be overcome by using a combination of hydroxychloroquine and mepacrine.

Thalidomide

Thalidomide inhibits tumor necrosis factor (TNF) and various other cytokines, and decreases lymphocyte proliferation and neutrophil activity. It is not commonly used due to its potentially significant side effects, but it may be useful in the following.

- Aphthous ulceration—especially due to Behçet disease or in HIV infection.
- Pruriginous conditions—in which it may in part work by causing neuropathy (e.g. nodular prurigo).
- Erythema nodosum leprosum.
- Others—for example graft-versus-host disease, chronic discoid lupus erythematosus, and pyoderma gangrenosum.
  Side effects include the following.
- Teratogenicity—common and severe, so pregnancy must be avoided.
- Neuropathy—nerve conduction studies are a required part of monitoring.
- Other common effects—sedation, mood disturbance, nausea, decreased thyroid function, and rashes.

Careful monitoring and application of precautions to avoid pregnancy are mandatory and reduce the usefulness of this agent.

PRACTICE POINTS

- Avoidance of pregnancy is critical in women treated with thalidomide; also, neuropathy is a common and important issue requiring long-term monitoring.
- Colchicine commonly causes diarrhea that may be dose limiting.
- Dapsone can be very effective for neutrophilic or eosinophilic disorders but may cause dramatic early fall in blood parameters; careful monitoring is required, especially in the first 6 weeks of treatment.
- Patients treated with antimalarials for collagen vascular diseases must stop smoking to get good benefit; doses must be adjusted to address the long-term issue of retinopathy.

Interferons

Interferons are cytokines that have antimicrobial, antitumor, and anti-inflammatory actions. They are administered by subcutaneous injection. The major uses in dermatology (although usually administered by oncologists) are for melanoma or cutaneous T-cell lymphoma. HIV-related Kaposi sarcoma may also be treated, and interferon-alpha is part of the regimen for hepatitis C infection (which may present to dermatologists as cryoglobulinemia). Other infections, such as warts, and proliferations, such as epithelial tumors or hemangiomas, have been treated; experience in inflammatory diseases such as lupus erythematosus or immunobullous disorders is mixed.

Side effects of interferons (mostly documented with interferon-alpha) include the following.

- General—malaise, flu-like symptoms, and gastrointestinal upset.
- Hematologic—neutropenia and thrombocytopenia.
- Liver—raised hepatic enzymes.
- Cardiac—hypotension and arrhythmias.
- Neurologic—lethargy, sleepiness, depression, and seizures.
- Other—rash, rhabdomyolysis, and autoimmune disease.

Monoclonal antibodies and cytokine inhibitors

A number of agents termed monoclonals or (immuno)biologicals are being introduced into dermatology, notably for the treatment of severe psoriasis and for some lymphomas, although they will undoubtedly have numerous applications in immunologic diseases (atopic dermatitis and alopecia areata) and in immunotherapy of tumors. These agents are manufactured to target key cytokines in the relevant disease, such as TNF in psoriasis or cell surface receptors (such as basiliximab for lymphomas).

The agents with which there is most experience to date in psoriasis are as follows.

- Etanercept—a TNF receptor–immunoglobulin fusion protein, with anti-TNF activity; subcutaneous administration.
- Infliximab—a chimeric antibody, also with anti-TNF activity; intravenous administration.
- Alefacept—a lymphocyte function-associated antigen-3 receptor–immunoglobulin fusion protein that binds to CD2 on T cells; intramuscular administration.
- Efalizumab—an anti-CD11a antibody; subcutaneous administration.

Use of such agents is limited to treatment of chronic moderate or severe disease (generally, patients who might be considered for other systemic therapies or for photochemotherapy) due to high cost and some risks, for example risks of infection, especially reactivation of tuberculosis (discussed below). Most of these drugs are new, and there is therefore an uncertain risk of malignancy in the long term, as occurs with more commonly used immunosuppressive agents. None should be used in conjunction with immunosuppressive therapies or photochemotherapy. Antinuclear antibodies may occur in patients treated with TNF blockers, and rarely overt lupus erythematosus. All require monitoring of either CD4+ lymphocyte counts or platelet counts during therapy.

The main side effects that occur with this group of agents, most being applicable to several such drugs, include nausea, anaphylaxis or hypersensitivity reactions, fever, headache, blood dyscrasias (including thrombocytopenia and aplastic anemia), worsening of cardiac failure, and infection (especially reactivation of tuberculosis or development of septicemia, listeriosis, or varicella zoster). Some may cause injection site reactions: hypersensitivity reactions are a significant concern. Infliximab may also cause hepatitis, gastrointestinal bleeding, pneumonitis, arrhythmias, vasospasm, bleeding, rashes, and alopecia. Various anti-TNF drugs have been identified as possibly causing a demyelination disorder.

Many of the agents in use for systemic lymphomas have a potential role for cutaneous lymphomas as well, for example denileukin diftitox (which kills cells that express interleukin-2, e.g. in cutaneous T-cell lymphoma) and basiliximab (for B-cell lymphoma); again there are some potentially important side effects, such as vascular leak syndrome with denileukin diftitox.

Intravenous immunoglobulins

Aside from their original role in replacement therapy for hypogammaglobulinemias, intravenous immunoglobulins (IVIG; generally at higher doses than those used for replacement therapy) have an immuno-modulatory role. They have been used with variable success in disorders such as the following.

- Bullous disease—especially pemphigus and other severe autoimmune bullous disorders; toxic epidermal necrolysis.
- Connective tissue disease—dermatomyositis.
- Vasculitis and related disorders—especially Kawasaki disease.
- Other autoimmune disease—idiopathic thrombocytopenic purpura and the autoimmune type of chronic urticaria.

This treatment is expensive and has a risk of transmitting infection, as it is derived from pooled donor blood. Side effects include the following.

- Severe—anaphylaxis, severe hypotension, and acute renal failure. (Note: exclude anti-IgA antibodies in IgA-deficient patients, as these increase the risk of severe reactions.)
- Neurologic—headache, migraine, and aseptic meningitis (may be delayed onset).

- Skin—urticaria and eczematous rash.
- Milder reactions related to the infusion—nausea, flu-like symptoms, milder blood pressure changes; treat by slowing the infusion rate.

Plasmapheresis

This is really a physical therapy but is pertinent here as it is (rarely) used in many of the diseases discussed as potentially responding to immuno-suppressive therapy, such as immunobullous diseases, connective tissue disease, or vasculitis in which there are circulating antibodies or immune complexes that can potentially be decreased in titre by removal of plasma. Using a continuous circuit from the patient to the centrifuge machinery, blood is extracted and centrifuged, plasma removed, and fresh plasma replaced, before the blood is reinfused into the patient. It is relatively time consuming, and care must be taken to avoid hemodynamic instability or alteration of blood clotting.

FURTHER READING

Lebwohl M, et al. Treatment of Skin Disease. London: Mosby, 2002
Levine N (ed) Systemic dermatologic therapy. Dermatol Clin 2001; 19: 1–197
Wakelin SH. Handbook of Systemic Drug Treatment in Dermatology. London: Manson Publishing, 2002

Wolverton SE. Comprehensive Dermatologic Drug Therapy. Philadelphia: Saunders, 2001

INTRODUCTION

A number of physical therapies are used in dermatology. These include freezing (cryotherapy), numerous surgical techniques, laser treatments, radiotherapy, and different forms of phototherapy for a variety of inflammatory dermatoses and skin lymphomas. This brief overview is not exhaustive; some treatments with specific applications will be discussed in chapters relating to individual diseases.

CRYOTHERAPY

Cryotherapy, the therapeutic use of controlled cold injury, is widely used in dermatology (Fig. 5.1). Rapid freezing, usually using a liquid nitrogen spray, can achieve a temperature drop in the skin down to −20 to −40°C. Such freezing causes ice crystals to form in cell organelles, which then rupture on thawing and cause local damage. For many lesions, the effect of cryotherapy involves not only damage to the lesional cells, but also damage to local vasculature and the creation of an inflammatory response.

The main indications are as follows.

- Benign lesions—viral warts, seborrhoeic keratoses, other keratoses (e.g. porokeratosis), simple lentigo; less commonly pyogenic granuloma, venous lake, chondrodermatitis nodularis, other benign lesions.
- Premalignant epidermal lesions—actinic keratosis and Bowen disease.
- Epidermal malignancies—basal cell carcinoma.
- Other malignancies—lentigo maligna melanoma (in situ).

Several other lesions may be treated, usually by more experienced practitioners or with special techniques such as thermocouples to monitor the degree of freezing. Some dermatologists treat nevi with cryotherapy, but it should be borne in mind that this is a destructive technique that does not allow histologic evaluation.

Recording cryotherapy treatments should include a record of the cryogen (e.g. liquid nitrogen), the number of freeze–thaw cycles (typically one for benign lesions and two for basal cell carcinoma or lentigo maligna), and their duration in seconds.

Cryotherapy has several side effects. It is generally painful and may cause blistering (Fig. 5.2) or erosion, pigmentary disturbance (beware of hypopigmentation, especially in colored skin), hypoesthesia, delayed healing (especially on the elderly or oedematous lower leg), and incomplete response. Less commonly, deeper nerve or tendon damage may occur. These side effects are related to freeze duration and depth, and are minimized by appropriate choice of lesions and technique. Despite these potential disadvantages, for appropriate lesions the technique is quick, generally well tolerated, and leads to good cosmetic results without scarring.

SURGICAL TREATMENTS

A detailed discussion of surgical treatments is beyond the scope of this book, but a brief outline is provided.

Materials

It is essential when performing skin surgery to have adequate facilities, lighting, biopsy equipment, cautery, resuscitation facilities, etc. It is assumed that the reader will be familiar with these issues. This section on biopsy materials will therefore be limited to a brief discussion of local anesthesia and suture materials.

Local anesthetic

For some superficial procedures, such as destroying molluscum contagiosum lesions, topical local anesthesia may suffice. Agents that are used include amethocaine and a mixture of lidocaine and prilocaine.

For most procedures, injectable local anesthetics are used. These include agents such as lidocaine, bupivacaine, ropivacaine, and prilocaine (note that the latter is an ester and does not cross-react with amide anesthetics such

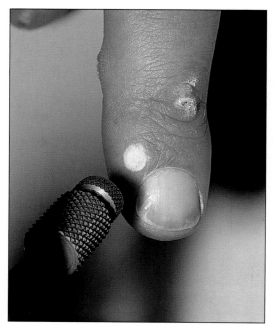

Figure 5.1 Cryotherapy of warts. Cryotherapy using the liquid nitrogen (LN2) spray technique. For warts or actinic keratoses, it is usual to perform a single period of freezing (one freeze–thaw cycle, FTC), whereas for malignancies two FTCs are usual, to increase the degree of damage. It is usual to record the cryogen, and the number and duration of treatment cycles, for example LN2, 2 × 20 s FTC.

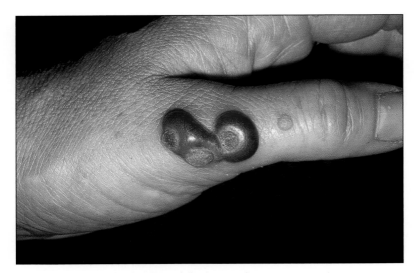

Figure 5.2 Hemorrhagic blisters following cryotherapy.

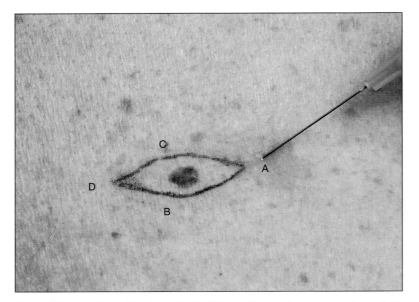

Figure 5.3 Injection of local anesthetic. Using a fine needle, local anesthetic (LA) is first infiltrated along one edge of the planned ellipse. Typically, the needle would be advanced from its insertion point A to point B, then LA injected as the needle is slowly withdrawn but without fully removing it from the skin (thus avoiding the discomfort of a second needleprick at point A). This is repeated from point A to C to give a V- or wedge-shaped area of anesthesia. After waiting a couple of minutes the LA is infiltrated from B to D and then from C to D, areas B and C at this point being anesthetized and therefore avoiding needleprick discomfort. Although the LA itself may sting, this method involves a single perceived needleprick, and avoids distorting the lesion itself with injected fluid. Note that the lesion shown is a simple seborrheic keratosis that required no intervention, and no needleprick was involved in this demonstration photograph.

as lidocaine, a point that is useful in rare patients with true local anesthetic allergy). These may be combined with vasoconstricting agents for use at most parts of the body, for example lidocaine with adrenaline (epinephrine) or prilocaine with octapressin. Vasoconstrictors not only reduce surgical bleeding but also slow absorption of the anesthetic so that less is required, anesthesia lasts longer, and the drug is less likely to cause toxicity by systemic absorption.

Many local anesthetics sting when injected. This can be reduced by using lower concentrations, by warming the solution, by slow injection using a fine 27-G needle (Fig. 5.3), and by using nerve blocks for tender areas such as nose or digits.

For the technique of liposuction, large volumes of very dilute local anesthetic are used (tumescent anesthesia).

Suture materials

While simple skin surface sutures are adequate for small wounds without tension, many dermatologic procedures benefit from additional use of

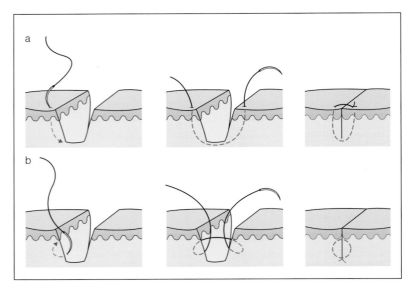

Figure 5.4 Suture placement. Each picture shows initial needle entry with planned pathway (in red), position of stitch before knotting, and final position of knotted suture. (**a**) Placement of simple non-absorbable suture: note the slightly flask-shaped placement, which causes some eversion of the wound edge during healing. (**b**) Subcutaneous suture: note the placement of the knot at the deeper aspect of the tied suture.

subcutaneous sutures to improve wound strength (Fig. 5.4). For either surface or deeper sutures, a huge array of different brands and materials are available. These vary in terms of absorption (fast, slow, or non-absorbable), filament type (monofilament or braided, coated or uncoated), diameter, and color. They also vary in their physical properties, for example in ease and strength of knotting.

Absorbable sutures include polyglycolic acid (Dexon), polyglactin 910 (Vicryl), polydioxanone (PDS), polyglyconate (Maxon), and poliglecaprone 25 (Monocryl). Commonly used non-absorbable suture types include nylon (e.g. Ethilon), polyester (e.g. Ethibond), polybutester (Novafil), and polypropylene (e.g. Prolene).

More recently, tissue glues such as cyanoacrylate have increased in popularity, both for simple wound closures and to adhere skin grafts to recipient sites.

Types of procedure

Dermatologists may perform a wide range of diagnostic or therapeutic procedures, including the following.

- Incisional biopsies for diagnosis—ellipse and punch biopsy.
- Curettage—a technique for scraping off superficial lesions; generally combined with cautery for hemostasis, occasionally with chemical hemostatics such as aluminum chloride.
- Shave biopsy—a superficial form of biopsy particularly suited to benign lesions such as ordinary nevi, but also used for diagnosis or treatment of small neoplasms, such as basal cell carcinoma, and as a treatment for broader areas of abnormal skin, such as rhinophyma.
- Cautery without tissue removal, for example to small angiomas.
- Excisional biopsy—the main method for removing skin neoplasia; includes specialized excisional procedures such as Mohs micrographic surgery, in which the tumor extent is mapped by special histologic processing (discussed and illustrated later in this chapter).

The choice of technique, and indeed consideration of alternatives such as cryotherapy or radiotherapy, takes into account many factors, including the following.

- Patient factors—age, general health and medications, body site affected (this may influence healing or scarring), ability to attend for treatment, ability to care for a wound, etc.
- Lesion factors—clinical or incisional biopsy diagnosis, subtype (e.g. morpheic basal cell carcinoma has higher local recurrence risk than in other types), size and rate of growth (may influence what is technically achievable or perceived aggression of the lesion).
- Other factors—availability of treatment and skills of the clinician.

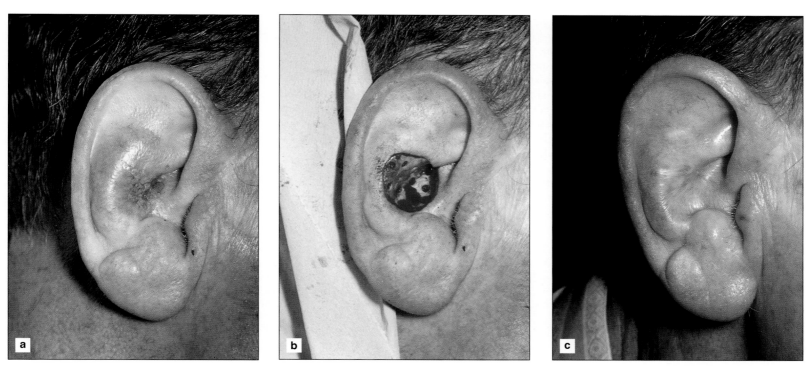

Figure 5.5   Healing by second intention. In this case, a basal cell carcinoma at the edge of the concha of the ear (**a**) has been excised as a disk down to cartilage. Making 3-mm punch biopsy holes through the cartilage, known as fenestration (**b**), allows granulation tissue to extend from the posterior skin of the ear to provide a base for epithelialization. Individual holes in this fashion preserve the rigidity of the cartilage (like a colander), and healing (**c**) is excellent, without distortion of the shape of the ear.

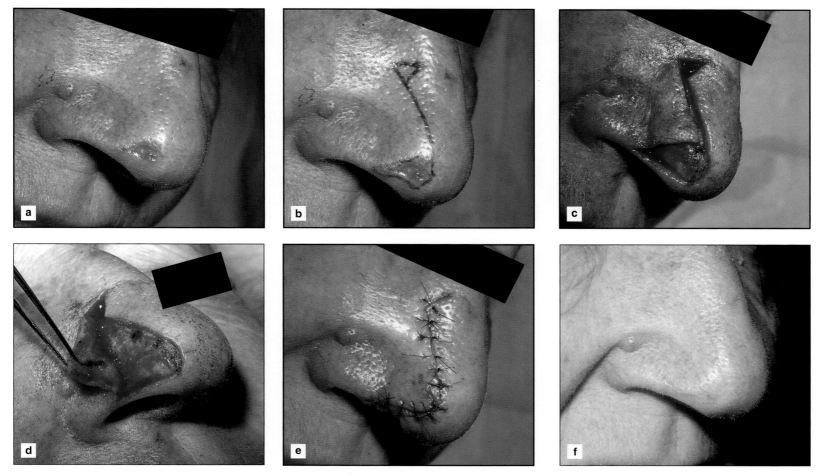

Figure 5.6   Rotation flap closure. (**a**) Basal cell carcinoma on the tip of the nose (the lesion in the nasolabial fold is a simple dermal nevus). (**b**) The edge of the tumor and the proposed flap design have been marked: the line of the proposed wound is along a ridge that separates nasal subunits. (**c**) The tumor has been excised with a margin of normal skin, and the flap is being prepared; note that the small wedge at the upper end of the wound (known as a Burow triangle) has been excised and discarded, a process that prevents puckering of the wound tip. (**d**) The flap is undermined to create mobility. (**e**) Flap sutured into place. (**f**) Final result.

Repair of excised wounds may involve a number of techniques. Elliptic wounds can generally be repaired by side-to-side closure, but other commonly used techniques include the following.

- Healing by second intention—a useful technique but slow to heal, and may produce contracture of the skin. Particularly useful on the ears where it may be combined with fenestration of the cartilage to improve granulation (Fig. 5.5).
- Skin grafting—split thickness or full thickness; the latter is especially used on the face to match the donor skin and recipient grafted site. Grafting is also used in treatment of leg ulcers, vitiligo, and other disorders.
- Various flap repairs—advancement, rotation, transposition, island pedicle, etc. (Figs 5.6 and 5.7). In some instances, if the wound is large and the area is tight, additional preliminary techniques such as tissue expansion may be applied.

Pitfalls

It is pertinent to briefly consider some potential pitfalls of surgery for the less experienced practitioner. These include the following.

- Unnecessary operation—for example of a lesion erroneously thought to be malignant or of a rash that could be clinically diagnosed.
- Wrong operation or technique—for example shave excision of a melanoma.
- Poor healing or infection—may be unavoidable but can be predicted if operating on infected lesions.
- Damage to other structures—especially nerve transection.

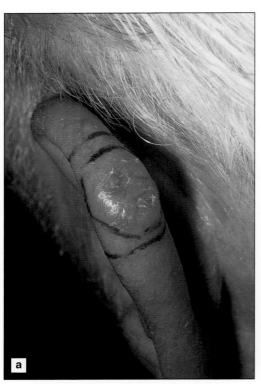

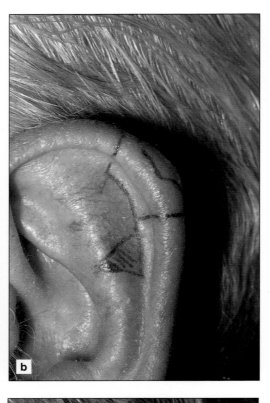

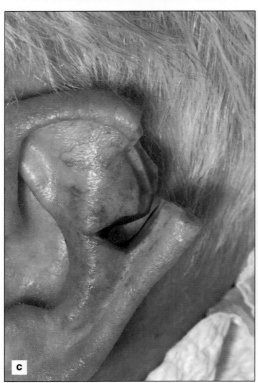

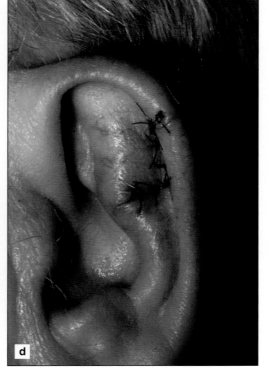

Figure 5.7 Flap on the rim of the pinna. (**a**) Basal cell carcinoma of the pinna. (**b**) Planned excision, with a sliding wedge repair (the aim of this, rather than a simple wedge resembling a slice of cake, is that it avoids a linear wound along which the cartilage can fold). (**c**) Tumor excised; note that both the lesion excision and the Burow triangle involve the full thickness of the ear. (**d**) Flap sutured into place; the final result is a slightly smaller but essentially normally shaped ear.

- Issues of scarring—stretched scars (Fig. 5.8), keloid scars, and effects of scar contracture (e.g. ectropion).
- Histology issues—lack of histology on some samples, surprise results, and interpretation of reports.
- Inadequate excision—for example incomplete removal of a malignant neoplasm.
- Inadequate records—a major cause of problems.

Many of the above are technical issues that can be avoided by appropriate training, and by attention to the local anatomy and to surgical options for operating at specific body sites. It is of importance to have some understanding of laboratory issues: adequate information for the pathologist is crucial, correct samples are required (e.g. frozen tissue for direct immunofluorescence), and reports must be read in the context of what has been performed. For example, a report indicating complete excision of a lesion that has been routinely 'bread loaf'–processed will just be an assessment of the adequacy of excision in the section(s) that have been examined (Figs 5.9 and 5.10). This problem is avoided by the micrographic surgical method, in which the whole of the deep and lateral margin of each specimen is examined and any residual tumor can be mapped; however, this technique is time consuming for both operator and pathologist, and is therefore usually reserved for large or indistinct tumors, recurrent lesions, tumors associated with scar tissue, or tumors at sites where maximum preservation of non-lesional skin is important (Figs 5.11 and 5.12).

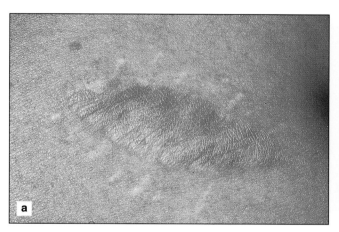

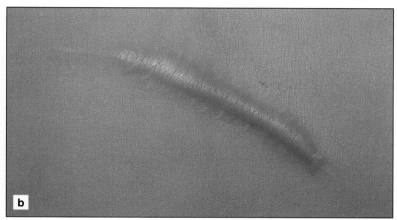

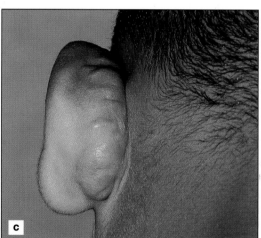

Figure 5.8   Complications of surgery include a stretched scar (**a**; note the stretched freckles), suture marks and hypertrophic scar (both shown in **b**), and keloid formation, which particularly occurs on the head and upper trunk, and is shown here following an otoplasty operation (**c**). (Panel a from Lawrence CM, Cox NH. Physical Signs in Dermatology, 2nd edn. London: Mosby, 2002.)

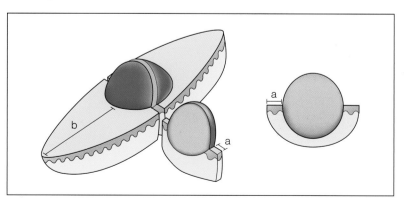

Figure 5.9   Methods used to take histopathologic sections of an excised localized lesion. An ellipse of skin containing a tumor is cut across the middle of the tumor nodule in the middle of the ellipse. At least in theory, this samples the tumor at the site of its closest lateral margin (compare distances marked 'a' and 'b'). Further slices may be taken parallel to this one ('bread loaf' technique) or from each end of the specimen at right angles to the section drawn. Compare with biopsy of a rash (Fig. 2.26). Explaining to the laboratory workers what has been sampled helps them to make the correct decision about tissue processing. (After an original drawing by Dr. N. H. Cox.)

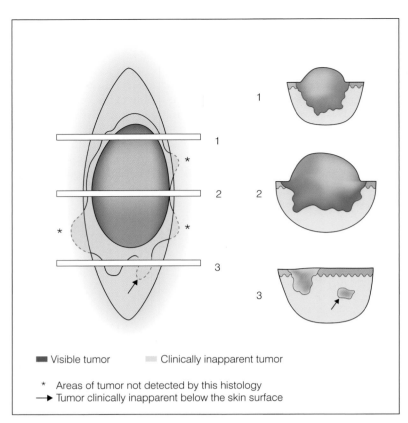

Visible tumor   Clinically inapparent tumor

*   Areas of tumor not detected by this histology
→ Tumor clinically inapparent below the skin surface

Figure 5.10   Limitations of histology reporting. Even with multiple sections from a tumor, it may be impossible to comment with complete accuracy on the excision. In this example, the visible tumor nodule is in dark blue and the clinically invisible extent is pale blue, with a solid border representing clinically unapparent tumor that will fall within the planned ellipse and a dotted border where tumor lies in skin outside the ellipse (asterisks) or below the skin surface (arrow). All three sections taken appear to have a margin of normal skin around the tumor, but three areas (asterisks) have not been excised. This is the rationale for micrographic surgery (Figs 5.11 and 5.12) in poorly defined lesions. (After an original drawing by Dr. N. H. Cox.)

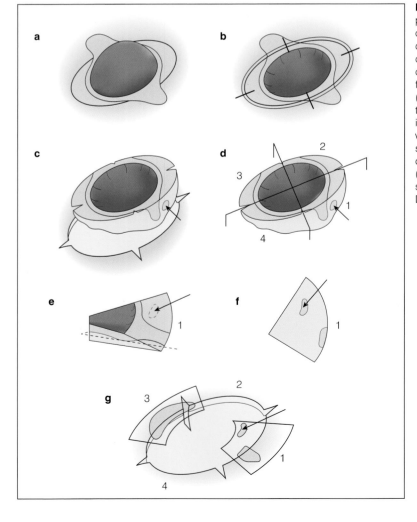

Figure 5.11   Mohs micrographic surgery. (**a**) Tumor nodule, with clinically visible portion in dark blue and clinically invisible portion in pale blue; the latter lies partly outside the planned circular excision. (**b**) The central nodule is debulked (this helps to determine the extent and creates a thinner skin specimen) and an excision line is created; nicks are made in the specimen and in the adjacent skin, so that the sample can be oriented and the tumor mapped histologically. (**c**) The specimen of skin is freed; in this diagram, a further, clinically unapparent extension of the tumor is shown (arrow) on the undersurface of the specimen. (**d**) The specimen is divided according to the premarked nicks at its edges, and the samples numbered to correspond to an identifiable quadrant of the surgical site. (**e**) Each quadrant is placed flat, so that the whole of the undersurface and the most peripheral margin will be sampled in a tissue section from this deep aspect (dotted line). (**f**) The location of tumor at the margin or deep surface of each specimen is documented and drawn on to a diagram.
(**g**) Further surgery can then take place at the sites where there is residual tumor, sparing areas where a clear margin has been identified. (After an original drawing by Dr. N. H. Cox.)

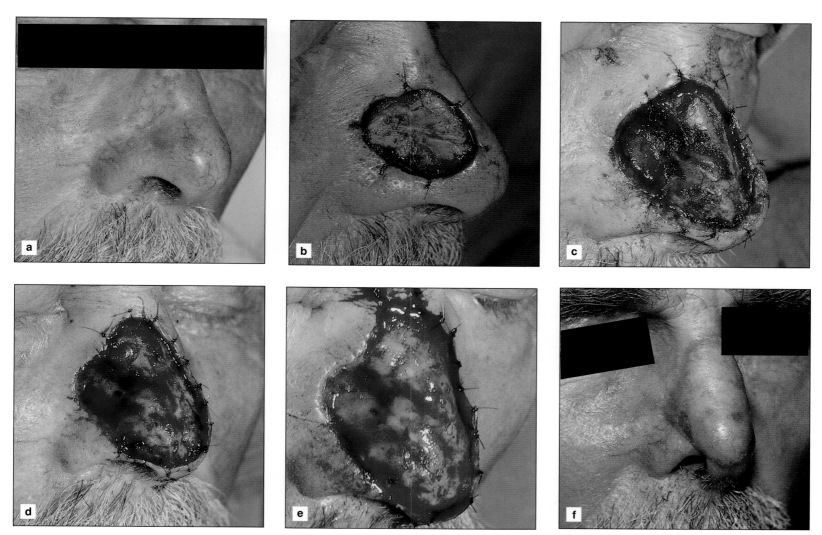

Figure 5.12 Micrographic (Mohs) surgery to a nasal basal cell carcinoma. (**a**) Initial poorly defined basal cell carcinoma. (**b**) Stage 1 excision. (**c**) Stage 2 excision. (**d**) Stage 3 excision. (**e**) Stage 4 excision. (**f**) After repair. (Courtesy of Dr. C. M. Lawrence.)

PRACTICE POINTS
- Cryotherapy is painful and may cause edema or blistering; always consider whether it is appropriate for the lesion and site.
- Always consider whether an operation is necessary, and whether the choice of procedure is the correct one.
- Stretched scars and effects of scar contracture (e.g. ectropion) can usually be avoided by consideration of tension lines and use of subcuticular sutures.
- Inadequate records are a major cause of medicolegal problems.

PHOTODYNAMIC THERAPY

Photodynamic therapy is a relatively new technique in dermatology. The basic principle relies on the fact that the porphyrin precursor aminolevulinic acid (ALA), or a derivative such as methyl-ALA, is selectively taken up into neoplastic cells. When activated by light (usually red light at about 630 nm, but sometimes other wavelengths), the ALA is converted into protoporphyrin IX (PPIX), which produces cytotoxic oxygen radicals and thus cellular damage.

The ALA or derivative may be administered systemically, but more commonly for dermatologic indications is applied topically under light-shielded occlusion for 3–4 h before photoactivation. The light source may be by laser, xenon arc, or diode; most commonly in dermatology, the safer non-laser sources are used.

Typical indications are as follows.
- Premalignant epidermal lesions—actinic keratosis and Bowen disease (Fig. 5.13).

- Epidermal malignancies—basal cell carcinoma (usually thin lesions).
- Benign dermatoses (less commonly)—some use for localized psoriasis, lichen planus, and porokeratosis; research continues in areas such as acne.
- Other malignancies (less commonly)—localized cutaneous T-cell lymphoma (CTCL) and metastases from some internal tumors.
- Photodynamic diagnosis (less commonly)—the fluorescence produced by PPIX has been used to identify sites of neoplasm.

The technique causes some discomfort, usually a burning pain, but is generally well tolerated. Treated lesions heal with crusting; cosmetic results are good, and healing is generally satisfactory even at areas such as the lower leg.

LASERS

Numerous different types of laser are used in dermatology. All share the principle on which the acronym laser is based: light amplification by stimulated emission of radiation. By excitation of various gases or crystals, lasers produce a coherent beam of monochromatic light such that all the light waves are in phase, in the same direction, and do not diverge. This intense light causes a number of effects on skin tissue, which will vary according to the wavelength, power, and duration of laser pulse. Some of the more commonly used lasers are summarized in Table 5.1.

Lasers may cause tissue damage by many means. For example, the carbon dioxide laser vaporizes water to produce relatively non-specific destruction, while a blue-green argon laser interacts with red chromophores, of which the most important is hemoglobin, to (relatively) selectively damage vasculature (Fig. 5.14). The energy produced causes heating in the region of the target chromophore; the energy density

53

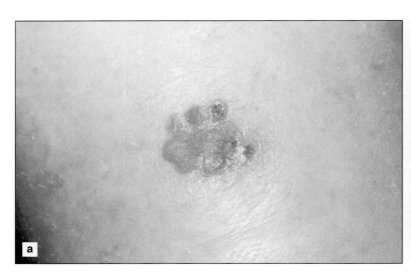

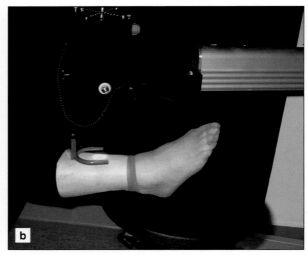

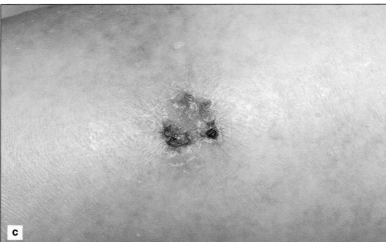

Figure 5.13 Photodynamic therapy. (**a**) Lesion of Bowen disease on the leg, before treatment. (**b**) Exposure to red light after pretreatment with methyl-aminolaevulinic acid for 3 h under occlusion. (**c**–**e**) Appearances at 1 week, 1 month, and 3 months after treatment.

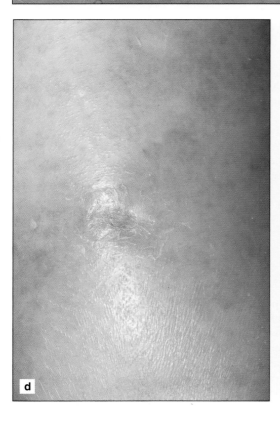

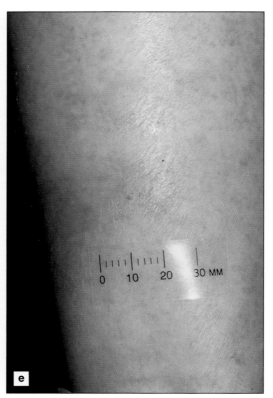

Table 5.1 SOME TYPES OF LASER

Type of laser	Light emitted	Some uses
Carbon dioxide (conventional-type continuous wave)	Infrared, 10 600 nm	Cutting (focused mode), coagulation (defocused)
Carbon dioxide (short-pulse types)	Infrared, 10 600 nm	Resurfacing (see text)
Neodymium:YAG[a]	Infrared, 1064 nm	Cutting, coagulation, black tattoo pigment, blue-colored veins
Neodymium:YAG (frequency doubled using KTP[b])	Green, 532 nm	Red and yellow tattoo pigment, pigmented epidermal lesions, vascular lesions
Erbium:YAG	Infrared, 2940 nm	Resurfacing
Argon	Blue-green, peaks between 488 and 514 nm	Coagulation, port wine stains (darker lesions, adults), pigmented lesions, black tattoo pigment
Pulsed dye	Orange, 585 nm	Telangiectasias, paler vascular lesions
Pulsed dye	Green, 510 nm	Vascular lesions, red tattoo pigment
Argon-pumped tunable dye	Variable, 488–638 nm	Depends on wavelength
Q-switched ruby	Red, 694 nm	Brown-pigmented lesions, nevus of Ota, black and green tattoo pigments
Copper vapor and copper bromide	Green/yellow, 510/578 nm	Vascular lesions, red tattoo pigment, epidermal pigmented lesions
Alexandrite	Near infrared, 755 nm	Black tattoo pigment, pigmented lesions, hair removal
Excimer	193 nm	Resurfacing (see text)
Excimer	308 nm	Localized psoriasis
Diode	Various, around 800 nm	Tissue ablation, small vessels, hair removal, powering solid-state lasers
Diode	532 nm	Small vascular lesions, pigmented lesions

[a]Yttrium–aluminum–garnet.
[b]Potassium–titanyl–phosphate.

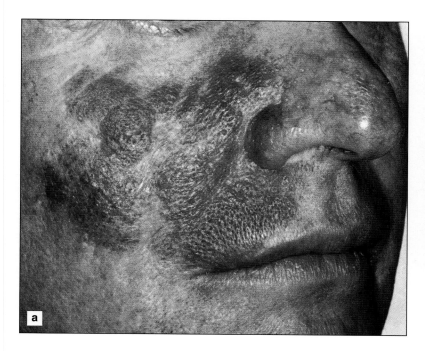

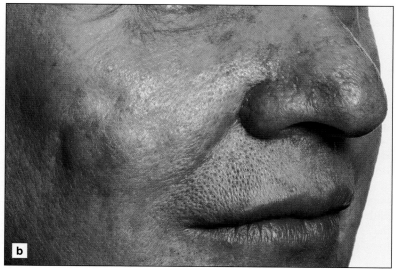

Figure 5.14 Laser therapy of a port wine stain on the face. (**a**) Before treatment, (**b**) 3 years after treatment (8 sessions of treatment were required). Courtesy of Dr. C. M. Lawrence.

(fluence) in the skin is the product of the power output and the pulse duration. Secondary effects, such as heating of adjacent tissue or interaction with other chromophores, may limit the benefit; for example, spread of tissue heating outside the blood vessel may damage other structures and lead to scarring, but may be minimized by short pulse duration and longer intervals between pulses at the same site (typically achieved by a variety of scanning devices). An important concept in this regard is that of thermal relaxation time and selective photothermolysis. To increase specificity of damage, pulse durations should be shorter than the time taken for the chromophore to lose heat to its surroundings. This will vary according to the size of the chromophore; it is shorter, for example, for a melanosome than for an ectatic vessel.

Uses of lasers are numerous, and more are being discovered. Different types of carbon dioxide laser, for example, may be used for various depths of lesion, depending on the pulsing and number of passes performed. To minimize tissue damage, the lasers used for resurfacing use either short pulses, or a system of moving the laser beam so that individual areas receive only brief exposure. Thus they are used cosmetically for aged skin; therapeutically for actinic keratoses and superficial tumors; for destruction of warts, rhinophyma, xanthelasma, syringomas, adenoma sebaceum, and the like; and for treatment of melasma. Less obvious applications include carbon dioxide laser treatment of Hailey–Hailey disease (Ch. 19), and various lasers are being investigated in treatment of localized psoriasis and of acne. Hair removal lasers are increasingly popular, but work best on dark hair, may lead to depigmentation in dark skin, and have uncertain long-term benefit at present.

Laser sources (usually red light types) may also be used in photo-dynamic therapy (as discussed). Various non-laser intense light sources are used for some similar applications, such as the infrared coagulator for vascular lesions and the intense pulsed light (IPL) source that produces intense light from 500–1200 nm.

COSMETIC INTERVENTIONS

The emphasis of this textbook is on dermatologic disorders, but a brief overview of cosmetic procedures may be helpful. Skin aging is inevitable, but it is augmented by photodamage; chronically exposed sites such as the face are therefore mostly affected, and the changes that occur are a source of cosmetic concern. Some specific features of photoaging are illustrated in Chapter 17. Other factors, notably cigarette smoking, also contribute to facial skin aging.

Facial peels and resurfacing

A variety of methods are used to remove the skin surface, and thereby achieve a degree of smoothening and removal of minor superficial blemishes. The approaches may be chemical (facial peels) or physical (dermabrasion and laser resurfacing); several may be combined for different facial sites.

Facial peels are performed with varying degrees of aggression to achieve different depth of peeling, using peeling agents that vary from relatively mild (alpha-hydroxy acids such as glycolic acid), through medium, to severe (phenol). Different concentrations and durations, pretreatment measures (e.g. use of solid CO_2), and concurrent use of occlusion or of other drugs (such as 5-fluorouracil) all alter the effects; for example, different concentrations of trichloroacetic acid (TCA) may be used at different sites depending on the depth of peeling required. Different disorders are treated with different depths of peeling (Table 5.2).

The increased spectrum and availability of lasers has reduced the use of peeling. Many dermatologists who do not practice cosmetic procedures will utilize some aspects of peeling agents, for example localized TCA to xanthelasma. Adequate training is necessary, as peeling may lead to pigmentary disturbance, scarring, or secondary infection (notably herpes simplex infection).

Botulinum toxin

Botulinum toxin is an irreversible neurotoxin. Known for many decades as a potentially fatal toxin from dietary contamination with *Clostridium botulinum*, it was relatively recently used to block the nerve fibers involved with various dystonias such as blepharospasm. Subsequently, it was realized that it could also block the nerve fibers causing contraction of facial muscles, such blockade thereby reducing frown lines that lead to facial creases (dynamic wrinkles). Common areas for treatment are glabellar creases, forehead creases, and lateral canthus 'crow's feet'. The toxin has no effect on wrinkles due simply to skin laxity. There are eight serotypes, of which types A and B are used therapeutically.

Botulinum toxin has also found a role in treatment of hyperhidrosis, by blocking the stimulatory autonomic nerve supply; use is generally restricted to localized sites such as the axillae, palms, or localized areas on the face (e.g. as in Frey syndrome). Because of local pain of injections on the palms, nerve blocks are generally required to treat this site. It can also be useful in treating anal fissures.

In all situations, growth of adjacent new nerve fibers leads to recurrence of symptoms, and treatment needs to be repeated. For example, the effect in hyperhidrosis generally lasts about 4–9 months. Adverse effects include injection site reactions such as bruising or urtication, and excessive nerve blockade leading to muscle weakness (notably ptosis of the eyelid when treating strabismus, or weakness of small muscles of the hand when treating hyperhidrosis).

Collagen and tissue fillers

Fillers that can be injected into the skin to increase bulk include autologous fat; modified proteins such as bovine collagen; polysaccharides (hyaluronic acid); and synthetic agents such as silicone, polymethyl methacrylate, or expanded polytetrafluoroethylene (ePTFE or Gore-Tex).

Fat is mainly used for deeper contour defects; it is popular for injection of the lips but generally does not last well.

Collagen is the most widely used agent. It may be injected into wrinkles to fill them out, or into areas such as the lips to enlarge them. Bovine collagen is most commonly used but may cause allergic reactions, which present as granulomatous inflammatory nodules; skin testing is required prior to treatment to identify individuals for whom this is a likely complication. Treatment of bovine collagen with glutaraldehyde increases cross-linking and improves the duration of the treatment.

Most fillers need to be injected in excess, but the degree of this over-treatment differs between agents and requires experience. Most are transient, lasting in the region of 6–18 months; silicone is permanent. Side effects are mainly local, but embolic problems, including blindness, have been reported due to injections around the eyelids and glabellar region.

Liposuction

Liposuction is mainly used for cosmetic purposes to remove fat from areas such as the buttocks, thighs, lower abdomen, and flanks, and to provide a source of autologous fat to use as a tissue filler. It is usually performed using tumescent anesthesia (described earlier). However, it may also be useful in treatment of lipomas and abnormal lipohypertrophies, and for large neurofibromas, and it has been used in lymphedema and in treatment of axillary hyperhidrosis.

Sclerotherapy

Sclerotherapy may be used to treat prominent veins of various sizes. Larger vessels are more likely to be treated by a vascular surgeon than by dermatologists. However, it is important to recognize that the benefits of injecting small vessels will be limited unless related larger vessels are also treated.

Table 5.2	CHEMICAL PEELS		
Type of peel	**Depth**	**Agents used**	**Uses**
Superficial	Epidermis	Alpha-hydroxy acids, salicylic acid, Jessner solution[a], TCA[b] < 25%	Aged skin, fine wrinkles, mild solar damage, ephelides, melasma
Intermediate	Papillary Dermis	TCA 25–35% Phenol	More prominent age or actinic changes, moderate wrinkles, actinic keratoses, lentigines
Deep	Reticular Dermis	TCA > 35% Phenol	Acne scars, lentigines, xanthelasma, deep wrinkles, severe actinic damage

[a]Contains resorcinol, salicylic acid, and lactic acid in ethanol.
[b]Trichloroacetic acid.

Reticular veins of 1–4 mm in diameter may be associated with deeper truncal varicosities, or may present as arborizing telangiectasia. They have a bluish color and may be treated with neodymium:yttrium–aluminum–garnet (Nd:YAG), diode, or alexandrite laser, or with sclerosants such as sodium tetradecyl sulfate, polidocanol, or hypertonic saline. They are often fragile, bruise easily, and may be associated with residual pigmentation.

Telangiectasia and venulectasia, vessels of about 2 mm, are typically treated with sclerosants.

Smaller vessels of less than 2 mm are less easy to cannulate but may be treated with sclerosants (usually at a lower concentration than that for wider diameter vessels), or with lasers such as pulsed dye, potassium–titanyl–phosphate (KTP), or copper vapor types.

Hair and scalp

Laser hair removal is discussed briefly earlier in this chapter.

Cosmetic surgical procedures for the scalp include excision of bald areas (which may be combined with tissue expansion to create loose skin for closure of the wound) and various hair-grafting techniques. Details of these will not be provided here. All rely on the principle that the occipitoparietal hair is relatively resistant to androgenic balding, and that this is maintained if hairs from these regions are transplanted into sites of common balding. The excisional techniques in particular may also be used for other causes of hair loss, such as traumatic or burn scarring, or for static localized areas of scarring due to dermatoses such as morphea en coup de sabre.

IONTOPHORESIS

This is a technique that is applied in various situations.

- Direct therapeutic effect—as treatment for localized hyperhidrosis (mainly palms or soles).
- Indirect therapeutic effect—to enhance penetration of topically applied drugs such as some local anesthetics, cytotoxic agents (e.g. 5-fluorouracil and methotrexate), and others (e.g. ALA, tretinoin, and antiviral agents).
- Investigative—for example, using iontophoresis of histamine in the investigation of mechanisms of itch.

The technique classically involves generation of H^+ ions by use of an electric current; this is generally achieved by using two containers of tap water, one hand (or foot) in each, one being connected to the anode and the other to the cathode of a direct current source. There are several modifications, some using alternating current (AC) rather than direct current (DC) sources, and sometimes using an anticholinergic chemical such as glycopyrronium in the solution.

Side effects are generally few, usually a burning or irritation if anything, but use of anticholinergic solutions is accompanied by systemic absorption, which may cause dry mouth, visual blurring, and other anticipated symptoms. The benefits are transient, but machines for home use are relatively inexpensive, and the tap water method is generally satisfactory.

RADIOTHERAPY

Although it was at one time used to treat or prevent benign dermatoses such as chronic hand dermatitis or keloid scars, the role of radiotherapy in dermatology is primarily for treatment of primary or metastatic tumors; non-melanoma skin cancers account for the majority of treatments. For either a primary lesion or for tumor-related lymphadenopathy, radiotherapy may at times be used as the primary treatment, in an adjunctive role (e.g. if incomplete excision is suspected), or in a palliative role. Radiotherapy is useful in the following conditions.

- Non-melanoma skin cancer and precursors—basal cell carcinoma, squamous cell carcinoma, and Bowen disease.
- Lymphomas—localized B-cell or tumor-stage CTCL, and total skin electron beam therapy for CTCL.
- Sarcomas—for example angiosarcoma and Kaposi sarcoma.
- Others—cutaneous metastases, Merkel cell carcinoma, and lentigo maligna.

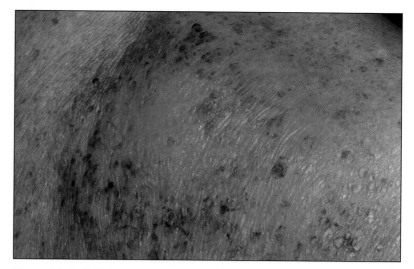

Figure 5.15 Radiotherapy to skin or deeper structures may cause a burn in the skin, as shown here.

Factors that might favor use of radiotherapy over other treatments have been discussed in the surgical section of this chapter. Often, the rationale for use of radiotherapy will include several issues, such as a broad lesion at a technically difficult site in a patient with poor general health, in whom a complex surgical procedure may be daunting.

Radiotherapy, in most situations, has the advantage of simplicity. Treatments are usually brief and painless, although larger lesions treated with many fractions will become tender, and healing usually involves a degree of erythema and desquamation. The need to shield the eyes for eyelid lesions, and the inevitable epilation, may be a relative contraindication on eyelids and at hair-bearing sites, respectively.

Radiotherapy may cause acute skin reactions (Fig. 5.15) and, in the longer term, radiotherapy wounds may show pigment variation and telangiectasia (Fig. 5.16). However, the most important late effect of radiotherapy is soft tissue necrosis. This is generally avoided by fractionation of doses. For example, basal cell carcinomas can usually be treated with a single treatment, or with two treatments about 6 weeks apart; for squamous cell carcinoma, treatment is more labor-intensive, as this is often treated with 10–20 daily treatments. The radiation source and type (e.g. superficial or orthovoltage), energy, number of fractions, and dose per fraction (usually in cGy) of radiation administered should be recorded.

Necrosis is more likely if larger fractions are used; it is also particularly likely if the same area of skin is treated twice. Thus marginal recurrences or nearby tumors cannot usually be treated with radiotherapy due to the likelihood of overlapping fields. Some sites, such as the lower leg, are also at particular risk of poor healing or late necrosis. These late effects mean that radiotherapy is generally more likely to be used for treating lesions in older patients than those in the younger age group.

PHOTOTHERAPY

Phototherapy of various types is widely available in dermatology departments. Most phototherapy utilizes different wavelengths of ultraviolet (UV) radiation; the nomenclature for wavelengths is discussed further in Chapter 17. The source for all these is fluorescent lamps, but different coatings on the tubes allow filtering of different wavelengths. Dosimetry is generally determined by initial tests to determine the minimal erythema dose, and subsequent gradually increasing doses are applied.

Disorders that may benefit are numerous, but they include the following main indications.

- Commonly treated inflammatory dermatoses—psoriasis, eczema (especially atopic but also others, such as pompholyx), and polymorphic light eruption.

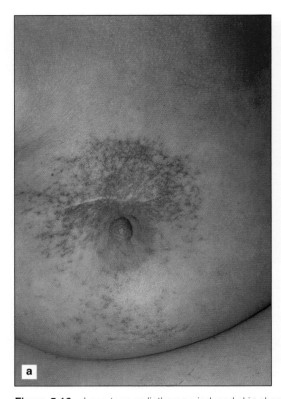

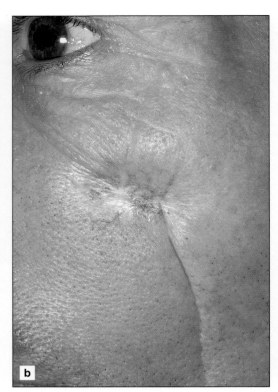

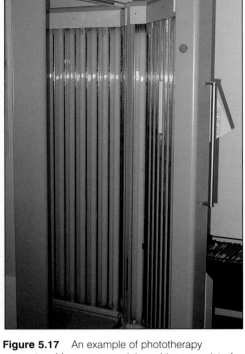

Figure 5.16 Long-term radiotherapy–induced skin change includes atrophy and telangiectasia (**a**). Necrosis may cause ulceration or, many years after treatment of a basal cell carcinoma, some contraction that has created new facial crease lines (**b**).

Figure 5.17 An example of phototherapy apparatus. Many commercial machines consist of about 40 vertically oriented fluorescent tubes in a stand-up cabinet style as shown; the door panel includes apparatus to set exposure doses. The main difference between a PUVA machine (as shown) and those for UVB is the type of fluorescent tube fitted, requiring a different output sensor and generating a different range of exposure times.

- Cutaneous lymphomas, precursors, and related conditions— poikiloderma, parapsoriasis, mycosis fungoides, and pityriasis lichenoides chronica.
- Less commonly treated inflammatory dermatoses—pityriasis rubra pilaris, acne, graft-versus-host disease, vitiligo, urticaria, solar urticaria, actinic reticuloid, urticaria pigmentosa, and scleroderma.

Some of the specifics of phototherapy in these disorders are discussed in relevant disease chapters if they differ from the general approach outlined here.

UVB

UVB is the simplest form of phototherapy, as it involves light exposure alone without additional chemicals. Broadband UVB consists of radiation of 280–315 nm, but the lower wavelengths contribute significantly to burning (UVB is the burning component of natural sunlight, which is well known to have useful benefit for many dermatoses). In the past decade, use of different coatings on the fluorescent tubes allowed development of narrow-band UVB with a narrow emission peak at 311 nm; this is more effective in depleting infiltrating T cells and results in faster clearance of psoriasis, with less risk of burning. This technique is generally used before considering PUVA for the more commonly treated dermatoses. It is particularly useful for patterns such as guttate psoriasis (Ch. 7). Test doses are read after 24 h, and treatment is usually given two or three times weekly. Courses are usually limited to one or two courses of up to 6 weeks annually, as all UV exposure carries risks of skin aging and carcinogenesis if used excessively.

PUVA

This uses UVA (315–400 nm) to activate chemicals known as psoralens, hence psoralen ultraviolet A (PUVA) (Fig. 5.17). The usual psoralens are 5- or 8-methoxypsoralen or trimethylpsoralen. Oral administration of psoralen with UVA 2 h later was used for many years, but various forms of topical administration are increasingly used, such as bath PUVA. This avoids some of the systemic effects of oral psoralen, notably nausea and uptake by the cornea (such that protective glasses are required for 24 h after oral PUVA therapy).

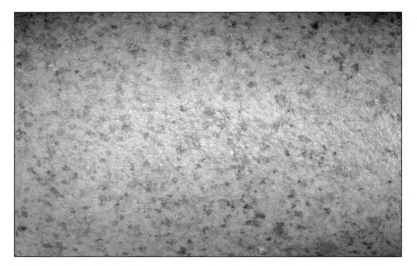

Figure 5.18 PUVA freckles are common in patients receiving long-term PUVA. The freckles often have a stellate shape and involve covered as well as sun-exposed skin.

Test doses are generally read at 72 h, but peak erythema varies from 2 to 4 days; the faintest test dose is termed the minimal phototoxic dose, as it relies on UV radiation and a photosensitizer. PUVA is generally administered less often than UVB (twice- or just once-weekly clearance, 2–3-weekly maintenance), so may be more suitable for patients who live a long distance from the treatment center. However, long-term PUVA has significant carcinogenesis risks and may cause marked lentiginosis (Fig. 5.18). A summary of disorders that respond to PUVA is given in Table 5.3.

Table 5.3   DISORDERS THAT MAY RESPOND TO PUVA[a]

Type of disorder	Usually respond	Variable response
Papulosquamous	Psoriasis Palmoplantar pustulosis	Pityriasis rubra pilaris
Immunologic	Atopic dermatitis Graft-versus-host disease	Pompholyx eczema Alopecia areata Vitiligo Lichen planus
Lymphocytic infiltrates	Parapsoriasis Mycosis fungoides (patch, thin plaques)	Lymphomatoid papulosis Mycosis fungoides (thicker plaques) Pityriasis lichenoides
Photodermatoses	Polymorphic light eruption Chronic actinic dermatitis	Hydroa vacciniforme Solar urticaria
Miscellaneous		Nodular prurigo Urticaria pigmentosa Urticarias Granuloma annulare

[a]Psoralen ultraviolet A.

Other types of light

UVA1 (340–400 nm) is not widely available but appears to be useful for atopic dermatitis and for scleroderma spectrum disorders. Various types of visible (red and blue) or laser light, as well as UVB, have been used in acne.

Extracorporeal photopheresis (ECP) is a technique used in treatment of erythrodermic CTCL and in scleroderma. It essentially combines the methods of plasmapheresis with PUVA: the patient takes psoralen, and this is then irradiated outside the body in a plasmapheresis machine and returned to the circulation. This technique is not widely available.

FURTHER READING

Alster TS, Lupton JR (eds) Update on lasers. Dermatol Clin 2002; 20: 1–176

Ammirati CT. Advances in wound closure materials. Adv Dermatol 2002; 18: 313–38

Bennett ML, Henderson RL. Introduction to cosmetic dermatology. Curr Probl Dermatol 2003; 15: 35–83

Grekin RC, Auletta MJ. Local anesthesia in dermatologic surgery. J Am Acad Dermatol 1988; 19: 599–614

Lawrence CM. An Introduction to Dermatological Surgery, 2nd edn. Edinburgh: Churchill Livingstone, 2002

Salasche SJ (ed) Dermatologic surgery, parts I and II. Curr Probl Dermatol 2001; 13: 1–60, 61–132

Sheridan AT, Dawber RPR. Curettage, electrosurgery and skin cancer. Austral J Dermatol 2000; 41: 19–30

6 Eczema and Related Disorders

INTRODUCTION

Eczema spans a large area in dermatology, including atopic dermatitis, contact dermatitis, and various eczematous disorders. It represents a category of diseases in which the skin is inflamed, usually due to a topical allergy or irritant, and in which host factors such as an atopic tendency may also play a part. The skin surface barrier is disrupted and water is lost. The underlying skin dries out, and more irritants or allergens are able to make their way into the skin. Pruritus is typical. Scratching further disrupts the water barrier and protective function of the skin, worsening the condition. Note that the terms *eczema* and *dermatitis* in common usage are synonymous and do not imply internal or external causation.

The clinical appearance of eczematous skin should be differentiated from that of papulosquamous conditions such as psoriasis. Both conditions are red and scaly, but the edges of eczema are less well defined, and the entire area is not significantly raised compared with papulosquamous conditions. Scales are generally larger in papulosquamous conditions compared with the scaling in eczemas.

Allergic contact dermatitis is an entire area unto itself. Not only is it an important area clinically, but it is a model for the skin's participation in the immune system. Indeed, the skin plays an active role in the body's immune system, with Langerhans cells playing a key role in antigen processing and presentation to T cells.

One should suspect a cutaneous allergy when the eruption is acutely eczematous or bullous and the lesions are linear, streaky, or in unusual shapes. An eczematous condition on certain parts of the body should raise at least the consideration of allergy (e.g. the earlobe in a woman, the hands, or the periorbital area). If not obvious by history, patch testing can be invaluable in determining the exact offending agent. It should be noted that different types of eczema may coexist, for example a patient with atopic eczema may also have an irritant dermatitis (e.g. from exposure to detergents) or an allergic contact dermatitis. Although the risk of allergic contact dermatitis may be reduced in atopic eczema due to altered T-lymphocyte responses (discussed later), patients with atopic eczema may be more exposed than the general population to some topical agents that can cause allergy (e.g. preservatives or even corticosteroids in treatment creams).

Finally, it appears that atopic dermatitis is often either caused or aggravated by a type of cutaneous allergy. After epidermal penetration, aeroallergens bind to allergen-specific IgE on Langerhans cells and are subsequently presented to T lymphocytes. Interleukins (IL–4 and IL–5) seem to be important in the migration and maintenance of eosinophils in the area (which do not appear in standard allergic contact dermatitis). It appears that the eosinophils release their granular contents in the epidermis and damage it, resulting in altered barrier function. This allows

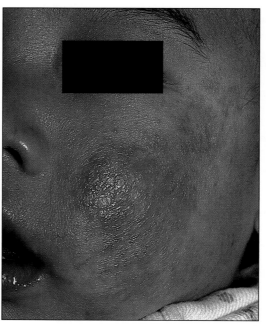

Figure 6.1 Infantile atopic dermatitis (AD) on the cheeks. The patient with AD often has a personal or family history of asthma or hay fever. The infant often presents with bilaterally symmetric, red, scaly, chapped, dry, glazed cheeks. An irritant dermatitis from saliva may be contributory.

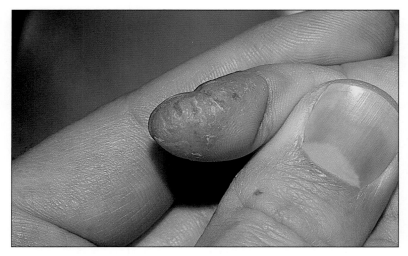

Figure 6.2 Fingertip eczema. Eczema of the fingertips in a child can be very difficult to treat. Any sucking or biting must be stopped.

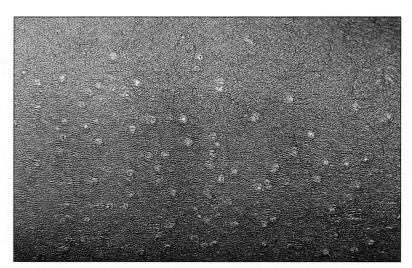

Figure 6.3 Follicular eczema in a dark-skinned patient. Such patients with atopic dermatitis often show follicular accentuation. At times, only the follicles are involved, as shown here.

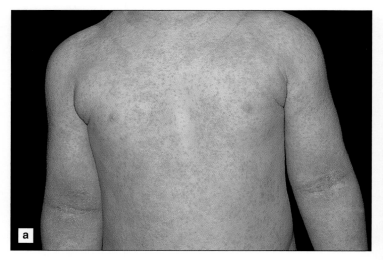

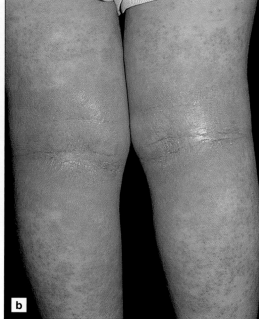

Figure 6.4 (**a,b**) Diffuse atopic dermatitis (AD). The red, scaly rash of AD may spread to cover much or all of the body. The child scratches incessantly and sleep may be significantly disrupted, both for the child and for the parents. In children, the rather follicular pattern shown may signify secondary infection.

for the vicious cycle of increased epidermal permeability to aeroallergens, more epidermal damage, etc.

ATOPIC DERMATITIS

Etiology and pathogenesis

Atopic dermatitis (AD) is an extremely common condition, especially during childhood. The prevalence of AD peaks in infancy and tapers gradually thereafter. Studies from the UK show that as many as 20% of infants have AD, while only 5–15% of prepubertal children are so affected. Patients with AD and their relatives are more likely to have asthma and/or allergic rhinitis (hay fever).

Atopic dermatitis is caused by both a defective barrier function of the skin and by altered immune responses that include allergy to a variety of environmental and dietary allergens. IgE levels tend to be quite high. Treatment involves restoring the skin barrier function, reducing the exposure to allergens, and decreasing the patient's immune response.

Experimental work using an atopy patch test (APT), or aeroallergens dissolved in cream and applied for 48 h, has demonstrated a type of epidermal immune reactivity different from that of allergic contact dermatitis. The APT is more likely to be positive if the patient's eczema-tous lesions predominate on skin not covered by clothing (e.g. hands, forearms, head, neck, and ankles). In one study, the APT was positive for house dust mite (HDM) in 80% of patients, for grass pollen in 50%, and for cat dander in 3%, although there is wide variation: HDM gave positive results in only 36% and grass pollen in 16% in another study. In general, positive reactions to HDM are most frequent. The APT may correlate with antigen-specific IgE results by radio-allergo-sorbent test (RAST), but neither reliably correlates with patient history of HDM-related clinical problems.

With regard to food allergy in children with AD, prick tests tend to correlate with acute skin reactions (e.g. pruritus, urticaria, and exanthema), whereas the patch test tends to correlate with delayed reactions (eczematous); this is as expected, as the former evaluate the more immediate IgE-mediated type I hypersensitivity. Milk is more frequently a problem in children than in adults. Prick tests or RAST results to animal dander do not reliably correlate with patient's experiences when in contact with animals.

A further contributory factor is colonization of atopic skin with *Staphylococcus aureus*, and also increased nasal carriage. This can play a major part in exacerbations of the disease, as it produces superantigens that bypass the normal antigen-presenting mechanisms and directly activate T lymphocytes. Weeping of the skin and scratching allow increased

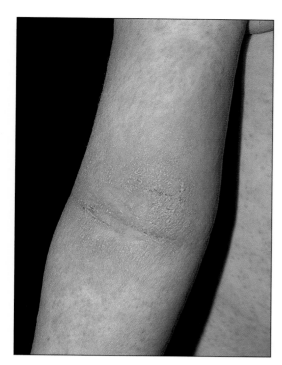

Figure 6.5 Atopic dermatitis, diffuse, with accentuation in the folds. Often there is accentuation of the flexures, as illustrated here.

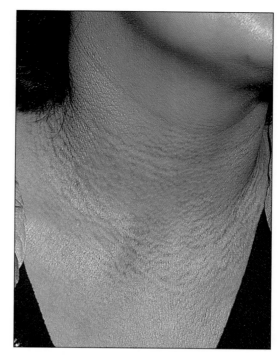

Figure 6.6 Atopic 'dirty' neck. The neck of an atopic may take on a brown, 'dirty' appearance.

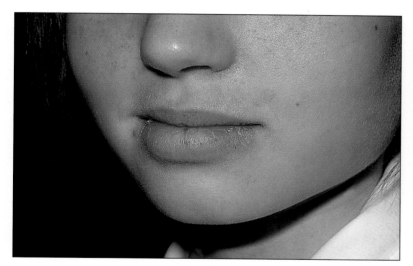

Figure 6.7 Atopic dermatitis of the lips.

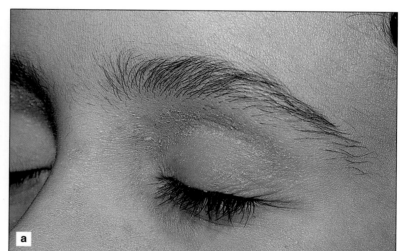

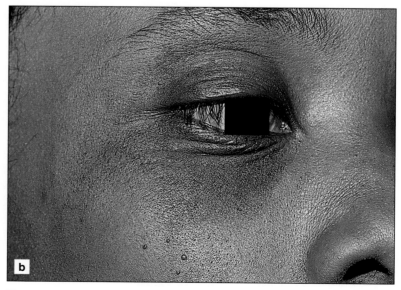

Figure 6.8 (**a**) Periorbital atopic dermatitis. The skin about the eyes is prone to eczema. A dry environment predisposes to an outbreak. Many patients rub and scratch (although this patient has not). (**b**) Atopic eyelids. Any chronic dermatitis about the eyes can cause multiple creases of the lower eyelid. In an atopic patient, these have been called Dennie–Morgan folds. Chronic rubbing may cause hyperpigmentation, as seen in this patient.

staphylococcal colonization, hence more T-cell activation, and a vicious cycle is set up. Thus antibacterial measures may also be important in therapy.

Environmental tobacco smoke aggravates AD. Parents of children with AD should be encouraged to stop smoking.

Clinical

Infants with AD may develop red, scaly lesions anywhere (Figs 6.1–6.3). In severe cases, the entire body may be affected (Fig. 6.4). As the child ages, eczematous lesions gravitate toward the flexures (Fig. 6.5), for example the antecubital fossa, the popliteal fossa, the neck (Fig. 6.6), and the posterior gluteal cleft. In older children, wrists and ankles may be the most prominent site of involvement. AD may persist into adulthood as frank, diffuse eczema. More often, however, the patient is affected by localized disease, for example lip (Fig. 6.7), eyelid (Fig. 6.8), retroauricular, facial, or hand dermatitis (Fig. 6.9).

Early lesions of AD are red and scaly. Chronic lesions that have been scratched may appear as lichenified plaques with excoriation (Figs 6.10 and 6.11); chronic scratching or rubbing, as well as the inflammation of the disease itself, may lead to pigmentary disturbance (Fig. 6.12). Secondary bacterial infection is a complicating factor (Fig. 6.13), as discussed earlier. Chronic scratching precipitates and exacerbates both the dermatitis and

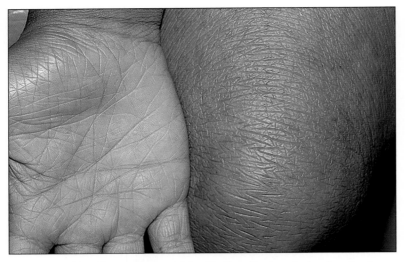

Figure 6.9 Hyperlinear palms and lichenification. Atopic patients often develop accentuation of the palmar creases.

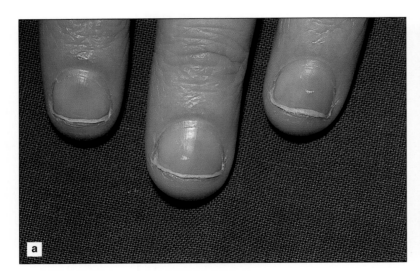

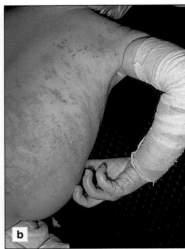

Figure 6.10 Scratching. (**a**) The nails of an atopic patient are often polished, with a beveled edge, as a result of constant scratching. (**b**) Stopping a child from scratching is next to impossible. Many patients will scratch many times during a short visit to the doctor.

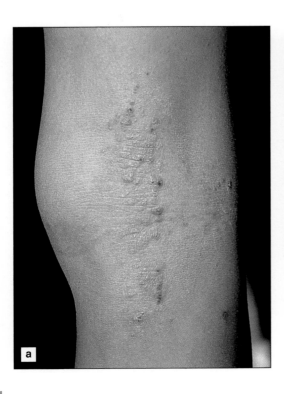

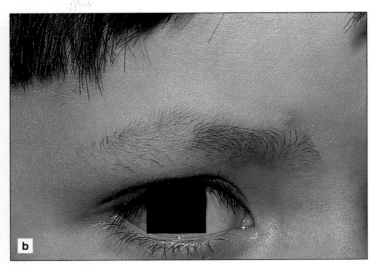

Figure 6.11 (**a**) Flexural atopic dermatitis with lichenification. Much of the skin changes are secondary to scratching. Linear lichenification, as shown here, and excoriations are typical. (**b**) Hertoghe sign: loss of the outer eyebrow may occur in the atopic patient, as a result of chronic rubbing.

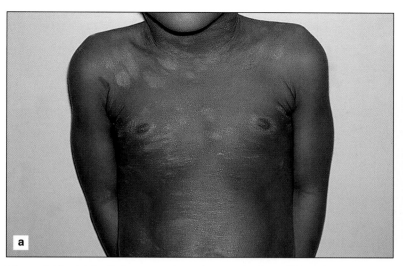

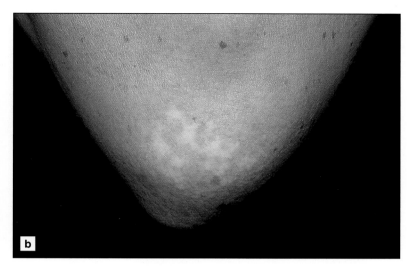

Figure 6.12 (**a**) Postinflammatory hypopigmentation in an African-Caribbean patient. Temporary hypopigmentation may develop at sites of previous eczema, as shown here. (**b**) Postinflammatory depigmentation. Uncommonly, as in this case, pigment loss may be complete and permanent.

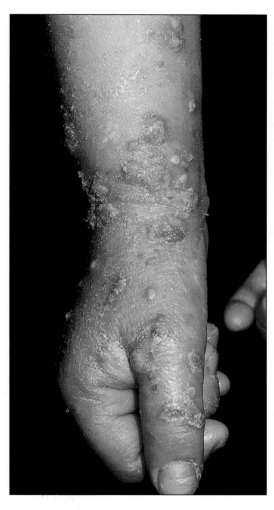

Figure 6.13 Bacterial secondary infection in atopic dermatitis. Atopic skin often harbors significant numbers of bacteria. Overt infection is common and is manifested by areas of erosion, crusting, or oozing. Superinfection by *Staphylococcus* is most common. This patient developed a secondary infection by *Streptococcus*.

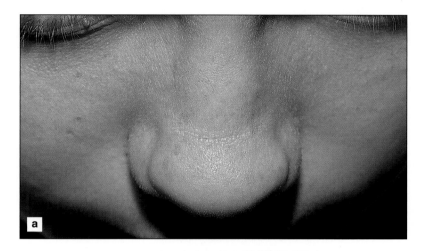

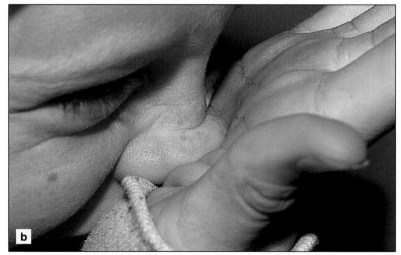

Figure 6.14 (**a,b**) Atopic salute. Atopy combines atopic dermatitis, asthma, and allergic rhinitis. Children with allergic rhinitis often rub their nose straight up, which, over time, creates a crease.

the infection. Features of associated asthma or hay fever may be present (Fig. 6.14), usually in slightly older children, and vascular hyperreactivity may occur (Fig. 6.15).

A persistent red face pattern has been described in adult AD, and probably has various causes. In some this may represent HDM exposure (e.g. in pillows), in some it is probably due to *Pityrosporum* sensitivity or seborrheic dermatitis, in some it is at least in part a corticosteroid-induced rosacea, and in others it may represent a contact allergy (e.g. due to topical corticosteroids that may have been applied long term).

Various criteria for diagnosing AD have been proposed. One of the most recent is by the UK working party and is outlined in Table 6.1. Minor diagnostic criteria include nipple eczema (Fig. 6.16).

Trigger factors
House dust mite

There seems to be sufficient evidence now to implicate the HDM, *Dermatophagoides pteronyssinus*, as a trigger factor for AD. However,

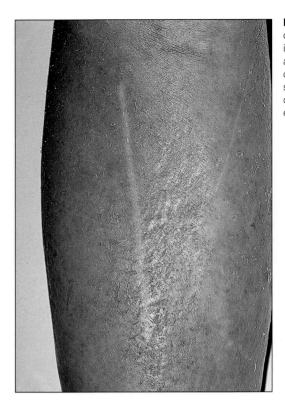

Figure 6.15 White dermatographism. There is a vascular reactivity in atopic patients that can create a white line on scratching. It may also occur in other erythrodermas.

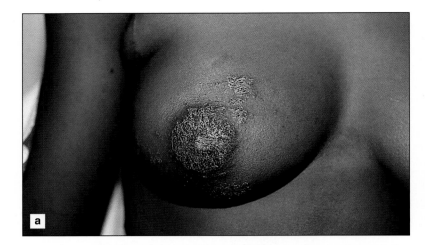

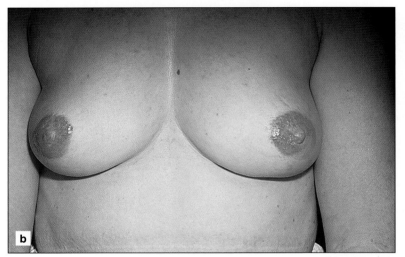

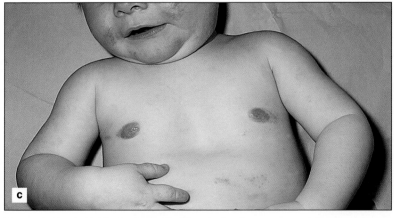

Figure 6.16 (**a,b**) Nipple dermatitis. The nipple of a woman not infrequently develops an eczematous dermatitis. Rubbing on a bra or clothing, or scratching by the patient, are common here. Nipple eczema is sufficiently common in atopic patients that it is part of Hanifin's diagnostic criteria. (**c**) Nipple eczema in an atopic child.

thorough avoidance of HDM is difficult, and there are conflicting results of trials of avoidance (especially in adults).

Food

Various foods can exacerbate AD, especially in children, the most common being eggs, peanuts, milk, fish, soybeans, and wheat. Adults may give a history of their disease being exacerbated by foods. In adults, milk-inducible eczema and casein-specific T cells are commonly found. Often, the flare is delayed—occurring 24 h after consumption of the offending food—and this should be distinguished from immediate urticarial reactions, which, while they may aggravate AD by leading to increased scratching, are not dermatitis and require oral antihistamine therapy rather than topical corticosteroids or other immunomodulators. Unfortunately, there is no reliable test to establish such a cause and effect role for dietary agents, short of a double-blind, placebo-controlled food challenge; RAST positivity, for example, does not always correlate with actual sensitivity (although prick tests or RAST are more reliable in the urticarial pattern of food reactions, as they measure type I hypersensitivity). Such tests are more valuable in excluding the presence of IgE-mediated food allergy than in proving a link with eczema or for predicting severity.

It is clear that clinically relevant food-induced worsening of eczema is more likely in those with moderate or severe disease than in those with mild AD. If there is a clear history of reactions to specific foods, then there is evidence that avoidance may be helpful; however, undirected elimination diets should be avoided. It is also important to be aware of the effects of dietary restriction on nutritional status, and especially on growth in children. Usually, clinical testing and decisions about dietary intervention are made by the allergist, those who are most likely to benefit being children with moderate to severe AD that responds poorly to conventional therapy, or those with a clear history of dietary triggering.

There is no unanimous evidence about the role of maternal avoidance of dietary agents or of aeroallergens during pregnancy or during breast-feeding, in terms of either the likelihood of the child having atopic eczema or of the severity if the child is affected. Prolonged breast-feeding may delay onset of clinical eczema, as may probiotic therapy with *Lactobacillus*, but probably have little protective effect on development of the disorder. The same uncertainty surrounds the role of supplements such as oil of evening primrose or its purified formulations.

Contact allergens

In an intriguing study, 25 of 39 children less than 2 years of age admitted to a hospital for AD tested positive for a contact allergen (standard allergic contact dermatitis allergens). Allergen avoidance was very helpful in the therapy of most of these children. However, this was probably a very selected group. In general, type IV contact hypersensitivity is unusual in children, especially if their clinical pattern is typical of AD for the age group, but those children not responding to standard therapy may benefit from patch testing.

Other factors that aggravate eczema

These include the following.

- Clothing—wool or other rough clothing may be irritating (Fig. 6.16); cotton clothing is better tolerated.
- Airborne irritants—exacerbation of eyelid involvement by chlorine or cigarette smoke has also been reported, although this pattern may also occur due to habitual rubbing (especially if there is associated watering of the eye due to allergic atopic conjunctivitis).
- Hormonal—premenstrual flaring is common, and pregnancy, parturition, or menopause may also be trigger factors.
- Stress—whether stress alone can cause a flare of AD is unclear.
- Sweating—in some patients, sweating can cause pruritus, scratching, and thus more eczema; in a recent study, activities that provoked sweating were viewed by patients as the most important factor in aggravation of their eczema. Most patients' conditions are worse during dry, cold winters, but some may experience exacerbations during the summer.
- Others—the season of birth, animal exposure during the first few months of life, and exposure to viral infections have all been proposed to influence incidence or severity of AD.

Differential diagnosis

A list of differential diagnoses is given in Table 6.2.

A red, scaly, itchy rash in an infant is most commonly AD, but infantile seborrheic dermatitis should be considered if the rash predominates in the scalp, axillae, and groin, or if the appearance of the rash is florid while the degree of itch is less prominent. Scabies should always be considered and the presence of burrows excluded.

In a child, except for scabies, the differential possibilities are few. Rarely, pityriasis rubra pilaris, psoriasis, and cutaneous T-cell lymphoma (CTCL) will present in a similar fashion.

When an adult presents with the recent onset of an eczematous rash, one should exclude scabies and contact dermatitis. Patch testing is usually necessary. Excessive water contact may precipitate asteatotic eczema. Occasionally, drugs will cause a drug eruption with an eczematous morphology. Tinea corporis may be suggested by annular, raised edges.

Table 6.2	DIFFERENTIAL DIAGNOSIS OF ATOPIC DERMATITIS[a]
Patient	**Differential diagnosis**
Neonate	Seborrheic dermatitis Irritant dermatitis (especially napkin area) Candidiasis (especially napkin area or flexures) Rarities: non-bullous ichthyosiform erythroderma, Netherton syndrome, and other ichthyoses; Leiner disease; Langerhans cell histiocytosis; immunodeficiencies with eczema (e.g. Wiskott–Aldrich syndrome, hyper-IgE syndrome, selective IgA deficiency, chronic granulomatous disease, biotin deficiency, essential fatty acid deficiency)
Infant	Seborrheic dermatitis Scabies Irritant dermatitis (especially napkin area) Infantile psoriasis Tinea corporis (especially confused with discoid or annular pattern atopic dermatitis) Ichthyosis vulgaris Rarities: as for neonate
Child	Seborrheic dermatitis Scabies Irritant dermatitis (especially hands) Allergic contact dermatitis Psoriasis Pityriasis rubra pilaris Tinea corporis (especially confused with discoid or annular pattern atopic dermatitis) Ichthyosis vulgaris Keratosis pilaris, keratosis pilaris atrophicans faciei Drug eruptions (rarely confused, as most are acute) Rarities: immunodeficiencies mainly as for neonates
Adult	Seborrheic dermatitis Scabies Irritant dermatitis Allergic contact dermatitis Asteatotic eczema Nummular (discoid) eczema Psoriasis Pityriasis rubra pilaris Tinea corporis Acquired ichthyoses Keratosis pilaris, keratosis pilaris atrophicans faciei Drug eruptions (rarely confused, as most are acute) Mycosis fungoides

[a]Note that at all ages, infections, either of the skin itself (staphylococcal, herpetic, candidal) or systemic infections causing an exanthema (viral, streptococcal, etc.) may be confused with a flare of eczema in a patient with known atopic dermatitis but are unlikely to be confused with this diagnosis otherwise.

Table 6.3	OVERVIEW OF THERAPY FOR ATOPIC DERMATITIS
Area	**Therapy**
General	Education and treatment demonstration by a nurse specialist
	Written information and sources of literature, self-help groups, patient associations, etc.
	Occupational advice (adults and older children)
Prevention	Avoid irritants, especially soaps, detergents, etc., also cigarette smoke, excessively low-humidity environment
	Cotton or silk rather than wool in contact with the skin
	Dietary restriction if relevance has been proved
	Avoid grass pollens, animal dander, etc. if clearly relevant
	?House dust mite avoidance
	?Prolonged breast-feeding
Therapy	Plentiful use of emollients
	Bandaging, wet wraps
	Combined emollient and antiseptic if clinically indicated
	Topical corticosteroids
	Topical immunomodulators
	Other topical therapies: mild tars, doxepin
	Treat secondary bacterial or herpetic infection
	Oral antihistamines
	Consider patch testing (especially adults or if unusual patterns)
	Phototherapy: UVB, PUVA (mainly adults), UVA1 (not readily available)
	Systemic medications (all especially in adults): corticosteroids (avoid), ciclosporin, azathioprine, (?interferon-gamma,
	?mycophenolate mofetil, ?Chinese herbal medicines)
	Psychotherapy, behavior modification, hypnotherapy, etc.
	?Phosphodiesterase inhibitors
	?Probiotics
	?Evening primrose oil
	Consider short-term hospital admission, alternative diagnosis (Table 6.2), or compliance if unresponsive

Treatment

An overview of treatment is provided in Table 6.3.

Basic skin care and approach to therapy

The singular admonition to not scratch is of paramount importance and should be reinforced during every visit. When the child is very young, such intervention is unrewarding; only older children may follow such direction. Daily bathing is useful, but patients should avoid baths or showers lasting longer than 5 min, avoid unduly hot water, and pat dry. A mild soap (e.g. non-deodorized and uncolored) or a soap substitute should be used to avoid the irritant effects of soaps and detergents; patients should avoid harsh shampoos or any use of bubble bath products. Topical emollients and medicines should be applied to the skin within minutes of the bath or shower to lock in the moisture, for example an emolliating cream or ointment to the non-inflamed skin plus either a topical immunomodulator or steroid to the active, eczematous areas. Because of their high water content, lotions are less effective. Bath emollients, with or without an antiseptic as determined by the clinical picture, appear to be helpful in some instances but generally have limited emollient effect.

Topical steroids

Topical steroids have been the mainstay of therapy for decades. They should be used when emollients are not sufficient. However, it is important that patients or parents do not use them for the emollient effect of the base. A useful rule is to use emollients for dry skin but steroids for red skin. Often, steroids are needed for thicker-skinned areas such as the trunk and extremities of adults, and some patients need to use different potencies for different sites, or different frequency of application for different sites. In general, studies suggest that once-daily application is as effective as more frequent use, with emollients at other times. Medium-potency topical steroids such as triamcinolone are appropriate for mild to moderate disease, with higher-strength steroids reserved for severe disease.

As discussed in Chapter 3, there are several potential local side effects of steroids, and even the potential for systemic absorption and hypothalamic–pituitary axis suppression. However, such effects in normal use are very uncommon; some relate mainly to the enthusiasm that followed introduction of high-potency fluorinated steroids. The greatest risk of systemic problems is in young children with severe eczema, but it should be noted that AD in itself may lead to growth retardation. The best way to avoid excessive use of steroids is by experience of judging eczema severity combined with elimination of triggers (food allergy and secondary infection); use of adjunctive therapy (emollients, topical immunomodulators, bandaging, appropriate clothing, oral antihistamines, etc.); and adequate time, explanation, and demonstration of treatment application by a dermatology-trained nurse.

Topical immunomodulators

Topical pimecrolimus and tacrolimus have made a dramatic impact on the therapy of AD. They both appear to be safe and effective, and most significantly lack the potential for cutaneous atrophy inherent with topical steroids. Pimecrolimus and 0.03% tacrolimus equate to hydrocortisone potency, and 0.1% tacrolimus to moderate steroid potency, in terms of clinical effectiveness. They are particularly helpful for eczema of the face and neck in both adults and children, and should probably be used as the foundation of therapy for active eczema of the face, neck, and flexures. However, they are contraindicated in the presence of infection, may cause initial burning or stinging, are much more expensive than equivalent-potency steroids, and their longer-term skin cancer risks are unknown (they are similar to drugs used for systemic immunosuppressive therapy, in which skin tumor risk is significant).

Other therapies

The primary method for decreasing the itch of eczema is to decrease the eczema. Scratching, of course, makes the eczema worse, but some patients seem unable to stop scratching and need more intervention than just topical steroids. Hydroxyzine is a time-honored intervention. When given routinely (e.g. 2 mg/kg per day every 6 h while awake and before sleeping), it can help decrease the itch. It should be noted that antihistamines are not thought to improve the rash directly, but they merely decrease scratching. Much of the evidence suggests that they do this through sedation, and are thus especially indicated for patients with night-time itch. Bandaging, either with tar- or emollient-impregnated bandages, or with wet wraps, may be useful, especially for acute flares of AD or to occlude lichenified areas where scratching has become habitual. Mittens, especially in bed at night (even sewn to pajamas) may be helpful to reduce scratching.

Topical doxepin is very helpful for reducing the itch in localized areas. If applied over a large area, sedation may result. The use of special silk fabric improved AD compared with use of cotton clothing in one study of 46 children.

Many other therapies have been suggested but have limited or conflicting evidence; some are listed in Table 6.3.

Sleep difficulties

One study found that children with AD who have sleep difficulties usually experience them during AD flares and may keep their parents up for 2–3 h a night on average. Those strategies rated by the parents as most successful were putting creams on the child, using cotton clothes, keeping the room cool, using wet wraps, putting very few blankets over the child, and cuddling the child. Bringing the child into the parents' bed seemed only to prolong the problem (Fig. 6.17).

Treatment for severe atopic dermatitis in a child

For children with moderate to severe AD, unresponsive to topical therapies, the following may be considered.

- First, make sure an oral antistaphylococcal antibiotic has been tried. A course of an antibiotic is helpful for a short period if there appears to be a secondary infection, but a prolonged course in the absence of signs of infection does not seem to be helpful.
- Hospitalization for intensive therapy. This is often of value: it can be used to reinforce educational issues, may possibly remove the child from allergens at home, and gives the parents a deserved rest.
- Systemic therapies. Generally, these are avoided in children due to the risk of side effects. If necessary, ciclosporin, started initially at 5 mg/kg per day and tapered to 5 mg/kg given every 5 days, is one effective approach. In another study of ciclosporin for children, 5 mg/kg per day given for 6 weeks was well tolerated and safe. Another author recommended 3–3.5 mg/kg per day for 1–3 months. Although very effective, ciclosporin has many side effects, including immune suppression and nephrotoxicity. The clinician must also be aware of various drug interactions. Oral or intramuscular corticosteroids may have a role if itch is severe but are best avoided, as flare-up after stopping treatment is common, and the side effects preclude ongoing use.
- Other therapies that may be helpful in some children with severe disease include phototherapy (usually narrow-band UVB or PUVA, sometimes UVA1 or combined therapies). Because of the associated photodamage and risk of cutaneous cancer later in life, PUVA should be reserved for disabling disease.

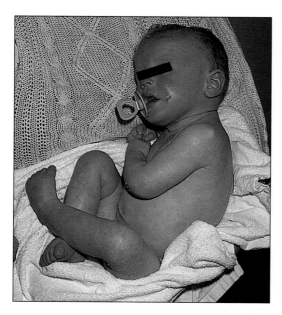

Figure 6.17 Atopic infant. The infant with atopic dermatitis is often quite unhappy, the skin is very itchy, and sleeping is difficult.

Treatment for severe atopic dermatitis in an adult

All the above measures for children should be considered. Systemic therapies and phototherapy are more likely to be tried in adults, due to disease chronicity and the fact that adult AD often affects the whole body. Measures listed in Table 6.3, such as consideration of patch testing, are also important, particularly if there has been a change in clinical pattern.

Treatments that may be considered in adults include the following (see Table 6.3 for a fuller list).

- Azathioprine—several studies have shown significant benefit, but side effects may limit treatment.
- PUVA and narrow-band UVB—phototherapy and photochemotherapy can be very helpful in the treatment of severe AD. In one study, a single episode of PUVA or UVB treatment reduced *S. aureus* numbers by 70–80%. Thus it may be that the effect of UV therapy is mediated partially by its antimicrobial effect.
- Ciclosporin—this can be very effective, but potential side effects make it a drug to use only in the most severe of cases, especially as an exacerbation usually follows rapidly after the drug is stopped, hence maintenance treatment may be required.

Role of the dermatology nurse

Anecdotally, for many years, dermatologists have utilized the skills and knowledge of their nursing staff to help in management of AD and other eczemas. The benefits of this approach are now supported by scientific study. There is a huge amount of information for patients and parents to assimilate regarding causation and treatment, and many of these issues relate to practicalities regarding bathing, how and when to use treatment, strengths of treatment, how to apply bandages, how to cope with itch or flares, etc. This cannot be taken in at a single clinic visit, no matter how prolonged. Using a nurse to reinforce the discussion and to demonstrate treatment and bandage application is immensely useful. In the UK, many nurses in hospital departments have extended this educational role and now run eczema clinics, are trained to prescribe, and can take on treatment of many children with AD. A similar process in primary care is entirely feasible, particularly with good links with the local hospital for shared care, but is rather more limited to enthusiasts rather than being the accepted norm.

Prognosis

Generally, it has been thought that most infants or young children with AD outgrow it over several years. However, one recent study found that, after 20 years, 72% of patients were still affected by micromanifestations (e.g. perlèche, eyelid dermatitis, retroauricular dermatitis, and dry, cracked fingertips). Nummular dermatitis was not seen in this population. Thus parents should be told that their child's skin disease will most likely improve, but that he or she may always have a tendency toward dry skin and eczema. In particular, older children need advice about occupations that might cause aggravation or recurrence of their eczema; hairdressing is the notable culprit but any irritant exposure may be relevant. Armed forces may not accept applicants with atopic disease.

PRACTICE POINTS

- Always consider secondary infection as a reason for a flare of atopic dermatitis (AD), especially infections due to *Staphylococcus aureus* (or less commonly, see below, herpes simplex).
- For the adult who presents with 'new onset' eczema, inquire about any eczema as a child, as adults with a history of AD may have experienced a recurrence in cold weather, when water exposure is high (e.g. when taking a water aerobics class or showering multiple times per day), or if exposed to an offending allergen (e.g. from dog or cat).
- In adults with known AD but with a change of pattern or severity, consider the possibility of a contact allergy (always include treatment agents in the test series).
- Patients with AD (and their parents) need ample discussion of bathing, soaps, emollients, itching, sleep time, clothing, pets, etc. A trained nurse who can provide this care is a major asset.

ECZEMA HERPETICUM

Etiology and pathogenesis

This widespread infection by herpes simplex, previously called Kaposi varicelliform eruption, is most common in patients with AD but may also occur in patients with other forms of dermatitis (including seborrheic, neuro-, and photosensitivity dermatitis), as well as in Darier disease, pemphigus foliaceus, CTCL, benign familial pemphigus, second-degree burns, and congenital ichthyosiform erythroderma. Ocular involvement (as evidenced by slit-lamp examination) is uncommon, even though there may be a concentration of lesions periorbitally and a conjuctival swab may be positive (Fig. 6.18). Kaposi varicelliform eruption has occurred rarely in atopic patients secondary to cowpox infection.

Clinical

Any age group can be affected. The rapidly progressive, widespread, crusted papules, vesicles, and erosions are characteristic (Fig. 6.19). Monomorphic 'punched out' lesions are very suggestive of this diagnosis. Secondary bacterial infection may occur (Fig. 6.20). Many patients with AD will present with crusted lesions, and the etiology (viral versus staphylococcal) is impossible to determine without a culture (Fig. 6.21). Thus both viral and bacterial cultures are essential when vesicles (Fig. 6.22) are not apparent.

Differential diagnosis

Superinfection of AD by *S. aureus* can appear very similar, with the acute onset of crusting, eroded skin. However, the monomorphous, circular vesicles that are commonly seen in eczema herpeticum are absent, although the later punched out lesions can occasionally occur with primary staphylococcal infection or even in very acute eczema.

Treatment

Oral or intravenous aciclovir, or a related antiviral agent, should be given. Twice-daily soaks can be helpful for removing crust. A topical antiseptic or antibiotic ointment may also help speed healing.

PRACTICE POINT

- If you get a phone message saying that one of your patients is experiencing a significant flare of his or her eczema, especially if around the head and neck or accompanied by systemic symptoms, see them urgently: it may be eczema herpeticum. The authors make no apology for repeating this point.

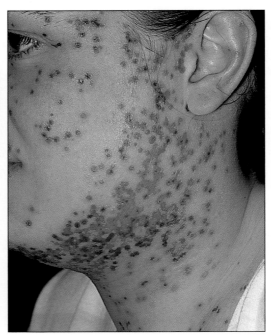

Figure 6.20 The face of a patient with eczema herpeticum. The patient with atopic dermatitis is predisposed to infection not only by *Staphylococcus aureus* but also by herpes simplex. Rapidly progressive, widespread, crusted papules, vesicles, and erosions are characteristic of this viral infection.

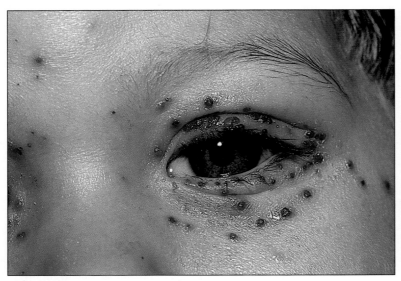

Figure 6.18 Eczema herpeticum in a child. A periorbital distribution is not infrequent.

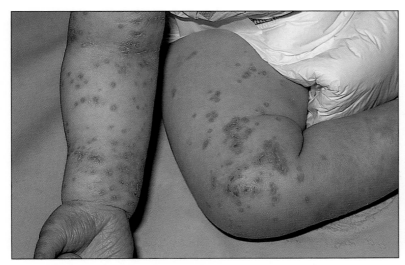

Figure 6.19 Eczema herpeticum in a child.

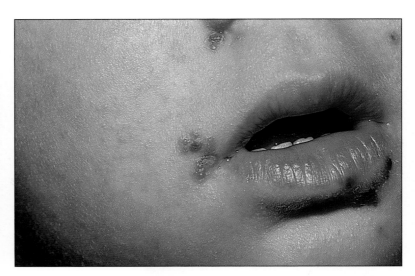

Figure 6.21 Close-up view of eczema herpeticum. Crusted lesions in the atopic patient may represent bacterial or viral infection. At times, only culture will distinguish between the two.

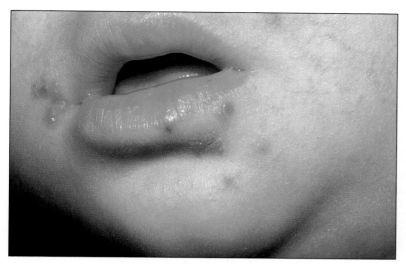

Figure 6.22 Close-up view of eczema herpeticum, showing classic umbilicated vesicles.

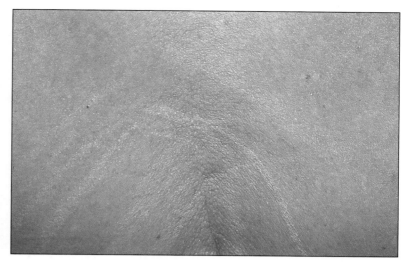

Figure 6.23 Xerosis and scratching. An atopic background; dry, cold weather; frequent water contact; advanced age; and irritants predispose to dry skin, also known as xerosis. Dry skin itches, as illustrated by the scratch marks here.

OTHER ECZEMAS

Xerosis

Etiology and pathogenesis

The surface of the skin is composed of a lipid–rich layer that provides a barrier to evaporation of water. When this layer loses lipid, the skin becomes more scaly and flaky. Lay people will say their skin is 'dry'. Some parts of the body are more prone to xerosis as a result of either a low density of sebaceous glands (e.g. the shins) or due to exposure; additionally, there may be an inherent tendency to dry skin. Individuals with diabetes may have a propensity to develop xerosis on the shins, which correlates with palmar cheirarthropathy (see Ch. 12).

Clinical

Dry, scaly, itchy skin is a common occurrence on the shins in an older individual during the winter, and in those with AD (Fig. 6.23).

Differential diagnosis

The various forms of genetically determined ichthyosis appear similar, but their scales are larger and often plate-like.

There are a large number of disorders in which an acquired ichthyosis may occur, at various ages. Some of these are listed in Table 6.4.

Treatment

Application of petrolatum or other greasy emollients within minutes of the bath or shower is very effective. Ammonium lactate (12% or 5%) and emollients containing either urea or lactic acid have also been used. One study suggested that estrogen use in older women was protective against

dry skin, but the longer-term disadvantages of hormone replacement therapy outweigh any such benefit.

Asteatotic eczema

Etiology and pathogenesis

In the setting of xerosis, the underlying skin may become inflamed and red. This is called asteatotic eczema or winter itch (Figs 6.24–6.27). It is most common in the cold, winter months in the elderly. Always inquire

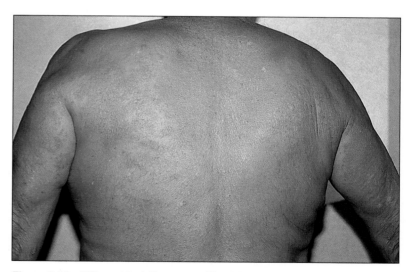

Figure 6.24 Diffuse asteatotic eczema. The older patient is commonly affected during the winter.

Table 6.4 SOME CAUSES OF ACQUIRED ICHTHYOSIS	
Category	**Cause**
Mechanical or irritant	See this chapter's section on *Xerosis*
Endocrine, metabolic and deficiency diseases	Hypothyroidism, hyperparathyroidism, chronic renal failure, malnutrition generally and specific deficiencies (e.g. essential fatty acid deficiency, niacin deficiency)
Malignancy	Especially systemic lymphomas, also mycosis fungoides, various cancers
Infections	HIV, human T-cell leukemia virus (HTLV)-I, leprosy, tuberculosis
Drugs	Hydroxymethylglutaryl-CoA reductase inhibitors (statins), retinoids
Inflammatory and autoimmune	Sarcoidosis, systemic lupus erythematosus, graft-versus-host disease

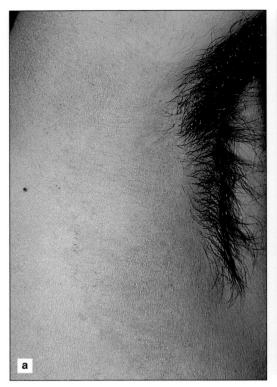

Figure 6.25 Asteatotic eczema. (**a**) An eczematous dermatitis on the posterior axillary line is not uncommon. (**b**) Close-up view.

Figure 6.26 Eczema craquéle. At times, the fissures are quite red and prominent, giving a cracked appearance to the skin, much like some porcelain vases.

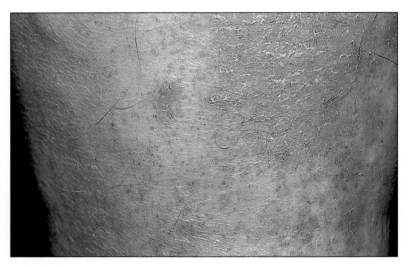

Figure 6.27 Eczema of the leg, with purpuric changes. Some degree of purpura is common in eczema of the lower leg, especially if the onset is acute, if the patient is elderly, or if there is associated swelling of the leg.

about water exposure, such as bathing several times per day, swimming, or water aerobics. What emollient is being used? Ironically, some patients seem to precipitate their condition by using a lotion multiple times per day.

Clinical

The skin appears thin, erythematous, and cracked, with wide but superficial fissures, the overall appearance resembling crazy paving.

Differential diagnosis

Other eczemas should be considered, especially venous disease and contact allergy to medicaments that have been applied. Nummular lesions may coexist (see differential diagnosis discussed below).

Treatment

A steroid or emollient in a cream or ointment form applied immediately after the bath or shower is curative. Patients may need to maintain this emolliation, especially during the winter months.

Nummular eczema (discoid eczema, nummular dermatitis)
Etiology and pathogenesis

Nummular eczema, also termed discoid eczema, is a specific variant of eczema in which the lesions occur in round or oval shapes, like a coin. Risk factors include excessive bathing (e.g. more than 10 min) or other prolonged water exposure (e.g. swimming). Some studies have found it to be common in atopic individuals, while others have not. Lesions usually occur in crops, and adults are more commonly affected than children. There is an association with dry skin.

Less commonly, nummular eczema may occur as a variant of drug eruption, although it is hard to explain the morphologic distribution; several studies (usually selecting those with resistant disease or with clinical suspicion) have demonstrated positive patch test reactions in some patients.

Clinical

Coin-shaped (nummular), red, eczematous areas are characteristic and common on the arms and legs. The surface may be oozing and crusted or dry and scaly. As in AD, the border of the lesions is not as sharply defined as seen in some of the differential diagnoses discussed here. Pruritus may be significant (Fig. 6.28).

Differential diagnosis

This commonly includes the following.

- Psoriasis—this has more sharply demarcated lesions, silvery scale rather than crust, and much less itch.
- Venous eczema—this is usually localised medially on the lower leg above the malleolus, or has a more extensive stocking-like distribution compared with the anterior skin pattern of nummular eczema.
- Bowen disease—this is common on the lower legs of older women in particular, but usually as solitary or few lesions with a more lobulated border, sharply defined, and often no itch.
- Seborrheic keratosis—on the older lower leg, a pattern of seborrheic keratosis termed clonal may give rise to diagnostic confusion; it is usually sharply defined, red-brown-colored, and not weepy or itchy.

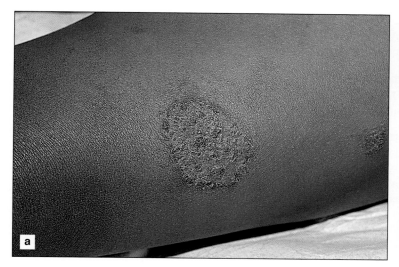

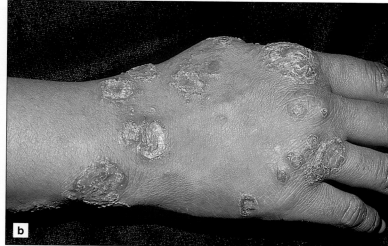

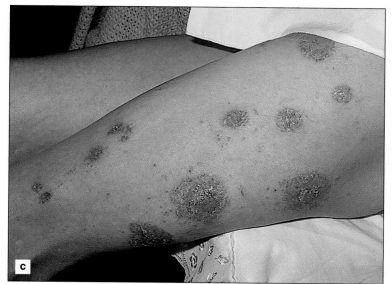

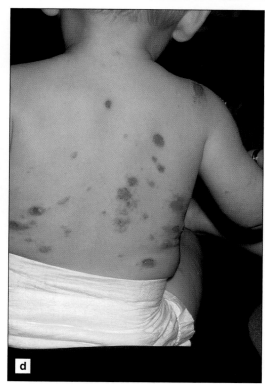

Figure 6.28 Nummular eczema. (**a**) The appearance of this lesion is *not* that of ringworm (Fig. 26.27). The redness and inflammation are uniformly distributed throughout. An active border is not seen. As was typical in this patient, multiple lesions tend to erupt on the arms and legs. Pruritus is usually significant. (**b**) Circular lesions with signs of scratching. (**c**) Multiple red, scaly lesions on the arms and legs are typical. (**d**) Nummular eczema in an infant.

- Tinea corporis—this often has a raised, red, scaly border with a sharper border and a clearing center, whereas nummular eczema is usually uniformly affected throughout.
- Drug reaction—as discussed earlier.
- Contact allergy—as discussed earlier.

Treatment

Prolonged water exposure should be avoided. A medium- to high-potency topical steroid ointment should be applied after the bath or shower; use of inappropriately mild agents for the degree of itch are a common reason for treatment failure in primary care, but the response to therapy should be rapid for individual lesions. Systemic steroids may be given if the lesions are widespread or resistant to topical treatment. Secondary infection should be considered. Petrolatum or a heavy cream applied to the skin immediately after the bath or shower helps prevent future outbreaks; note that patients are often elderly, and that inability to apply treatment adequately is a cause of therapeutic failure. It is also helpful to warn patients that they may get outbreaks from time to time, as this will encourage prompt treatment and shorter duration of episodes.

Patients with resistant nummular eczema should be patch tested, and occasionally treatments such as phototherapy may be required.

PRACTICE POINTS

Treatment of nummular (discoid) eczema involves the following.
- Regular use of emollients.
- Short-term use of an adequately potent topical steroid ointment for the degree of itch.
- Education that there may be further outbreaks from time to time, as this will encourage prompt treatment and shorter duration of episodes.
- Patch testing for those with therapeutically resistant disease.

Infectious eczematoid reaction
Etiology and pathogenesis

In this variant of eczema, a progressive, moist, eczematous process seems to result from a combination of eczema and superficial bacterial infection with *S. aureus*.

Clinical

The skin is erythematous, wet, and oozing. At the edge, small circular lesions appear and coalesce as the condition spreads (Figs 6.29 and 6.30).

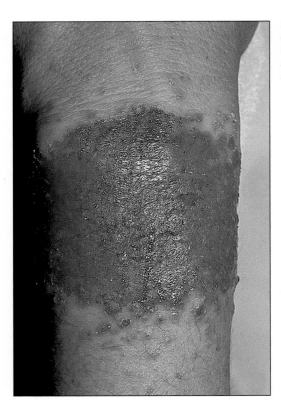

Figure 6.29 Infectious eczematoid reaction. This reaction responds best to a potent topical steroid and an oral antibiotic.

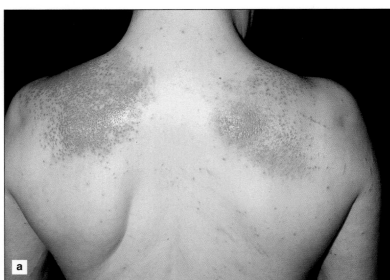

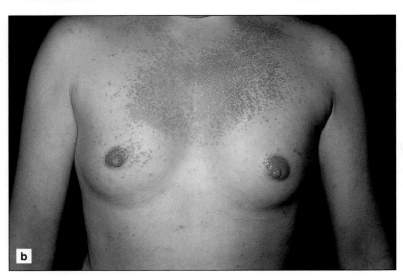

Figure 6.30 Acute eczema. (**a**) Acute eczema showing an infectious eczematoid reaction with moist circular lesions at the edges, which coalesce as the condition spreads. (**b**) One must always consider eczema herpeticum when small circular lesions are present. Compare for example with Figure 6.21.

Differential diagnosis

Allergic contact dermatitis should be excluded, as it also may be acute, moist, and inflammatory.

Treatment

Treatment should involve both a potent topical steroid and an oral antistaphylococcal antibiotic.

Pompholyx (dyshidrotic or vesicular eczema)
Etiology and pathogenesis

Patients with this condition appear to fall into three main groups. In the majority, the condition seems to be idiopathic but often aggravated by environmental conditions or activities that provoke sweating. In some, the condition is confined to the summer months or to working in hot, humid conditions. Less commonly, there may be an atopic background or the condition may occur due to contact allergy (irritant or allergic, although the latter is usually more florid).

Several studies, especially from Scandinavia, have demonstrated an aggravation of vesicular hand eczema by cigarette smoking. Additionally, a subset of patients with recurrent vesicular hand dermatitis may experience flares due to nickel ingestion. Helpful criteria for these patients include a positive patch test to nickel, and a flare of their dermatitis within 3 days of oral challenge with 2.5 mg of nickel, but not by placebo.

Rare patients may have their disease induced by sun exposure, with UVA being the action spectrum. In individual cases, palmar vesicles may occur as an id reaction due to tinea pedis or active foot eczema.

Clinical

Tiny 'tapioca' vesicles on the sides of the fingers but also the fingertips, palms, and soles occur in this syndrome, which is also called dyshidrotic or vesicular eczema (Fig. 6.31).

Areas may become red, scaly, and weeping, and the patient usually complains of intense itching. A mild form may occur in which small vesicles rupture to form enlarging collarettes of scale (Fig. 6.32). A severe form may occur with large palmar and plantar bullae (Fig. 6.33). For pompholyx of the feet, the amount of sweating should always be addressed. For some patients, it seems that the wearing of occlusive shoes and increased sweating contribute to the problem.

Differential diagnosis

When recurrent, tiny, pruritic vesicles occur on the sides of the fingers, the diagnosis is clear. The following should also be considered.

- Acute onset may represent allergic contact dermatitis.
- Scabies should always be considered for an itchy and possibly vesicular rash on the hands.
- Drug eruptions may cause acral inflammatory eruptions.
- Palmoplantar pustulosis (Ch. 7) may be particularly difficult to differentiate—although characterized by larger and varied color pustular lesions, small vesicles may also occur in this condition.
- Consider the state of the feet as well, to exclude any fungal infection. Patients may be more concerned about their hands.
- Some eruptions may cause small lesions that are solid but that resemble vesicles, notably lichen nitidus and some cases of lichen planus on the hands or feet.

Treatment

One should always try to elicit any trigger factors from the patient. Does contact with chemicals, friction, or specific items cause the breakout? Is the patient a cigarette smoker? Other than in mild transient cases, or those that are clearly provoked by heat and humidity, it is prudent to perform patch testing, as a contact allergy cannot be excluded by the morphology alone. Shoe dermatitis can mimic pompholyx of the soles. Usually no trigger factors are found, but this exercise is always important.

High-potency topical steroids are the mainstay of treatment, and should be applied before sleeping or twice daily to the volar surface. Application on the dorsal surface may cause atrophy in the long term. When there is more scale than erythema, keratolytics may be prescribed. If excessive sweating is thought to be related, use of a topical antiperspirant may be

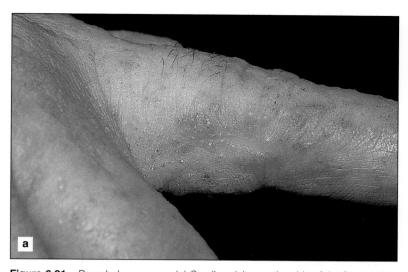

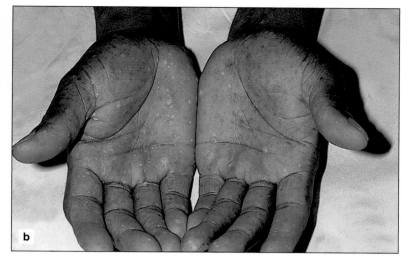

Figure 6.31 Pompholyx eczema. (**a**) Small vesicles on the side of the fingers, (**b**) Acute pompholyx in an African-Caribbean patient.

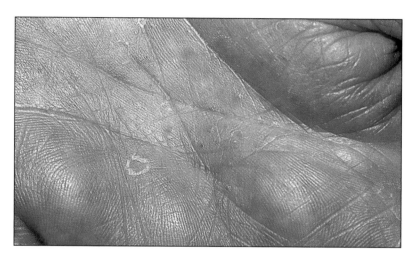

Figure 6.32 Keratolysis exfoliativa. Deep-seated vesicles that rupture to form spreading collarettes of scale.

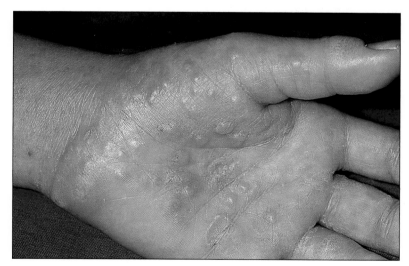

Figure 6.33 Pompholyx. Deep-seated vesicles and bullae.

helpful; this is best applied at night (see *Hyperhidrosis*, Ch. 23). Patients with pompholyx, as with any other form of hand dermatitis, should be instructed about avoidance of irritants that may aggravate the situation.

For severe cases, oral or intramuscular steroids may be indicated. PUVA and UVB have been used. Disulfiram (200 mg/day) and disodium cromoglycate have been tried in those suspected of having nickel allergy. Ciclosporin (2.5–5.0 mg/kg per day) and azathioprine (50–150 mg daily) appear to be effective.

Hyperkeratotic eczema
Etiology and pathogenesis
This condition, which is most frequent in middle-aged men, can be a very persistent and bothersome problem. There may be significant interference with ability to work. The clinical appearance is somewhere between that of eczema and that of a keratoderma. Patch testing and mycology are important for excluding other causes. In some patients, this condition may be a type of lichen simplex chronicus of the palms. In such cases, any friction (e.g. work-related friction) should be minimized (Fig. 6.34).

Clinical
A diffuse, thickened, fissured hyperkeratosis of the palms occurring in a middle-aged man is characteristic.

Differential diagnosis
The main considerations are as follows.
- Allergic contact dermatitis—should always be excluded by patch testing.
- Psoriasis—this may appear similar and can be very difficult to differentiate, even histologically, although classically psoriasis hyperkeratosis is rather more silvery (see Ch. 7); psoriatic lesions elsewhere on the body should be sought.
- Fungal infection—this is usually less keratotic, more red, and unilateral; always inspect the feet, where there may be bilateral involvement (see Ch. 26).
- Palmar keratodermas—hyperkeratosis is usually more uniform and smoother, with cut-off at the wrist creases (see Ch. 7).

Treatment
The disease is usually resistant to treatment. Lubrication and keratolytics are essential. Potent topical steroids may be tried. Hand PUVA may be of some benefit if the keratotic component has been addressed. Acitretin or ciclosporin can be effective in some cases.

Secondary (autosensitization) eczema
Etiology and pathogenesis
This condition (also termed an id reaction) is an eczematous reaction pattern to inflammation at other skin sites. It may be widespread or may be clinically identical to pompholyx. Such reactions have occurred after nummular eczema, stasis dermatitis, lichen simplex chronicus, allergic contact dermatitis, radiation dermatitis, tinea, or scabies.

Clinical
A diffuse, symmetric, eczematous rash may occur after a flare of a localized eczematous eruption; the primary eruption is often on the legs or feet.

Differential diagnosis
The key to this diagnosis is the presence of another eruption of sufficient inflammation to induce an id response. Without such an eruption, the

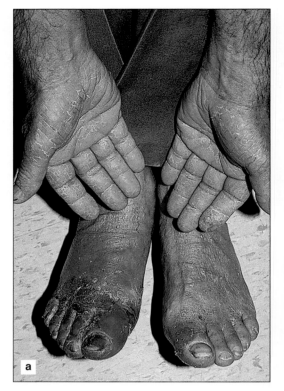

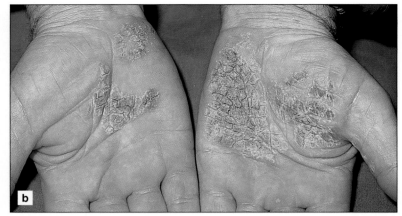

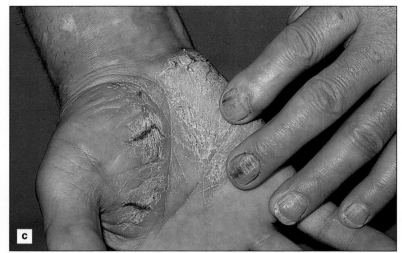

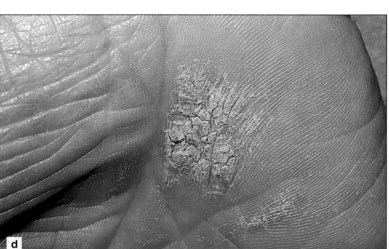

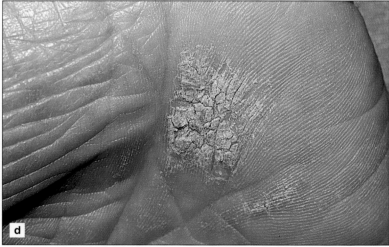

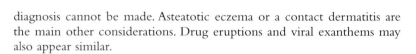

Figure 6.34 Hyperkeratotic eczema. (**a**) Diffuse, thickened, fissured hyperkeratosis of the palms occurring in a middle-aged adult is characteristic. Fissuring, as illustrated here, can be quite painful. Often, the initial sign of hyperkeratotic eczema is a plaque of scale and hyperkeratosis in the central palm or ulnar eminence. (**b**) This pattern affecting the central palm is probably caused by friction, but does not usually signify an external allergic cause. (**c**) Hyperkeratotic eczema made worse by scratching. This patient also picks his fingernails to create a typical morphology of habit tic dystrophy. (**d**) Close-up view of hyperkeratotic eczema.

diagnosis cannot be made. Asteatotic eczema or a contact dermatitis are the main other considerations. Drug eruptions and viral exanthems may also appear similar.

Treatment

The inciting eczematous or infected eruption should be treated; bear in mind that this may include use of antibacterial or antifungal agents to the primary area in some cases, but these are not necessary for the more widespread eruption which is eczematous rather than itself being infected. Topical, or sometimes systemic, steroids may be used to treat the secondary eczema.

Pityriasis alba
Etiology and pathogenesis

An eczematous patch occurs first, followed by loss of pigment (Fig. 6.35). The patient typically presents with a patch of lighter-colored skin at the malar eminence. Usually the preceding eczema has already resolved (Fig. 6.36) and may have been so mild that it has not been noticed (see Ch. 21 and Fig. 21.13). In white skin, patients may have a disproportionate tendency to present after the summer period, as the pale areas are often apparent only after the normal skin has tanned. Residual fine scaling is typically present.

Exfoliative erythroderma

The skin is diffusely red and scaly (Fig. 6.37). Various conditions may cause this (see Ch. 7), including drugs, pityriasis rubra pilaris, psoriasis, and CTCL.

CONTACT DERMATITIS

There are two types of contact dermatitis: irritant and allergic. Irritant contact dermatitis results from damage to the skin from topically applied liquids or chemicals, etc. in the absence of an allergic mechanism, and it includes both acute damage as well as more chronic disease due to repeated exposure. Hand dermatitis is the most common example, but lip-licking dermatitis and various other conditions, where frequent water or chemical contact occurs, are included (Figs 6.38 and 6.39). By contrast, allergic contact dermatitis is mediated through a type IV hypersensitivity or allergic mechanism (Fig. 6.40). Patients are allergic to a specific allergen, and whenever their skin comes in contact with that allergen (in sufficient concentration), an eczematous rash will occur. From a practical point of view, the two types may not only be impossible to distinguish clinically but may even coexist; for example, a building laborer may have irritant dermatitis from cement and 'wear and tear', but may additionally be allergic to chromate in cement and plaster.

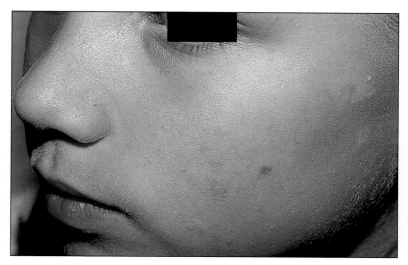

Figure 6.35 Pityriasis alba. Initial eczematous patch.

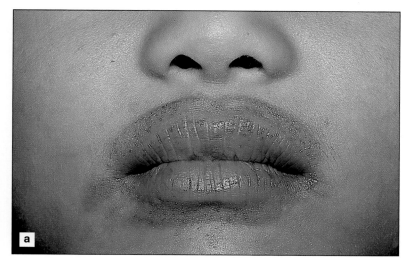

a

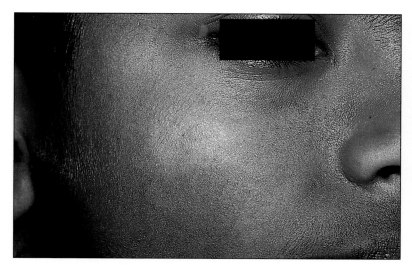

Figure 6.36 Pityriasis alba. Typical presentation of pityriasis alba; the preceding eczema has already resolved.

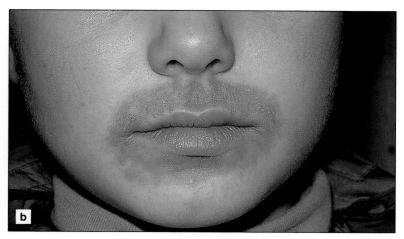

b

Figure 6.38 (**a**,**b**) Lip-licking dermatitis. An eczematous eruption occurs periorally and covering only those parts of the skin the tongue can reach. This represents a type of irritant contact dermatitis from saliva.

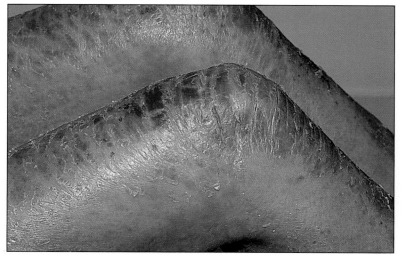

Figure 6.37 Exfoliative erythroderma.

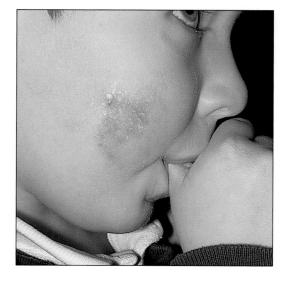

Figure 6.39 Irritant dermatitis to saliva. Saliva may pool in contact with the cheek during sleep.

Irritant contact dermatitis
Etiology and pathogenesis

The hands are the most important site, both numerically as they are a common site for contact dermatitis, and in terms of impact for the patient because hands are so important for function. Patients with hand eczema usually have some precipitating or contributing factor. They may have a history of AD, or their work may expose them to irritants. Housewives may develop a hand dermatitis from housework. The work-up requires an inquiry about a history of AD; occupational activities; exposure to potential irritants and allergens; and daily activities that involve the hands, for example hand washing, cleaning, cold exposure, and wet work (exposure of the hands to water for at least 2 h per day). Patients with obsessive-compulsive disorders may wash their hands excessively (Fig. 6.41).

77

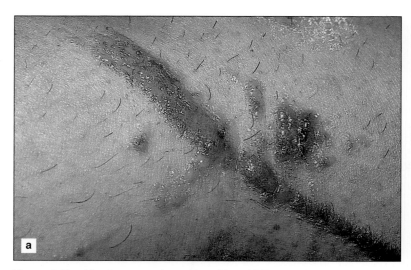

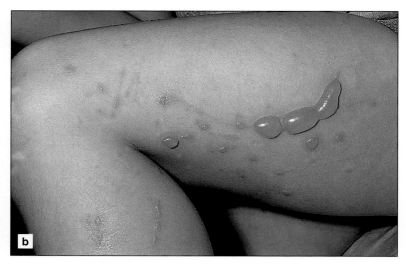

Figure 6.40 Allergic contact dermatitis to *Rhus*. (**a**) The classic appearance of allergic contact dermatitis is illustrated in this patient, who came into contact with poison oak. The lesions are linear but not following Blaschko lines. The eruption is microvesicular and extremely pruritic. (**b**) *Rhus* dermatitis. Linear bullae are characteristic of an allergic contact dermatitis. (Courtesy of O. Dale Collins III.)

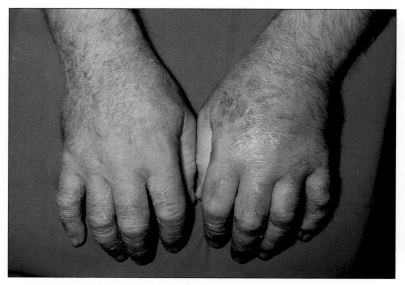

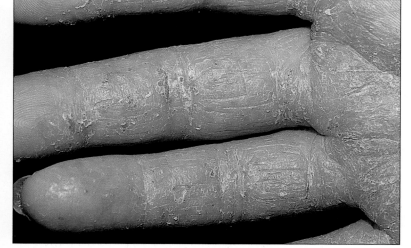

Figure 6.42 Irritant dermatitis. This woman developed an irritant hand dermatitis soon after having her first baby.

Figure 6.41 Hand dermatitis. Irritant chronic hand dermatitis can pose a significant problem for patients, their doctors, and their employers. Inquiry should be made regarding the patient's occupation and hobbies, the frequency of hand washing, and exposure to chemicals or irritants. Allergic contact dermatitis should be excluded.

Clinical

Red, scaly areas, often with fissuring, can affect any part of the hands in irritant hand dermatitis (Figs 6.42 and 6.43). Patterns do not necessarily correlate with cause; for example, while involvement of finger webs is common in those using detergents or whose condition is related to frequent hand washing, it does not preclude the possibility of reaction to an allergen. Secondary staphylococcal infection is common. Deep and painful fissures typically indicate such a superinfection (Fig. 6.44). If left untreated, multiple pustules may develop. AD has been found to increase the risk of hand dermatitis in women.

Differential diagnosis

The main differential diagnosis is from allergic contact dermatitis. Patch testing may be appropriate, particularly in those without any obvious history of exposure to irritants or if the disorder is resistant to standard therapies.

Tinea manus, psoriasis, and scabies are the main other differentials. Tinea of the hands is usually unilateral, but either irritant or allergic

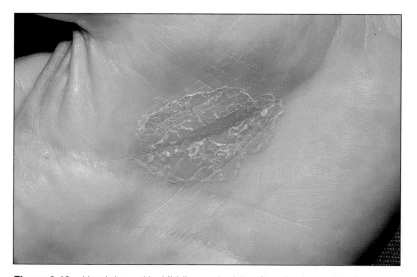

Figure 6.43 Hand dermatitis. Middle-aged adults often develop a chronic eczematous dermatitis of the palms. Some have called this variant hyperkeratotic eczema.

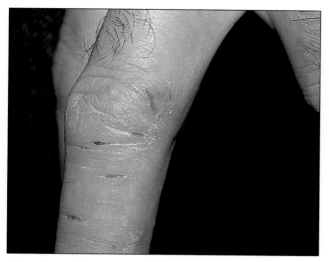

Figure 6.44 Hand dermatitis with fissures. Eczematous skin is not as supple as normal skin, and instead of bending, may break. This causes a fissure, which is usually quite painful. Bacteria are usually abundant. A topical antibacterial ointment and a bandage overnight are helpful for limited lesions. An oral antibiotic (antistaphylococcal) may be necessary for multiple lesions.

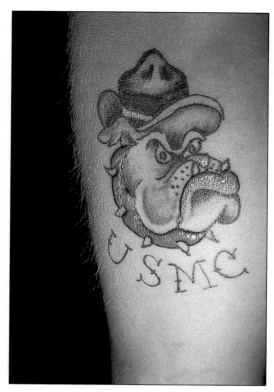

Figure 6.45 Tattoo allergy. Rarely, a patient will be allergic to the tattoo pigment. Reaction to the red pigment, cinnabar (mercuric sulfide), is most common. (Courtesy of Michael O. Murphy.)

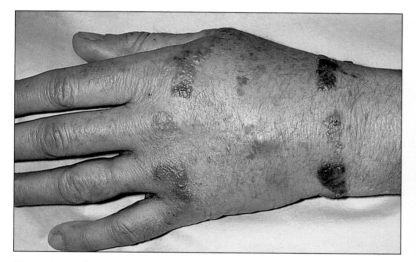

Figure 6.46 Colophony dermatitis to the adhesive in tape. Colophony, or rosin, is common in a variety of sticky things (see Figs 6.54 and 6.58).

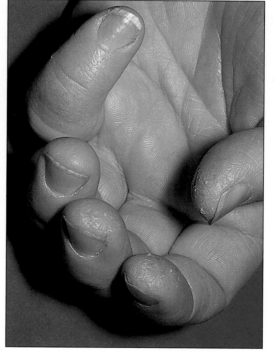

Figure 6.47 Garlic allergy. Allergy to foods may cause a hand dermatitis. Here, the offending food was garlic, which is typically held between the thumb, index, and middle fingers of the non-dominant hand.

contact dermatitis may be (e.g. dermatitis may be asymmetric in hairdressers, who hold scissors in the dominant hand but wet, chemical-loaded hair between the fingers of the non-dominant hand).

Treatment

The patient should decrease repeated hand washing, and reduce exposure to water, cold air, and irritants as much as possible. Gloves should be used as necessary to protect the hands (e.g. heavy-duty vinyl gloves for contact with water or when handling fruits or vegetables, cotton gloves for dry housework, and leather gloves for outdoor work). Wash the gloves, not the hands!

A topical steroid ointment morning and night is helpful for the erythema and itch, usually medium- to high-potency for the palms and low to medium for the finger webs or dorsum. Occlusion may be added if needed. Some patients prefer a cream, especially during the day. Frequent emolliation with a heavy cream or ointment is critically important. Because of their high water content, lotions are less effective. A hand cream should be carried conveniently for frequent use during the day, especially after water exposure and hand washing. If there is significant roughness, ammonium lactate (12% lotion) combined with a potent steroid cream can help.

Painful fissures may be occluded overnight with an antibiotic ointment if infection is a consideration. Oral antibiotics (e.g. erythromycin for

7 days) may be helpful, especially when fissures or other signs of bacterial infection occur. Sometimes, treatment-resistant hand dermatitis, even without overt signs of bacterial infection, will respond to oral antibiotics.

Allergic contact dermatitis
Etiology and pathogenesis

Allergic contact dermatitis occurs through an allergic mechanism in which a topically applied allergen incites an allergic response. A variety of allergens may be implicated (Figs 6.45–6.52). Table 6.5 lists the most common allergens and their most likely source. When faced with a patient with an eczematous or even vesicular eruption, the possibility of allergic contact dermatitis should be considered (Fig. 6.53).

When cutaneous allergy is suspected, patch testing may be helpful (Figs 6.54–6.55). A standard tray of allergens, and, if necessary, selected allergens based on the history of exposure, are applied to the back for

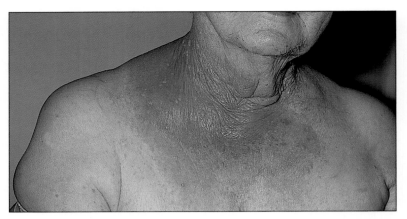

Figure 6.48 *Perfume and medicament allergy. Multiple allergies are often found. This patient developed a reaction first to a perfume and then to a topical medication applied to soothe the initial rash.*

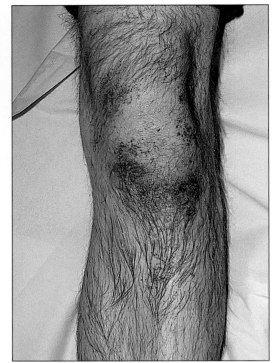

Figure 6.49 Cement burn. This occurs due to the highly alkaline pH of wet cement. It should be distinguished from allergy to chromates, which are present in cement and are allergenic in the powdered form. After the cement sets and hardens, it is no longer allergenic.

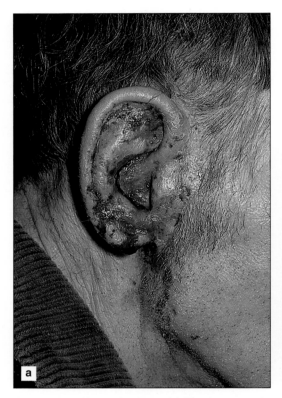

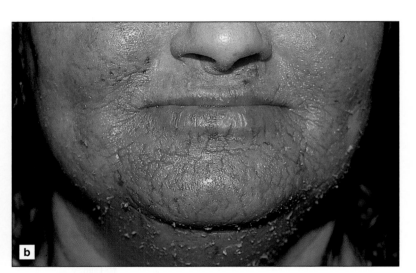

Figure 6.50 *Neomycin allergy.* (**a**) *Allergic contact dermatitis to neomycin in eardrops is not uncommon.* (**b**) *This woman applied neomycin, hoping to cure a rash about the mouth. Instead, a rash 10 times worse developed.*

48 h. Conventionally, readings are performed at 48 h, and a second reading after a further 1–3 days is useful, as some tests may produce a delayed positive reaction. Unfortunately, the standard patch test trays available in the USA are becoming more and more inadequate at finding most clinically relevant contact allergens. In one study, the US standard allergy patch test kit and the Thin-Layer Rapid Use Epicutaneous Test kit (TRUE Test) identified less than a third of patients with allergic contact dermatitis. Oftentimes, the testing must include over 80–100 allergens. Examples of allergens missed by standard trays are cocamidopropyl betaine (an ingredient in 'no more tears' shampoos that can cause a contact dermatitis on the forehead), bacitracin, and gold sodium thiosulfate (suspect in cases of woman allergic to gold jewelry).

In the UK and Europe, experts meet to determine the tests that are likely to be most appropriate for routine screening, as this may vary with the introduction of new chemicals; for example, increased use of new preservatives may be associated with a rise in the reports of contact allergy, while older agents may be used less often and therefore problems with allergy diminish. The current (2004) European series is known as the Extended European Standard Battery and contains 35 agents.

Clinical

Lesions are either eczematous (Fig. 6.56), microvesicular, or frankly bullous. Lesions may be linear (Fig. 6.57) or in streaks (Fig. 6.58), and may be asymmetric depending on the allergen and the mechanism of exposure. Certain sites suggest certain allergens (Figs 6.59–6.64). For example, the scalp (also the neck and face) are affected by black hair dye (Fig. 6.65); rubber causes problems with shoes, gloves, and elasticated garments (Figs 6.60 and 6.66); nickel affects several sites (Figs 6.67–6.69); and nail polish may be transferred to the head and neck (Fig. 6.70).

Differential diagnosis

A huge range of differential diagnoses may apply, depending on the site affected; full discussion of all possibilities would be impossible. The main eczematous disorders to consider are as follows.

- Irritant contact dermatitis—this presents similarly, as discussed earlier.
- Photosensitivity—this may mimic a contact dermatitis due to an airborne allergen, or one that is applied to exposed sites (e.g. a sunscreen or moisturizer). Sometimes, an allergen may cause a reaction only when also sun-exposed (photoallergic contact dermatitis). A combination of

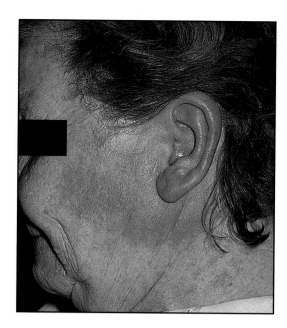

Figure 6.51
Hydrocortisone allergy. Surprisingly enough, allergic contact dermatitis may occur from topically applied topical steroids.

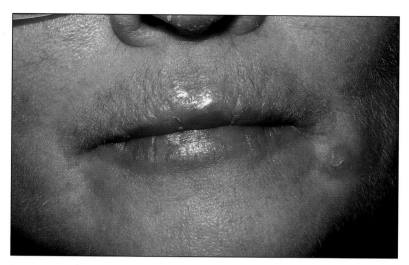

Figure 6.52 Allergic contact dermatitis to quaternarium-15.

Table 6.5 ALLERGENS COMMONLY INVOLVED IN ALLERGIC CONTACT DERMATITIS

Allergen	Comments
Antiseptics and antimicrobials	Include thimerosal (thiomersal, merthiolate), quinolines (clioquinol), and chloxylenol. Thimerosal is notable for inclusion in eyedrops, contact lens solutions, vaccines and toxoids. Quinolines are used as an additive in some topical steroid preparations, and impart a yellow color when exposed to air.
Balsum of Peru	A crude test for perfume allergy; also reacts with various essential oils in foods. Present in fir trees.
Benzocaine and related agents	These are local anesthetics used topically; benzocaine is the prototype but others also cause reactions, so a mixture such as Caine Mix III is often used for patch testing. The patient should study the list of ingredients of any medication meant to anesthetize or 'soothe' the skin, mucosa, or gums; for example, medications to soothe sore throats, teething babies' gums, and preparations for insect stings or hemorrhoids.
Carba mix	A rubber allergen (e.g. polyurethane foam rubber).
Cetoaryl alcohol	Emulsifier in creams and cosmetics; check ingredient lists, including those of medical products.
Cinnamic alcohol or aldehyde	Cinnamon flavor and fragrance; some toothpastes, cassia oil, some colas and chocolates.
Cobalt	Mainly found in the same sources as nickel (see below).
Colophony	Also known as rosin, sap of pine trees. In glues, adhesives—anything sticky; Scotch tape, polish for furniture, floors, cars; printer's ink, solder, violin bow resin, and occasionally eye cosmetics.
Epoxy resin	Two-part glues that must be mixed just before using. Some dental material; some plastics.
Ethylene diamine	Stabilizer in some creams. Cross-reacts with aminophylline when given intravenously. May cross-react with meclizine, tripelennamine, or hydroxyzine.
Formaldehyde	Some photographic chemicals, embalming fluid, fumigants, industrial disinfectants, automotive fluids, manufacturing of plastics and plywood. Some finishes of fabric. Note that some other preservatives release formaldehyde, so they may need to be avoided; many are also allergenic in their own right.
Fragrance mix	A mix of the eight commonest perfume bases; picks up about 75–80% of patients with contact allergy to perfumes.
Fusidic acid	Antibiotic; allergy to topical preparations may occur.
Latex	Latex gloves such as those prevalent in medical offices, latex balloons, latex-containing condoms. Foods that tend to cross-react and may cause clinical allergic reactions include avocado, banana, tomato, chestnut, and kiwifruit.
Mercaptobenzothiazole (MBT) and related agents	Rubber allergens: both MBT and a 'mercapto mix' are tested (see rubber, below). Pet and veterinarian products.
Para-tertiary butyl phenol formaldehyde resin	Adhesive used in footwear, chipboard, etc.
Plants	Primin (primula family) and sesquiterpene lactone (many plants) are routinely tested in Europe, as well as Compositae (daisy family) in selected cases. See also *Rhus*.

Table 6.5	ALLERGENS COMMONLY INVOLVED IN ALLERGIC CONTACT DERMATITIS—*cont'd*
Allergen	**Comments**
Preservatives	Preservatives are widely used in cosmetics, especially water-based (shampoos, liquid soaps, etc.), as well as in industrial settings (cutting fluids, emulsion paints, etc.). Note that some may be in creams (but not usually ointments) applied to the skin, so patients need to check ingredient listings if an allergy is identified. Relevant agents that are often tested include parabens (hydroxybenzoates), imidazolidinyl urea (Germall 115), diazolidinyl urea (Germall 111), quaternium 15 (Dowicil 200), isothiazolinones (Kathon CG), chlorocresol, bronopol, and methyldibromo glutaronitrile (Euxyl K).
Neomycin (Neosporin)	A topical antimicrobial agent. Common in triple antibiotic ointments.
Nickel	The most common offending metal allergen. Most costume jewelry, necklaces, fasteners on jeans, safety pins, etc. Dimethylglioxime is used to test metals for nickel content. There is debate as to the significance of nickel in the diet. Some experts recommend a nickel-free diet in nickel-sensitive patients who continue to experience 'flare'.
Para-phenylenediamine (PPD)	Black dye: most common in hair dye. Not allergenic once set. Some rubbers cross-react, as might *para*-aminobenzoic acid (PABA), sulfa drugs, or benzocaine.
Potassium dichromate	Causes cement dermatitis, as chromates are found in the powdered form of cement. Leather may contain chromates. Coatings for rust, yellow and green paints, other green items, match heads.
Rhus	Poison oak and ivy. Their leaves have a distinct three-leaflet design from a common node: 'leaves of three, let them be'.
Rubber	Rubber gloves, polyurethane foam rubber, elastic in clothing, shoes, hoses, belts, adhesives, and tapes. See mercaptobenzothiazole, thiuram mix, and carba mix. The European battery also tests PPD black rubber mix.
Sunscreens	Many sunscreen chemicals can cause allergy. However, the commonest reason for reaction to sunscreen product is perfume allergy, followed by allergy to preservatives in the base cream.
Topical steroids	Allergy to these may be difficult to spot. The usual screening tests are to pixocortol pivalate (hydrocortisone allergy) and budesonide (several cross-reactions).
Wool alcohols	Patients should inspect the ingredient list of anything put on skin. Also known as wool wax alcohol or wool alcohol. Derived from sheep's wool. The cause of allergy to lanolin.

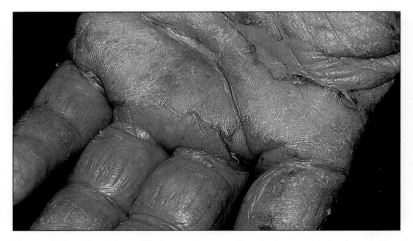

Figure 6.53 Hand dermatitis from a cleanser. The doctor should always consider allergic contact dermatitis in a patient presenting with an eczematous eruption. The hands are a common site for both allergic and irritant contact dermatitis, because they come into contact with so many things. This patient was allergic to an ingredient in the cleanser used at work.

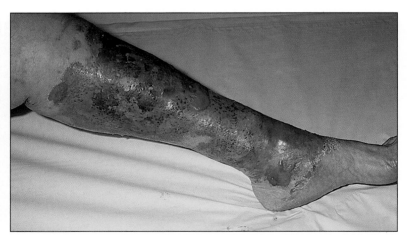

Figure 6.54 Contact dermatitis in a patient with a leg ulcer. There is a high prevalence of contact sensitivity in patients with stasis dermatitis or leg ulcers. Patch testing is often indicated.

patch testing and photopatch testing (Ch. 17) may help to distinguish between these conditions and others, such as chronic actinic dermatitis.

- Atopic dermatitis—AD may coexist; always consider contact allergy if there is an odd pattern, new pattern, flare after a prolonged trouble-free period or related to a new occupation, or resistance to therapy (remember topical steroid allergy).

Treatment

Obviously, the offending agent should be identified and eliminated. If left untreated and exposure to the allergen is removed, allergic contact dermatitis will run a 2–3-week course. If limited in scope and sufficiently severe, a potent topical steroid is appropriate. Lesser strengths are often not sufficient. For widespread disease, a systemic corticosteroid is sometimes

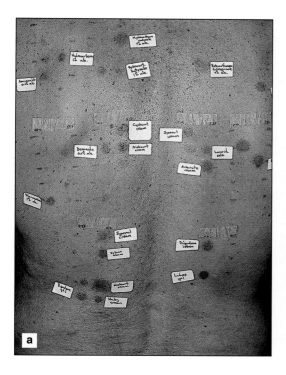

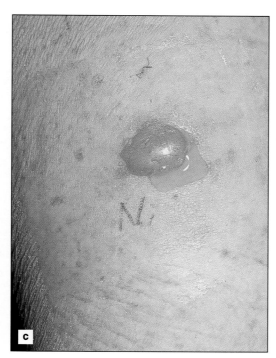

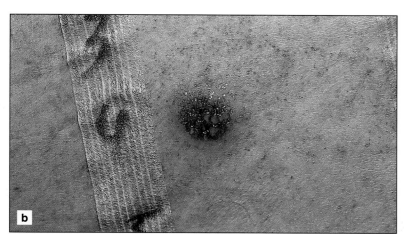

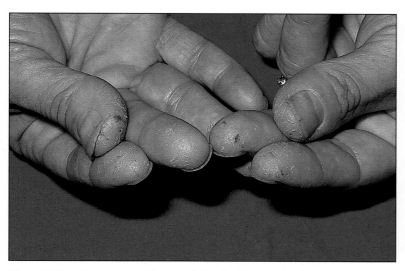

Figure 6.55 (**a**) Patch testing. Patch tests detect type IV reactions to external allergens. Batteries of common allergens pertinent to the clinical situation are applied to the back for 48 h. In this case, there were multiple reactions to medicament agents including several topical steroids. (**b**) Patch test, positive reaction. In this case, allergen 4 (paraphenylenediamine) reacted. Paraphenylenediamine is a black dye, and it is the only patch that leaves a black color. In addition to the black coloration, multiple vesicles and a surrounding erythema are seen. (**c**) In extreme sensitivity, bullous test reactions may occur even to standard test agents, in this case to nickel. (Panel a courtesy of Daniel W. Shaw, M.D.)

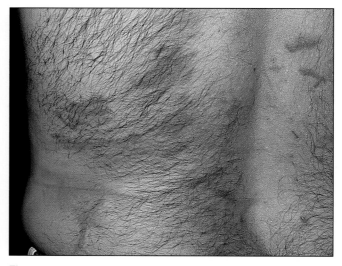

Figure 6.56 Colophony reaction in a florist. Florists may develop an eczematous reaction of the fingertips to a variety of plant components (see also Fig. 2.24).

Figure 6.57 Rash due to contact with a fig tree. This patient, without a shirt, was pruning a fig tree. The lesions are linear and haphazardly arranged. The area on the lower left suggests that a liquid allergen ran down the back.

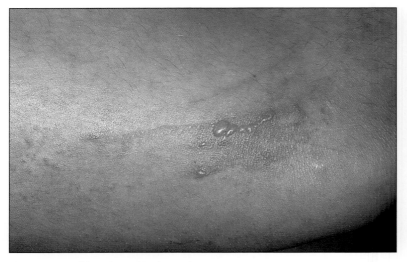

Figure 6.58 Plant dermatitis. A streaky pattern suggests an exogenous cause, which in this case was a plant.

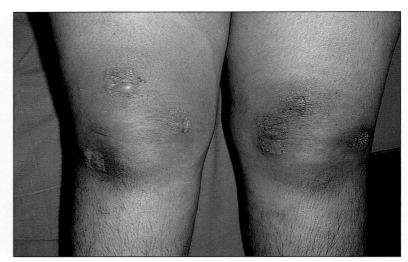

Figure 6.60 Colophony reaction. Square blisters have developed in this patient with sensitivity to colophony (see also Figs 2.24 and 6.43). These lesions were due to adhesive dressings.

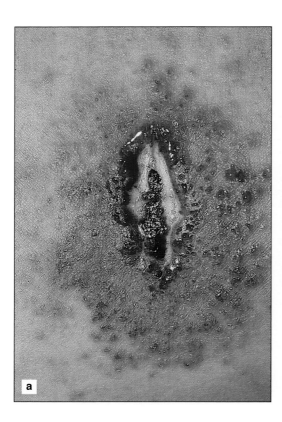

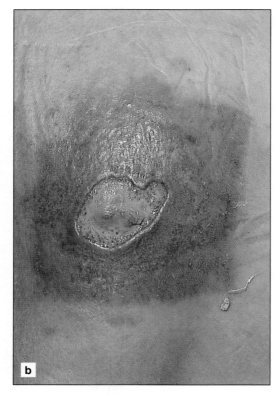

Figure 6.59 Contact allergy complicating wounds. (**a**) Bacitracin allergy. This patient developed redness, inflammation, and dehiscence 10 days after a minor surgical excision. Allergic contact dermatitis to bacitracin was the cause. Always consider an allergy when the patient returns with a 'wound infection'. (**b**) Adhesive allergy. Allergy about a wound site may also occur in response to the adhesive of the dressing. Note the square shape.

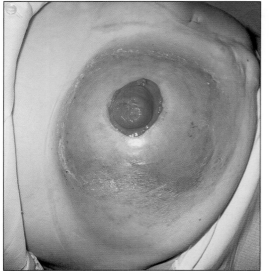

Figure 6.61 Adhesive dermatitis. Reaction to the adhesive in an ostomy bag.

used (e.g. prednisone 1 mg/kg for several days and then tapered over 2–3 weeks). Shorter 'pulses' will usually lead to relapse. In chronic cases, where allergen avoidance is difficult to achieve (e.g. some airborne contact dermatitis, as discussed later), treatment options are as for AD.

Airborne contact dermatitis
Etiology and pathogenesis

Allergens in the air can cause a dermatitis in the exposed areas of the face, neck, and arms. Causative agents include pollens, dust, ragweed, sawdust, airborne household sprays, animal hairs, occupational volatile chemicals, Compositae plants, epoxy resin, chrysanthemums, and glutaraldehyde (occupational). In India, airborne contact dermatitis to the weed *Parthenium hysterophorus* has become widespread.

Clinical

A dry, lichenified, and rarely vesicular eruption occurs in the exposed areas.

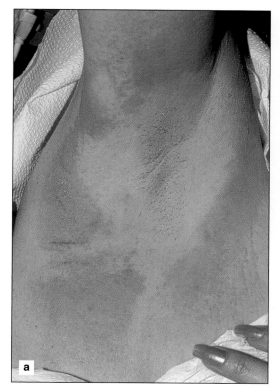

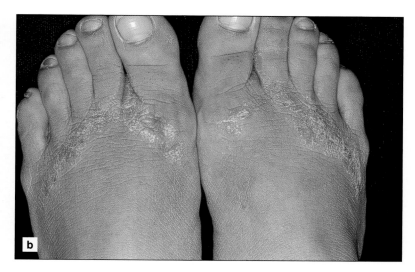

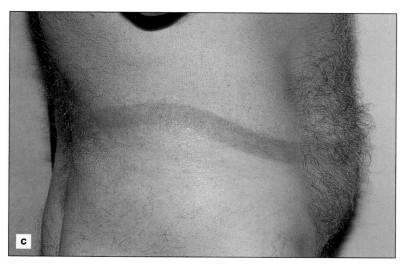

Figure 6.62 Allergic contact dermatitis to clothing. (**a**) An eczematous eruption about the axilla but sparing the inner vault is typical of an allergic contact dermatitis to clothing. Usually, the offending material is newly purchased and was not washed before being worn, and the condition does not recur after the clothing is washed. (**b**) Allergic contact dermatitis to thongs. The diagnosis is easy when the distribution of the rash replicates the shape of the offending item. (**c**) Elastic (waistband) dermatitis. This red, pruritic eruption is unmistakably related to elastic in the patient's underwear. The eruption did not develop until the patient's wife bleached his underwear, a classic history. This is also known as the bleached rubber syndrome.

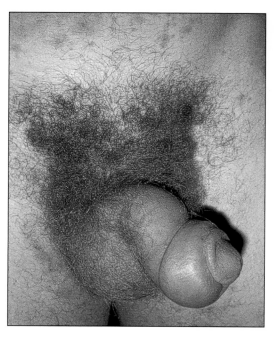

Figure 6.63 *Rhus* dermatitis. Men working outdoors may carry the *Rhus* antigen to their penis while urinating. Tremendous edema may result. (Courtesy of Michael O. Murphy, M.D.)

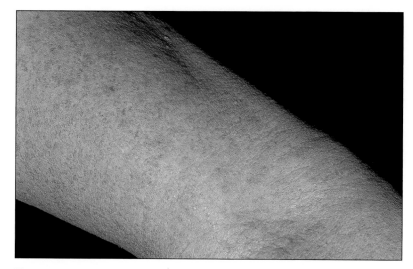

Figure 6.64 Allergic contact dermatitis to a body lotion. A diffuse allergic reaction to a topically applied lotion may mimic a drug eruption.

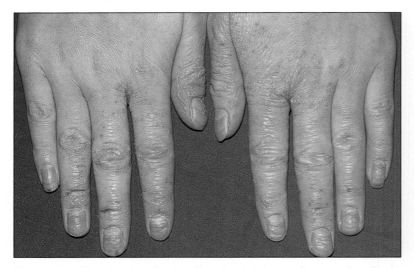

Figure 6.65 Paraphenylenediamine allergy in a hairdresser. Paraphenylenediamine is most commonly found in black hair dye. Hairdressers are prone to this allergy. The non-dominant hand is more severely affected in this patient, because it is in greater contact with the wet hair (and any allergens) as a result of holding hair between the non-dominant fingers while holding implements such as scissors in the dominant hand.

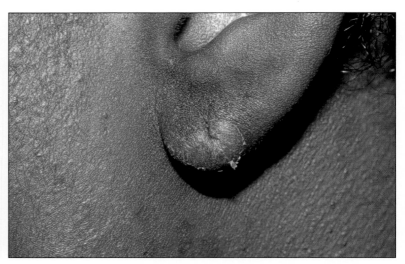

Figure 6.67 Nickel dermatitis from earrings. Nickel allergy is very common in women. The earlobes become pruritic, inflamed, and eczematous. Lichenification may result from chronic rubbing. Other areas in contact with nickel-containing metal may react. When told they have an allergy, patients often protest, saying they have used the item for years without trouble. However, this is the typical story; usually it is only after years of exposure that the patient develops the allergy.

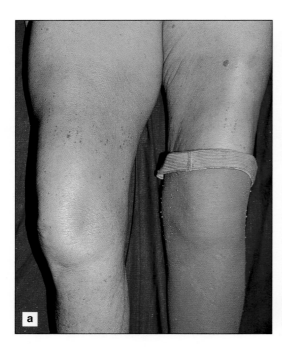

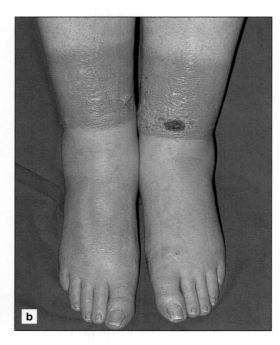

Figure 6.66 Allergic contact dermatitis to rubber. (**a**) The patient has developed an eczematous eruption on the thighs at the contact point of the elastic support band of the stocking. The classic rubber allergens are mercaptobenzothiazole, carba mix, and thiuram. (**b**) Elastic dermatitis to socks. Note the tremendous reaction to the elasticated portion of sports socks.

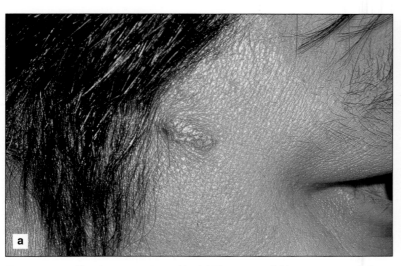

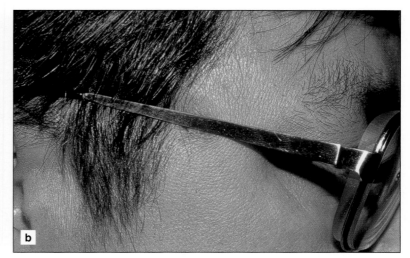

Figure 6.68 Allergic contact dermatitis. (**a**) The cause of this eczematous rash was not obvious until (**b**) the patient put on his glasses.

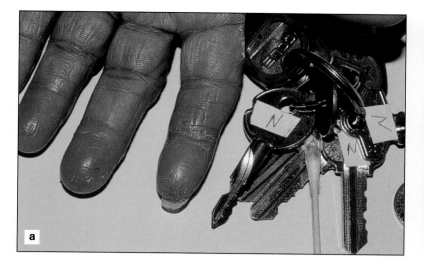

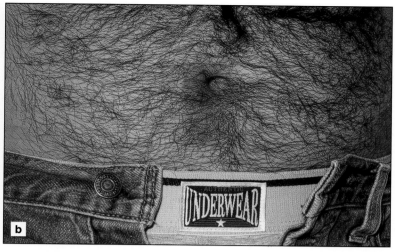

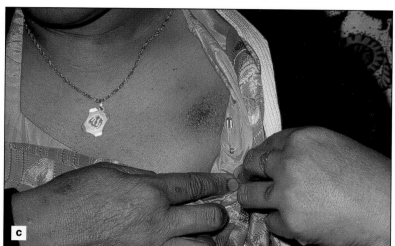

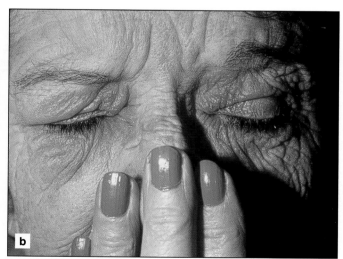

Figure 6.69 Nickel allergy. (**a**) Patch testing in this patient showed a nickel allergy. Three of her keys tested positive to dimethylglyoxime. Changing keys greatly improved the eruption. (**b**) This patient with an allergic sensitivity to nickel has developed a reaction on the lower abdomen to the inner metal fastener of jeans. (**c**) This patient developed a reaction at the site of contact with a safety pin.

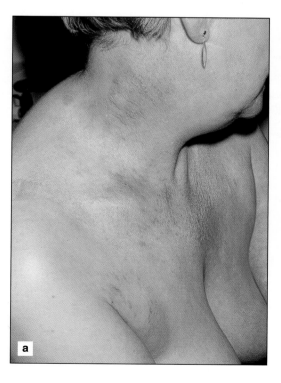

Figure 6.70 Nail polish allergy. (**a**) Note the streaky pattern of erythema on the neck. Material on the nails is not infrequently carried to the neck and face by the hands. (**b**) A periorbital eczematous dermatitis in a woman is not infrequently caused by allergy to material on the nails. Patch testing is usually in order, along with removal of all nail coatings. (Courtesy of Michael O. Murphy, M.D.)

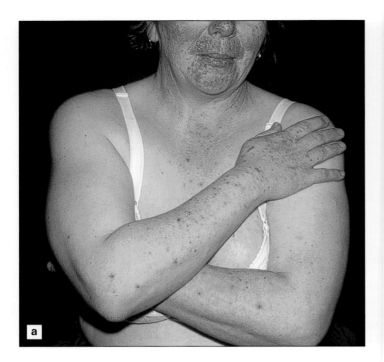

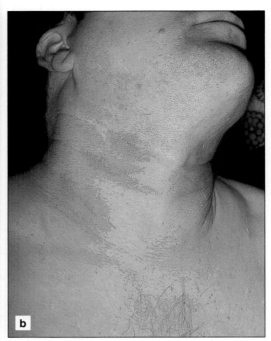

Figure 6.71 Airborne allergic contact dermatitis. (**a**) The pattern of airborne allergic contact dermatitis may resemble a photodistribution, in that it affects the exposed areas. However, areas typically spared UV exposure, such as the upper eyelids and the anterior neck, are usually affected by airborne contact dermatitis. (**b**) Airborne allergic contact dermatitis to balsam. Note the involvement of the anterior neck, which would not be seen in a photodistributed dermatitis. Also, the creases are involved, suggesting an airborne dust.

Differential diagnosis

- Atopic dermatitis may show a preference for the head and neck.
- Photodermatitis of several types, including photodistributed drug eruptions, may appear similar; however, airborne contact allergy typically affects the upper eyelid and anterior neck under the chin, whereas these photoprotected areas are spared, at least in the early stages, in a photodistributed eruption (Fig. 6.71).

Treatment

The offending allergen should be identified and avoided. Topical steroids should be prescribed. Narrow-band UVB therapy can be very effective for difficult cases.

SEBORRHEIC DERMATITIS

Etiology and pathogenesis

This is a very common dermatosis, mainly affecting the face and scalp. It is probably the single most common scalp problem for which a patient seeks medical attention. While the hair is normal, the scalp is scaly and mildly erythematous. Seborrheic dermatitis is also common on the oily areas of the face (e.g. the nasolabial fold and eyebrows). Diffuse, fine, non-inflammatory scaling of the scalp (pityriasis capitis or dandruff) is also a form of seborrheic dermatitis. If there is both scaling and erythema, the term seborrheic dermatitis is used.

The leading theory as to the cause of seborrheic dermatitis is that the fungus *Pityrosporum ovale* (*Malassezia furfur*) overgrows and causes irritation of the skin. It may do this directly or by secretion of a toxin or other mediator. This irritation causes hyperproliferation, scaling, and erythema of the skin, i.e. an eczematous response. Infrequent shampooing is thus a contributing factor as it allows overgrowth of *P. ovale*, and antifungal 'medicated' shampoos help by reducing the numbers of *P. ovale*.

Seborrheic dermatitis occurs in a high percentage of HIV-positive patients. Whether *Pityrosporum* occurs in higher numbers in such patients or whether the immune system responds abnormally to its presence is unclear.

Seborrheic dermatitis of the face is commonly exacerbated by cold and dry air, as is typical for other eczematous conditions.

Clinical

Erythema and scale may affect the scalp (Fig. 6.72), the ears (including the external auditory canal, causing otitis externa), the nasolabial folds

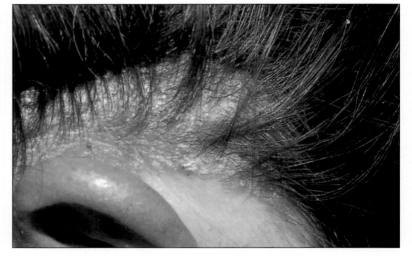

Figure 6.72 Sebopsoriasis. Severe seborrheic dermatitis may resemble psoriasis. In such cases, the term sebopsoriasis is often used.

(Fig. 6.73), the glabella, the eyebrows (Fig. 6.74), and even the entire face (Fig. 6.75). Patients often have an oily complexion, thus the term seborrhea. Men with a beard or hairy chest (Fig. 6.76) may develop seborrheic dermatitis in these areas. Sometimes the rash may extend to the mid-back, eyelid margin (seborrheic blepharitis), axillae, gluteal cleft, perianal area, and umbilicus.

In black skin, the scaling is prominent but the erythema may be masked (Fig. 6.77). Often, postinflammatory hypopigmentation is seen. Sometimes, the changes of seborrheic dermatitis in the black patient blend with lesions of tinea versicolor on the neck and upper trunk.

Differential diagnosis

This will depend on the site affected; discussion is limited to the commonest face and scalp sites.

For the scalp, the following should be considered.

- Other patterns of dermatitis—AD and contact dermatitis may affect the scalp.
- Psoriasis—the scale of scalp psoriasis is usually much thicker and may often be hyperkeratotic.
- Pityriasis amiantacea—this is a description of asbestosis-like scalp scaling for which there are many causative conditions, of which

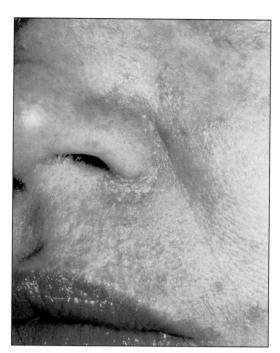

Figure 6.73 Seborrheic dermatitis of the nasolabial fold. Redness and scale along the nasolabial fold is a classic sign of seborrheic dermatitis.

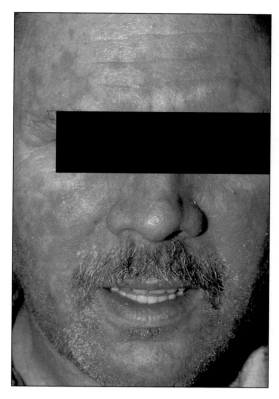

Figure 6.75 Diffuse seborrheic dermatitis of the face. Seborrheic dermatitis is the most common cause of a red, scaly facial rash.

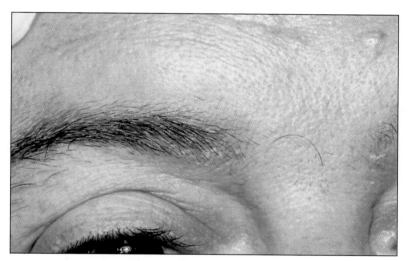

Figure 6.74 Seborrheic dermatitis of the eyebrow. Note the redness and scale.

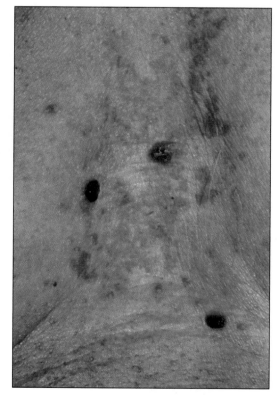

Figure 6.76 Seborrheic dermatitis of the chest. Seborrheic dermatitis commonly occurs on the mid-chest of an adult man.

seborrheic dermatitis is one. The scales are larger than in typical seborrheic dermatitis, forming white adherent plates.

- Pityriasis rubra pilaris—this may start in the scalp as a red, scaly rash but quickly progresses to other areas of the body.
- Lupus erythematosus—may produce redness and scaling, usually well demarcated. The redness tends to be perifollicular, and scarring often ensues.
- Lichen planus—perifollicular redness, often rather purple in color, and follicular scaling.
- Dermatophyte fungal infection—rarely affects scalp, other than with cattle ringworm; it is more localized than typical seborrheic dermatitis, and may have a pustular component.
- Dermatomyositis—scalp redness and scaling are probably under-estimated.

  For the face, the following should be considered.
- Other patterns of dermatitis—AD (usually whole face or sites of rubbing such as the eyelids) and contact dermatitis (many patterns). Contact dermatitis may be localized to eyelids, ears, etc. but does not usually have the 'full house' of sites affected by seborrheic dermatitis.
- Psoriasis—facial involvement is common and tends to correlate with severity, but rarely occurs in the absence of psoriasis at other sites. Scalp

margin and ears are often affected. Some patients seem to have an overlap condition sometimes termed sebopsoriasis.

- Pityriasis rubra pilaris—facial involvement occurs at an early stage.
- Rosacea—a common mid-facial rash, mainly affecting cheeks, chin, and central forehead rather than nasolabial folds and scalp margin. Involvement of the scalp and ears would not be expected, and the rash has papules and pustules. However, it can be difficult to distinguish and may coexist in some individuals, as both are common conditions.
- Lupus erythematosus—discoid lupus erythematosus may produce redness and scaling of individual areas such as the ear or eyebrow. Systemic lupus erythematosus is in the differential of mid-facial

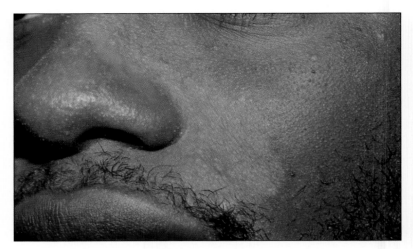

Figure 6.77 Seborrheic dermatitis in a black patient. Note the scale and postinflammatory hypopigmentation.

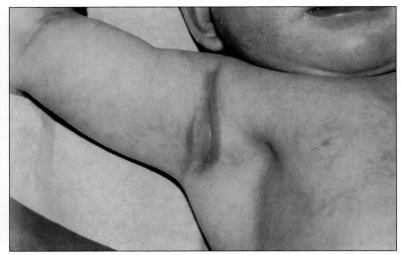

Figure 6.78 Seborrheic dermatitis in the axillary fold in a child.

(butterfly) rash but affects the cheeks rather than the nasolabial folds, and is associated with systemic symptoms.

- Dermatophyte fungal infection—uncommonly affects the face; if it does, then it is typically asymmetric.

Treatment

For the patient who shampoos only once a week, shampooing daily or every other day may be sufficient. Otherwise, daily use of a medicated shampoo (e.g. selenium sulfide 2.5%, zinc pyrithione, and tar) is recommended. One of the best shampoos is ketoconazole (Nizoral shampoo), which contains an imidazole antifungal agent to kill *Pityrosporum* yeasts. It is highly effective and more cosmetically acceptable to patients than more abrasive tar shampoos. Use of any of these shampoos may be followed by the use of another shampoo or conditioner of the patient's choice. Ketoconazole 1% shampoo is available over the counter; although less effective than the 2% solution, it is helpful in mild cases.

If itching of the scalp is a persistent problem, a topical steroid should be added (e.g. betamethasone diproprionate solution, triamcinolone 0.1% lotion, and fluocinonide solution) or, in the most stubborn cases, clobetasol propionate solution. Alternatively, fluocinolone 0.01% shampoo (patients lather the scalp, leave 5 min, and rinse daily) is very effective at clearing the itch. For the rare patient with a persistent lesion in the same area of the scalp, excessive scratching may be a contributing cause.

When seborrheic dermatitis is present on the face, the patient can lather the face daily or every other day with the medicated shampoo or can use topical ketoconazole cream. A topical steroid (e.g. hydrocortisone 1% cream) is usually recommended as well to treat the eczematous response; for convenience, a combined imidazole–hydrocortisone preparation may be used.

For seborrheic dermatitis of the eyelids, daily gentle shampoo with ketaconazole shampoo (or baby shampoo if irritation occurs) should be tried. For lid margin seborrheic blepharitis, carefully apply combined miconazole–hydrocortisone cream to the base of the lashes from the cutaneous rather than from the mucosal aspect: imidazoles are irritant to the conjunctiva. For seborrheic dermatitis of the ear, a low-potency topical steroid or imidazole–corticosteroid combined product applied twice a day for the pinna and a corticosteroid otic preparation for the ear, are effective. Daily use of a medicated shampoo is also recommended.

Due to the hair type of most African-Caribbean patients, medicated shampoos (e.g. ketoconazole 2% shampoo) should be recommended and the patient instructed to let the shampoo sit on the scalp (contact with the hair is not necessary) for approximately 15–20 min twice a week. For those with significant itching or inflammation, a topical steroid should be added. A steroid ointment applied after shampooing is usually best, and is appropriate for any type of hair: processed or hot-combed. It may also be used as a substitute for hair oils.

PRACTICE POINTS
- Always ask the patient with seborrheic dermatitis how often they shampoo and if they shampoo their face. It may be helpful to tell them they have 'dandruff of the face' to help motivate treatment.
- Stress the need for using a medicated shampoo daily or every other day. Many patients will paradoxically shampoo less often, as they think they are irritating the skin.
- For best results in seborrheic dermatitis, treat both the causative yeast (with topical imidazole) and the eczematous response (with hydrocortisone).

INFANTILE SEBORRHEIC DERMATITIS

Etiology and pathogenesis

The existence of infantile seborrheic dermatitis as a distinct entity has been questioned recently, although some authors have reported changes in density of *Pityrosporum* yeasts, as in the adult variant. Cradle cap may be a form of seborrheic dermatitis. The onset is from 2 weeks to 6 months.

Clinical

In seborrheic dermatitis of infants, the groin is red and scaly, with prominent involvement of the flexures (in contrast to diaper dermatitis). The scalp is frequently red and scaly. Axillary involvement may be seen (Fig. 6.78). Facial involvement may be prominent, and there is often greasy yellowish scalp scaling, termed cradle cap. In severe cases, the entire body may be affected (Fig. 6.79).

Differential diagnosis

This varies according to the sites affected. Intertrigo, napkin candidiasis, primary irritant dermatitis, AD, infantile psoriasis, Leiner syndrome, and Langerhans cell histiocytosis are all in the differential diagnosis. Involvement of the scalp helps confirm the diagnosis of seborrheic dermatitis, although this is also a feature of the (very rare) condition Langerhans cell histiocytosis.

Atopic dermatitis is an important differential diagnosis, usually present on other areas of the body and sparing the folds in neonates but becoming more flexural later. By contrast to AD, itch is relatively less prominent in seborrheic dermatitis; a useful question is whether the rash is mainly bothering the child (atopic, miserable, and scratching) or the parents (happy child, but 'something must be done'). However, both conditions are common, and their age group of predilection overlaps, so they may coexist (especially in about the second month of life), in which case the differential diagnosis is clearly impossible.

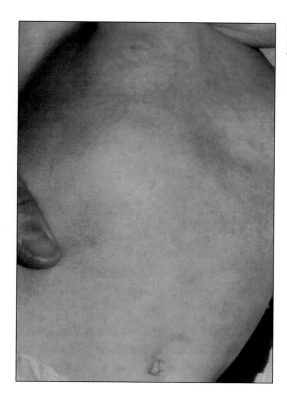

Figure 6.79 Diffuse seborrheic dermatitis in a child.

An irritant contact dermatitis usually accompanies diarrhea in the diapered infant, but skin folds are relatively spared.

Treatment

A daily bath with the use of a medicated shampoo, followed by application of hydrocortisone 1% cream to the flexures and hydrocortisone 1% ointment to the body, is recommended. Alternatively, ketoconazole cream may be applied daily.

RELATED CONDITIONS

Intertrigo
Etiology and pathogenesis
The term intertrigo describes an inflammation of the skin that results from chronic wetness and maceration. Almost any skin at a body fold may be affected, although the groin and inframammary areas are most typically involved.

Clinical
The skin of a body fold becomes red and scaly. Itching is typical. In severe cases, the skin may become macerated. Obese women with large breasts exposed to hot humid climates, or men whose groin stays hot and sweaty, are typical patients. Secondary infection by candida is very common, and its presence is indicated by satellite pustules.

Differential diagnosis
Differential diagnoses are as follows (see also Table 2.4, p. 24).
- Candidiasis of flexures, especially inframammary, may mimic intertrigo or occur as a secondary event. Satellite lesions, sometimes pustular, should suggest this possibility.
- Bacterial infection (staphylococcal or streptococcal) in flexures may occur secondary to intertrigo and should be considered, as it may be misdiagnosed and erroneously treated as a simple 'flare' of known intertrigo.
- Erythrasma will affect the flexures but is red-brown in color, with less inflammation. A Wood's light examination may be performed to exclude erythrasma.
- Tinea cruris contains scale and a raised, scaly border, and concurrent tinea pedis is almost always present.

Treatment

Patients must be educated on the cause of the rash. Specifically, they must understand that any skin does best if kept cool and dry. Typical discussion points include the following. Does the affected skin stay hot and sweaty? What can be done to keep the affected skin cool and dry? What is the patient's profession? (Prolonged sitting on plastic seats, for example, creates a hot sticky environment.) How hot does the patient get during the day? Does the patient have air conditioning at work? At home? What sort of underclothes are worn? Would boxers be better than briefs?

Initially, a topical steroid cream or solution is needed to reduce the inflammation. Cool soaks b.i.d. may help dry a moist, oozing eruption. A steroid cream with added nystatin is helpful in areas where *Candida* is common, for example the inframammary area or the corners of the mouth. Long term, to prevent recurrences, the area *must* be kept dry. A superabsorbant powder (e.g. Zeasorb) two or three times daily is helpful. Some of these products have miconazole or other antifungal powders included. In extreme cases, a strip of an old white sheet or other cloth may be placed in the folds to absorb moisture.

For maintenance therapy, have patients shower every day, use a blow-dryer to completely dry the area, and then apply a roll-on antiperspirant.

Some athletes can get an irritation in the groin from the friction that occurs with exercise. Olive or other oil applied before workouts to decrease friction may be tried.

> **PRACTICE POINT**
> - For the patient with intertrigo, recommend for maintenance the use of a blow-dryer followed by an antiperspirant daily.

Grover disease
Etiology and pathogenesis
Grover disease, also known as transient acantholytic dermatosis, is of unknown etiology. Some view it as a type of heat rash, as it is often associated with increased sweating. Women may develop it at menopause as a result of hot flushes. It may occur in the winter (e.g. after Christmas in a patient given flannel pajamas and a new comforter). The patient should always be asked about increased sweating, particularly at night. A Grover disease-like rash has resulted from interleukin-4 administration.

Clinical
Discrete, truncal pruritic papules and papulovesicles in a middle-aged or elderly person are characteristic (Fig. 6.80). The rash is usually symmetric across the chest, with an increased involvement just below the breasts in both men and women. Although originally described as a transient phenomenon (weeks to months), the disease may last years.

Differential diagnosis
This may include the following.
- Acne—an acneiform condition may occur acutely and diffusely on the trunk, but the lesions are follicular with scattered pustules.
- Miliaria—lesions are smaller, clear or red, and very transient.
- Seborrheic keratoses—tiny lesions of this type may resemble the brownish scaling that occurs in established lesions of Grover disease.
- Itchy red bump disease—a condition of unknown etiology, very itchy, that also tends to affect the trunk in older men mainly.
- Eczemas—the lesions of nummular or of asteatotic eczema are larger.

Treatment
Patients should avoid heat, as it may contribute to an outbreak. Air conditioning or a ceiling fan may help, as may emollients or topical steroids. Dapsone, PUVA, and isotretinoin have been useful but are usually not needed.

Papuloerythroderma of Ofuji
Etiology and pathogenesis
Papuloerythroderma of Ofuji is a term used to describe a rash with a characteristic sparing of folds known as the 'deckchair' sign (Fig. 6.81). It

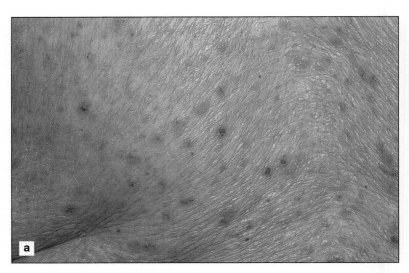
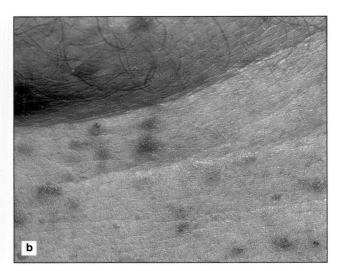

Figure 6.80 Grover disease. (**a**) This older man presented with very pruritic papulovesicles on the abdomen and trunk, which proved to be Grover disease. (**b**) Close-up view of the crusted erythematous papules.

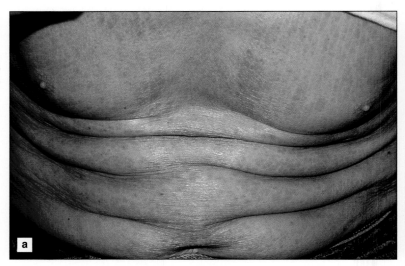
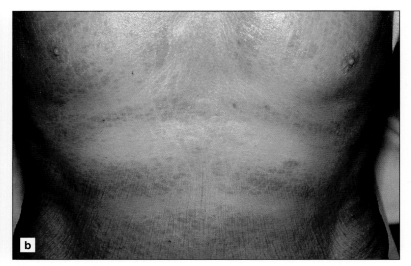

Figure 6.81 Papuloerythroderma of Ofuji. (**a,b**) The 'deckchair' sign is the appearance of horizontal bands of erythema separated by normal skin. The normal skin occurs in the folds made by bending forward.

has been argued that this disease is not a single entity but instead a pattern of expression of, or association with, various inflammatory dermatoses, including lymphoma, hypereosinophilic syndrome, cancers, AD, pityriasis versicolor, and drug reactions. The work-up should include the exclusion of the above-mentioned entities, especially lymphoma. Localized or abortive forms have been described.

Clinical

There is diffuse, papular erythroderma that spares the skin folds, creating the deckchair sign. This condition typically occurs in older patients, many of whom have a peripheral eosinophilia and some lymphadenopathy.

Differential diagnosis

This eruption has a very characteristic appearance and the clinical label is usually not in doubt, although the underlying cause is often uncertain.

Treatment

If no specific cause is found, topical or oral corticosteroids (e.g. 30–60 mg of prednisone every day) may be tried. PUVA and interferon-alpha have been used. Ciclosporin has been reported to be very effective.

FURTHER READING

Bourke J, Coulson I, English J. Guidelines for care of contact dermatitis. Br J Dermatol 2001; 145: 877–85

Hanifin J (ed) Management of atopic dermatitis: current status and future possibilities. Dermatol Ther 1996; 1: 1–103

Hanifin JM, Cooper KD, Ho VC, et al. Guidelines of care for atopic dermatitis. J Am Acad Dermatol 2004; 50: 391–404

Rietschel RL, Fowler JF. Fisher's Contact Dermatitis, 5th edn. Philadelphia: Lippincott Williams & Wilkins, 2001

7 Psoriasis and Related Disorders

PSORIASIS

Psoriasis (Fig. 7.1) is a common skin disorder with a prevalence of about 2% in white populations. The severity varies from a minor, intermittent, localized skin eruption through to total skin involvement and associated systemic effects. It may develop at any age (the oldest recorded age of onset is 108 years), but is most frequent in young adults, in whom the psychologic effects of skin disease are often considerable. Both sexes are affected equally. Although psoriasis rarely causes severe symptoms, its high prevalence and psychologic impact make it one of the most important skin diseases.

Pathology

Psoriasis is not often biopsied for diagnostic purposes, as the diagnosis is usually clinical. When it is biopsied due to atypical clinical features, this may be reflected in the pathology report; in the differential between palmar dermatitis versus psoriasis, it is not uncommon for reports to describe the same dilemma that arises clinically (as a psoriasiform dermatitis versus an eczematized psoriasis). None the less, it is helpful to know the main features of psoriasis, bearing in mind that processes such as psoriasiform drug eruptions that mimic psoriasis may show some, but often not all, of these pathologic features. Psoriasis itself is characterized by the following features.

- Epidermal proliferation—the epidermis is thickened and hyper-keratotic, and mitoses occur above the normal basal layer. However, the epidermis above the papillae is thin (suprapapillary thinning), a feature that is absent from many other causes of psoriasiform epidermal thickening.
- Loss of epidermal differentiation—in particular, being manifest as retention of nuclei in keratinocytes (known as parakeratosis, when it is visible in cells in the stratum corneum). There is also a decrease in the granular cell layer, with a corresponding alteration in epidermal cytokeratin patterns.
- Vascular proliferation, typically seen as tortuosity of papillary vessels; immunologic methods can show up-regulation of endothelial cell markers.
- Inflammation—the T lymphocyte is the main early infiltrating cell, and is important in pathogenesis. Influx of neutrophils typically causes small microabscesses or pustules within the epidermis and stratum corneum (Munro microabscesses; their presence strongly suggests a diagnosis of psoriasis, and they are particularly prominent in the pustular and erythrodermic variants of psoriasis).

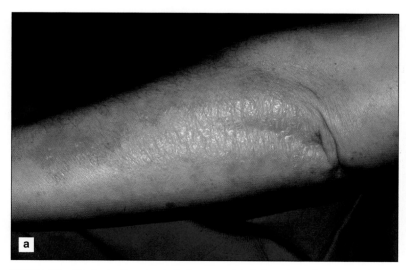

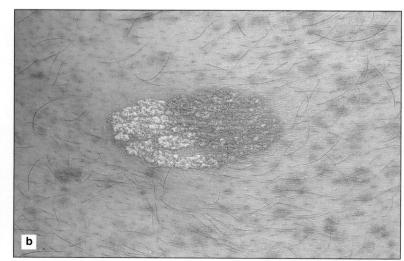

Figure 7.1 Psoriasis. The classic lesions consist of discrete erythematous plaques with flakes of silvery scaling, shown in (**a**) at a typical site on the extensor aspect of the forearm near the elbow. The scaling can be accentuated by gentle scratching, a process known as grattage (**b**).

Etiology and pathogenesis

The pathogenesis of psoriasis has been studied in great detail but is still not fully understood. Some involved factors are discussed here.

Genetics and human leukocyte antigen (HLA) associations

Genetic factors are important. There are two main peaks of onset age: in the late teens to twenties, and in the sixth and seventh decades. In the younger age group in particular, a familial tendency is common (present in 40–50%, up to 75% if onset is before 20 years), which is usually consistent in age of onset. The earlier age of onset is associated with HLA-Cw6, B13, and B17, whereas the older age of onset is associated with HLA-Cw2 and B27. There is high concordance in monozygotic twins and lesser (15–20%) concordance in dizygotic twins. Several putative psoriasis genes have been identified; the most convincing to date is *PSOR1*, which lies within the HLA gene coding region. Psoriasis is relatively uncommon in black or Asian skin (Fig. 7.2a).

Inflammatory mediators and epidermal proliferation

Several interrelated factors are involved.

- Epidermal proliferation. Psoriasis is characterized by rapid epidermal maturation and turnover. The cell cycle time of epidermal cells is much shorter than normal, such that movement of cells from the basal layer to the stratum corneum is about 10-fold faster than normal (3 days instead of 30 days). In conjunction with this, altered epidermal differentiation causes pathologic changes, as described earlier. This process involves calcium and calmodulin (hence the effect of vitamin D analogs therapeutically), and retinoids.
- Prostaglandins. Prostaglandin metabolism has in the past attracted considerable interest in psoriasis; the clinical correlate is that some non-steroidal antiinflammatory drugs, which inhibit cyclooxygenase and therefore increase metabolism toward leukotrienes, may provoke psoriasis.
- Neutrophils. Influx of neutrophil polymorphs is also a characteristic histologic feature, as described earlier.
- Lymphocytes and cytokines. T lymphocytes probably have a central role in the pathogenesis of psoriasis, due to their ability to generate active cytokines. Among the cytokines, tumor necrosis factor (TNF) is probably pivotal: new monoclonal anti-TNF antibodies (see Ch. 4) are very powerful treatments for psoriasis. The cytokine pattern in psoriasis is termed TH1, and differs from the TH2 pattern of atopic dermatitis.

Disease associations

Psoriasis occurs with increased frequency in association with the following.

- Reiter syndrome.
- Palmoplantar pustulosis (discussed later in this chapter).
- Subcorneal pustulosis (Ch. 16).
- Inflammatory bowel disease, notably Crohn disease.
- Other autoimmune diseases, for example vitiligo (Fig. 7.2b), pemphigus, and pemphigoid.
- HIV infection—probably not a true association, but (like seborrheic dermatitis and Reiter syndrome) psoriasis may be particularly severe and difficult to manage in this situation.

Provocative factors

Provocative factors in psoriasis include the following.

- Drugs—notably lithium, antimalarials, and beta-blockers (see also psoriasiform drug eruptions, Fig. 18.52).
- Streptococcal infection—particularly linked with guttate psoriasis (discussed later in this chapter).
- Alcohol—a complex relationship; alcohol excess seems to be associated with an adverse effect on psoriasis, with more inflamed plaques and with poorer treatment compliance, and it may contraindicate some of the systemic treatment options. However, the precise nature of the relationship with alcohol is difficult to determine: while there are arguments in favor of a causal relationship, the counterargument is that severe psoriasis is stressful and leads to increased drinking.
- Cigarettes—there is a particularly strong link with palmoplantar pustulosis (discussed later). There is also a modest increase in the proportion of patients with psoriasis who smoke cigarettes compared with in the general population; the same cause or effect argument applies as for alcohol consumption.
- Local trauma—psoriasis is one of the disorders that classically exhibits the Koebner phenomenon (see Ch. 2 also); minor skin injury such as scratches or burns are the most common trigger (Fig. 7.3), but other rashes, such as sunburn or contact dermatitis, may be viewed as a form of injury and act as a trigger (Fig. 7.4). Psoriasis may develop in such areas a few days after the insult, especially in patients with unstable or increasing psoriasis at the time.

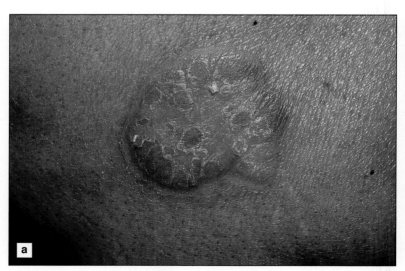

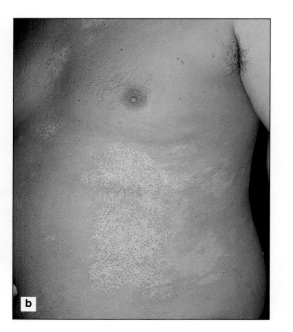

Figure 7.2 Skin color and psoriasis. (**a**) Psoriasis is relatively uncommon in black or Asian skin. (**b**) Psoriasis coexisting with vitiligo. This association is not uncommon; the psoriasis may colocalize with vitiligo, as shown here, or the two may have totally independent body site distribution. In either case, the association can be a problem: it can be difficult to distinguish vitiligo from postinflammatory hypopigmentation, and phototherapy can cause burning of the vitiliginous skin.

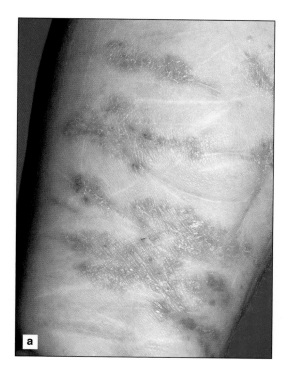

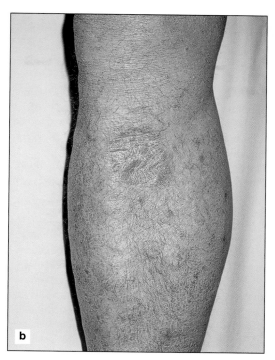

Figure 7.3 The Koebner phenomenon. (**a**) Psoriasis occurring at the site of self-inflicted cuts on the wrist. Note that older, healed cuts are unaffected; this process affects only new wounds, usually when psoriasis is in a phase of exacerbation. (**b**) An interesting variation of the Koebner phenomenon, in which psoriasis has localized to a skin graft recipient site below the knee. (**c**) The Koebner phenomenon causing localized psoriasis around the nipple in a mother with a breast-fed baby. Treatment options are limited due to the risk of chemical ingestion by the baby. (**d**) The Koebner phenomenon, localizing psoriasis to a recent abdominal scar and ostomy site, with more scattered plaques elsewhere.

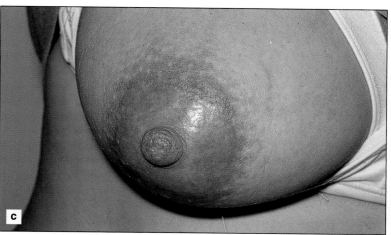

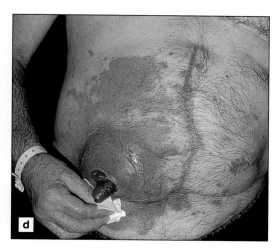

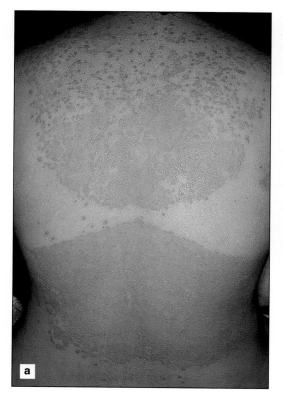

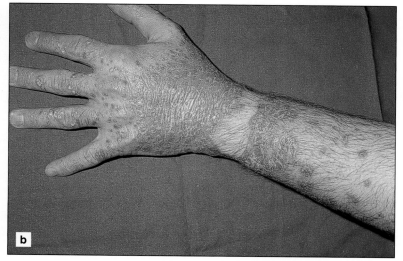

Figure 7.4 The Koebner phenomenon, in these two cases being apparent by virtue of areas that have been spared. (**a**) Extensive small-plaque psoriasis triggered by sunburn and sparing the covered sites. (**b**) This patient appears to have a photosensitivity reaction sparing the watch strap area. In fact, the rash was psoriasis, occurring as a Koebner reaction into an area of contact dermatitis to a rubber glove but sparing the area under the watch.

Table 7.1   MAIN CLINICAL PATTERNS AND SITE-RELATED VARIANTS OF PSORIASIS

Variant	Description
Main pattern	
Plaque psoriasis	Usually chronic, often familial; plaques or annular lesions
Guttate psoriasis	Typically eruptive small spots, mainly trunk; associated with streptococcal sore throat
Generalized pustular psoriasis	Severe, usually rapid onset; often with systemic symptoms; a medical emergency
Palmoplantar pustulosis	Chronic; pustules of different colors and sizes, due to progressive new lesions evolving over time
Acropustulosis of Hallopeau	Subungual and distal digit pustules
'Unstable' psoriasis	Rapidly increasing in extent and degree of inflammation; often itchy
Erythrodermic or exfoliative	Severe, variable speed of onset; often with systemic symptoms
Subacute annular (Lapière)	Rare, diagnostically difficult
Linear	Rare; usually lower leg, and associated with plaques at other sites
Specific sites	
Elbows and/or knees	Common site(s), may be affected in isolation but usually symmetric
Hands and feet	On palms and soles has important diagnostic and therapeutic issues
Scalp	Common site, may be affected in isolation or just with elbows or knees
Flexures and genital	Not uncommon, may not be volunteered; therapeutic differences from ordinary plaques
Nails	Usually in patients with known psoriasis; may occur in isolation (usually adults)
Face	Underestimated; usually in patients with psoriasis elsewhere

Table 7.2   DIFFERENTIAL DIAGNOSIS OF PSORIASIS BY CLINICAL PATTERN

Clinical pattern	Differential diagnosis
Plaque psoriasis *Discoid lesions*	Discoid eczema (which is less well demarcated, much more itchy, often on legs) Subacute cutaneous lupus erythematosus (usually photosensitive) Bowen disease (if limited plaques on the legs) Lichen simplex (usually solitary lesion and overtly itchy) Lichen planus (main difficulty in diagnosis is on legs; remember to look for oral lesions)
Annular lesions	Tinea corporis Subacute cutaneous lupus erythematosus Sarcoidosis Parapsoriasis or mycosis fungoides
Guttate psoriasis	Viral exanthem or pityriasis rosea Drug eruption Eruptive lichen planus Infections (e.g. syphilis, scabies), less commonly
Generalized pustular psoriasis	Folliculitis (especially bacterial, yeast, eosinophilic) Acute generalized eruptive pustulosis (a drug reaction, Ch. 18) Extensive miliaria or areas of macerated keratin
Palmoplantar pustulosis	Tinea manuum or pedis (suspect especially if single foot or non-smoker) Pompholyx eczema
Acropustulosis of Hallopeau	Fungal nail disease Acute bacterial infection (paronychia) Herpetic whitlow
'Unstable' psoriasis	Drug reactions Viral exanthem or pityriasis rosea
Erythrodermic or exfoliative	Any differential diagnosis of erythroderma (Table 7.4), especially pityriasis rubra pilaris
Subacute annular (Lapière)	Tinea corporis Lupus erythematosus Cutaneous lymphoma Drug reactions
Linear	Lichen striatus Linear lichen planus or rarities such as linear porokeratosis

Table 7.3   DIFFERENTIAL DIAGNOSIS OF PSORIASIS BY BODY SITE

Body site	Differential diagnosis
Elbows and/or knees	Thick skin (normal variant or occupational friction, usually below the knee over the tibial tubercle) Granuloma annulare (common at these sites) Dermatomyositis (elbow and knee involvement is underestimated, and often quite psoriasiform)
Hands and feet	Dermatitis (especially lichen simplex or hyperkeratotic dermatitis of palms) Tinea (beware: it can coexist with psoriasis) Pityriasis rubra pilaris Palmoplantar keratodermas Bazex acrokeratosis paraneoplastica (rare, distal fingers)
Scalp	Seborrheic dermatitis (often affects ears also, as does psoriasis) Lichen simplex (usually affects nape of neck, a common site for psoriasis also) Actinic keratoses (bald scalp) Collagen vascular disease (lupus erythematosus or dermatomyositis), less commonly
Flexures and genital psoriasis	Flexures and female genital: seborrheic dermatitis, candidal or bacterial intertrigo, tinea (especially groin flexures), contact dermatitis, lichen simplex, erythrasma, Hailey–Hailey disease; also note that psoriasis of the nipple may need to be differentiated from dermatitis or from Paget disease Male genital: sexually transmitted diseases, bacterial or candidal infection, lichen planus, erythroplasia of Queyrat
Nails	Fungal disease (note: may coexist with psoriasis, especially toenails) Dermatitis: nail fold involvement may cause pitting or transverse ridging Chronic paronychia: causes transverse ridging Trachyonychia: surface changes may resemble psoriatic pitting Disorders causing onycholysis (see Ch. 29)
Face	Dermatitis: especially seborrheic, allergic contact dermatitis Lupus erythematosus Bazex acrokeratosis paraneoplastica (rare, nose and ears)

Clinical types and sites of psoriasis

The main clinical patterns and sites of psoriasis, and their differential diagnosis, are summarized in Tables 7.1–7.3.

Plaque psoriasis

This is the common pattern of psoriasis (Figs 7.1 and 7.5). Plaques may occur at very localized areas or may be widespread, usually with a symmetric body site distribution. Some body sites, notably elbows, knees, scalp, and sacrum, are common areas for plaque psoriasis. Central clearing of plaques is a common feature, leading to an annular morphology. Silvery scaling is typical but may not be apparent in flexures or if emollients have been used; massive hyperkeratotic scaling may occur (rupioid psoriasis, Fig. 7.6).

Guttate psoriasis

This variant of psoriasis (Fig. 7.7) is often triggered by streptococcal upper respiratory tract infections (Fig. 7.8). The psoriasis appears about 7–10 days later, and may arise de novo or in patients with a background of preexisting plaque psoriasis.

Guttate psoriasis is a common pattern of psoriasis in children, about a third of whom have a negative family history and 30–40% of whom never develop ordinary psoriasis at a later age. The pattern is a sudden eruption of numerous tiny spots (Fig. 7.7), and may be associated with the Koebner phenomenon. It is difficult to treat because of the scattering of lesions, but often responds well to sunlight or phototherapy, or to mild topical steroids, and even, if untreated, will generally resolve over a period of a few months. In individuals with recurrent episodes associated with streptococcal sore throats, some will respond to prophylactic low-dose penicillin, or to tonsillectomy. If required in such cases, the streptococcal trigger may be proved by bacteriology swabs at the time of the sore throat or serologically for several weeks afterward.

Generalized pustular psoriasis

The most common type of generalized pustular psoriasis (GPP), known as the von Zumbusch type, is a severe and progressive disorder in which there are inflammatory red patches with irregularly shaped borders, studded with small pustules that are usually 1–2 mm in size (Figs 7.9 and 7.10). Affected patients have sore skin, fever, and malaise; hypoalbuminemia, hypocalcemia, and leukocytosis are frequent. Some cases are drug-induced, and abrupt withdrawal of systemic corticosteroids in a patient with known psoriasis is a significant risk factor. For this reason, use of oral or very potent topical steroids in patients with psoriasis is best avoided, although this approach may be used by specialists on occasions to achieve rapid reduction of inflammation while introducing other systemic therapy.

The pustules are sterile, but secondary infection of preexisting psoriatic plaques should be excluded by culture of pustule contents and blood cultures. Occasionally, tiny areas of macerated keratin within plaques of psoriasis (especially in flexures or under occlusion) may mimic pustular psoriasis, usually in patients without the obvious malaise of true GPP.

Oral lesions of fissured tongue or geographical tongue (migratory glossitis) occur with increased frequency in patients with generalized pustular, erythrodermic, and other actively increasing psoriasis (Fig. 7.11).

Variants of GPP include subacute forms (Fig. 7.12), and an essentially identical eruption can occur de novo in pregnancy, known as impetigo herpetiformis. It recurs in subsequent pregnancies but remits after delivery. GPP can also occur in children, usually resembling a severe seborrheic dermatitis initially. Bullous lesions may occur in pustular and other forms of psoriasis (Fig. 7.13).

Palmoplantar pustulosis

This disorder and acropustulosis of Hallopeau may be grouped together as localized pustular psoriasis. However, it is a matter of debate whether palmoplantar pustulosis (PPP) is a form of psoriasis or a closely related disorder. It has a different age of onset (mostly over 50 years), a female predominance (equal sex incidence in ordinary psoriasis), different HLA associations, and a strong link (about 90%) with cigarette smoking (compared with about 50% in plaque psoriasis). However, about 20–30% of patients have ordinary plaque psoriasis, far more than expected by

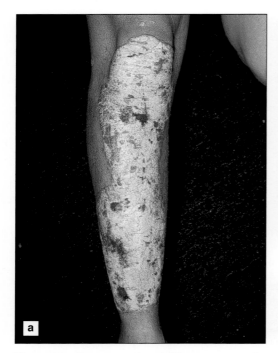

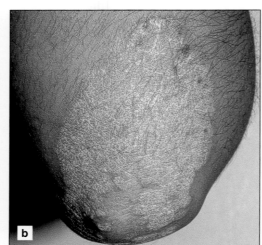

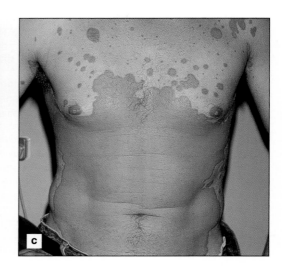

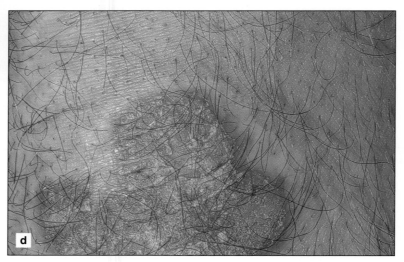

Figure 7.5 Some examples of different patterns of psoriasis. (**a**) Plaque psoriasis, with very marked silvery hyperkeratosis. Topical therapies and UV treatments are unlikely to be useful unless a keratolytic is used initially. (**b**) Plaque psoriasis affecting the elbow, a typical site and one that may be affected in isolation. (**c**) Extensive plaque psoriasis in which lesions have gradually merged, producing a large confluent erythematous plaque on the abdomen. (**d**) Psoriatic plaques (and, less commonly, some other localized inflammatory lesions) may have a narrow band of vasoconstriction around the plaque, an appearance known as a Woronoff ring.

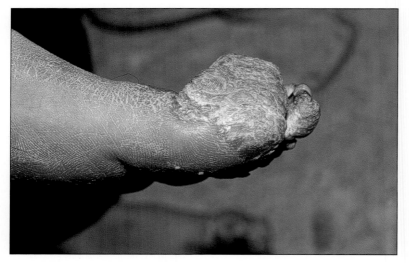

Figure 7.6 A massively hyperkeratotic plaque of psoriasis on the toe. This pyramidal pattern of hyperkeratosis may affect many lesions, and is known as rupioid psoriasis.

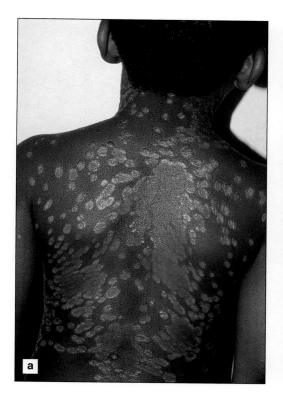

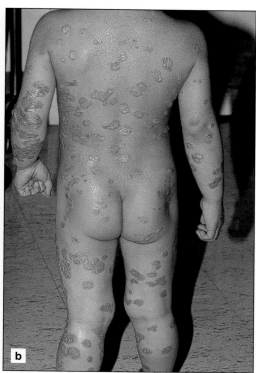

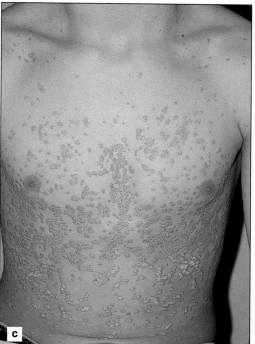

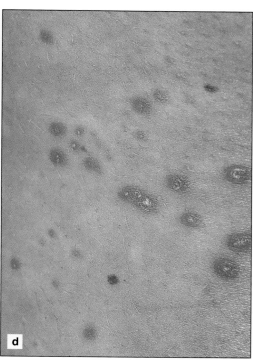

Figure 7.7 Guttate psoriasis. (**a**) In an African-Caribbean child: the typical scattered small lesions look white due to the visible scaling but essentially invisible erythema. (**b**) Psoriasis in a 3-year-old child. In most instances of psoriasis in this age group, psoriasis has eruptive onset and resolves in a few months. However, the presence of rather larger plaques than usual for guttate psoriasis should cause some reservation about the prognosis for recovery. (**c**) Extensive tiny spots of guttate psoriasis on the trunk in a young adult. This pattern may be confused with a viral exanthem but is scalier and lasts longer. (**d**) Close-up view of guttate psoriasis lesions.

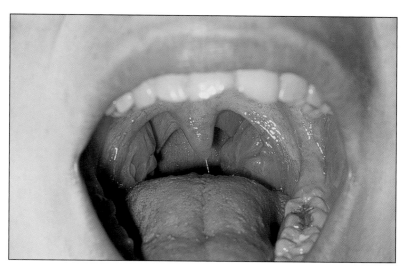

Figure 7.8 Enlarged tonsils in a patient with guttate psoriasis triggered by a streptococcal sore throat. This can often be diagnosed in retrospect by serologic tests (antistreptolysin titer).

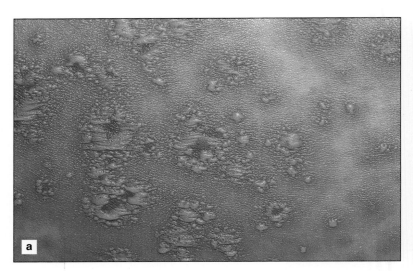

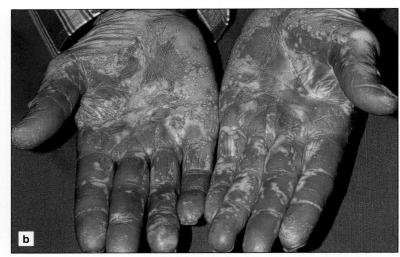

Figure 7.9 Generalized pustular psoriasis (GPP). (**a**) Demonstrating semiconfluent, grouped, tiny, superficial pustules. Patients usually have significant malaise and often pyrexia, so primary infections and severe pustular drug eruptions (Ch. 18) may need to be excluded, especially if systemic immunosuppressive therapy is likely to be required. (**b**) Palmar involvement in a patient with GPP, demonstrating confluent erythema and pustulation with skin shedding.

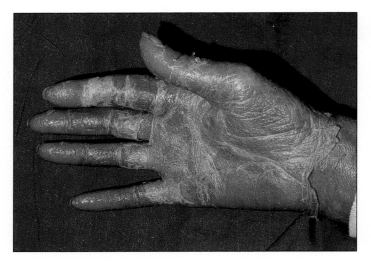

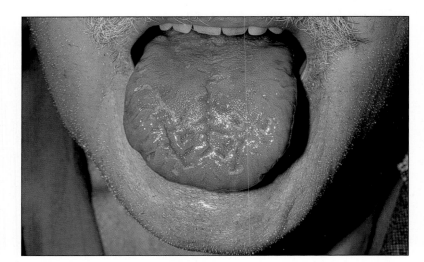

Figure 7.10 Marked palmar desquamation in the resolving stage of acute generalized pustular psoriasis.

Figure 7.11 A red, fissured tongue may be associated with generalized pustular psoriasis.

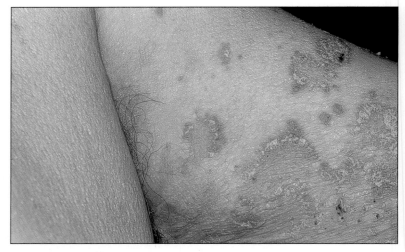

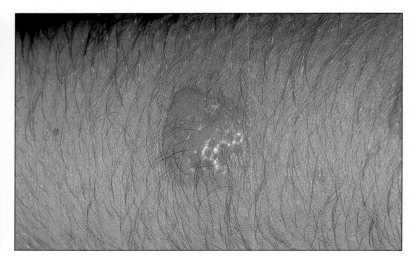

Figure 7.12 A less aggressive form of generalized pustular psoriasis can occur and is known as the subacute annular variant (of Lapière), shown here on the thigh; these patients are not usually systemically unwell, and the eruption progresses over several weeks.

Figure 7.13 Bullae may occur in patients with psoriasis exposed to excessive sun.

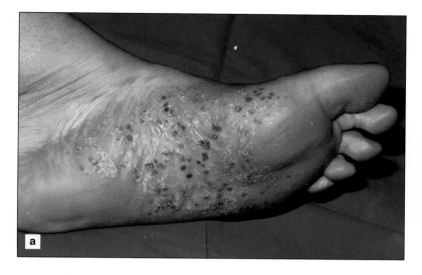

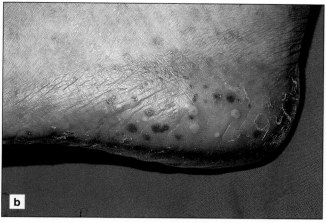

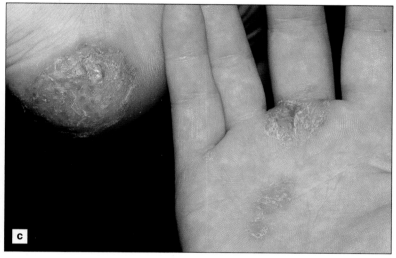

Figure 7.14 Palmoplantar pustulosis. The precise relationship of this disorder to psoriasis remains debatable, but the physical signs are typical. (**a**) The pustules are fairly large (often 5 mm in diameter), on a well-defined erythematous scaly background. (**b**) Closer view of pustules, demonstrating the mixture of different colors (yellow, green, and 'dried up' brown) that are typically present. (**c**) The palm lesions in this patient are very suggestive of 'ordinary' psoriasis, despite the more pustular appearance on the heel. (Panel b from Lawrence CM, Cox NH. Physical Signs in Dermatology, 2nd edn. London: Mosby, 2002.)

chance, suggesting that it is a psoriasis variant rather than a separate disorder.

Palmoplantar pustulosis usually presents as a localized scaling erythematous plaque on one or both feet, or (less commonly) on the palms of the hands, or at both sites. The heel, instep, and central palm are the most common sites. Characteristically, the pustules are large (usually about 5 mm), and several stages of evolution of pustules are present concurrently (Fig. 7.14). When there is a solitary plaque on one foot, it is important to exclude fungal infection; in symmetric disease, pompholyx eczema (especially with secondary infection) may resemble pustular psoriasis but usually occurs at a younger age and causes much more prominent symptoms.

Unfortunately, PPP is difficult to treat; stopping smoking does not reverse the disorder, and it usually runs a chronic course.

Acropustulosis of Hallopeau

This disorder resembles PPP in morphology of pustules but affects one or more (usually several) distal digits. The subungual pustules that occur may result in transient or permanent loss of nails (Fig. 7.15). It is most troublesome on the fingers due to the potential for irreversible damage to the nails, and due to the functional deficit that it causes.

Unstable psoriasis

This is not usually viewed as a specific variant of psoriasis, but it has important implications. The term is used to describe psoriasis that is rapidly increasing in extent; is often very red, inflamed, and pruritic; and often exhibits areas of Koebner reaction (Fig. 7.16). Sometimes, there is a trigger such as a recent infection, or Koebnering of psoriasis into a drug rash. The important issue is to avoid potentially irritant treatments such as anthralin or vitamin D analogs, as these may further inflame the lesions. Generally, use of a potent topical corticosteroid with gradual decrease in

potency, while concurrently introducing more specific agents, will allow the psoriasis to settle to a less inflamed state, but careful supervision is required, as some patients will progress to subtotal or total erythroderma.

Erythrodermic and exfoliative psoriasis

Erythrodermic psoriasis (Fig. 7.17) is an uncommon form of psoriasis that usually occurs in patients with known and deteriorating psoriasis, but it can occasionally present de novo. In the latter case, it is important to differentiate other causes of erythroderma (Table 7.4) because, although some of the treatments for erythroderma are common to all causes, certain treatments are more psoriasis-specific. In particular, in erythrodermic psoriasis, systemic corticosteroids are best avoided (due to the risk of pustular psoriasis on withdrawal), but agents such as systemic retinoids or methotrexate, which would not usually be used for most other causes of erythroderma, may be appropriate. It is also important to consider factors that may have provoked erythroderma, such as withdrawal of corticosteroids or other systemic therapies, UV burns, drug reactions, and so on.

The systemic consequences of erythroderma are listed in Table 7.5. Thermoregulation is impaired due to central effects of interleukins and other cytokines, the huge cutaneous blood flow causing heat loss, and impaired sweating. Shedding of scale, and the malabsorption that occurs in erythrodermic states, leads to loss of protein and of folate, of which body stores are low; ankle edema may occur due to hypoproteinemia or high-output cardiac failure. The high epidermal turnover causes hyperuricemia.

Exfoliative psoriasis (Fig. 7.18; see also Fig. 18.52) is considered with erythroderma, as it usually arises in similar situations. However, some patients have profound shedding of scale without a prominent erythrodermic component; they are less unwell systemically but may still have the metabolic consequences of erythroderma (see Table 7.5), especially hypoproteinemia and folate deficiency.

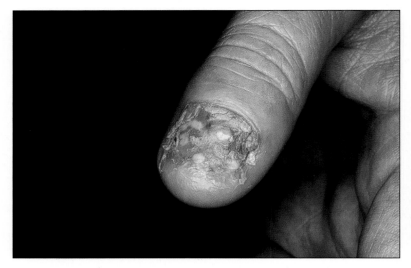

Figure 7.15 Acropustulosis of Hallopeau, showing the nail destruction that may occur. The pulps of the digits may also be affected.

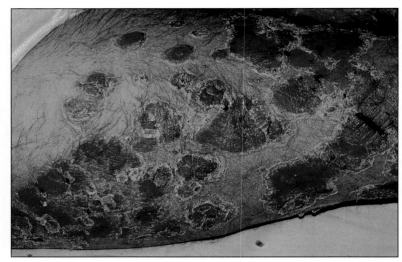

Figure 7.16 Unstable psoriasis on the thigh: widespread, bright-red, inflammatory psoriasis with silvery but rather loose scaling and some fissuring.

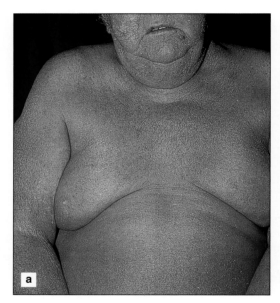

a

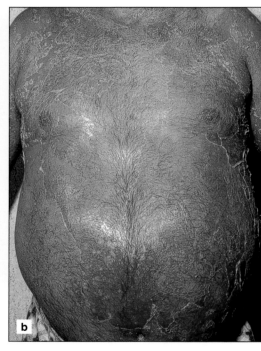

b

Figure 7.17 Erythrodermic psoriasis. (**a**) Erosive areas on the trunk in a patient with a long history of psoriasis, which had rapidly become 'unstable' and inflamed. (**b**) Erythrodermic psoriasis. The differential diagnosis includes drug eruptions, dermatitis, and cutaneous lymphoma. A previous history of psoriasis or the presence of typical nail changes may be useful, but biopsy may be required.

Table 7.4 CAUSES OF ERYTHRODERMA	
Cause	**Approximate frequency (%)**
Eczema (atopic, contact allergies, seborrheic)	40
Psoriasis	30
Drug eruptions (allopurinol, sulfonamides, anticonvulsants, penicillins, imatinib)	15
Cutaneous lymphomas, Sézary syndrome	10
Others (pityriasis rubra pilaris, ichthyosiform erythrodermas, severe dermatophytosis or infestations)	5

Table 7.5   SYSTEMIC EFFECTS OF ERYTHRODERMA

Malaise, fever, shivering
Insensible heat loss from the skin, impaired sweating
Hypovolemia, hypoproteinemia
High-output cardiac failure
Leukocytosis
Anemia, folate deficiency
Hyperuricemia
Malabsorption

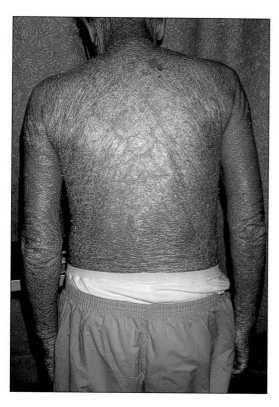

Figure 7.18 Exfoliative psoriasis in a patient taking lithium, a known trigger for psoriasis.

Specific sites of psoriasis

The main sites affected by psoriasis, with their features and differential diagnosis, are summarized in Tables 7.1 and 7.3. A few site-specific differential diagnostic and therapeutic issues are discussed here; more general aspects of both issues are discussed and summarized later.

Hands and feet

The hands and feet can be affected by ordinary plaque psoriasis or by PPP (discussed earlier). Plaque psoriasis of the palms or soles (Fig. 7.19) can occur without psoriasis at other sites, in which case it can be extremely difficult to distinguish from a chronic dermatitis in some individuals. A frictional dermatitis known as hyperkeratotic dermatitis of the palms is particularly difficult to differentiate with confidence, and even histologic examination of a biopsy specimen may show mixed features (see Fig. 6.34).

Features that may help to establish a diagnosis include the following.
- Hyperkeratosis—silvery hyperkeratosis strongly suggests psoriasis.
- Sharp demarcation of lesions—strongly suggests psoriasis.
- Significant itch—favors dermatitis.
- Nail changes—in dermatitis, usually consist of shallow irregular pits, rippled appearance, transverse ridging if there is paronychia; in psoriasis, usually see more sharply defined pits, onycholysis and distal thickening, pinkish yellow subungual color.
- Vesicles—may occur in palmar psoriasis, but large numbers favor dermatitis.
- Pustules—if sterile, favor psoriasis.
- Psoriasis elsewhere—favors psoriasis but may need to be looked for.

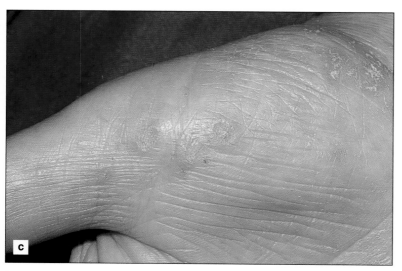

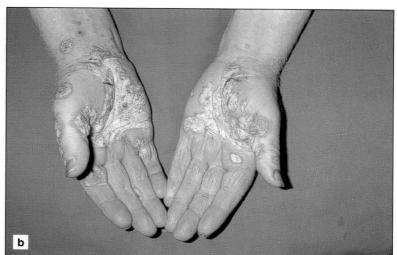

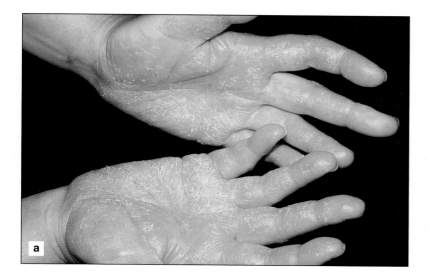

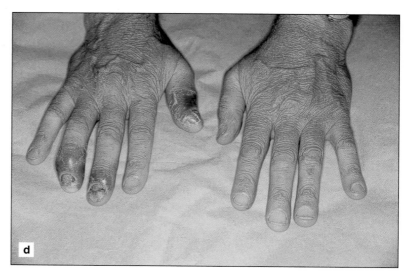

Figure 7.19 Psoriasis of the hands. (**a**) This patient had nail changes, which may be helpful in the differential diagnosis from dermatitis. (**b**) Discrete, well-demarcated silvery plaques on the hands, a pattern typical of psoriasis. This type of palmar involvement may be very limiting, despite the small proportion of body area involved. (**c**) The Caro–Senear ridge, a pattern of psoriasis that is useful to distinguish this from dermatitis. The lesions are usually on the sides of the fingers or border of the hand, and have central umbilication. (**d**) Psoriasis of hands with a predominantly acral distribution, marked nail dystrophy, and terminal interphalangeal joint arthritis.

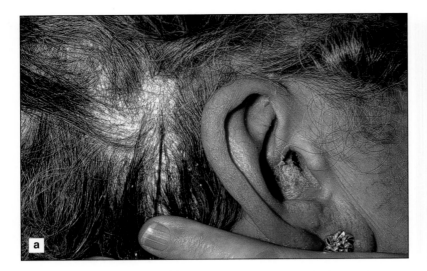

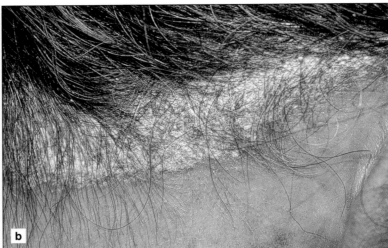

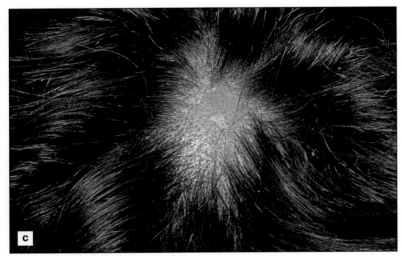

Figure 7.20 Scalp psoriasis. (**a**) Demonstrating the typical silvery scaling and the commonly associated involvement of the ears. Scalp involvement in isolation causes diagnostic confusion. (**b**) Involvement of scalp psoriasis: involvement of the lateral scalp margin, extending on to the nape, is a common pattern. (**c**) Alopecia may occur due to severe inflammation in scalp psoriasis. If treated promptly with keratolytics and antiinflammatory measures such as corticosteroids, there is usually full regrowth. In this example, intact follicles capable of regrowth are clearly visible.

Where the diagnosis of psoriasis can be made with confidence, it allows a large number of topical and systemic treatment options that would not typically be used for dermatitis (e.g. strong tars, anthralin, vitamin D analogs, systemic retinoids, and methotrexate). Palm and sole psoriasis tends to be more keratotic than typical psoriatic plaques, and a keratolytic agent is an important component of the therapeutic regimen. It is also disproportionately disabling for the surface area involved, and may be a reason to use systemic therapies. Finally, a clear distinction from dermatitis may be important for the patient's occupation.

Palmoplantar pustulosis can likewise be difficult to distinguish from fungal infection, especially if only one palm or sole is affected.

Scalp

The scalp is commonly affected by psoriasis (Fig. 7.20). The typical pattern is one of well-demarcated erythematous plaques with thick silvery scaling, affecting the area above the ears or the occipital region. Involvement of the frontal scalp margin is also common but usually less scaly. The differential diagnosis is predominantly from seborrheic dermatitis (especially frontal scalp margin and around the ears, see Ch. 6) and from lichen simplex (occipital).

Treatment is affected by the presence of hair, which limits use of ointments and may be stained by some treatments.

Flexures and genital psoriasis

Flexural psoriasis (Fig. 7.21) may occur in isolation (sometimes termed inverse psoriasis), especially in children. Umbilical involvement is common, usually in those with psoriasis at other sites but occasionally as the presenting feature.

Flexural psoriasis differs from psoriasis found at more typical sites, as the moist, warm, thin skin of the flexures tends to be erythematous but not particularly scaly. It is frequently misdiagnosed as candidiasis or erythrasma. Napkin psoriasis in infants resembles seborrheic dermatitis. Treatments for the flexures should be relatively mild compared with those for other body sites.

Genital psoriasis also causes diagnostic and therapeutic difficulty (Fig. 7.22). In women, vulval skin may require short-term potent steroid applications to achieve symptomatic control of psoriasis; distinction from candidiasis is important. In men, genital involvement not infrequently occurs in isolation and causes diagnostic difficulty, but rarely causes significant symptoms other than anxiety about the diagnosis.

Nails

The nails are frequently involved in patients with psoriasis, and can provide useful support for an uncertain diagnosis (Fig. 7.23). In patients with psoriatic arthropathy, nail involvement occurs in about 80%, and is almost inevitable in distal interphalangeal joint arthropathy. However, psoriatic nail dystrophy can also occur in isolation, in which case it is typically confused with fungal infection; note also that fungal infection may occur in the already damaged psoriatic nail, especially thickened toenails.

The features of nail psoriasis are often striking and specific, allowing a confident diagnosis even in the absence of psoriasis at other sites. They include well-defined pits of the nail plate, onycholysis, subungual hyperkeratosis, oil drop appearance, and salmon-pink subungual patches.

Other sites and variants

The face is said to be uncommonly affected by psoriasis, although this is not true of the patients with psoriasis of severity requiring hospital referral (Fig. 7.24). Linear variants of psoriasis may occur in isolation or with psoriasis at other sites, and are relatively resistant to treatment (Fig. 7.25).

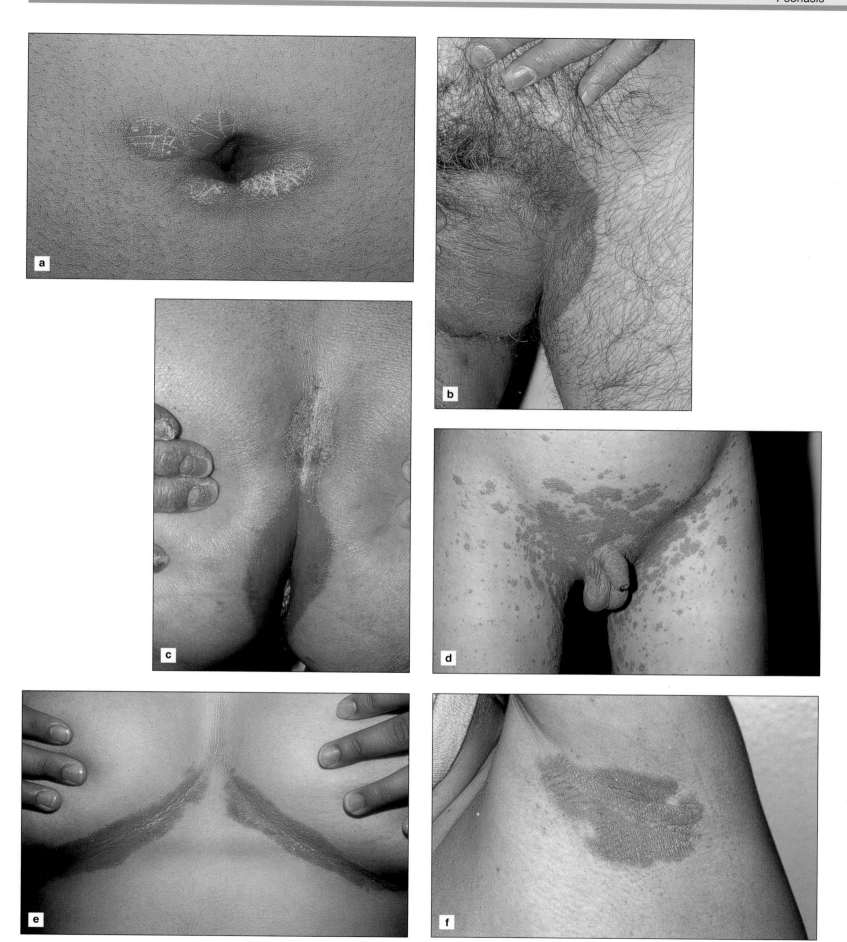

Figure 7.21 (**a**) Flexural psoriasis affecting the umbilicus is common. It has a more moist erythematous appearance, with less scaling, compared with plaques at non-flexural areas. (**b**) Flexural psoriasis affecting the groin of an adult man. Treatment options may be limited by irritancy. (**c**) Flexural psoriasis of the sacrum and perianal skin. The sacrum in particular is a common area for psoriasis, but symptomatic lesions and diagnostic problems are more likely with the perianal lesion. (**d**) Flexural psoriasis, in this case in the groin area, is a common variant of psoriasis in children. (**e**) Flexural psoriasis of the inframammary area is common, and may require treatments with an antiseptic or anticandidal component to deal with secondary infection. (**f**) Flexural psoriasis in the axilla of an adult may be difficult to distinguish from seborrheic dermatitis.

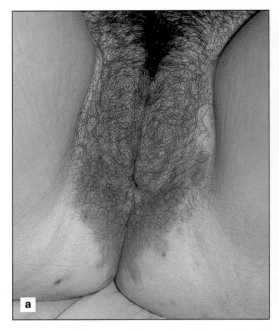

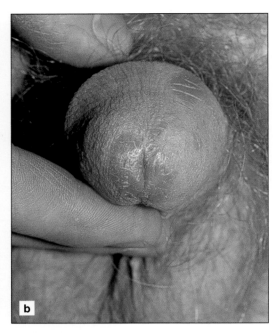

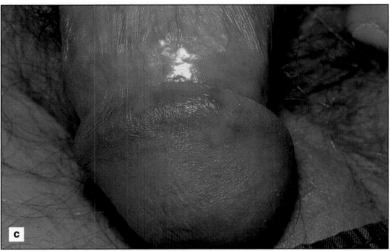

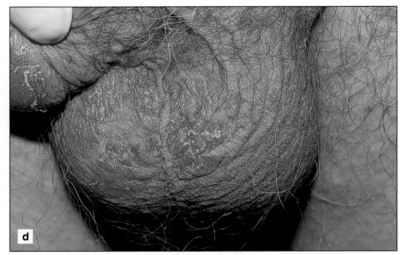

Figure 7.22 Genital psoriasis. (**a**) Vulval psoriasis in an adult, which had been treated unsuccessfully as candidiasis. The confluent erythema might occur in either disorder, but the degree of inflammation, lack of satellite lesions, and lack of therapeutic response make candidal infection unlikely. (**b**) Penile psoriasis, with typically psoriatic morphology of discrete plaques. Genital lesions of psoriasis are often less distinct than in this case. (**c**) Penile psoriasis with an annular morphology, known as a circinate balanitis. This patient also had HLA-B27-positive ankylosing spondylitis. A similar morphology occurs in Reiter syndrome (Fig. 7.30). (**d**) Scrotal lesions of psoriasis. The glans penis is also affected.

Differential diagnosis of psoriasiform disorders

Ordinary plaque psoriasis is usually clinically characteristic, but atypical lesions, less common patterns, or psoriasis at less common sites (especially if in isolation) may cause diagnostic difficulty. The differential diagnosis depends on the pattern and site; the main considerations are listed in Tables 7.2 and 7.3. Some specific issues that cause problems have been discussed in the earlier sections.

In general, the disorders most likely to be confused with psoriasis, and their chapter cross-references, are as follows.

- Dermatitis (Ch. 6)—more inflammatory plaques may be difficult to distinguish from discoid eczema; seborrheic dermatitis may be very similar to psoriasis, especially in flexures and on the face, scalp, and ears; hand dermatitis can be very difficult but important to differentiate.
- Viral exanthems (Ch. 25)—these are commonly in the differential of guttate psoriasis and sometimes of unstable psoriasis.
- Drug eruptions (Ch. 18)—also commonly in the differential of guttate psoriasis and sometimes of unstable psoriasis.
- Lichen planus (Ch. 8)—may resemble several types of psoriatic lesion; the eruptive generalized pattern is particularly likely to be confused with the more common guttate psoriasis.
- Fungal infection (Ch. 26)—may resemble plaque psoriasis; it is particularly in the differential of palm, sole, or nail involvement (including PPP).
- Bowen disease (Ch. 32)—may closely resemble psoriasis, especially if there are just a few lesions on the legs; it is mainly a consideration in older patients.

- Secondary syphilis (Ch. 20)—an important, albeit uncommon, mimic of psoriasis.
- Photodermatoses (Ch. 17)—some (usually female) patients have photo-aggravated psoriasis, a pattern that may cause confusion (Fig. 7.26).

PRACTICE POINTS

- Psoriasis is usually a clinical diagnosis; if there is doubt, a specialist opinion is usually more valuable than a skin biopsy.
- The fact that a patient has psoriasis does not mean that non-specific toenail dystrophy is due to psoriasis; fungal infection may coexist.
- If there is uncertainty about hand dermatitis versus psoriasis, inspect the elbows, knees, sacrum, and scalp before considering more complicated investigations.
- Guttate psoriasis may be difficult to distinguish from viral exanthems or pityriasis rosea; the classic psoriatic silvery scale may take a while to appear, and may not be apparent if emollients are being used.
- Always send skin scrapings for mycology from apparent palmoplantar pustulosis if only one foot is involved or if the patient is a non-smoker.
- Erythrodermic, and especially generalized pustular, forms of psoriasis may develop abruptly, cause systemic symptoms, and may required urgent hospitalization.

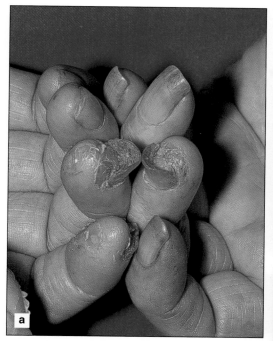

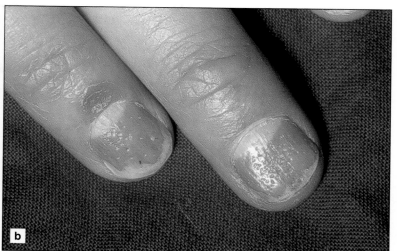

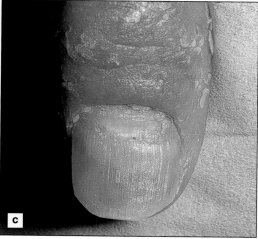

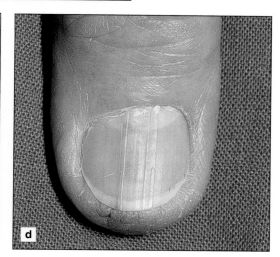

Figure 7.23 Nail psoriasis. (**a**) Subungual hyperkeratosis and onycholysis also occur in dermatophyte infections. (**b**) Nail pitting in psoriasis. The pits are more discrete and regular compared with pits affecting the nail plate in dermatitis. (**c**) Onycholysis due to psoriasis, with associated cutaneous psoriasis. (**d**) The oil drop appearance in psoriasis, a diagnostic sign of this disorder.

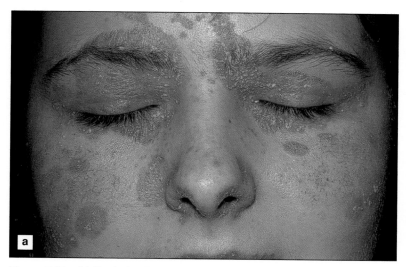

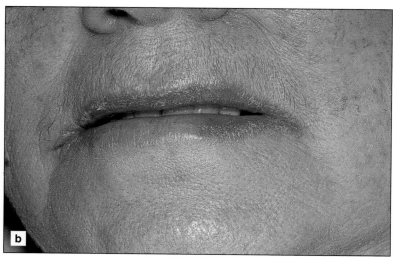

Figure 7.24 (**a**) Psoriasis affecting the face. This extent of facial involvement would be unlikely in the absence of significant psoriasis at other sites. (**b**) Psoriasis of the lips. This is an uncommon site, and the patient had little psoriasis at other, more typical areas.

Psoriatic arthropathy

On average, psoriatic arthropathy occurs in about 5% of patients with psoriasis (Fig. 7.27), but it is more common (about 35%) in those with more severe psoriasis. It has been divided into five subtypes (Moll and Wright classification), but other forms can probably be added (Table 7.6). However, patterns may co-exist, evolve to include others, and vary in different countries, so a simpler three-pattern classification has recently been proposed, consisting of asymmetric oligoarthritis, symmetric polyarthritis, and spondyloarthropathy, and a even a two-pattern classification of peripheral arthritis and axial (with or without peripheral) arthritis. The axial patterns are more common in men, and the acral type in women. Skin involvement precedes arthropathy in two-thirds of patients; the remainder are equally divided into those with concurrent onset and those in whom the joint disease occurs first. The most common pattern is the oligoarticular asymmetric pattern, in which the digits are often affected by a symmetric polyarthropathy of medium-sized joints.

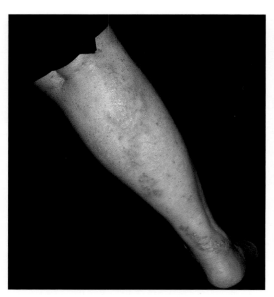

Figure 7.25 Linear psoriasis, associated with ordinary chronic plaque psoriasis at other sites. There remains debate about whether some such cases represent a Koebner reaction into an inflammatory linear verrucous nevus. An identical distribution pattern may occur in lichen planus (Fig. 8.16).

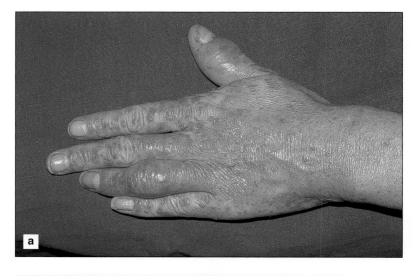

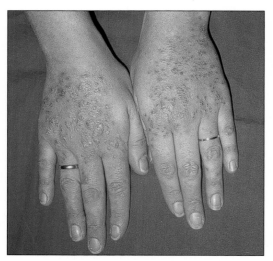

Figure 7.26 Photoaggravated psoriasis. Most patients with psoriasis improve in sunlight, but some (usually women) clearly have photoaggravated lesions, as shown here in sun-exposed skin. Some of these conditions are provoked mainly by long-wavelength UVA, and may respond to UVB or PUVA.

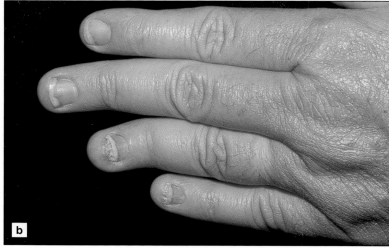

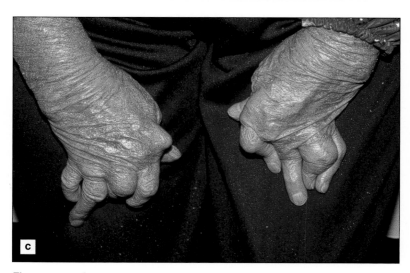

Figure 7.27 Psoriatic arthropathy. (**a**) Affecting the terminal interphalangeal joint of the thumb and the proximal interphalangeal joint of the ring finger, in this case obviously associated with extensive psoriasis of the skin also. (**b**) Psoriatic arthropathy of the terminal interphalangeal joint. Adjacent psoriasis is not seen, but the nail changes are suggestive of psoriasis. (**c**) Arthritis mutilans, a typically psoriatic pattern of arthritis, which is associated with a characteristic 'pencil in cup' radiographic appearance of the digits.

Table 7.6   SUBTYPES OF PSORIATIC ARTHROPATHY

Subtype[a]	Description
1	Asymmetric oligoarthritis, affecting fewer than five joints (often digits)
2	Symmetric polyarthritis, mainly wrists, ankles, feet, and knees (resembles rheumatoid arthritis)
3	Spinal (axial) form, affecting any part of spine, sacrum, and sacroiliac joints
4	Distal interphalangeal joints
5	Arthritis mutilans, a severe destructive form affecting fingers and toes
6	SAPHO: the combination of synovitis, acne, pustulosis, hyperostosis, and (sterile) osteomyelitis; this pattern often affects the clavicles and the manubriosternal region
7	Onychopachydermoperiostitis: a painful inflammatory pattern of distal periostitis

[a]Subtypes 1–5 according to the classification of Moll and Wright.

Table 7.7 FEATURES THAT DISTINGUISH PSORIATIC AND RHEUMATOID ARTHRITIS

Feature	Psoriatic arthropathy	Rheumatoid arthritis
Symmetry	Asymmetric	Symmetric
Hand involvement	Distal interphalangeal	Metacarpophalangeal
Joint changes	Ankylosis	Narrowing of joint space
Periarticular change	Osteolysis	Osteoporosis

Nail psoriasis is common in patients with psoriatic arthropathy, especially of acral pattern (associated with HLA-B38), and ocular symptoms such as uveitis are associated with the axial pattern (often in patients who are HLA-B27-positive). The most difficult differential diagnosis, especially in the absence of skin lesions, is rheumatoid arthritis (Table 7.7).

REITER SYNDROME, KERATODERMA BLENNORRHAGICUM, AND CIRCINATE BALANITIS

Reiter syndrome consists of arthropathy, iritis, urethritis, and skin lesions (Figs 7.28 and 7.29). It is typically provoked by non-gonococcal urethritis or by bowel infection with *Yersinia* or other organisms. The urethritis pattern has a strong male predominance. Patients are often HLA-B27-

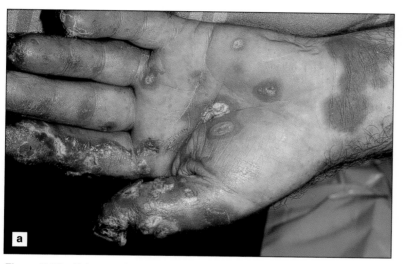
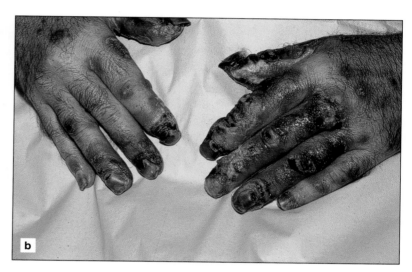

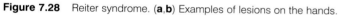

Figure 7.28 Reiter syndrome. (**a**,**b**) Examples of lesions on the hands.

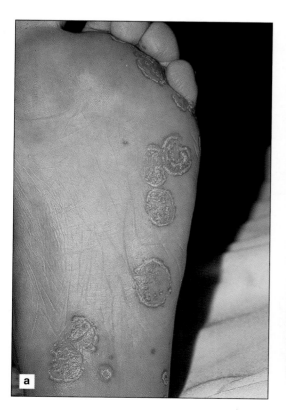
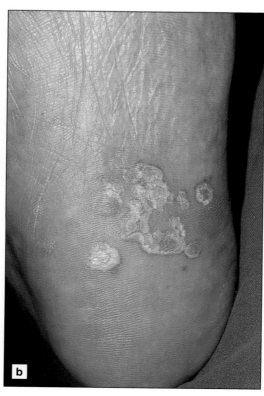

Figure 7.29 Reiter syndrome. (**a**,**b**) Examples of lesions on the soles; these annular lesions are typical of keratoderma blennorrhagicum.

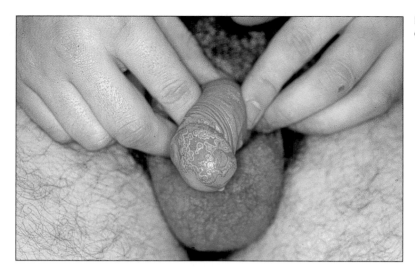

Figure 7.30 Reiter syndrome. Circinate balanitis, with urethral discharge. (Courtesy of Dr. B. Stanley.)

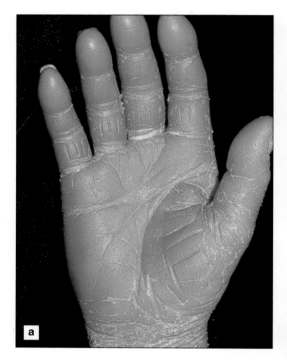

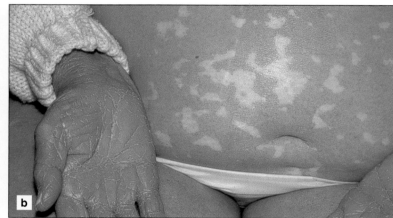

Figure 7.31 Pityriasis rubra pilaris (PRP). (**a**) Confluent orange-colored palmar hyperkeratosis. (**b**) Islands of sparing. (**c**) Psoriasiform lesions. (**d**) Scaling with a more unusual rippled pattern. (**e**) Follicular papules, semiconfluent in places.
Continued.

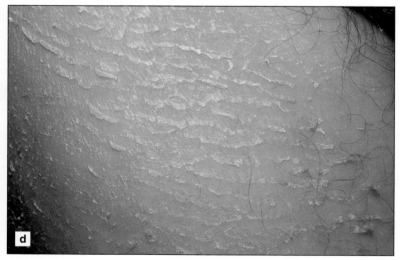

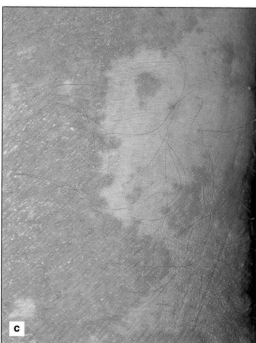

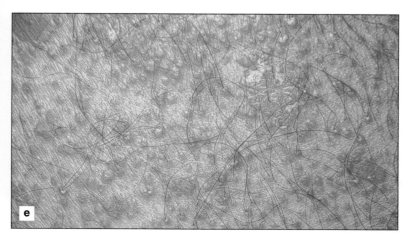

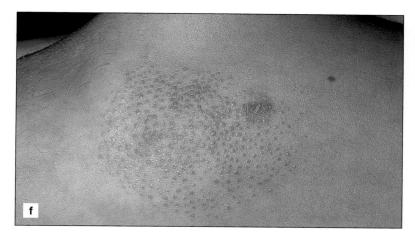

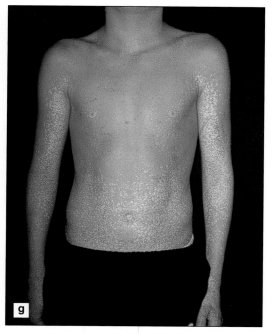

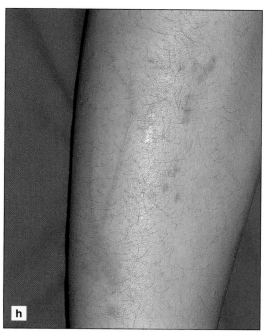

Figure 7.31, *cont'd* Pityriasis rubra pilaris (PRP). (**f**) Localized PRP in a child. (**g**) Confluent and follicular PRP of acute onset in a child. (**h**) The Koebner reaction also occurs in this condition, as shown here in a teenaged patient.

positive, and a similar pattern of skin lesions can occur with axial arthritis in the absence of an overt infective trigger.

The skin lesions consist of localized patches of plantar psoriasiform hyperkeratosis, and penile patches that may form a characteristic circinate balanitis (Fig. 7.30). Psoriasiform lesions may occur at other body sites, especially digits and nails. Like psoriasis, Reiter syndrome may be particularly severe in HIV infection. However, the 10-fold increased frequency of Reiter syndrome in homosexual or bisexual men may be related to other infections, as it does not appear to be specific to HIV status.

The main differential diagnosis, if the trigger is asymptomatic, is psoriasis or dermatitis of palms or soles. Primary skin infections are sometimes considered in more crusted examples.

Treatment is that of the underlying cause plus treatments as for psoriasis.

PITYRIASIS RUBRA PILARIS

Etiology and pathogenesis

Pityriasis rubra pilaris (PRP) is an uncommon but often characteristic dermatosis of unknown etiology. Most patients present in mid-childhood or in late middle age.

Clinical features

Pityriasis rubra pilaris resembles psoriasis in many respects, and many of the treatments are similar. Useful features that help to distinguish PRP (Fig. 7.31) from psoriasis are the follicular prominence (especially in the localized types and the initial lesions of the generalized types), the orange color of the palmar involvement, the islands of sparing that occur in the generalized types, and the absence of typical psoriatic pits in the thickened nails.

Pityriasis rubra pilaris has classically been divided into five types (Griffiths), with more recent addition of HIV-associated PRP.

   I. Classic adult type
  II. Atypical adult type
 III. Classic juvenile type
 IV. Circumscribed juvenile type
  V. Atypical juvenile type
 VI. HIV-associated type

Differential diagnosis

The differential diagnosis is that of psoriasis (see earlier discussion of clinical features), of erythroderma (Table 7.4), or of acquired palmoplantar keratodermas (see later in this chapter), depending on the mode of presentation. Note that many of the palmoplantar keratodermas are inherited and develop in early years of life with a positive family history, thus distinguishing them from PRP.

The islands of sparing that occur in generalized PRP are not a feature of other erythrodermas, although this may be difficult to determine in the evolving suberythrodermic patient. A useful diagnostic feature is that PRP tends to spread from the head downward, often over a few weeks; although the head may be involved initially in generalized seborrheic dermatitis, this often involves flexures also, evolves less rapidly, and spares the palms and soles.

Treatment

Treatment is generally similar to that for psoriasis (see following section), but PRP is often both widespread and relatively refractory to therapy, so there is a much greater likelihood that systemic therapies will be required. In adults, acitretin is often used; other options include UVB, PUVA, methotrexate, or ciclosporin. Photoaggravation may limit use of UVB. In young women, the need to avoid pregnancy for 2 years after taking acitretin is a major limitation, and isotretinoin has been used as an alternative in this group. The juvenile-onset types often resolve in the teenage years, and systemic therapy may not be required, but the prognosis in individuals who develop PRP in the second half of childhood is less predictable.

TREATMENT OF PSORIASIS AND RELATED DISORDERS

Numerous agents may be used with success in the treatment of psoriasis (Figs 7.32–7.41, Tables 7.8–7.10). However, there are important considerations in choice of therapy, which must be tailored to the individual patient. Several of the topical agents are potentially irritant if used on thin skin (face and flexures) or on very inflamed lesions (unstable psoriasis), while all the systemic agents have (at least potentially) severe toxicity and would therefore be inappropriate for milder psoriasis that might respond to safer treatments. Body site(s) affected, clinical pattern, chronicity, response to initial treatment choices, social aspects for the patient, and ability to use treatments effectively may all influence the choice of treat-ment and the progression from one to another. Some of these issues are summarized in the following sections on topical and systemic therapies.

There are a few fundamental issues that are worth considering.

- Treatment is likely to work only if it is used—a treatment that is too messy (Fig. 7.32), too irritant for the type of psoriasis (Figs 7.33 and 7.34), too time consuming, cosmetically inelegant (Fig. 7.35), or inadequately explained may therefore fail. Using an expert nurse to demonstrate treatment is greatly appreciated by many patients.

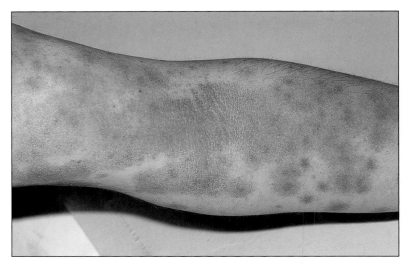

Figure 7.34   Vitamin D analogs are a potentially useful and clean therapeutic agent, but may irritate psoriasis if used on 'unstable' inflamed lesions, as in this case.

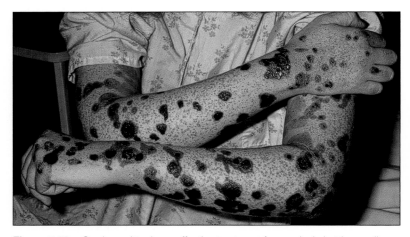

Figure 7.32   Crude coal tar is an effective treatment for psoriasis but is usually too messy for home use.

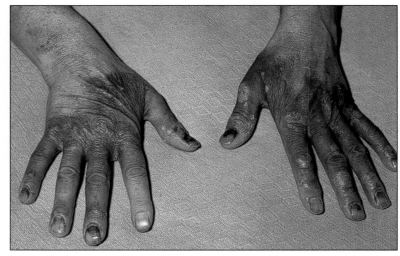

Figure 7.35   Treatment with anthralin (dithranol): residual brown staining after treatment. This lasts only a week or so after lesional clearance, but some patients may not wish to use it on exposed sites such as the hands.

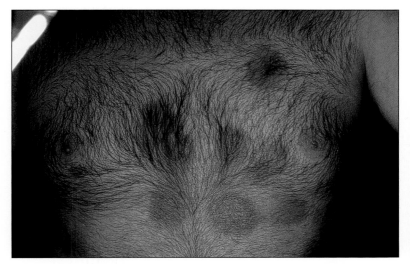

Figure 7.33   Treatment with anthralin (dithranol): erythema around treated lesions. If symptomatic, this usually resolves by omitting treatment for a day or two, then using a lower concentration, but it may limit treatment in some patients.

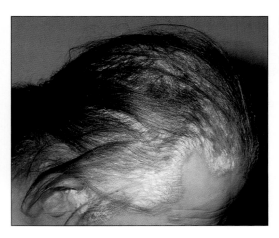

Figure 7.36   Scalp hyperkeratosis. This often requires treatment with a keratolytic agent.

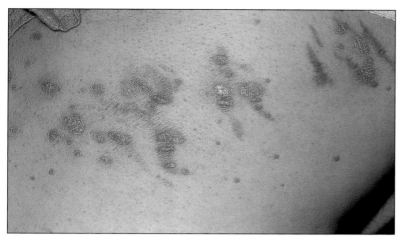

Figure 7.37 Topical corticosteroids are useful for psoriasis, but are often best used either as a preliminary treatment to control inflammation, or in conjunction with other more specific therapy. Use in isolation carries the risks of tachyphylaxis and rebound, resulting in increased strengths being required, and increased risk of side effects such as striae, as shown here around the plaques of psoriasis.

- Patients who are admitted to hospital, or who attend a day treatment center, respond faster than those performing treatment at home, although the reasons for this are often unclear.
- If there is significant scaling, use of a keratolytic agent is important at the start of therapy (Fig. 7.36), as other topical agents will otherwise fail to penetrate and will thus be ineffective. This simple measure can often resurrect 'failed' treatment, and is particularly important for the palms, soles, and scalp.
- Strong topical corticosteroids have significant side effects, especially at thinner skin areas (Fig. 7.37); if the need for higher potency is increasing, it may be best to combine treatment with another, more specific, antipsoriatic agent.
- It is technically difficult for patients to treat widespread small lesions such as those of guttate psoriasis, particularly with messy or irritant treatments; UVB phototherapy is often a better option, a short course over 4–6 weeks generally being adequate.
- Systemic therapies such as methotrexate or retinoids have potentially significant side effects (Figs 7.38 and 7.39), as does PUVA (Figs 7.40 and 7.41).

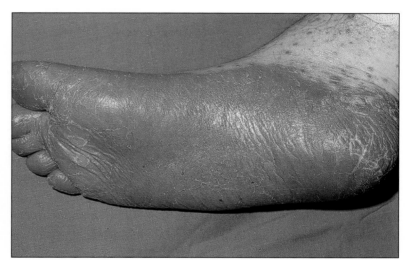

Figure 7.39 Systemic retinoids are helpful for hyperkeratotic psoriasis of palmoplantar skin, but treatment involves a balance between excessive keratosis due to the disease and excessive peeling (leaving a rather red, thin, glazed-looking skin) due to the treatment.

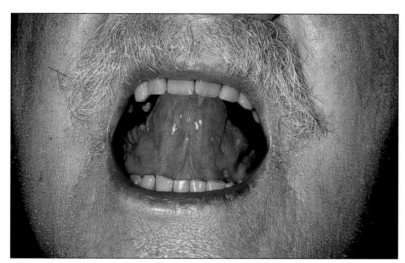

Figure 7.38 Mouth ulceration in a patient taking methotrexate for psoriasis. This is a warning of potential hematologic toxicity.

Figure 7.40 Psoriasis before (**a**) and after (**b**) treatment with PUVA photochemotherapy.

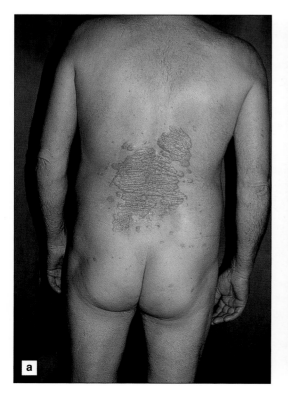

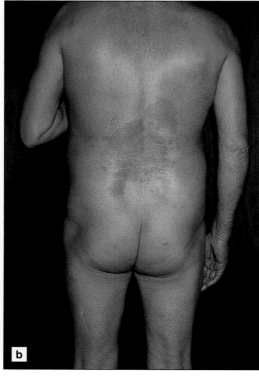

a

b

- Unstable psoriasis should not be treated with irritant agents—it is likely to get worse.
- The pattern or body site of psoriasis may significantly influence the best choice of treatment (Table 7.8).

Specific therapies that may be used are listed in Tables 7.9 and 7.10, and are discussed in more detail in the general therapeutic chapters (Chs 3–5).

Some individuals would recommend a therapeutic approach based on body surface area (BSA) involved. This can be useful as one method of guiding therapy, but it needs considerable flexibility depending on the pattern, sites, degree of inflammation, and other factors discussed in this section. For example, 2% BSA involvement may seem minor if it is a thin plaque on the buttock, but can be career threatening (and totally alter the therapeutic approach) if the 2% BSA happens to be 1% contributed

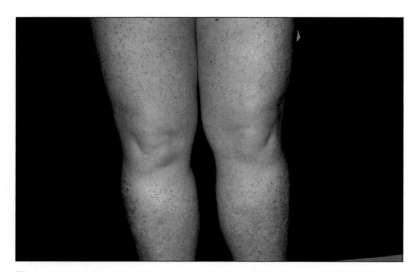

Figure 7.41 Marked lentiginosis may occur in patients treated with PUVA. The lesions are typically angular or stellate in shape, and affect the usually covered skin of the buttock by comparison with the (usually paler) lesions caused by sunlight exposure. In some instances, as shown here, lesions are confined to the distribution of a resolved plaque of psoriasis.

by each palm. Similarly, limited but very inflammatory psoriasis would require a different approach to that for pale, thin, chronic plaques of the same extent. Some possible options for plaque psoriasis based on BSA affected, and some limitations of the BSA approach, are provided in Table 7.11.

Topical therapies

These are summarized in Table 7.9, and a possible approach for plaque psoriasis in Table 7.11. In most patients (the majority have limited plaque psoriasis at body sites that do not influence treatment choice), most of the options listed in Table 7.9 are potentially suitable. However, several factors may influence the final choice of topical agents for the individual patient; note that some patients get the best results by combining different modalities to get the advantages, but reduce the disadvantages, of each. The main factors include the following.

- Pattern of psoriasis—using treatments that need to be applied accurately, such as anthralin, is difficult if there are lots of small lesions.
- Body site—for example, hyperkeratotic areas need a keratolytic as part of the regimen; a cosmetically inelegant preparation or post-treatment staining may preclude use of some agents on hands or scalp.
- Severity of the lesions—degree of inflammation and scaling; for example, beware of use of vitamin D analogs on inflammatory or unstable psoriasis.
- Extent of lesions—BSA involved may influence treatment choice (including the choice of topical versus systemic), but it is often poorly estimated (especially in guttate psoriasis, where involvement is overestimated). Note also that the site affected may be more important than the extent.
- Previous experience—for example, good or poor response with a specific agent.
- Patient wishes and lifestyle—influenced by treatment that is messy or time consuming, work or social aspects, and ability to perform treatment adequately.
- Patient motivation—for example, anthralin used well is very effective, but the need to vary strength and use of 30-min wash-off (short contact) treatment is off-putting for some patients.

Table 7.8   SOME THERAPEUTIC IMPLICATIONS OF THE DIFFERENT CLINICAL PATTERNS AND SITE-RELATED VARIANTS OF PSORIASIS

Variant	Therapeutic implications
Main pattern	
Plaque psoriasis	Most options potentially applicable, depending on extent and degree of inflammation
Guttate psoriasis	Self-limiting, but pattern makes it difficult to treat (especially if messy or irritant treatment); often treated with UVB phototherapy
Generalized pustular psoriasis	Usually requires hospitalization to monitor systemic effects, usually needs systemic therapy
Palmoplantar pustulosis	Chronic; usually treated topically initially, but often poor response
Acropustulosis of Hallopeau	Nail destruction often requires systemic therapy
'Unstable' psoriasis	Avoid potentially irritant topical agents, monitor carefully
Erythrodermic or exfoliative	Usually requires hospitalization to monitor systemic effects, usually needs systemic therapy
Subacute annular (Lapière)	Rare, may respond to simple topicals but often scattered lesions
Linear	Usually topicals as for plaque psoriasis, but response is usually incomplete and recurrence is expected
Specific sites	
Elbows and/or knees	Topicals as for plaque psoriasis
Hands and feet	Usually requires a keratolytic as well as other topical agent(s); thick skin, therefore use an adequate potency if using a corticosteroid; may warrant systemic therapy
Scalp	Usually requires a keratolytic as well as topical corticosteroid or other topical agent(s); thick skin, therefore use an adequate potency if using a corticosteroid, but beware of overuse at scalp margin and treat ears with milder agents; expert nurses can greatly influence success of scalp treatment
Flexures and genital	Mild agents, avoid irritant treatments
Nails	Difficult; may respond to strong corticosteroids to nail fold; may need intralesional steroid to nail matrix or bed (but painful); may respond to systemic therapy, but usually only used if severity of skin involvement warrants this
Face and ears	Mild agents as for flexures

Table 7.9 TOPICAL DRUG THERAPY FOR PSORIASIS

Agent	Comments
Emollients and keratolytics	Emollients are important, should be used in most patients, and may be all that is required in some. Keratolytics include salicylic acid, coconut oil. An important part of therapy of psoriasis: failure to remove scaling or hyperkeratosis (especially on the scalp and palmoplantar surfaces) before using other topicals is a common reason for poor treatment response.
Corticosteroids	Antiinflammatory and antiproliferative actions; effective and widely used, but potential disadvantage of tachyphylaxis and of rebound exacerbation of psoriasis if strong agents are suddenly discontinued. This can lead to ever-increasing strengths being applied, with the attendant risks of skin atrophy. Useful as first-line therapy for localized plaques, areas where other treatments may irritate (e.g. flexures) or stain (e.g. scalp), and also in 'unstable' psoriasis to allow introduction of more specific agents.
Vitamin D analogs	Antiproliferative, clean to use. Some irritate face or flexures. May worsen unstable psoriasis. In some patients, hyperkeratosis responds well but redness does not, therefore potential to use in conjunction with topical corticosteroid.
Anthralin (dithranol)	A potent antipsoriatic agent, which has disadvantages of staining and skin irritation; only suitable for stable disease. Very effective if used carefully, usually as 30-min 'wash-off' regimen in conjunction with other agents. Benefits from demonstration to the patient.
Tars	Antimitotic and antiinflammatory, also help to remove scale. Preparations vary considerably in strength and cosmetic suitability. Mild preparations are useful for areas such as the ears. Used in conjunction with UVB in the Goeckerman regimen.
Vitamin A analogs	Used systemically for psoriasis, more recently topically. Useful for descaling.

Table 7.10 SYSTEMIC DRUG THERAPY AND PHOTOTHERAPY FOR PSORIASIS

Agent	Comments
Methotrexate	Usually effective for skin or joints, cheap. Nausea may limit treatment. Given once weekly, often with folate supplementation. Myelosuppression (Fig. 7.38) and liver side effects are important. Less popular than it was, due to additional new agents plus need for liver biopsy; newer monitoring methods (PIIINP[a]) may help.
Acitretin	Especially useful for hyperkeratotic psoriasis, palms and soles. Pregnancy must be avoided for 2 years, so use is limited in younger women. Rarely useful for joints. May cause dry lips, peeling palms and soles (Fig. 7.39), hair loss, arthralgia, hyperlipidemia. Expensive.
Ciclosporin	Useful for skin and joints, but nausea is common. Main adverse reactions are hypertension and renal impairment (risk increases with time) and numerous drug interactions.
Mycophenolate mofetil	Less experience in psoriasis than ciclosporin, but can be useful; the two may be used together. See Chapter 4 for additional details.
Hydroxyurea	Generally safe. Causes myelosuppression, but rarely severe and is reversible. May cause gradually increasing anemia, often paralleled by a gradually decreasing efficacy over some years.
Systemic corticosteroids	Avoid due to risk of pustular psoriasis on withdrawal.
Azathioprine	Infrequently used in psoriasis.
UVB phototherapy	Often used for guttate psoriasis or for widespread, essentially stable, plaque psoriasis, generally for intermittent courses. Narrow-band 311 nm is now usually used in preference to broadband UVB.
PUVA photochemotherapy	Effective (Fig. 7.40), relative lack of short-term side effects. However, has a skin-aging effect, increased risk of squamous cell carcinoma and lesser risk of melanoma. Severe lentiginosis may occur (Fig. 7.41). Concurrent use of retinoids can be helpful.
Anti-tumor necrosis factor monoclonals	A new treatment for severe psoriasis. Effective but hugely expensive; several potentially important side effects (see Ch. 4) and uncertain long-term side effects.
Lasers	Excimer laser 308 nm has been used but can treat only small areas, and often causes burning or blistering.
Intralesional corticosteroid	Occasionally used for thick, stubborn, localized plaques; also used in severe nail disease, but painful, usually needs ring-block anesthesia.

[a]Amino terminal peptide of type III procollagen.

Table 7.11   A POSSIBLE APPROACH TO PLAQUE PSORIASIS, AND SOME LIMITATIONS OF THE BODY SURFACE AREA (BSA) APPROACH[a]

BSA involved (approximate %)[b]	Usual options	Non-responders	Limitations and comments
< 10%	Initial treatment: topical corticosteroid and/or vitamin D analog. May need pretreatment with an emollient or keratolytic if very scaly, and ongoing concurrent use of emollient is generally helpful. If starting with a topical corticosteroid to reduce inflammation, try to combine with other agents after 2–3 weeks, such as tars, anthralin, vitamin A analog (usually one treatment at either end of the day, but some are available in combination formulations, and short-contact anthralin can be added in with other treatments).	Try other topicals in the first instance, or combining agents if not already tried. If doing home treatment, day center attendance with nurse supervision may improve response. Combine topicals with phototherapy (usually narrow-band UVB initially) or consider admission (and possible use of messier options, such as stronger tars, or stronger anthralin preparations). Possibly use systemic agents if still poor response.	Purely flexural psoriasis is usually in this BSA range, but requires a different approach (e.g. some vitamin D analogs may be irritant). Guttate psoriasis is often in this BSA range if assessed accurately (often overestimated), but requires a different approach with an early move to UVB phototherapy potentially being more useful than trying multiple topicals. The same may apply to widespread, scattered, stable, small-plaque disease. Localized hand or foot plaques will be in this BSA range but typically require use of a keratolytic with other topical options, and may warrant an early move to systemic therapy. Toxicity of systemic agents should limit their use in patients with BSA involvement at this level without careful consideration of, and usually failure of, simpler options.
10–20%	Topicals as above; phototherapy is often used at an earlier stage (the two approaches would generally be used together).	Hospital admission or systemic treatments, as above.	Widespread small plaques amounting to 10–20% BSA are a more valid indication for phototherapy than a small number of larger plaques, as topical therapy is more difficult and time consuming. Hospital admission may avoid the need for systemic therapy if side effects (especially long term) are an issue: rate and severity of relapse may be more important in making this decision than the initial extent of psoriasis.
> 20%	Phototherapy is often suggested as first-line treatment, but there is actually no good reason not to use topicals as first-line therapy, especially on a supervised treatment center or inpatient basis.	UVB phototherapy if not already tried. PUVA or systemic agents if UVB plus topicals has failed.	Patients with BSA involvement over 20% are often those with more inflammatory psoriasis; choice of topicals is important. Phototherapy takes time to work (weeks), so may not be the best option in isolation unless plaques are stable. The > 20% BSA option covers a huge range; an additional group are therefore considered below.
Semiconfluent plaques and suberythrodermic	May need topical corticosteroid to decrease inflammation (with close outpatient supervision or inpatient management, usually the latter); early use of a systemic agent.	Responders to topical therapy may still need to be considered for systemic therapy for ongoing control. If systemic therapy fails, then combination with topicals or with other systemic agents, or a different systemic agent, may be needed.	Phototherapy with UVB or PUVA is generally not appropriate for this group: the psoriasis is usually inflammatory, and phototherapy is too slow to work anyhow.

[a]The subject of this table is plaque psoriasis of varying extent; erythrodermic and pustular psoriasis are not considered.
[b]Advice is usually based on < 10%, 10–20%, and > 20% but has been extended for this table.

Phototherapy

The beneficial role of sunlight is a feature in about 90% of patients with psoriasis, and some patterns, such as the guttate form, respond almost universally. For many patients, this is an intermediate treatment between topical therapy and systemic therapies, although it may be a first-line treatment (e.g. in guttate psoriasis). It can be used in conjunction with many topical treatments, although some can interfere with penetration of UVB (notably vitamin D analogs and some emollient bases), so topical agents should generally be applied at least 6 h before, or any time after, phototherapy. A small proportion of patients (usually women) clearly worsen in sunlight or with artificial UV sources (Fig. 7.26).

The beneficial part of sunlight is the UVB wavelengths from 280 to 320 nm. A smaller group of patients gets some benefit from the UVA wavelengths (320–400 nm) that are produced by standard tanning beds, but this benefit is usually less reliable and the UVB wavelengths are used therapeutically. A narrow-band UVB lamp with a narrow wavelength peak at 311 nm (the TL01 lamp) is used with increasing frequency and has superseded photochemotherapy (PUVA) as the treatment of choice for many patients. This may be used alone or in conjunction with topical therapies, but each treatment course is usually limited to a month or two in order to minimize skin cancer and skin-aging risks. The duration of experience with narrow-band UVB is less than that with PUVA, so the risks and the limitations that should be placed on treatment duration are less clear.

Systemic therapies

The main systemic therapies used in psoriasis are summarized in Table 7.10. They are discussed in more detail in Chapter 4 regarding other indications and side effects.

All systemic therapies have some, at least potential, side effects and require careful monitoring. In patients with psoriasis, a disease that clearly has a major impact but is rarely dangerous, several factors need to be considered in making the decision to treat systemically. These include the following.

- Chronicity and severity of disease—for example, acute severe forms of psoriasis generally need systemic treatment.
- Ability to use topical treatment effectively—for example, an elderly patient without help at home may be unable to use topical treatment adequately.
- Response to and relapse rate after topical therapy—in routine practice, this rather subjective area is the main determinant of the type of therapy that may be required.
- Associated problems—such as psoriatic arthropathy (patients more likely to use systemic therapy) or medical conditions that may contra-indicate some systemic options.
- Other drug treatment—several systemic agents for psoriasis have important drug interactions.
- Patient wishes and lifestyle—the patient's wishes are clearly important, but it would be irresponsible to use potentially dangerous drugs for mild psoriasis; the patient's lifestyle may influence treatment (e.g. work commitments may preclude hospital admissions; high alcohol may contraindicate methotrexate or may raise concerns about the reliability of the patient).
- Treatment options that are available to the physician (PUVA may be available only at larger departments, funding for monoclonal agents may have to be individually negotiated, etc.) or to the patient (e.g. due to cost or insurance limitations if working in a healthcare system where these apply).

PRACTICE POINTS

- The best way to explain treatment application is to use an expert nurse to demonstrate what to do.
- Don't forget to treat scaling with a keratolytic before moving to more specific therapy.
- Beware of using gradually increasing strengths of corticosteroids to treat psoriasis, especially if extensive or at thin skin sites; consider combining treatment with another more psoriasis-specific topical agent.
- Be gentle in treatment of unstable psoriasis, and review progress regularly.
- There are significant therapeutic issues relating to specific patterns and body sites affected in patients with psoriasis.
- Palmoplantar pustulosis treated topically often seems to respond best if different agents are combined (e.g. one morning, one at night).
- Patients who require systemic therapy need careful discussion of the potential side effects.

PALMOPLANTAR KERATODERMAS

Etiology and pathogenesis

A variety of different disorders are considered under this broad heading. Some are inherited, others acquired, but the inherited types may be clinically manifest only later in life; many are therefore presumed to represent an inflammatory dermatosis such as psoriasis.

There are many eponymous types of hereditary palmoplantar keratoderma (PPK), of which the most common (Thost–Unna type) has autosomal dominant inheritance. These may be subdivided into diffuse, localized, and punctate types. The mechanism of keratin defect is known in many cases, such as epidermolytic PPK (Vörner syndrome), which is due to defects in keratin type 9 (a keratin that occurs only in palmoplantar skin).

Keratoderma climactericum is a moderately common keratoderma of the feet that typically develops in women around the menopause, although a causal relationship with the menopause is by no means definite; most patients are overweight, which may be more relevant.

A diffuse keratoderma secondary to malignancy (tylosis) is rare, but palmar keratoses and pits occur in several malignancy syndromes.

Keratodermas that are eczematous in nature are discussed in Chapter 6, but can be very difficult to distinguish from psoriasis (especially hyper-

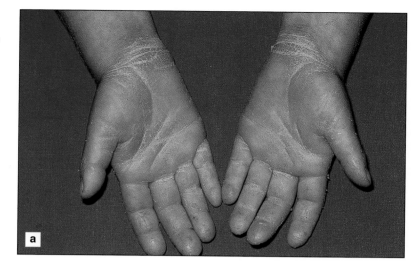

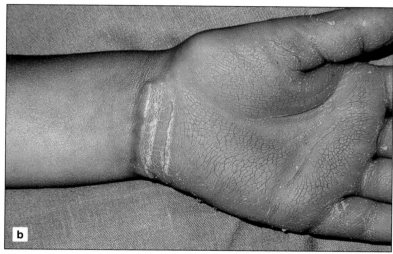

Figure 7.42 Diffuse palmoplantar keratoderma of Thost-Unna type. (**a**) This is not inflammatory enough to be psoriasis, and the cut-off is too sharp for a dermatitis of the palms. (**b**) Although the bulk of the affected area just has the appearance of thickened keratin, an erythematous border is often apparent.

keratotic dermatitis of palms, which is usually frictional in etiology and represents a form of lichen simplex).

Hypothyroidism may cause a degree of keratoderma, as well as a yellowish color (due to carotenemia) that resembles the color of thickened keratin.

Clinical features

The Thost–Unna type of hereditary PPK can usually be distinguished from psoriasis by the family history (autosomal dominant), young age of onset, and the morphology (Fig. 7.42). It affects the whole of the palms and soles, often with spread on to the dorsum of the fingers distally and over the joints (known as the transgrediens pattern), and consists of yellowish-colored formed hyperkeratosis with a mildly red border (see Fig. 7.42b). However, some other diffuse PPKs can be excluded only by biopsy. Occasionally, less confluent PPKs, or milder cases of Thost–Unna PPK, can be difficult to distinguish from psoriasis or a primary dermatitis.

The other relatively common hereditary types are focal PPK (Fig. 7.43) and punctate keratoderma (keratosis punctata), which consists of tiny, umbilicated, keratotic papules (see Ch. 19 and Fig. 19.58).

Keratoderma climactericum is distinguished by its characteristic distribution, affecting mainly the border of the heels and to a lesser extent the other weight-bearing areas of the feet or toe pulps (Fig. 7.44).

Differential diagnosis

The differential diagnostic issue with most keratodermas is usually that of distinguishing between different inherited types, to provide genetic

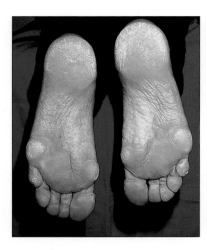

Figure 7.43 Focal palmoplantar keratoderma: this may be confused with simple callosities, but the degree of the keratoderma is more marked in this genodermatosis. (From Lawrence CM, Cox NH. Physical Signs in Dermatology, 2nd edn. London: Mosby, 2002.)

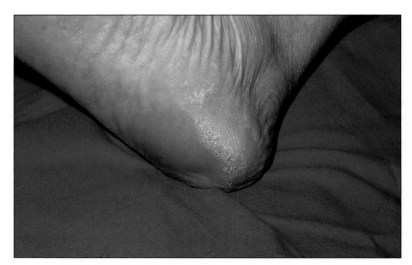

Figure 7.44 Keratoderma climactericum may be difficult to distinguish from dermatitis or psoriasis. It occurs around the border of the heels and sometimes on the toes in middle-aged women; despite the name, a hormonal basis is not proved.

counselling. However, other diagnostic areas that need to be considered include the following.

- Diffuse pattern—distinguish from psoriasis (as discussed earlier) or dermatitis (usually itchy), and consider hypothyroidism. Associated malignancy (of the esophagus) is relevant only in families known to have this association.
- Focal pattern—distinguish from simple thick skin (it is often noticed over weight-bearing areas of the foot), and sometimes from dermatitis or psoriasis. On palms, consider hyperkeratotic dermatitis or lichen simplex of palms in late-onset thickening. On soles, consider keratoderma climactericum if it is mainly around the margin of the heel in a female patient; this pattern is perhaps the most likely to be confused with psoriasis.
- Punctate pattern—lesions may be confused with viral warts, with arsenical keratoses (Ch. 32), with palmar porokeratosis, or with the pits

and keratoses of Cowden syndrome or nevoid basal cell carcinoma syndrome (although these are usually much smaller than the lesions in keratosis punctata). Tiny pits and keratotic papules also occur in the crease lines of the palm and fingers in some individuals, without any specific inheritance or associated features.

Treatment

The milder forms may require no treatment, or emollients or keratolytics such as salicylic acid, urea, or lactic acid. Topical retinoids and topical vitamin D analogs may both be useful. More severe cases may require acitretin (discussed earlier).

FURTHER READING

Callen JP, Krueger GG, Lebwohl M, et al. AAD consensus statement on psoriasis therapies. J Am Acad Dermatol 2003; 49: 897–9

Camisa CA. Psoriasis. Boston: Blackwell Scientific Publications, 1994

Christophers E, Wolff K (eds) Treatment of psoriasis. Dermatol Ther 1999; 11: 1–119

Clayton BD, Jorizzo JL, Hitchcock MG. Adult pityriasis rubra pilaris: a 10-year case series. J Am Acad Dermatol 1997; 36: 959–64

Gawkrodger DJ (ed) Current management of psoriasis. J Dermatol Treat 1997; 8: 27–55

Henseler T. The genetics of psoriasis. J Am Acad Dermatol 1997; 37: 1–11

Koo J, Lebwohl M. Duration of remission of psoriasis therapies. J Am Acad Dermatol 1999; 41: 51–9

Lebwohl M, Ali S. Treatment of psoriasis. Part 1. Topical therapy and phototherapy. J Am Acad Dermatol 2001; 45: 487–98

Lebwohl M, Ali S. Treatment of psoriasis. Part 2. Systemic therapies. J Am Acad Dermatol 2001; 45: 49–61

Roenigk HH, Maibach HI. Psoriasis, 3rd edn. New York: Marcel Dekker, 1998

THE LICHENOID ERUPTION

The lichenoid eruptions are those that resemble lichen planus. However, the term is used for both clinical and for histologic resemblance. Clinically, lichenoid conditions all tend to have flat-topped and rather shiny lesions, often with a violaceous or brownish color. However, some lesions that carry the term *lichen* (such as lichen sclerosus) bear little clinical resemblance to lichen planus, although they have a strong histologic resemblance. The term *lichenoid*, as applied to the histologic pattern, describes a band-like interface dermatitis; the features of this reaction pattern are listed in Table 8.1, and some disorders that may have lichenoid histology are listed in Table 8.2.

Conversely, some disorders having names that include the term lichen or lichenoid, on the basis of flat or flat-topped lesions, such as lichen aureus (a capillaropathy, Ch. 14) or pityriasis lichenoides (Ch. 33), are histologically distinct. Other disorders may be clinically very similar to lichen planus, having flat, purplish lesions, but are different in behavior and pathology; the rare condition of paraneoplastic pemphigus is an example (Ch. 16).

Lichen sclerosus does have lichenoid histology, especially in early lesions, but is discussed elsewhere in accordance with its two main clinical presentations, either as genital lesions (Ch. 20) or as areas of altered pigmentation and atrophy (Ch. 22).

Most of the lichenoid pathologic features are present to varying degrees in lupus erythematosus. Clinically, distinguishing lichen planus from discoid lupus erythematosus (Ch. 13) is not usually difficult, but at some sites in isolation (notably scalp, nail folds, and oral mucosa) the clinical and pathologic features may both be very similar. Direct immunofluorescence of a skin biopsy usually helps to resolve this issue, as deposition of IgG and complement C3 at the dermo–epidermal junction or in cytoid bodies favors lupus erythematosus, whereas prominent fibrin deposition favors lichen planus. IgM in cytoid bodies or at the dermo–epidermal junction occurs in both disorders.

LICHEN PLANUS

Etiology and pathogenesis

Lichen planus (LP) is a moderately common disorder with a prevalence of about 0.5%, and a slight female predominance but no racial predilection. It is generally viewed as an autoimmune disorder, and is more commonly associated with several other autoimmune disorders than would be expected by chance. Associated diseases include the following.

- Skin—alopecia areata, vitiligo, dermatitis herpetiformis, pemphigus, and sclerodermas.
- Gastrointestinal—primary biliary cirrhosis, chronic active hepatitis, and ulcerative colitis.
- Endocrine—thyroiditis and diabetes mellitus.
- Hematology—pernicious anemia and thymoma.

There are also associations with human leukocyte antigen (HLA)-A3, A5, B8, Bw35, and DR1. Familial cases may occur. In some countries, such as Italy, the association with hepatitis (especially chronic hepatitis C) infection appears fairly strong, but this has not been confirmed in other studies (e.g. in the UK). It may be that there is an interaction between HLA and infection that explains these geographic differences. However, treatment for hepatitis C virus (HCV) does not correlate with clearance of LP, and HCV is not found in lesional skin.

The pathogenesis of purely oral LP without skin involvement may be different, for example contact allergy frequently plays a part. This is discussed separately later.

Table 8.1 HISTOLOGIC FEATURES OF LICHENOID ERUPTIONS

Structure	Histologic features
Epidermis	Vacuolar (hydropic) degeneration of the basal layer Increased thickness of granular layer (hypergranulosis) Hyperkeratosis and acanthosis Eosinophilic-staining degenerate keratinocytes (known as cytoid, colloid, or Civatte bodies)
Dermis	Irregular, saw-toothed appearance of dermo–epidermal junction Deposition of fibrin and/or fibrinogen at the dermo–epidermal junction Cytoid bodies in the upper dermis Melanin pigment in macrophages (melanophages) Dense, band-like upper dermal lymphocytic infiltrate

Table 8.2 SOME DISORDERS THAT MAY HAVE LICHENOID HISTOLOGY

Disorder	Comments
Lichen planus (LP)	The prototype of this tissue reaction
Drug- or contact-induced lichenoid reaction	Usually more psoriasiform clinically; mixed infiltrate, including eosinophils histologically
Lupus erythematosus	Not usually clinically confused, but may be difficult at some sites; direct immunofluorescence of biopsy may distinguish the two
Erythema dyschromicum perstans (ashy dermatosis)	Resembles healing LP, may be a variant of LP
Lichen nitidus	May resemble guttate or follicular LP clinically; histologically, infiltrate is tightly compacted and often granulomatous
Keratosis lichenoides chronica	Clinically distinctive (also known as Nékam disease)
Lichen planus pemphigoides	Extreme basal epidermal degeneration in LP causes clefts (Max–Joseph spaces) that resemble the subepidermal bullae of lichen planus pemphigoides
Lichenoid actinic keratosis	Usually solitary, clinically a rather flat actinic keratosis; unlikely to cause a diagnostic problem if clinical and pathologic features are considered together
Lichen striatus	Clinically distinctive (see text for details)
Syphilis	May have lichenoid histology (may include plasma cells); secondary syphilis is in the clinical differential of generalized or palmoplantar LP
Lichenoid mycosis fungoides	A rare variant, usually plaques rather than the more isolated lesions of LP; histologically has epidermal component, atypical lymphocytes
Graft-versus-host disease	One pattern of this reaction, usually apparent from the clinical situation

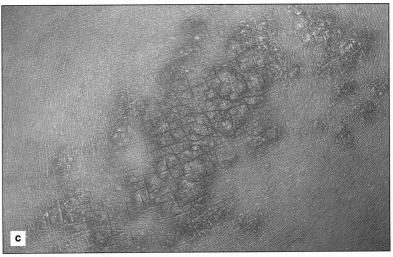

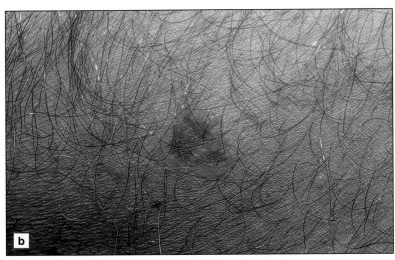

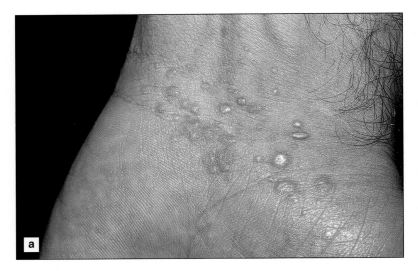

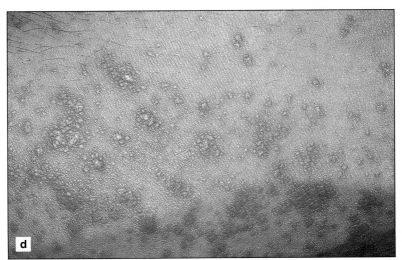

Figure 8.1 Lichen planus (LP): (**a**) typical, flat-topped, polygonal papules at a typical site on the wrist. (**b**) LP lesions with the typical purple color. (**c**) Semiconfluent papules of LP. (**d**) Multiple eruptive small spots of LP, with typical purple color.

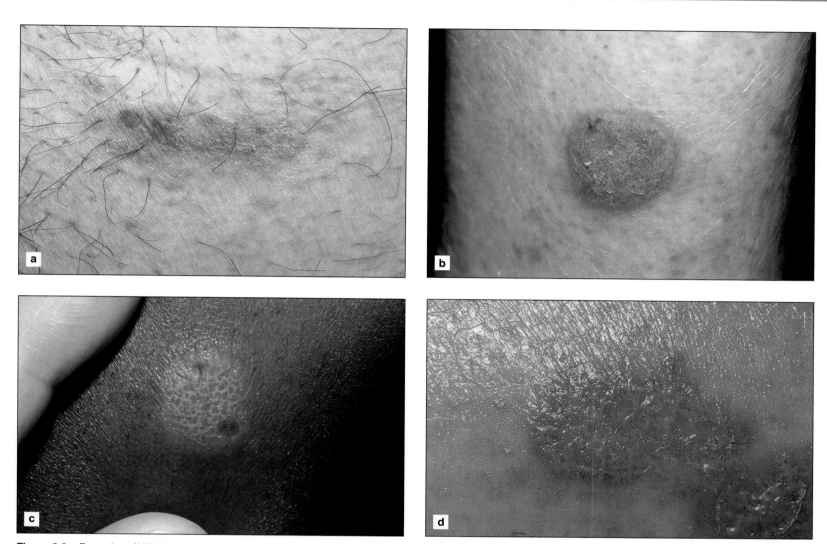

Figure 8.2 Examples of Wickham's striae in lichen planus (**a–d**). Note the annularity of the lesions in (a) (see also Fig. 8.8). If not readily visible, these can be accentuated by the application of oil (or even water) to the lesion, as shown in (d).

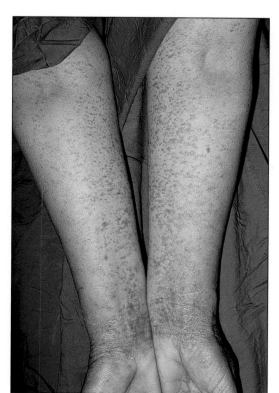

Figure 8.3 The volar aspect of the wrist is a typical site for lichen planus, and is an area where Koebner reactions are often seen.

Clinical features

Lichen planus may develop at any age, but men are typically affected at a younger age than women are.

The typical lesion of LP is a violaceous or purple, angulated (polyhedral), flat-topped papule or small plaque (Fig. 8.1). These are usually, but not invariably, extremely itchy; however, by contrast with eczemas, scratched lesions are unusual. The surface of the lesions, when viewed carefully, is notable for the presence of a white, lace-like patterning known as Wickham's striae (Fig. 8.2). Application of mineral oil to the surface of the lesion to fill air spaces in the keratin makes the striae more easily visible.

Lesions generally occur as crops, with a predilection for volar wrists or forearms (Figs 8.1a and 8.3) and around the shins and ankles. New lesions continue to appear for a few weeks to several months in most patients and, if untreated, the eruption generally lasts about 12–18 months.

Lichen planus is one of several disorders that exhibit the Koebner reaction, in which new lesions develop at the sites of minor injuries, such as scratches or burns (Fig. 8.4). A list of causes of this reaction is given in Chapter 1. A further notable feature, typically seen in resolving postinflammatory LP lesions but occasionally very prominent in new lesions, is a marked muddy-brown pigmentation (Fig. 8.5). This may be very intense at flexural sites.

Oral involvement is common, in about 75% of cases, but is asymptomatic in about 75% of those in whom it occurs; it is therefore incumbent on the physician to examine the mouth. The most common site for oral lesions is the buccal mucosa; the esophagus and other mucosae may be affected. These lesions have a white, lace-like pattern, and are discussed further with other oral lichenoid eruptions (later in this chapter).

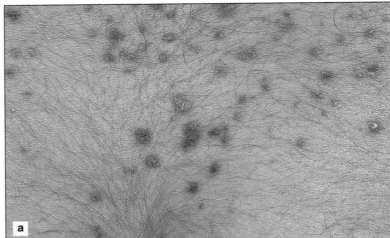

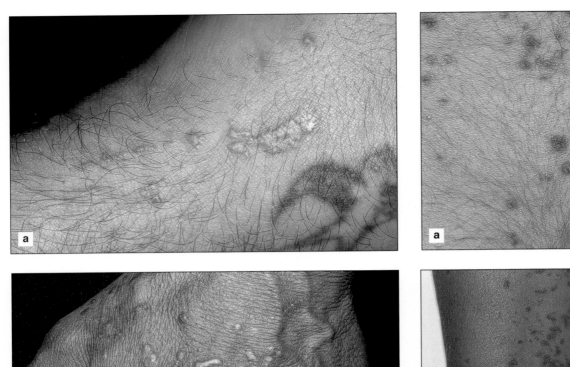

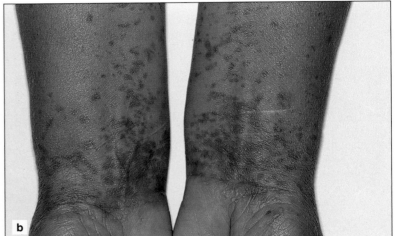

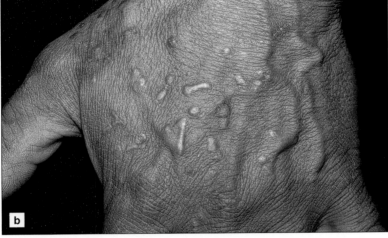

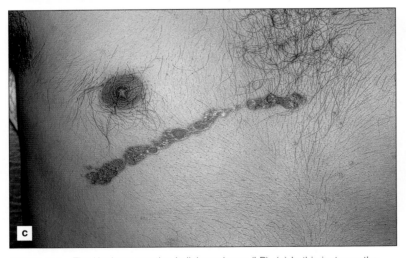

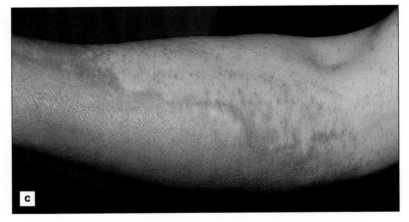

Figure 8.4 The Koebner reaction in lichen planus (LP). (**a**) In this instance the reaction followed a scratch on the arm. Lesions take about a week to appear, about the time the wound would normally take to heal. (**b**) Multiple small scratches on the dorsum of the hand, demonstrating the Koebner reaction in LP. (**c**) Pigmented Koebner reaction of LP due to an abrasion incurred while moving a heavy cabinet.

Figure 8.5 Postinflammatory pigmentation is often prominent in lichen planus (LP). (**a**) This illustration of the lower back (also a typical site) shows a mixture of newer purplish-red lesions and fading brown lesions. If using strong topical treatments, it is important to realize that the old lesions do not require treatment. (**b**) Old lesions of LP on the wrists, demonstrating postinflammatory dermal pigmentation. (**c**) Scattered and confluent heavily pigmented LP lesions.

There are a number of morphologic patterns and variants that appear different to classic LP; these are discussed here.

Specific patterns and sites of involvement
Generalized or guttate
In some patients, LP can be of dramatic and widespread onset, affecting any part of the body (Fig. 8.6). The lesions are often quite small papules and may not be readily recognized as LP, although they are generally purplish in colour. This pattern behaves rather like a viral exanthem, with which it may be confused.

Follicular (lichen planopilaris)
Follicular LP, consisting of tiny keratotic spots, also tends to be relatively widespread (Fig. 8.7) and has a tendency to involve the scalp, where it may cause alopecia.

Annular and atrophic
Annular lesions may be the main morphology present, usually in LP of rather limited distribution (Fig. 8.8). They are particularly common on the penis (Fig. 8.9). They may resolve with atrophy, although atrophic lesions of LP may occur de novo as well.

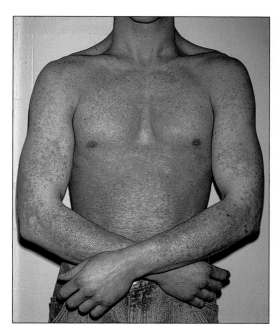

Figure 8.6 Generalized lichen planus, with abrupt, exanthem-like onset. This pattern is associated with hepatitis infection in some countries, but viral serology was negative in this case.

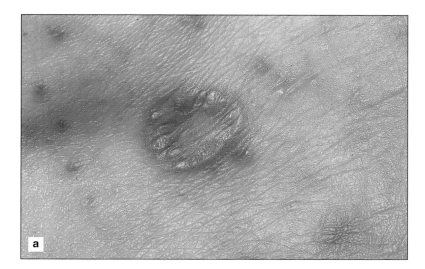

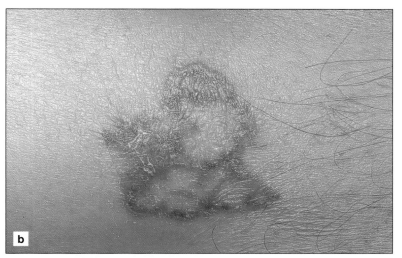

Figure 8.8 (**a**,**b**) Annular lesions of lichen planus may be confused with granuloma annulare or dermatophyte infections, but are usually small and have a narrower border than in either of these disorders.

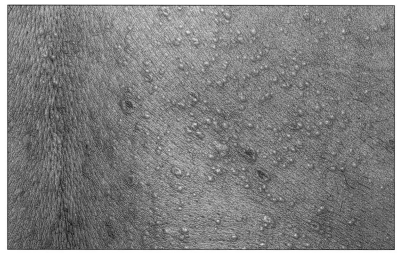

Figure 8.7 Follicular lichen planus, demonstrating multiple small conical papules centered on follicular orifices.

Localized or hypertrophic

In some patients, and at some body sites, lesions of LP may become grossly thickened and hypertrophic (Fig. 8.10). The shins are the most common site for this to occur. LP may occur as hypertrophic lesions on the lower legs in the absence of lesions at other sites, and may be confused with lichen simplex (Ch. 9). Rarely, keratoacanthoma or squamous cell carcinoma may arise on chronic hypertrophic LP.

Palm and sole

Lichen planus of palms or soles (Fig. 8.11) may be a very difficult diagnostic and therapeutic challenge, particularly if typical sites are un-affected. Lesions tend to be sheet-like rather than discrete, isolated papules, and are often hyperkeratotic and yellowish colored. They may resemble palmar psoriasis or even xanthomas. Less commonly, plantar LP may be severely erosive. Drug-related lichenoid reactions often involve palmoplantar skin (see later in chapter).

Nails and nail fold

Lichen planus may cause nail plate damage (Figs 8.9 and 8.12) or periungual inflammation (Figs 8.12b and 8.13). LP of the nail fold is important, as the inflammatory process may lead to scarring and adherence of the nail fold to the dorsal nail plate, a process known as pterygium. This is irreversible and warrants aggressive therapy to preserve the normal nail.

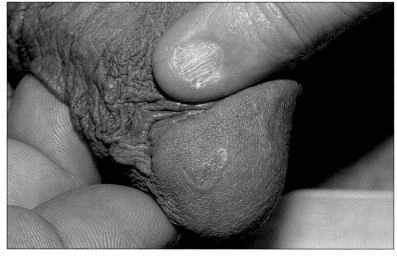

Figure 8.9 Annular lichen planus of the penis. Annular lesions are common at this site, and are usually asymptomatic. Note the nail involvement.

Scalp

Scalp involvement by LP is relatively uncommon but may occur in isolation (Fig. 8.14). It may be primarily around the follicles and hyper-keratotic, producing a nutmeg-grater-like feel to the scalp. This is known as lichen planopilaris. The clinical differential diagnosis is usually from discoid lupus erythematosus. Both of these are scarring disorders at this site, and carry a risk of permanent alopecia, so prompt diagnosis and aggressive therapy are required.

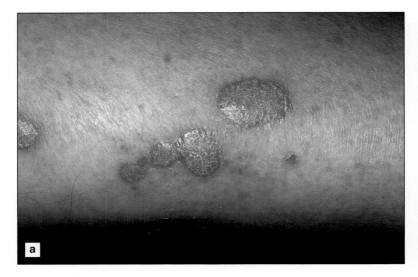

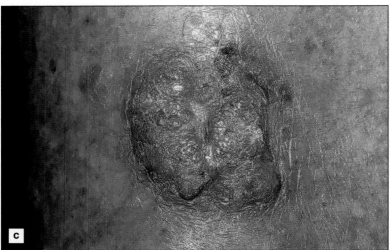

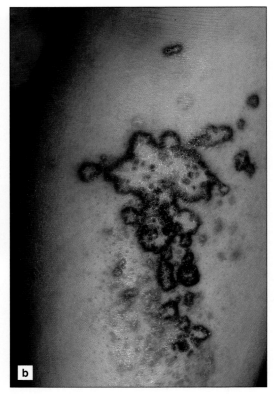

Figure 8.10 Hypertrophic lichen planus (LP). (**a**,**b**) The shins are a typical site and may be affected in isolation. This pattern tends to run a protracted course and is relatively unresponsive to therapy. Note the annularity and smaller follicular lesions in (b). (**c**) Hypertrophic LP, with a more keratotic surface, which may be difficult to distinguish from an epidermal neoplasm if the lesion is solitary.

Genital, perianal, and flexural

Genital involvement is frequent in LP, and often occurs in isolation. Again, this is often asymptomatic or less symptomatic compared with other sites, and may not be volunteered by the patient. Penile lesions often have an annular morphology (Fig. 8.9) but may be erosive (Fig. 8.15). Vulval LP (Fig. 8.16) may be of typical LP morphology, but may present as a moist, desquamative vaginitis, which may be confused with candidiasis or atrophic vaginitis; involvement of the female genital tract and the oral mucosa together (vulvovaginalgingival syndrome) is notoriously resistant to therapy.

Perianal LP (Fig. 8.17) may resemble a simple intertrigo; striae, if visible, may be confused with simple maceration of keratin. Flexural LP is diagnostically difficult; some cases are erosive, while others have pigmented macules without the typical surface changes of LP.

Other rarer patterns and sites

- Linear LP follows developmental lines, usually down the leg (Fig. 8.18), but it may be zosteriform or may erupt in a swirled pattern (Fig. 8.19) following the lines of Blaschko (see Ch. 2).
- Bullous LP may exist in two forms. One (termed bullous LP) is the development of blisters on lesions of otherwise typical LP (Fig. 8.20). The other form, in which blisters occur on normal skin as well as on LP lesions, has a close resemblance to bullous pemphigoid histologically (hence the name LP pemphigoides). This latter type may occur as a drug reaction to captopril, which may also cause a non-bullous lichenoid reaction.
- Actinic LP occurs in young people in the tropics; it is hyperpigmented and may resemble melasma or eczema.

- Lichen planus pigmentosus is seen mainly in India and Asia; it affects the face and upper trunk, causing a widespread pigmentary disturbance.

Very localized LP may cause diagnostic difficulty, for example on the lip or the eyelids (Fig. 8.21), where seborrheic or contact dermatitis are differential diagnoses.

Differential diagnosis

This varies according to the site and morphologic pattern (Table 8.3).

Treatment

The mainstay of treatment for LP is strong topical corticosteroids. Patients with less prominent itch may be treated with milder agents, and asymptomatic oral lesions require no active treatment. It is important to educate the patient in the use of stronger agents to minimize the risk of side effects. Treatments do not speed up resolution of postinflammatory pigmentation, so patients should be informed to treat new red-purple itchy lesions but not quiescent brown asymptomatic marks. In most patients, this will lead to resolution; further episodes are uncommon.

Resistant localized lesions, such as on the shins, may be treated with intralesional steroids or with steroids under occlusive dressings. Unfortunately, this is a body site where resolution is less easy to predict with confidence; prolonged treatment and incomplete clearance are frequent.

Lesions at critical sites such as scalp or nail folds should be treated aggressively, using very potent topical steroids or systemic therapy, because of the risk of scarring. Systemic treatment of LP has traditionally been with corticosteroids, usually at doses equivalent to 20–40 mg of prednisolone initially, reduced over a period of a few weeks. Other immunosuppressive agents have been used, of which ciclosporin appears to be the

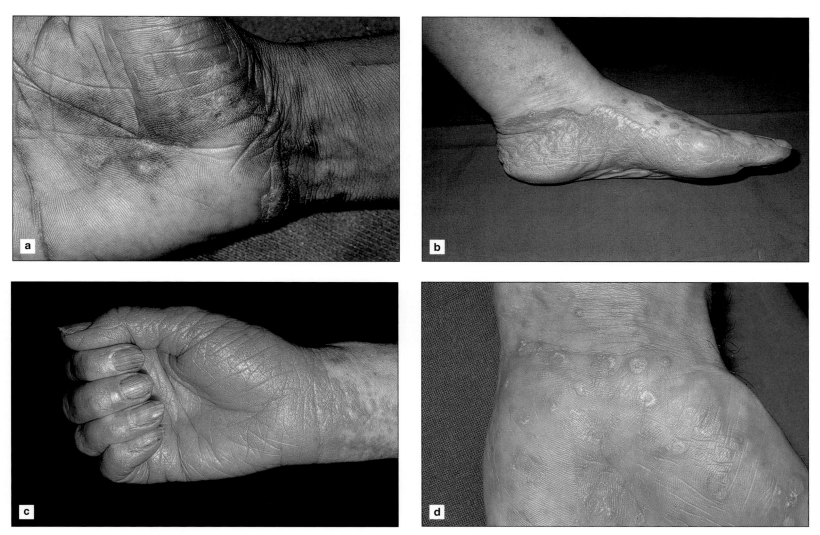

Figure 8.11 Palmar lichen planus (LP). (**a**) In African-Caribbean skin, demonstrating prominent pigmentation. (**b**) LP on the sole of the foot, with a more confluent pattern. A number of disorders may show this pattern of being confined to the skin below (occasionally above) the Wallace line, which runs a centimeter or so above the weight-bearing area of the true plantar skin. (**c**) LP of the palm with confluent lesions resembling psoriasis. (**d**) LP of the palm, in this case with discrete hyperkeratotic lesions that had a yellowish color reminiscent of pustules or xanthomas.

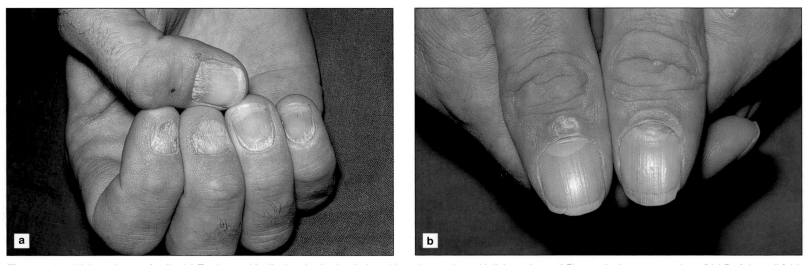

Figure 8.12 Lichen planus of nails. (**a**) Trachyonychia-like longitudinal nail plate ridges in a patient with lichen planus (LP) at typical cutaneous sites. (**b**) LP of the nail fold with proximal nail plate dystrophy; if not treated aggressively, this may cause permanent damage by scarring to the surface of the nail plate (see also Fig. 8.13).

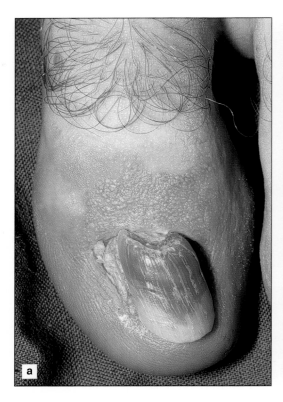

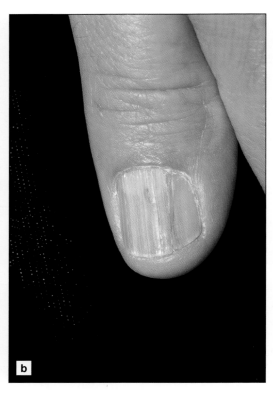

Figure 8.13 Lichen planus affecting the nails. In the patient shown in (**a**), treatment with systemic steroids avoided permanent nail dystrophy; normal nail growth is recommencing and just visible beyond the cuticle. (**b**) A permanent longitudinal nail dystrophy; old changes such as this may be clinically indistinguishable from a traumatic dystrophy.

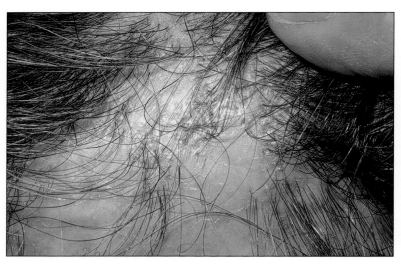

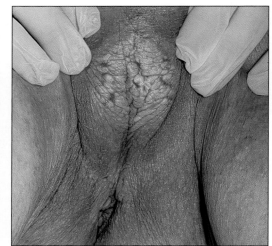

Figure 8.16 Vulval lichen planus, in this instance with macerated keratin producing a white color but still with a purplish background component.

Figure 8.14 Lichen planus of the scalp: scarring alopecia with purplish-colored perifollicular inflammation.

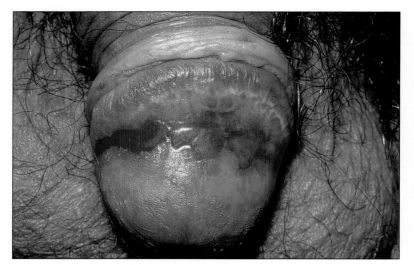

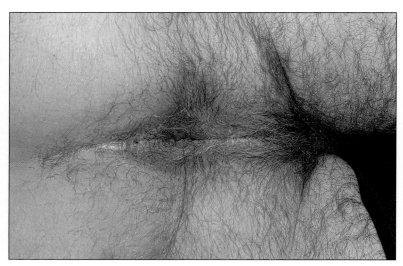

Figure 8.15 Erosive genital lichen planus may occur in either sex, in this case becoming apparent only following circumcision for treatment of chronic balanitis.

Figure 8.17 Perianal lichen planus may resemble intertrigo, seborrheic dermatitis, or psoriasis, due to the occluded skin at this site.

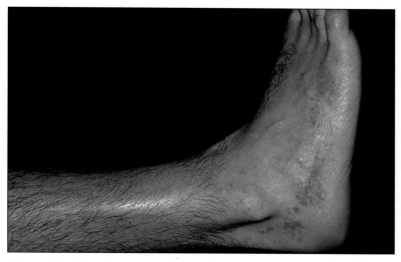

Figure 8.18 Linear lichen planus (LP), shown here along the lateral border of the foot in a patient with no evidence of LP at other sites. Linear LP usually develops as a broad band from the buttock down the posterior aspect of the leg to the foot. A similar pattern may occur with linear psoriasis. (Courtesy of Dr. L. Barco.)

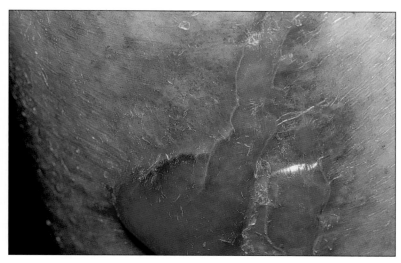

Figure 8.20 Bullous lichen planus (LP) on the leg, within a typically purplish-colored lesion. This variant also occurs in clinically normal skin with LP elsewhere, in the mouth, and occasionally on the scalp.

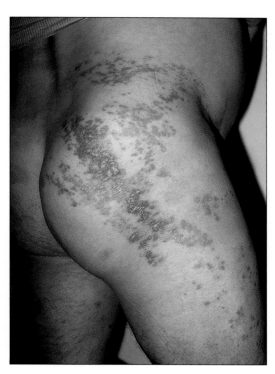

Figure 8.19 Lichenoid lesions in the lines of Blaschko: this eruptive pattern may be better termed lichenoid blaschkitis rather than lichen planus in Blaschko lines.

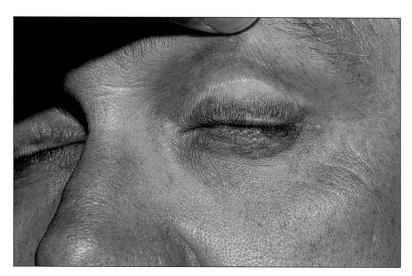

Figure 8.21 Lichen planus affecting the eyelids, in a pattern that could be misdiagnosed as a contact dermatitis. Note, however, that the lesions are sharply demarcated, which is unlikely in eczematous processes at this site.

most consistently useful. Heparin seems to be useful in some patients, for uncertain reasons. PUVA photochemotherapy can also be useful. All these agents have some risk of side effects, and they are generally reserved for patients with extensive lesions, refractory LP, or involvement at potentially scarring sites.

PRACTICE POINTS

- In any patient with a purplish-colored rash, think about lichen planus (LP) and look in the mouth.
- Penile LP is often atypical: annular lesions are common, and itch is often not a feature.
- Consider drug-induced lichenoid eruption in any patient with clinically atypical LP, and get a skin biopsy.
- Potent topical corticosteroids are often necessary for symptomatic control in LP.

ORAL LICHEN PLANUS AND THE ORAL LICHENOID ERUPTION

Etiology and pathogenesis

The oral lichenoid eruption is a less specific entity compared with LP of the skin. It is best considered as a reaction pattern of the oral mucosa to a variety of insults, including LP itself, contact allergy (especially to mercury in dental amalgam), trauma, and other inflammatory dermatoses (e.g. oral lupus erythematosus may look very lichenoid). Some cases related to dental fillings appear to be related to corrosion of amalgam or to use of mixed metal materials, creating a galvanic effect. Even patients in whom mercury allergy cannot be demonstrated may benefit from removal of fillings.

Clinical features

Oral lichenoid reactions resemble the Wickham's striae seen in the surface of skin lesions of LP. Fine, white streaking and reticulate patterning is

Table 8.3 DIFFERENTIAL DIAGNOSIS OF SOME MORPHOLOGIC AND SITE-SPECIFIC VARIANTS OF LICHEN PLANUS

Variant	Differential diagnoses[a]
Classic	Psoriasis, eczema, tinea, pityriasis rosea, scabies, lupus erythematosus, ashy dermatosis
Generalized or guttate	Viral exanthems, drug eruptions, guttate psoriasis, lichen nitidus, syphilis, lichenoid pattern of sarcoidosis
Annular	Granuloma annulare, tinea
Atrophic	Lichen sclerosus, guttate morphea
Hypertrophic	Lichen simplex, psoriasis, skin neoplasm, lichen amyloidosis
Palm or sole	Psoriasis (including pustular form), dermatitis, syphilis, scabies, warts, xanthomas, callosities
Nail	Psoriasis, tinea, 20-nail dystrophy, idiopathic onycholysis
Follicular (lichen planopilaris)	Body: keratosis pilaris or Darier disease Scalp: lupus erythematosus
Linear	Koebner reaction, herpes zoster, lichen striatus, linear psoriasis, inflammatory linear epidermal nevus
Oral	Leukoplakia, candidiasis, gingivitis, lupus erythematosus (especially lip), white sponge nevus
Male genital (usually annular)	Sexually transmitted disease, warts, Zoon balanitis (if erosive on glans)
Female genital	Candidiasis, lichen sclerosus, other causes of vaginitis
Flexural	Psoriasis, dermatitis (seborrheic, contact), simple intertrigo, erythrasma

[a]Drug-induced lichen planus is in the differential of most variants, but particularly lichen planus of generalized or predominantly acral distribution.

apparent in the mouth, and is usually most apparent on the buccal mucosa (Fig. 8.22). However, any part of the mouth can be affected, including the gums, lips, palate, and tongue (Fig. 8.23).

The most elegant, fine, lace-like pattern is seen in true LP (see Fig. 8.22), most other lichenoid reactions being rather coarser in pattern (Fig. 8.24). Erosive and pigmented LP also occur in the mouth (Fig. 8.25).

The site of lesions may give clues to the etiology. Repetitive trauma due to trapping of the buccal mucosa between the upper and lower molars produces a linear lichenoid lesion (bite line). Reactions to mercury in dental amalgam or other dental filling reactions are usually most prominent in proximity to filled teeth. Lupus erythematosus may affect the lips (Fig. 8.26) in isolation or in patients with discoid or systemic disease, and may be associated with lichenoid eruptions at other intraoral sites (Ch. 13).

Investigations

Biopsy may be required to exclude leukoplakia and confirm that the eruption is benign lichenoid change, especially if the changes are unilateral or asymmetric. Chronic candidal infection may require swabs and biopsy to distinguish it from oral lichenoid change. Special techniques such as immunofluorescence examination of biopsy specimens may be required in cases in which there is suspicion of mucous membrane pemphigoid, in which resolved blisters may leave a residual lichenoid change. Longstanding, especially erosive, oral LP carries a small risk of neoplastic degeneration and should be biopsied in cases where lesions deteriorate or become thickened.

In patients with oral lichenoid change and without skin signs of LP, about 20% have a contact allergy, which can be identified by patch testing. Lichenoid oral contact allergy can be to flavoring agents such as balsams or cinnamaldehyde, but most are to mercury in dental amalgam.

Differential diagnosis

This is listed in Table 8.3.

Treatment

Many patients with oral lichenoid appearance, due to LP or other causes, have no symptoms. In such instances, no treatment is required, although

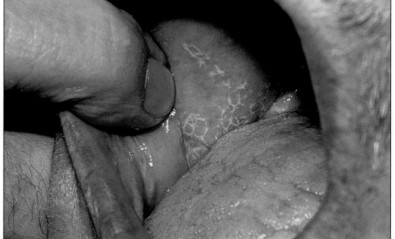

Figure 8.22 Buccal lichen planus showing the typical fine lace-like pattern.

follow-up has been advised due to the risk of subsequent oral squamous carcinoma.

In symptomatic patients, topical corticosteroids may be administered as ointments, dental pastes, aqueous sprays, or dental lozenges. Non-steroidal antiinflammatory mouthwashes, and antiseptic mouthwashes, may also be helpful. Topical ciclosporin as a mouthwash produces variable benefit, but may be limited by lack of penetration into the mucosa. Topical tacrolimus can be beneficial, but the response is not reliable in the author's experience.

Resistant lesions may require intralesional steroid injection, or systemic treatment as for LP. The combination of oral and genital or perineal LP, without lesions elsewhere, seems to be a particularly troublesome and resistant form of this disease.

In patients with allergy to mercury in dental fillings, most improve after their fillings are removed and replaced with composite materials. However, the release of mercury during the procedure, and the physical handling of the mouth, may cause transient deterioration in symptoms.

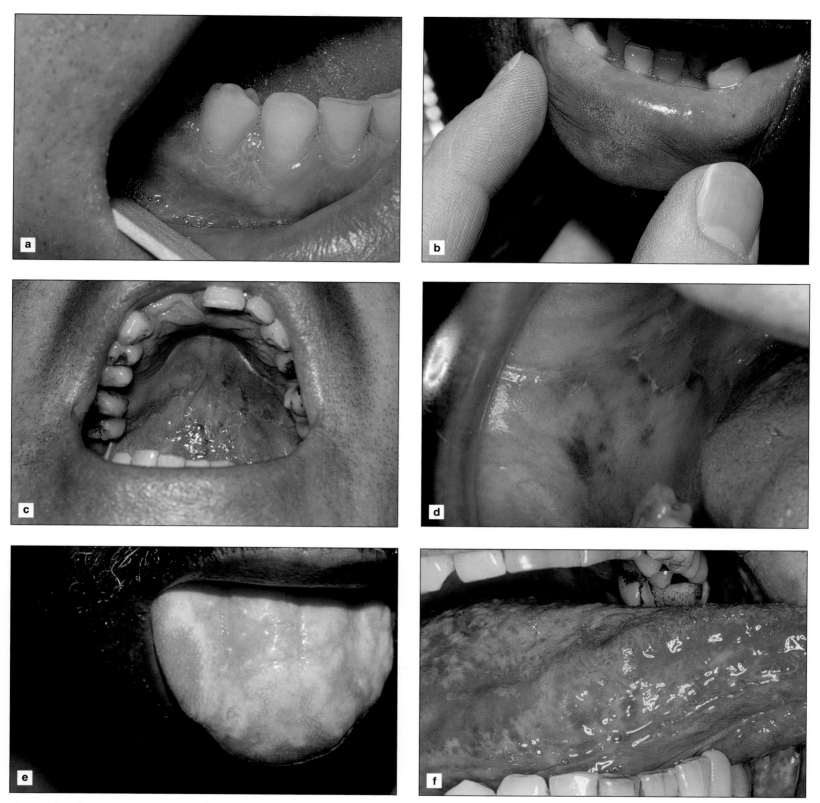

Figure 8.23 Patterns of lichen planus (LP) affecting the mouth. (**a**) LP of the gingival mucosa, again with typical fine, white striae. (**b**) LP of the lip. In this case, there are quite irregular teeth, which may have caused a degree of local trauma. In the absence of LP elsewhere, this should be biopsied to exclude leukoplakia. (**c**) Erosive LP of the palate. This was associated with perianal and genital LP, and was unresponsive to a wide range of topical and systemic medications, including ciclosporin, azathioprine, and thalidomide. (**d**) Pigmented LP in the mouth causes diagnostic concern but has no particular significance. It may occur in lichenoid drug eruptions. (**e**) Annular lesions of LP on the tongue may be confused with migratory glossitis or candidiasis. Secondary syphilis should also be considered. (**f**) LP of the lateral tongue border, a pattern that closely resembles leukoplakia and requires a biopsy.

PRACTICE POINTS

- If oral lichen planus (LP) is very localized, consider the possibility of reaction to amalgam fillings.
- Oral LP may persist long after the cutaneous component has resolved.
- Patients with erosive oral LP justify review due to the risk of malignancy.

OTHER LICHENOID CONDITIONS

Several other conditions are usefully discussed here. Most are clinically lichenoid (i.e. consisting of flat-topped papules or small plaques); some also have lichenoid histology.

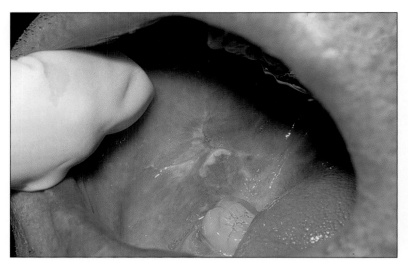

Figure 8.24 Lichenoid reaction due to dental amalgam, which produces a coarser pattern of white streaks (compare with Fig. 8.22). When the mouth was closed, this lesion was in close proximity to a filled tooth, just visible in the upper jaw. The patient had positive patch tests to mercurial chemicals.

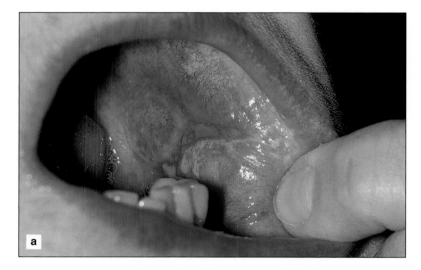

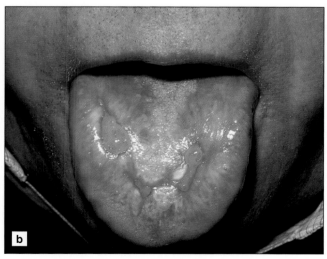

Figure 8.25 Ulcerative oral lichen planus (LP). (**a**) LP causing buccal erosion. By contrast to most oral LP, this pattern often causes significant soreness and difficulty eating. When it occurs as part of the eruption of cutaneous LP, it may persist long after the skin lesions have resolved. (**b**) Ulcerated LP of the tongue. The dorsal surface of the tongue is purplish in color, with myriad small, white striae and extensive ulceration.

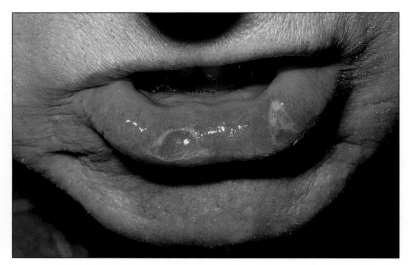

Figure 8.26 Lupus erythematosus of the lips may be more scaly and scarring, but in some patients produces prominent lichenoid change, as shown here (this patient had previous discoid lupus erythematosus on the cheek, and oral biopsies also favored this diagnosis).

Lichen nitidus

This is an uncommon disorder, of unknown etiology, which occurs predominantly in young adults, and which has a body site distribution similar to that of LP. However, the individual lesions are tiny (pinhead-sized), domed papules with a typical orange-brown color (Fig. 8.27). They are usually asymptomatic, not very visible, and no treatment is usually required. Koebner reactions are common (see Fig. 8.27a). Involvement of the palm and sole, or of the nails (Fig. 8.28), is extremely uncommon but may be relatively refractory and disabling due to hyperkeratosis at these sites.

Lichen striatus

This is an uncommon but characteristic eruption. It has an acute onset, and most commonly occurs as a solitary, long, thin lesion running down a limb (Fig. 8.29). It follows developmental lines known as lines of Blaschko. Occasionally, multiple lesions or truncal lesions may occur. In a minority of cases, there appears to be a temporal link with a recent infection, especially in children, and sequential development of lichen striatus in siblings has been reported, which supports the concept of an infectious trigger.

The close-up morphology may be strikingly lichenoid, but few patients report significant symptoms. A topical corticosteroid may be required to reduce the inflammatory component, and resolution usually occurs over a period of some months.

Frictional lichenoid eruption

This is a relatively uncommon disorder, but probably underdiagnosed, as it is often asymptomatic. It is most frequent in boys in the 5–10-year age group, and consists of clusters of tiny lichenoid papules, which occur predominantly over bony prominences on the limbs (Fig. 8.30). There is often an atopic background. Treatment is with emollients.

Lichen spinulosa

This poorly defined disorder resembles keratosis pilaris but occurs as closely grouped, spiky lesions, usually in children (Fig. 8.31). Treatment is with emollients if required.

Keratosis lichenoides chronica (Nékam disease)

This is a rare disorder, characterized by keratotic lichenoid papules and plaques with a streaky linear or reticulate patterning (Fig. 8.32). Any body site may be affected. The facial rash resembles seborrheic dermatitis.

Erythema dyschromicum perstans (ashy dermatosis)

An uncommon disorder, in which there are poorly demarcated blotchy areas of dermal pigmentation, typically with a slate-gray color, and usually

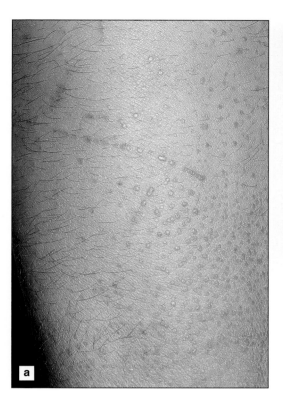

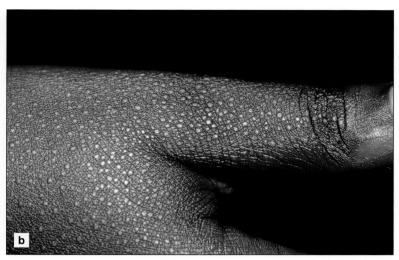

Figure 8.27 Lichen nitidus. (**a**) Small, orange-brown papules demonstrating the Koebner reaction. (**b**) Lichen nitidus on the hand of an African-Caribbean patient. In dark-colored skin, the papules of lichen nitidus look white and shiny.

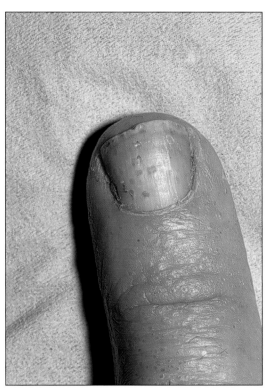

Figure 8.28 Lichen nitidus of the nail. Punctate red lesions are visible in the lunula, and nail pits. The patient had severe palmoplantar involvement with marked hyperkeratosis, a rare variant, and was treated with systemic retinoids.

Table 8.4 LICHENOID ERUPTIONS DUE TO DRUGS AND CHEMICALS	
Cause	**Agents**
Systemic drugs	
Cardiac	Beta-blockers, methyldopa, captopril, furosemide
Antimalarials	Mepacrine (Atabrine), chloroquine, quinine
Rheumatology	Gold, penicillamine, non-steroidal antiinflammatory drugs
Others	Phenothiazines, thiazides, tetracyclines
External contact	
Photographic	*Para*-phenylenediamine (PPD) color developers CD2, CD3
Car industry	Methylacrylic acid esters
Dental (oral lesions)	Mercury, rarely other filling materials
Others	Tattoo pigments (usually red), gold, topical aminoglycosides

Graft-versus-host disease

Graft-versus–host disease (GVHD) is a skin eruption that occurs in recipients of allogeneic tissues, in which donor immune cells attack host tissues due to histoincompatibility. It is discussed in more detail in Chapter 12. Chronic GVHD may cause a rash resembling LP, including oral lesions.

Drug-induced lichen planus or lichenoid eruption and other exogenous causes

Drugs may cause an eruption that is similar to LP (Fig. 8.34). A list of likely medications and external agents that may cause a lichenoid eruption or LP-like contact dermatitis is given in Table 8.4; a more detailed list of the drug triggers is provided in Chapter 18, along with a list of issues that contribute to difficulty in diagnosis.

Clinically, the possibility of a lichenoid drug eruption is suggested by the presence of lesions which have the violaceous or brownish color of LP, but which are clinically less well demarcated and usually lack classic Wickham's striae (see Fig. 8.3). The lesions are often larger plaques or macules compared with those of typical LP, and may have psoriasiform scaling. The rash is often generalized but may be predominantly acral; oral

occurring on the trunk in children or young adults (Fig. 8.33). In some cases, there is some preceding erythema and histologic evidence of basal cell vacuolization, but clinically there are no discrete lesions as seen in LP. It is the histology that resembles resolving LP; some view this as a variant of LP rather than as a separate disorder. Topical treatments are unhelpful.

Annular lichenoid dermatitis of youth

It is uncertain whether this recently described condition is a specific entity. Twenty-three patients, mean age 10 years, were described with an annular lichenoid dermatitis, with central hypopigmentation, resembling mycosis fungoides, morphea, or annular erythema. Treatment was with topical or oral steroids, or with phototherapy.

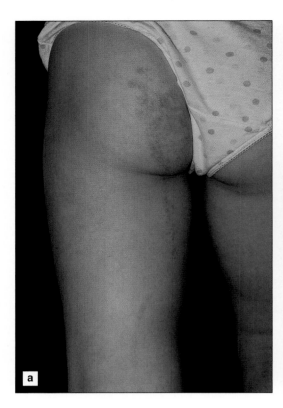

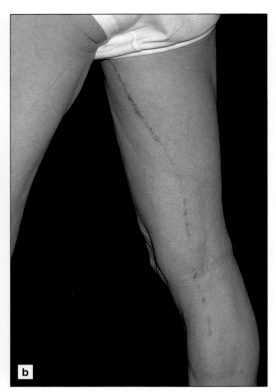

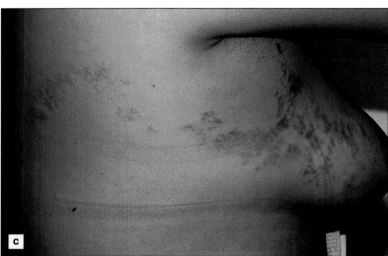

Figure 8.29 Lichen striatus. This is most common in children (**a**) but can occur in adults (**b,c**). Both (a) and (b) show a narrow band extending down the posterior aspect of the leg. Limb lesions of this disorder are usually solitary, whereas truncal lesions may be multiple and more arciform in distribution, following Blaschko lines (**c**). (Panel a courtesy of Dr. L. Barco.)

lesions occur with several drugs and do not necessarily imply idiopathic LP. Histologically, the inflammatory infiltrate may be mixed rather than purely lymphocytic (eosinophils may be prominent), and is usually less tightly aggregated below the dermo–epidermal junction than is seen in true LP.

Lichenoid reactions to tattoo pigments are uncommon with modern pigments, but may occur several years after a tattoo has been performed (Fig. 8.35).

Lichen planus-like rash due to color developers is now rare due to automated processing.

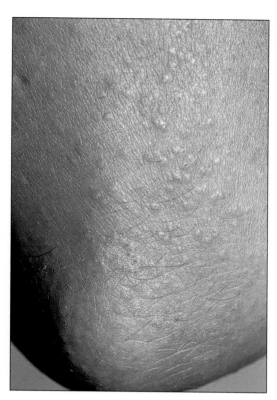

Figure 8.30 Frictional lichenoid eruption. Grouped, small, flat-topped papular lesions on the elbow, a typical site.

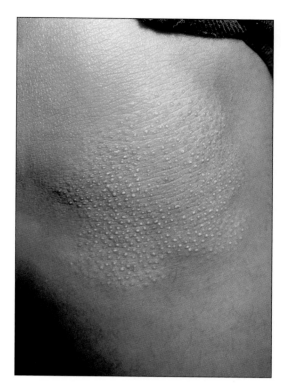

Figure 8.31 Lichen spinulosa. Closely grouped, spiky, keratotic lesions resembling keratosis pilaris but with a more discrete arrangement of lesions.

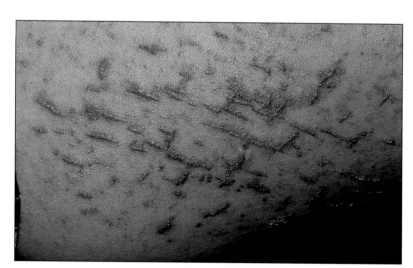

Figure 8.32 Keratosis lichenoides chronica (Nékam disease). Typical reticulate and linear arrangement of chronic inflammatory keratotic lesions. (Courtesy of Gerald Weinstein.)

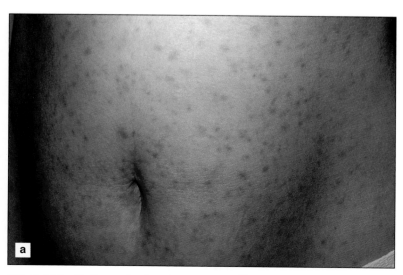

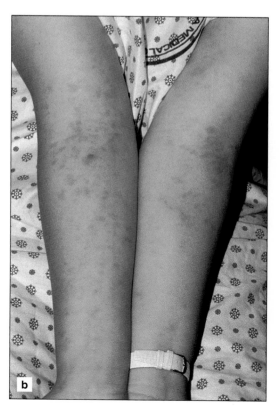

Figure 8.33 Erythema dyschromicum perstans. The reason for the alternative name, ashy dermatosis, is apparent from the grayish color of the lesions. The poorly defined blotchy appearance on the trunk (**a**) and arms (**b**), as seen here, is typical.

133

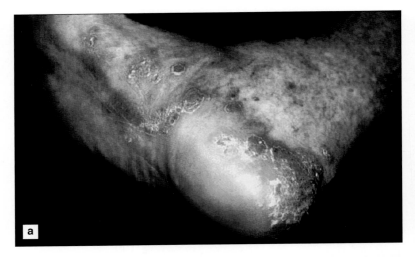

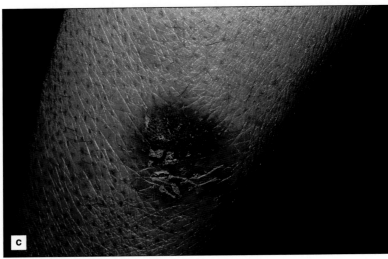

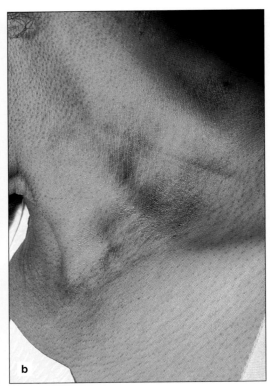

Figure 8.34 Examples of drug-induced lichenoid eruptions. Some occur due to a drug in isolation, such as this eruption on the foot (**a**) due to a beta-blocker. Acral sites are often affected in lichenoid drug eruptions. In other cases, the reaction may be photolichenoid, occurring on sun-exposed skin, such as the eruptions in (**b**) and (**c**), which were both due to the antimalarial drug hydroxychloroquine. (Panel a courtesy of Dr. G. Dawn.)

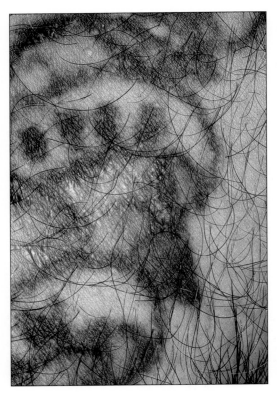

Figure 8.35 Lichenoid reaction to red pigment in a tattoo. This can sometimes be treated with topical or intralesional steroids, but may require removal of the tattoo.

FURTHER READING

Boyd AS. Update on the diagnosis of lichenoid dermatitis. Adv Dermatol 1996; 11: 287–315

Breathnach SM, Black MM. Lichen planus and lichenoid disorders. In: Burns DA, Breathnach SM, Cox NH, et al (eds) Rook's Textbook of Dermatology, 7th edn. Oxford: Blackwell Publishing, 2004: 1–32, 42

Chen W, Schramm M, Zouboulis CC. Generalized lichen nitidus. J Am Acad Dermatol 1997; 36: 630–1

Cribier B, Garnier C, Laustriat D, et al. Lichen planus and hepatitis C virus infection: an epidemiologic study. J Am Acad Dermatol 1994; 31: 1070–2

Dunsche A, Frank MP, Luttges J, et al. Oral lichenoid reactions associated with amalgam: improvement after amalgam removal. Br J Dermatol 2003; 148: 741–8

Gilhar A, Pillar T, Winterstein G, et al. The pathogenesis of lichen planus. Br J Dermatol 1989; 120: 541–4

Sánchez-Pérez J, Rios Buceta L, Fraga J, et al. Lichen planus with lesions on the palms and/or soles. Prevalence and clinicopathological study of 36 patients. Br J Dermatol 2000; 142: 310–4

Urticaria and Pruritus

INTRODUCTION

Itch is a prominent feature of many skin diseases. But what does it mean to itch? Some have defined pruritus as 'a sensation that, if sufficiently strong, will provoke scratching or the desire to scratch'. Poetic commentary is more entertaining, for example ''tis better than riches to scratch where it itches'. Many patients will present with itching but no rash, and it is the clinician's duty to ferret out the cause. Causes range from dry skin to scabies to Hodgkin lymphoma.

Urticaria is one of the commonest dermatoses that causes significant itch and is considered in this chapter. Itch is also typically prominent in eczemas (Ch. 6) and in lichen planus (Ch. 8). Finally, some people scratch for psychologic reasons. They may, for example, be convinced that bugs live in and on their skin, or that shards of glass or thorns from a plant are still embedded in their skin years after an injury. These patients, who are delusional (i.e. they hold on to a belief despite obvious evidence to the contrary), are perhaps the most difficult patients a dermatologist must deal with.

URTICARIA AND RELATED DISORDERS

Etiology and pathogenesis

The immune system has a complex task to perform. It fights off bacteria, viruses, and fungi, and yet it is supposed to leave the normal bodily tissue alone. Sometimes, the immune system fails to distinguish between self and non-self, and an autoimmune disease results. Many skin diseases can be said to fit into this category, including psoriasis, lichen planus, and some cases of urticaria. In the case of acute urticaria, the immune system is often using IgE-mediated mechanisms to attack transient things, such as food, medications, or viruses, and can thus be termed allergic urticaria. However, many cases of urticaria are not truly allergic, for example physical urticarias (Table 9.1) and some other non-immunologic urticarias (e.g. those due to some drugs, such as salicylates, radiocontrast media, and opiates).

The mechanism of wheal formation in urticaria typically involves the release of histamine, a vasoactive substance, from mast cells. Other changes in urticaria are due to other vasoactive substances, such as prostaglandins, and these changes may not respond to antihistamines. This explains why wheals may be prevented by antihistamines but erythema still occurs. In the usual urticaria, there is no damage to the vessels and the wheal resolves within 24 h. If the blood vessels are damaged, the lesions persist beyond 24 h and the term urticarial vasculitis is used.

The list of potential causes of urticaria is endless; some are apparent from the names of the individual disorders discussed (e.g. cold urticaria), others are discussed in the relevant sections. It is important to recognize that, other than in the case of episodic short-lived episodes of urticaria, a cause is often not apparent.

Solar urticaria is discussed in Chapter 17.

Dermatographism
Clinical
Patients with dermatographism develop linear wheals at the site of stroking of the skin (Fig. 9.1). Sometimes they note raised, red lines that occur soon after scratching, but some present with the chief complaint of intense itching and claim that there is no rash. Dermatographism may occur in various clinical situations, including the third trimester of pregnancy or after treatment for scabies, although, particularly when it is the sole morphology of urticaria, it is commonly idiopathic. The diagnosis

---

Table 9.1 SOME TYPES OF PHYSICAL URTICARIA

Dermatographism (dermographism)
Cholinergic urticaria
Cold urticaria
Solar urticaria
Heat urticaria
Deep pressure urticaria
Aquagenic urticaria
Exercise-induced urticarias or anaphylaxis (with or without preceding foods)

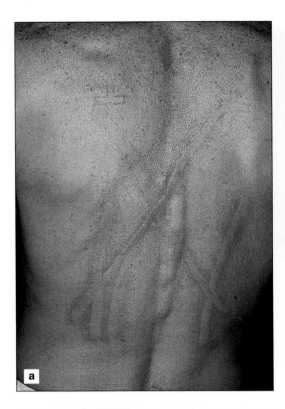

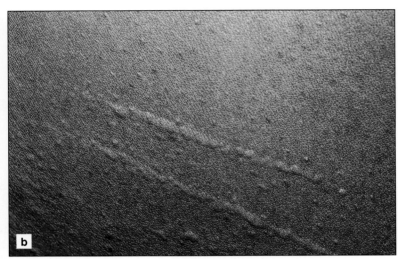

Figure 9.1 Dermatographism. (**a**) Stroking with a tongue blade can provide the diagnosis of dermatographism within minutes. Look not just for redness but whealing also. It is worth noting that many patients on antihistamines may get the flare without the wheal, as other mast cell mediators are involved in the erythema component. (**b**) In darker-skinned patients, the erythema is hidden but not the wheal. (**c**) Dermatographism from much scratching on a background of a florid urticarial eruption caused by antibiotic treatment.

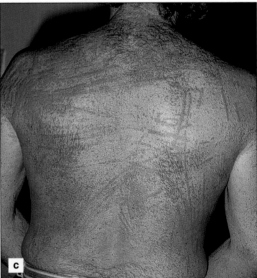

may be established by taking a tongue blade and stroking it several times across the back. Immediate redness will occur in most people, but true whealing will develop within minutes in patients with dermatographism. A dermatographometer can grade the pressure used to stroke the skin. Stroking the skin with a pressure of 3.5×10^5 Pa gives a positive result.

Treatment

As in any urticaria, a search for an allergen (e.g. recent antibiotic or infection) should be performed and, if found, eliminated. Most of the time, however, no allergen is found. Antihistamines are effective, with the non-sedating ones least objectionable to the patient (e.g. cetirizine 10 mg/day). Some advocate the addition of an H_2 blocker for dermatographism, but its effect appears minimal. Interestingly, the H_2 blocker famotidine has been reported to cause dermatographism.

Acute urticaria

Clinical

Urticaria of less than 6 weeks' duration is considered acute urticaria. If the duration is longer than 6 weeks, the term chronic urticaria is used. The deeper swellings of angioedema commonly accompany urticaria.

Itchy, edematous, raised, pink plaques without scale that move and change daily are characteristic of 'ordinary' acute or chronic urticaria (Fig. 9.2). Annular lesions resulting from central clearing and white halos (like the Woronoff ring of psoriasis) can occur due to vasoconstriction (Fig. 9.3). Persistence of urticaria for more than 24 h in the same location, or the presence of associated purpura, may indicate urticarial vasculitis (discussed later in this chapter). If there is any doubt about urticarial vasculitis, lesions should be circled and reexamined 24 h later. If the lesions

Table 9.2	KNOWN CAUSES OF NON-PHYSICAL URTICARIA	
Usually acute (lasting minutes to 1-2 days)	**Variable duration**	**Usually chronic, lasting weeks to months or longer**
Foods, vitamins[a] Bites and stings Local anaesthetics, intravenous drugs	Orally administered drugs Infections[b] (bacterial, viral, helminth, scabies) and vaccines	Autoimmune (with antibodies to IgE or the IgE receptor)

[a] Duration for foods and similar agents depends on whether ingestion continues
[b] Duration of infection triggered urticaria depends on duration to diagnosis; duration after treatment may be several weeks until immune reaction subsides

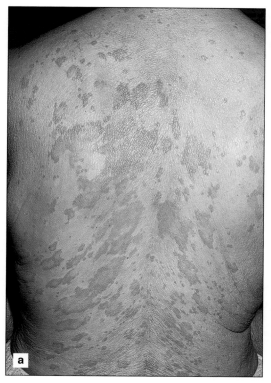

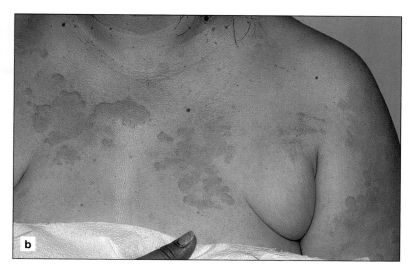

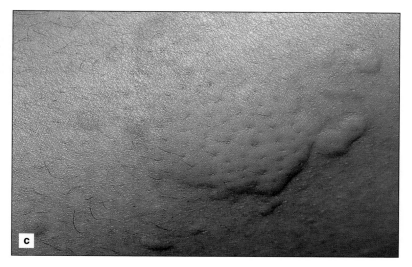

Figure 9.2 Urticaria. (**a,b**) Intensely pruritic wheals rise, migrate, and disappear, all within the course of a day. Often a transient antigen (e.g. nuts, a virus, or an antibiotic) is the cause. (**c**) The dermis swells with fluid. The surface balloons but is tented at the site of follicular orifices, like an orange peel.

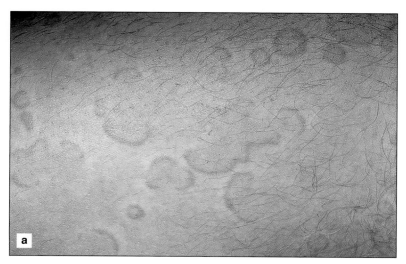

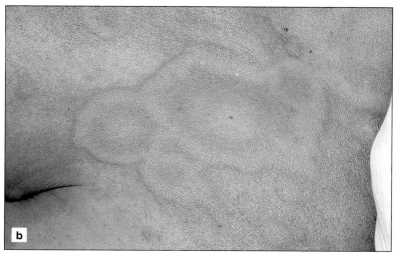

Figure 9.3 (**a,b**) Urticaria. These two cases illustrate a typical annular appearance caused by the pale center and red border.

are still in the circle, the patient may have urticarial vasculitis, although other diseases, such as erythema multiforme, should also be considered.

Causes, investigation, and treatment of acute or chronic urticaria

Table 9.2 lists the commonest categories of agents that cause urticaria (excluding physical urticarias). The physical urticarias should be excluded as the primary lesion. Delayed pressure urticaria and dermatographism may accompany urticaria. The diet, over-the-counter products, recent

infections, and medication history should be analyzed for any new potential allergens. The history may give useful clues; for example, most allergy to foods in adults relates to intermittently ingested items, and causes occasional brief episodes of rash lasting just a day or two. By contrast, presumably due to the immune response being activated and then gradually waning, urticaria triggered by infections typically lasts for several weeks.

Many would recommend that 'routine' screening tests are unlikely to be helpful in acute urticaria, other than to confirm suspicions from the clinical history (such as radio-allergo-sorbent test, RAST, to confirm a suspicion of allergy to shellfish, or serology to confirm a recent viral infection). This is because much urticaria is self-limiting over a couple of months, and also because the yield from non-directed tests is low.

If the urticaria becomes chronic, laboratory data may be obtained. The first set of tests may include complete blood count (CBC), antinuclear antibody (ANA), renal function, urine analysis, serum glutamate pyruvate transaminase (SGPT), creatinine, and hepatitis B and C serology. If these are unfruitful and the symptoms persist, the following might be helpful: cryoglobulins, chest radiography, complement C3 and C4, dental examination, stool for ova and parasites, biopsy, food diary, sinus radiographs, food elimination diet, and treatment for *Helicobacter pylori*. A simple food elimination diet is rice and water.

Some of the main triggers of urticaria are discussed in more detail here.

Food allergens

Food allergens have long been considered potential causes of urticaria. The exact incidence varies from 2 to 30% but is more likely to be lower in the range. Common potential offenders include fruits, nuts, eggs, soybeans, wheat, fish, seafood, tea, and food additives such as aspartame. Other rare cases have included caffeine (coffee and chocolate), ketchup, spices, vanilla, and peanut oil.

Diagnosis may be made by history, food diary, food elimination diet, and food challenge. Skin testing using the skin prick test may or may not be helpful. RAST is less beneficial but may be utilized. The gold standard for diagnosis of food allergy is a positive placebo-controlled oral challenge test.

Avoidance is the best treatment, with antihistamines as adjunctive therapy. Desensitization to food is not currently possible.

Food pseudoallergens

Note that several food constituents, such as salicylates, benzoates, or colorings, may act as so-called pseudoallergens that may cause or aggravate urticaria, causing mast cell degranulation by non-immunologic mechanisms (salicylates may also cause IgE-mediated immunologic urticaria). Some of these occur naturally, others are additives. Although probably not a major factor, their importance is threefold:

- they may occur in many different foods, and are therefore not suspected as a trigger;
- they do not give positive results on immunologic tests, or reliable results on skin tests; and
- their influence tends to be dose-related, therefore may vary from day to day.

While challenge tests to some of these are available, a period of dietician-supervised restriction of these agents can be worth trying for a few weeks. This is mainly applicable to those with chronic urticaria without other likely causes identified, and is likely to be capable of interpretation only if episodes are sufficiently frequent (at least every week) for an impact to be apparent.

Infection

Undoubtedly, various infections can cause urticaria, but the incidence is probably lower than the values given in early estimates, and the type of infection that can cause urticaria varies from region to region.

Examples include intestinal infection with *Citrobacter fructei*, as manifested by diarrhea; scabies; *Strongyloides stercoralis* associated with eosinophilia; giardiasis; *Toxocara canis*; cytomegalovirus; and hepatitis C. Chronic dental infection has in the past been felt to be a significant etiologic factor, but treatment of these foci usually does not improve the urticaria. Recently, *H. pylori* has been implicated.

In one study from France, 65% of patients with chronic urticaria versus 21% of control subjects had antibodies to *T. canis*. These patients were more likely to be in contact with pets. Some of them were cured or improved with thiabendazole or ivermectin treatment.

If *H. pylori* is suspected or implicated (e.g. by ^{13}C urea breath test), treatment may consist of, for example, amoxicillin 500 mg four times daily plus oral omeprazole 40 mg/day over a period of 2 weeks, followed by omeprazole alone for another 2 weeks. However, many studies do not show a clear difference in the frequency of *H. pylori* seropositivity in patients with urticaria compared with the background population frequency.

Medications

A huge number of medications may provoke urticaria. It is important to remember over-the-counter agents: aspirin can exacerbate chronic urticaria in a percentage of patients; other examples include multivitamins and wheat bran bath.

Sex

Urticaria developing after sex may occur in latex-sensitive patients after either partner uses a latex-containing condom. Rarely, a woman may react to her partner's semen.

Treatment

If a cause has been identified, then it should obviously be avoided (if possible). All patients should be instructed to avoid angiotensin-converting enzyme (ACE) inhibitors, aspirin, and other non-steroidal antiinflammatory medications, as these may exacerbate the urticaria. If the patient has had urticaria for months, or even years, and no obvious cause has been found, it is reasonably likely that an autoantibody is causing the mast cell degranulation. If so, the disease is unlikely to remit.

The foundation of therapy is antihistamines, with the newer, second-generation antihistamines being preferred, as they have lower sedating potential. These include (adult doses) cetirizine (10 mg/day), levocetirizine (5 mg/day), fexofenadine (120–180 mg daily), loratadine (10 mg/day), desloratidine (5 mg/day), acrivastine (8 mg t.d.s.), and mizolastine (10 mg/day). First-generation antihistamines are most helpful at night to help with sleep, for example chlorpheniramine 4 mg, hydroxyzine 10–25 mg, or doxepin 25–50 mg (the latter has the potential advantage of H_2 as well as H_1 blockade).

Pure H_2 blockers (e.g. cimetidine) may be given in conjunction with H_1 blockers, but the additional benefit is usually small. Similarly, avoidance of pseudoallergens may be tried; the best approach is strict avoidance for a few weeks, but abandoning the idea unless there is clear benefit.

Prednisone (30–60 mg/day) has been used in severe cases but is not something that can be continued for this condition, which often lasts years.

Acute urticaria in children
Clinical

In infants aged less than 6 months, urticaria is caused by allergy to cow's milk in 75%. For those aged 6–24 months, reactions to drugs (5-aminosalicylic acid, ASA, or amoxicillin) or to viral infections (e.g. hepatitis) are most common. Other causes include foods (milk, peanuts, seafood, and eggs), insect stings (e.g. bees and wasps), and bacterial infection (e.g. streptococci).

Treatment

Elimination of the offending agent if possible, plus diphenhydramine, hydroxyzine, or another antihistamine is appropriate (many adult antihistamines are either unlicensed in children or are unavailable in a suitable formulation, and the sedative effect of antihistamines is less limiting).

Chronic idiopathic urticaria
Clinical

It has been estimated that 15–20% of people will develop urticaria at least once in their lifetime. Many of these episodes will resolve within 6 weeks, but some will persist. In those cases where the urticaria lasts longer than 6 weeks and the cause is unknown, the term chronic idiopathic urticaria is used. The use of this term implies that physical urticarias (e.g. immediate dermatographism, delayed pressure urticaria, solar cholinergic urticaria, and cold urticaria) as well as urticarial vasculitis have been excluded. Mucosal angioedema may be associated.

Some patients have urticaria for years, seemingly unrelated to any allergen. Most large studies suggest that about one-third of these patients may have autoimmune mast cell disease in which an IgG autoantibody is directed against IgE or against the alpha chain of the IgE high-affinity receptor. Although research is still ongoing, current studies indicate that patients with chronic idiopathic urticaria are more likely than control subjects to have antithyroid autoantibodies, but not to have thyroid disease.

Treatment
See earlier text.

PRACTICE POINTS

- A diagnosis of urticaria can be made even in the absence of rash, as the individual lesions migrate and resolve within 24 h. If in doubt, draw around them with a suitable pen and review at 24 h. Some other dermatoses have lesions that expand, or that move, but not that move and resolve in this timescale.
- Identifying a cause of urticaria, unless it is immediately obvious from the history of recent events, is much more difficult than establishing the label of 'urticaria': in most patients with chronic urticaria, no cause can be identified.
- Always consider physical urticarias: they can usually be confidently diagnosed by appropriate provocation testing, which in turn means that extensive investigations for underlying causes are unnecessary.
- Urticaria is often self-limiting over a couple of months; in the absence of any specific clues of causation or any associated symptoms, 'routine' screening tests before this time are likely to have a low yield.

Aquagenic urticaria
Etiology and pathogenesis
Aquagenic urticaria is a rare physical urticaria in which urticaria develops after exposure to water. The lesions develop within 30 min of exposure. Patients with both aquagenic urticaria and cholinergic urticaria have been described.

Clinical
Urticarial wheals similar to those of cholinergic urticaria develop within 30 min of exposure to water, irrespective of temperature (e.g. washing one's hands, rain, or taking a bath). Sweat, saliva, and tears may induce the condition. Lesions persist for minutes to an hour. Usually the upper body is affected.

Differential diagnosis
Several other physical urticarias may be in the differential, highlighting the need for a careful history. These include the following.
- Cholinergic urticaria—due to hot water.
- Cold urticaria—triggered by cold water.
- Dermatographism—due to shower jets, or to toweling dry after water exposure.
- Heat urticaria—less common, due to hot water.

Non-urticarial water-related causes of itch include the pruritus of polycythemia rubra vera (after exposure) and aquagenic pruritus, a condition in which intense itching (without urticaria) occurs after contact with water of any temperature.

Treatment
Daily antihistamine use may be the best approach. PUVA was successful in one patient with aquagenic urticaria and polymorphous light eruption (PMLE). Preapplication of a barrier cream or ointment (e.g. petrolatum) can prevent development of the lesions.

Cholinergic urticaria
Etiology and pathogenesis
Cholinergic urticaria refers to a unique type of urticaria in which small wheals erupt in relationship to sweating. This may be due to exercise,

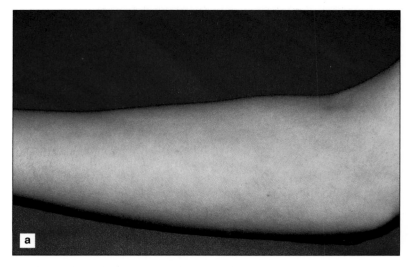

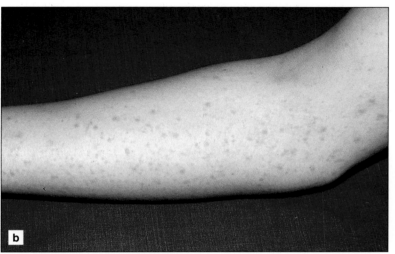

Figure 9.4 Cholinergic urticaria. The normal skin of the arm (**a**) in this patient has developed numerous lesions (**b**) shortly after a period of exercise. (From Lawrence CM, Cox NH. *Physical Signs in Dermatology*, 2nd edn. London: Mosby, 1993; courtesy of Dr. C. M. Lawrence.)

or due to external heat (e.g. a warm bath). One study of two men with cholinergic urticaria associated with hypohidrosis revealed histologic evidence of occlusion of the superficial acrosyringium. The researchers hypothesized that such a hypohidrosis due to occlusion of superficial sweat ducts may also play a role in other patients with cholinergic urticaria. Of note, cholinergic urticaria in these patients was exacerbated in winter, when sweating is not a frequent event.

Clinical
Urticarial papules, 1–4 mm in size, which occur within minutes of exercise, are characteristic (Fig. 9.4). In severe cases, they may be confluent, giving the skin a peau d'orange appearance. The patient can be made to exercise to the point of sweating to establish the diagnosis.

Differential diagnosis
This depends on the trigger; see earlier text for the differential diagnosis of urticaria involving warm water. More commonly, the trigger is exercise; this can sometimes aggravate ordinary urticaria, but postprandial or food-dependent exercise-induced anaphylaxis may also need to be considered. There are several types of exercise-induced urticarias or anaphylaxis, some of which are induced by certain specific foods followed by exercise and some by any food followed by exercise. The urticarial lesions in these conditions have a more typical urticarial morphology (i.e. are larger than lesions of cholinergic urticaria), and of course the patients progress to anaphylaxis.

Treatment

Antihistamines may be used prior to exercise in an attempt to ward off an attack, but this approach is not always successful. Some patients must reduce the amount they sweat to a minimum. If there is evidence that hypohidrosis is associated, for example in wintertime, a trial of frequent exercise or sweating to reduce symptoms may be tried.

Cold urticaria
Etiology and pathogenesis

Cold urticaria is a condition in which urticaria develops after exposure to the cold. It has been associated with acute viral infection, syphilis, drugs (e.g. penicillin, oral contraceptives, and griseofulvin), and HIV infection. It may be familial, presenting in infancy. Most cases are sporadic and idiopathic. Anaphylaxis may be associated. One study of children with acquired cold urticaria found a high association with asthma and allergic rhinitis, and a family history of atopic diathesis.

Clinical

Lesions may occur at any site that is exposed to cold, such as the fingers (Fig. 9.5). Fullness of the throat or swelling of the lips may occur with drinking cold liquids or eating ice cream. Swelling of the head, face, and ears may occur after coming indoors from the cold. Patients can drown if they swim in cold water, due to massive histamine release causing shock.

Differential diagnosis

The differential of water-triggered urticaria has already been discussed. Patients in whom the main trigger is cold wind may have swelling of exposed parts that resembles angioedema (see later in this chapter). To support the diagnosis, the ice cube test is performed as follows. Apply two ice cubes wrapped in thin foil or plastic (so as not to induce aquagenic urticaria) to the forearm for 10 min. Watch for whealing minutes after removal (Fig. 9.5). The presence of cryoglobulins, cryofibrinogens, and cold agglutinins should all be excluded. Familial cold autoinflammatory syndrome, formerly known as familial cold urticaria, is a rare condition characterized by fever, rash, and arthralgias elicited by exposure to cold.

Treatment

Antihistamines, both sedating and non-sedating, may be helpful. For example, desloratidine 5–10 mg/day was effective in a study of 12 patients. The combination of cetirizine 10 mg/day and zafirlukast 20 mg b.i.d. was more effective than either agent alone in one patient. The patient should be warned about the risks of anaphylaxis. Specific mention of the dangers of swimming or bathing in cold water should be discussed. An adrenaline (epinephrine) autoinjector may be prescribed.

Some patients are able to achieve desensitization by immersing parts of the body in cold water in turn, allowing the urticaria response to settle between each immersion (to avoid whole-body urticaria and the risk of histamine shock). This approach relies on the fact that there is a finite time for mast cell granules to re-form; the desensitization needs to be maintained with daily cool baths.

Delayed pressure urticaria
Etiology and pathogenesis

This condition is provoked by prolonged pressure; typical triggers include carrying a heavy bag (affects hands), prolonged walking or standing (feet), or tight clothing. It may coexist with other physical urticarias.

Clinical

The most important feature of this condition, as implied in its name, is the delay in onset of symptoms, often 6–8 h. It may also produce deep swelling at acral sites. In both of these respects, it therefore differs from most other urticarias.

Differential diagnosis

The two clinical factors just mentioned may mean that urticaria, and the relevance of the provocative stimulus, may not be suspected. The main differential is that of angioedema and disorders that mimic it (discussed later).

Treatment

Antihistamines should be tried but are often of limited benefit. Oral corticosteroids are helpful but usually only at doses that are unacceptable for long-term use. Avoidance of triggers is the best option.

Contact urticaria
Etiology and pathogenesis

Contact urticaria is usually mediated through IgE antibodies directed against protein peptides. It is more common in atopic individuals, and the classic situation involves the hands in response to contact either with specific foods or with latex. Note that some foods may cross-react with latex (Table 9.3) – particularly if there is a history of reaction to foods,

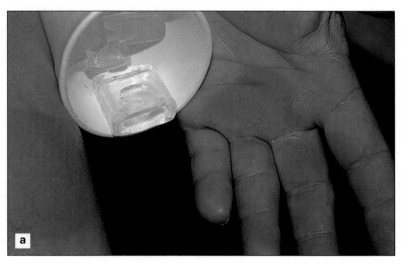

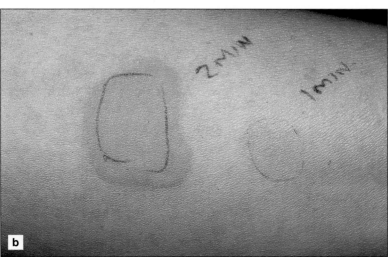

Figure 9.5 Cold urticaria. (**a**) Lesions on the hand and arm after an ice cube test. (**b**) Ice cube provocation test with dose response.

Table 9.3 CONTACT URTICARIA: SOME FOODS THAT MAY CROSS-REACT WITH LATEX	
Commonest	**Less common**
Avocado	Other exotic fruits (pineapple,
Banana	papaya, passion fruit, mango, fig)
Chestnut	Other fruits (apple, pear, peach,
Kiwifruit	cherry, tomato)
	Vegetables (turnip, potato, celery,
	spinach)

Table 9.4 SOME SOURCES OF LATEX

Household	Healthcare
Gloves	Gloves
Toys, balloons, erasers	Tubing (endotracheal, blood
Clothing (e.g. in elastic, shoes)	pressure cuff, stethoscope,
Swimming items (e.g. caps,	suction, drains, etc.)
goggles)	Anesthetic masks, bags, and circuits
Other sports items	Elasticated bandages, tourniquet
(e.g. racquet handles,	Rubber sheets etc.
tennis balls)	Dental dams and bite protectors
Car tires	
Condoms	
Infant pacifiers and	
bottle-feeding equipment	

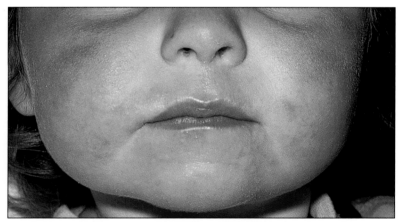

Figure 9.6 Contact urticaria to cheese. The reaction occurred on the hands and around the mouth immediately after eating a particular brand of cheese.

it is worth sending a RAST for latex even if latex itself is not clinically suspected as a cause of contact urticaria, as the food reaction may be a clue to latex allergy. Ingestion of offending foods can also cause otolaryngeal symptoms.

Latex allergy is particularly common in healthcare workers, who may be regularly exposed to sources of latex (Table 9.4); is more common in women than in men; and is more common in those with preceding hand dermatitis.

Clinical

The affected skin develops a wheal and flare after contact with the substance (Fig. 9.6). The hands may develop a vesicular or eczematous eruption with significant pruritus. Airborne latex may cause facial urticaria, for example due to powdered gloves.

The offending substance may be identified by history, RAST testing, scratch testing, or use test. Anaphylaxis may occur, and so great care must be taken.

Differential diagnosis

This includes the following.
- Other forms of urticaria.
- Angioedema—note that contact urticaria to foods may be manifest as oral swelling.
- Anaphylaxis—if there is laryngeal swelling; note, however, that shock is not a feature of contact urticaria per se, although items such as latex may also cause true anaphylaxis.

- Hand eczema—note that latex or foods may also cause eczematous reactions, so the contact urticarial component may be difficult to detect; it is prudent to check a RAST before performing patch tests to latex.
- Other facial dermatoses—these may be mimicked if there is a reaction to airborne latex.

Treatment

Avoidance of the offending substance is indicated. In the case of latex allergy, gloves are a major culprit: alternatives include nitrile, polythene, and PVC.

Angioedema
Etiology and pathogenesis

Angioedema refers to the acute swelling of tissue such as the lips or hands. The accumulation of fluid in the skin occurs at a deeper level than with the wheal of urticaria, although the latter is often associated. Mortality has occurred secondary to respiratory tract involvement. Several types occur, including the following.
- Hereditary angioedema—an autosomal dominantly inherited type (discussed in more detail later).
- Angioedema due to immediate hypersensitivity reaction.
- Drug-induced angioedema—especially that due to ACE inhibitors, which often occurs within the first week of treatment (it is a pharmacologic phenomenon due to altered bradykinin metabolism and is a non-immunologic class effect of this group of drugs).
- Angioedema due to acquired C1 inhibitor deficiency—this may be idiopathic, or associated with a B-cell lymphoma or with lupus erythematosus.
- Idiopathic angioedema.

Clinical

Almost any part of the body may be affected, but common sites are the eyes, lips, genitalia, hands, and feet (Fig. 9.7). These sites may swell to two or three times their normal size within hours. Resolution may occur that same day or several days later. Itching is usually minimal, but pain may occur if deep swelling occurs at 'tight' areas such as the sole of the foot.

Differential diagnosis

The main differential diagnosis issue is distinguishing hereditary angioedema from the other forms. Other differentials include the following.
- Contact urticaria of hands or face, as swelling at these sites may be more persistent than at other areas of the body.
- Delayed pressure urticaria, as this typically causes prolonged swelling and may affect hands (e.g. carrying a heavy bag) or feet (prolonged walking or standing).
- Rosacea—may cause facial edema without or with little erythema (Ch. 10).
- Early cellulitis—edema may precede redness but is usually associated with malaise.
- Lymphedema or venous edema—but these do not have the intermittent course seen in angioedema.
- Artifactual edema due to application of a tourniquet to a limb (Secretan syndrome).

Treatment

If the patient is on an ACE inhibitor, it should be stopped. Antihistamines should be given as for urticaria (see earlier). Danazol and stanozolol are effective for both the acquired and the inherited types. Acute, life-threatening attacks require more aggressive intervention. Adrenaline (epinephrine) and antihistamines are used for the immediate hypersensitivity type.

Angioedema, hereditary
Clinical

Episodic swelling of areas of the face, extremities, bowel (causing abdominal pain), and upper airway are characteristic. Attacks may be spontaneous, triggered by emotional stress or physical trauma. Inheritance is autosomal dominant. The cause is a congenital defect in C1 esterase inhibitor.

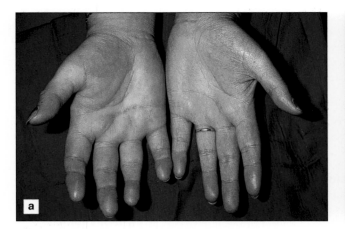
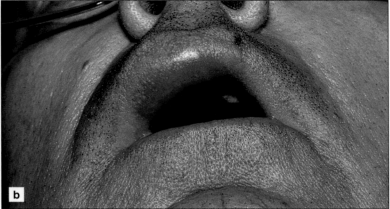
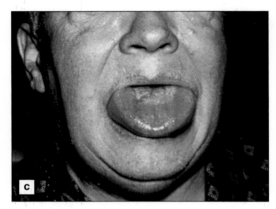

Figure 9.7 Angioedema. (**a**) Angioedema of the right hand. (**b**) Angioedema of the lip. This patient developed angioedema soon after starting an ACE inhibitor. (**c**) The tongue is a relatively common site in angioedema. If the mouth and lips are the only sites affected on a regular basis, then it is worth considering a contact urticaria to foods.

The majority of patients have low levels of C1 esterase inhibitor, but some have normal or elevated levels that are functionally inactive. The recurrent colicky abdominal pain results from submucosal swelling of the gastrointestinal tract.

Treatment

Attenuated androgens, especially danazol (which causes a rise in C1 esterase inhibitor levels), are used. The dose is 20–30 mg/kg per day, with a maximum dose of 800 mg/day. It may be used in children. Oxandrolone is another synthetic anabolic steroid that can be used to treat this condition in children. C1 esterase inhibitor may also be infused for treatment of acute episodes. The antifibrinolytic agents aprotinin, tranexamic acid, and epsilon-aminocaproic acid are useful for prophylaxis and treatment of angioedema, probably by inhibiting plasmin.

Anaphylaxis
Etiology and pathogenesis

Anaphylaxis consists of hypotension (shock), laryngeal edema, and bronchospasm, which may be accompanied by urticaria. Patients with acute urticaria and some facial swelling are somewhat overdiagnosed as having anaphylaxis by emergency services.

Triggers include the following main areas.

- Food allergies—especially to agents such as peanut, fish, shellfish, prawns, eggs, cow's milk, and nuts (e.g. brazil nut and almond; note that peanut is a vegetable rather than a nut).
- Exercise-induced anaphylaxis—exercise may be an isolated trigger, but food-dependent exercise-induced anaphylaxis is more common and may require careful history taking. It may require specific foods to have been eaten, or any food, depending on the individual, and it is often aggravated by concurrent aspirin ingestion. Omega-5 gliadin is particularly implicated as the major allergen in wheat-dependent, exercise-induced anaphylaxis. Rarer combinations may also trigger anaphylaxis, such as cold-dependent exercise-induced anaphylaxis.
- Drugs and iatrogenic—especially aspirin and non-steroidal anti-inflammatory agents, blood products, hyposensitizing agents, antibiotics, radiocontrast media, neuromuscular blockers, and local anesthetics (rarely, see Ch. 18).
- Others—such as latex and insect stings.

Clinical
The features are discussed earlier.

Differential diagnosis
This includes the following.
- Urticaria or angioedema without other features of anaphylaxis.
- Urticaria with hypotension but not the other features of anaphylaxis—for example histamine shock due to whole-body cold urticaria.
- Hereditary angioedema.
- Flushing with systemic symptoms due to food additives (e.g. monosodium glutamate), alcohol (especially with drug interaction also, e.g. metronidazole or Antabuse), mastocytosis (hypotension), or carcinoid syndrome (bronchospasm).
- Other food-related causes of shock—for example scombrotoxic shock.
- Other causes of collapse without a dermatologic component.

Dermatologists or immunologists may be consulted regarding identification of a cause. Generally, this is either evident from the history due to the close temporal relationship between the trigger and the response (often minutes, rarely more than a few hours), or a cause is never identified. A screening RAST for any suspect foods is safer than prick testing; it is worth including peanut, as it may be used in cooking and the fact that it has been ingested may not be obvious. Rechallenge is dangerous.

Treatment

This is not generally the province of the dermatologist but is briefly summarized here, as it is a rare complication of local anesthetic administration. Basic support includes lying the patient flat, administering oxygen, intubation if required due to laryngeal edema, etc.

Medications administered for acute management are adrenaline (epinephrine), corticosteroids, and an antihistamine. Adrenaline should be administered intramuscularly to ensure reliable absorption, and may need to be repeated at 5-min intervals depending on response; the adult and adolescent dose is 0.5 mg, which equates to 0.5 mL of 1:1000 (1 mg/mL) solution.

The other drugs are given intravenously, but take longer to act and may need to be continued for 1–2 days to prevent relapse. For those with repeated episodes or at high risk (e.g. those with severe peanut allergy), self-administration of adrenaline (epinephrine) using prefilled syringes may be taught.

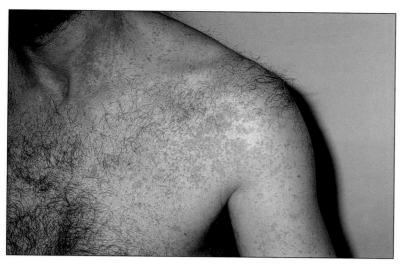

Figure 9.8 Familial Mediterranean fever. Multiple red, urticarial lesions are seen.

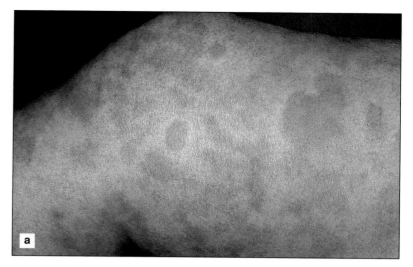

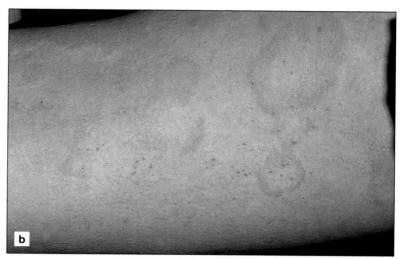

Figure 9.9 Urticarial vasculitis. (**a**) Active urticarial lesions are seen among non-blanching purpuric sites of prior activity. (**b**) Urticaria with purpura. Any residual purpura should prompt the consideration of urticarial vasculitis. In fact, the patient had purpura without any histologic evidence of vasculitis.

> **PRACTICE POINTS**
> - For anaphylaxis, adrenaline (epinephrine) should be administered intramuscularly at a dose of 0.5 mg: 0.5 mL of 1:1000 (1 mg/mL) solution (adult dose).
> - Further adrenaline may need to be administered at 5-min intervals, depending on response.
> - Intravenous adrenaline is potentially dangerous due to cardiac side effects; it also interacts with beta-blockers (may cause severe hypertension) and with tricyclic antidepressants (high risk of arrhythmias).
> - For patients with acute episodes of hereditary angioedema, C1 esterase inhibitor may also be infused.
> - Collapse that is not associated with injection site urticaria, facial angioedema, or respiratory symptoms, and especially if occurring after an uneventful procedure, is unlikely to be due to local anesthetic allergy.

Hereditary periodic fever syndromes

Etiology and pathogenesis

Familial Mediterranean fever (FMF), hyperimmunoglobulinemia D periodic fever syndrome (HIDS), and tumor necrosis factor receptor-associated periodic syndrome (TRAPS) are the hereditary periodic fever syndromes. FMF is caused by mutations in the Mediterranean fever gene *MEFV*, HIDS by mutations in the mevalonate kinase gene, and TRAPS by mutations in the tumor necrosis factor receptor superfamily 1A gene. Impaired function of the encoded proteins—i.e. pyrin in FMF, mevalonate kinase in HIDS, and the p55 tumor necrosis factor receptor in TRAPS—induce a dysregulated cytokine balance.

Clinical

Clinical manifestations are relapsing fever, serositis, arthralgia, myalgia, and miscellaneous forms of rash. In FMF, sharply bordered, 10–15-mm, red urticarial lesions occur, usually on the legs, especially the dorsal feet, over the ankle or over the knee (Fig. 9.8). The affected skin is hot, tender, and swollen, resembling erysipelas.

Differential diagnosis

From a dermatologic perspective, the differential is mainly from ordinary urticaria, although drug eruptions or viral exanthems may be considered in those with intermittent symptoms or less specific patterns of rash. Many other differential diagnoses, including lupus erythematosus, Behçet disease, and vasculitides, may need to be considered because of the systemic manifestations.

Treatment

The attacks and complications of FMF can be avoided by lifelong administration of colchicine. HIDS is treated symptomatically. Impaired tumor necrosis factor-α regulation in TRAPS can be treated with etanercept.

Urticarial vasculitis

Etiology and pathogenesis

Urticarial vasculitis (see also Ch. 14) is defined as urticarial lesions that persist at the same location for more than 24 h. This is most commonly associated with systemic lupus erythematosus (SLE), but also Sjögren syndrome, serum sickness, viral infections (e.g. hepatitis C and infectious mononucleosis), mixed cryoglobulins, a monoclonal IgM gammopathy (Schnitzler syndrome), IgA multiple myeloma, fluoxetine administration, and rarely neoplasm. Hypocomplementemia is common and, when it does occur, the association with SLE is highly likely. In one case, the lesions of urticarial vasculitis were induced by cold exposure, and an IgG was found on serum protein electrophoresis (SPEP).

Autoantibodies to vascular endothelial cells were found in 82% of patients with urticarial vasculitis and SLE, in 70% of patients with hypocomplementemic urticarial vasculitis, and in 14% of patients with urticarial vasculitis alone. They were found in only 32% of patients with SLE but without urticarial vasculitis.

Clinical

Urticarial lesions lasting more than 24 h at any given location are characteristic (Fig. 9.9). They may be painful rather than itchy. Diascopy may blanch much of the erythema, but purpura remains. Angioedema may occur. Histology shows a leukocytoclastic vasculitis. Systemic associations have included anemia, arthralgias, abdominal pain, glomerulonephritis, ocular inflammation, and pulmonary disease. Laboratory abnormalities may include elevated erythrocyte sedimentation rate (ESR), decreased complement levels, decreased or absent C1q, and C1q autoantibody. In one study, the C1q autoantibody was found in 100% of patients with hypocomplementemic urticarial vasculitis syndrome (HUVS), in 35% of patients with SLE, and in almost no control subjects.

Urticarial vasculitis is not a specific disease, but instead a clinical finding that is usually associated with a vasculitis that causes significant permeability of the dermal microvascular system. A search for a cause of the vasculitis should be undertaken. Work-up should include drug history (e.g. dexfenfluramine), skin biopsy, CBC, ANA, rheumatoid factor (RF), ESR, urine analysis, CH50, C3, C4, liver enzymes, hepatitis C serology, cryoglobulins, and SPEP.

Differential diagnosis
The most important differential diagnosis is from 'ordinary' urticaria; other issues are making the distinction between normocomplementemic urticarial vasculitis and HUVS, and searching for underlying causes such as SLE.

Treatment
If a specific cause is found, it should be treated directly. Otherwise, prednisone may be used (40–60 mg/day initially, then tapered). Azathioprine has been used (e.g. 50–100 mg/day). Other steroid-sparing agents include dapsone and hydroxychloroquine. Agents to try if these fail include indomethacin and colchicine. Urticarial vasculitis caused by hepatitis C has responded to interferon–alpha therapy.

Autoimmune progesterone dermatitis
Etiology and pathogenesis
Autoimmune progesterone dermatitis (APD), as the name suggests, is a condition in which the woman develops an immune response to her own circulating progesterone, resulting in a skin eruption.

Clinical
Patients with APD may present with an eczematous eruption, erythema multiforme, urticaria (Fig. 9.10), pompholyx-like, or a dermatitis herpetiformis-like rash. In some cases, anaphylaxis has been associated. The key diagnostic feature is that the skin changes tend to occur in the later half of the menstrual cycle and resolve within a day or two of the menses. A significant proportion of patients have a history of oral contraceptive use.

Differential diagnosis
In a woman who develops a cyclic rash with her menstrual cycle, autoimmunity to estrogen should also be considered. Patch and prick skin testing to both estrogen and progesterone may be done for diagnostic

Table 9.5   CAUSES OF ITCHING WITHOUT (MANY) SKIN CHANGES

Scabies

Dry skin

Dermatographism

Internal disorders (e.g. cholestasis, hepatitis C infection, see text)

Lymphoma

Drugs (e.g. codeine)

purposes. Both atopic and allergic contact dermatitis may also show premenstrual exacerbations.

Treatment
Anovulatory agents should be tried initially. Tamoxifen and buserelin (a gonadotropin-releasing hormone analog) have been successful. Oophorectomy has rarely been done.

PRURITUS AND RELATED DISORDERS

Generalized pruritus without skin changes
Etiology and pathogenesis
Some patients present with itching and very little rash. A variety of causes may be found (Table 9.5).

Clinical
To reach this diagnosis, a careful complete skin examination must be performed. Dry skin (xerosis) is a common cause of pruritus, especially in the elderly in the winter. Look for fine scale and accentuated skin lines, especially on the legs. Are there any signs of scabies (e.g. classic burrows in the web spaces)? Any new medications? Any new topical medications or exposures? Make sure to test for dermatographism.

Localized pruritus is a rather different issue: it may occur on the back (notalgia paresthetica) or arm (brachioradial pruritus), as discussed later. However, even localized itch may rarely be a manifestation of internal malignancy (e.g. severe nasal tip itch due to tumor of the fourth ventricle).

Differential diagnosis
If the patient is found to truly have pruritus without any skin changes, internal causes must be considered, including cholestasis, iron deficiency (even without anemia), rapid weight loss, renal disease, hypothyroidism, polycythemia rubra vera, and Hodgkin lymphoma. Delusions of parasitosis should be excluded, and depressive illness should always be considered; even if not the whole cause, it may aggravate the degree of symptoms. An appropriate work-up includes a history and physical examination with special emphasis on lymph nodes, plus CBC, serum bilirubin, alkaline phosphatase, antimitochondrial antibody, ferritin, thyroid function tests, creatinine, blood urea nitrogen (BUN), and chest x-ray. Screening for HIV may be appropriate. An interesting report found 39% of patients with unexplained itching to have evidence of hepatitis C infection.

Treatment
Treatment should be tailored to the cause. If no cause is found, a medium- to high-potency topical steroid applied after the shower to the itchiest areas, an emollient cream or ointment applied elsewhere, and a sedating antihistamine at nighttime may be tried. If this fails, doxepin before sleeping or UVB may be tried. Low-dose prednisone is occasionally helpful. HIV-associated pruritus can be treated effectively with UVB. Ondansetron (initially 8 mg/day, then tapered as possible), a competitive and selective antagonist of serotonin receptors, has relieved itching in a variety of situations (e.g. pruritus associated with cholestatic jaundice or chronic renal insufficiency).

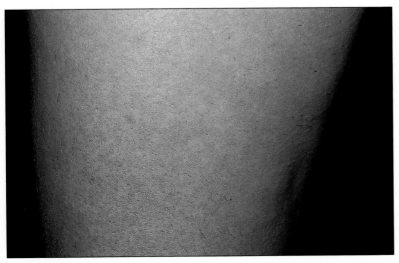

Figure 9.10   Autoimmune progesterone dermatitis. This woman broke out with a diffuse erythema each menstrual cycle.

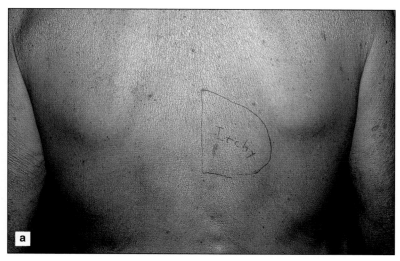

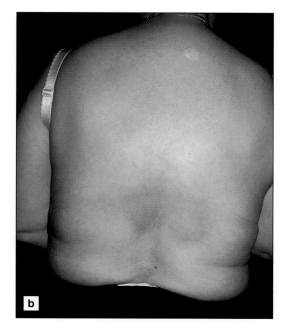

Figure 9.11 Notalgia paresthetica. (**a**) This middle-aged man was plagued by a very pruritic fixed area on his left back, outlined here in pen. As a cruel quirk of fate, this itch is often hard to scratch. (**b**) Note the prominent hyperpigmentation resulting from chronic scratching and rubbing in this patient with bilateral symptoms.

Notalgia paresthetica
Etiology and pathogenesis
Patients with notalgia paresthetica experience persistent itching in a fixed area in the middle of the back. Notalgia paresthetica is thought to represent a sensory neuropathy, as the cutaneous nerves take a right angle in their course to innervate that location. In one study, the striking correlation of notalgia paresthetica localization with radiographic degenerative changes in the spine suggests that spinal nerve impingement may contribute to the pathogenesis of this entity. In another report, a patient developed notalgia paresthetica of the right upper back and shoulder caused by a large osteophyte in the C3–C4 intervertebral space, impinging on the right C4 nerve root (visualized by magnetic resonance imaging).

Clinical
Middle-aged to elderly patients may present with a very pruritic, fixed spot on the back, just to one side of the midline (Fig. 9.11). Hyperpigmentation may be present, and in most patients is thought to be secondary to chronic scratching. Macular amyloidosis may be the cause of the hyperpigmentation in some cases.

Differential diagnosis
Idiopathic macular amyloid may be considered but typically involves the upper back. Generally, there is no meaningful differential: it is simply a matter of whether the physician has ever heard of this entity.

Treatment
Most of the time, the benefit of heroic interventions is not worth the effort. (The patient may merely be told to get a back scratcher.) Still, if therapy is desired, the following may be tried. Capsaicin applied topically 3–5 times/day for 2 months has been reported to decrease the pruritus. A eutectic mixture of local anesthetic (2.5% lidocaine, 2.5% prilocaine), applied twice a day with occlusion, has also been reported to be effective. In the case of the nerve impingement described earlier, cervical epidural steroid injection resulted in near-complete resolution of the symptoms. In another case, paravertebral block at D5–D6, and later at D3–D4, with 5 mL of bupivacaine (0.75%) combined with 40 mg of methylprednisolone acetate relieved all symptoms for 12 months.

Brachioradial pruritus
Etiology and pathogenesis
Patients with brachioradial pruritus experience chronic and persistent itching along the extensor forearm. There is ongoing debate regarding the etiology: it has long been viewed as a photodermatosis, but many authors feel that it represents a radiculopathy or some form of nerve entrapment.

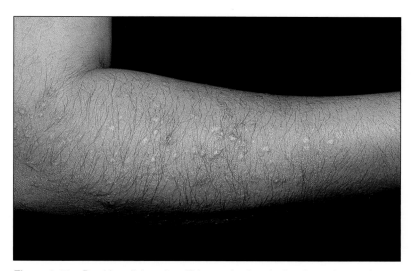

Figure 9.12 Brachioradial pruritus. This man had such chronic pruritus on the one arm that he could not resist scratching. Multiple excoriations and old white scars are shown.

The visible light spectrum was implicated in one report, and, because antihistamines helped in that case, it was suggested that some patients may experience degranulation of mast cells from visible light. Most cases do not fit one specific nerve distribution and radiographs are usually normal, which casts some doubt on the radiculopathy theory. Conversely, involvement of the non-driver's side forearm, or occurrence in those with minimal sunlight exposure, casts doubt on the idea of a photodermatosis, and several case series have documented features supporting a neuropathic component. Additionally, dramatic response to capsaicin in some cases is more supportive of this being a neuropathic process.

Clinical
Pruritus along the extensor forearm on one side is characteristic (Fig. 9.12). It may be worse in the summer with sunlight exposure. The classic patient is a professional driver whose arm hangs out the window while driving (a feature that might cause either solar exposure or neuropathy!), but any adult may be affected.

Differential diagnosis
As with nostalgia paresthetica, there is no meaningful differential if the physician has ever heard of this entity.

Treatment

Long-sleeved shirts to shield the arm from the sun may completely clear the symptoms (e.g. in 6 weeks). A medium- to high-potency topical steroid may be tried. In one report, cetirizine completely controlled a patient's symptoms. Topical capsaicin or oral gabapentin 300 mg t.i.d. has also produced marked benefit in various patients. Cervical spine radiology may be considered to rule out a radiculopathy.

PRACTICE POINTS
- Patients with generalized itch but no rash may have an internal cause; however, previously unappreciated dry skin, mild dermatographism, and subtle rashes are all more common than systemic causes of pruritus.
- Beware of interpreting scratch marks as a primary rash. Look at the central upper back to see if it is spared (the butterfly sign).
- Localized itch without rash typically occurs on the mid-back (notalgia paresthetica) or the dorsal forearm (brachioradial pruritus); both are underdiagnosed conditions.
- Even in those with minimal rash (especially the elderly), and especially in patients with nondescript scattered rash, always consider scabies as a cause of pruritus.

Itchy red bump disease
Etiology and pathogenesis

The diagnosis of itchy red bump disease is one of exclusion of the differential diagnoses described here. If no specific cause is found, the term itchy red bump disease may be used. It is unclear whether this is a specific entity, as no cause has been identified. Most patients are male and elderly.

Clinical

An adult with chronic pruritus and 1–2-mm erythematous papulovesicles scattered on the body is characteristic (Fig. 9.13).

Differential diagnosis

The patient with multiple itchy red bumps should have a careful drug history taken; should be carefully examined to exclude scabies; and should have patch testing, skin biopsy, and a trial of antibiotics. These maneuvers should exclude the most likely differentials of scabies, Grover disease, allergic contact dermatitis, drug rash, dermatitis herpetiformis, and folliculitis. Some patients have been found to have hepatitis B.

Treatment

Potent topical steroids before sleeping should be tried initially. If this fails, PUVA should be given. In one study, PUVA had the best chance of either helping (six out of nine patients) or clearing (three out of nine patients) itchy red bump disease. Antihistamines, UVB, intramuscular triamcinolone, and low-dose prednisone may be tried.

Delusions of parasitosis

Patients with delusions of parasitosis are convinced that some sort of parasite or 'bug' is living in or on their skin. This is discussed in more detail in Chapter 27.

Lichen simplex chronicus and prurigo nodularis
Etiology and pathogenesis

From an evolutionary standpoint, the occasional scratch is good, as it may dislodge a blood-sucking mosquito or tick, etc. However, chronic, daily, incessant scratching is bad. It damages the skin and exposes deeper tissues to infection. In response, the skin thickens in an attempt to protect itself. The term lichen simplex chronicus (LSC) refers to plaques of skin that have developed in response to repeated scratching, and the term prurigo nodularis refers to nodules.

The initial trigger may be one of the causes of generalized pruritus discussed in this chapter, particularly in those with widespread lesions of prurigo nodularis. Patients with atopic dermatitis may develop lichenification, usually at sites of otherwise obvious eczema but sometimes at distant sites.

In patients with LSC, it is always worth considering an underlying contact allergy, particularly if the vulva is affected or if LSC occurs at a site that is unusual.

Clinical

A chronic, hyperkeratotic, lichenified, excoriated plaque that the patient scratches daily is characteristic (Fig. 9.14). Often, the skin lines are accentuated within the lesion. Sometimes the skin is thickened relatively uniformly, in others the appearance has a more cobblestoned morphology: lesions may be relatively sharply defined or may be more diffuse at the

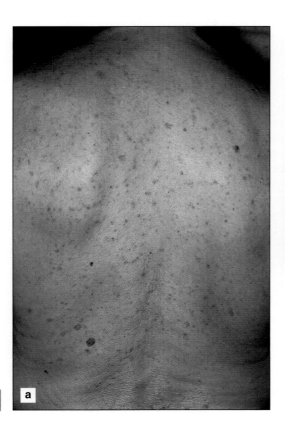

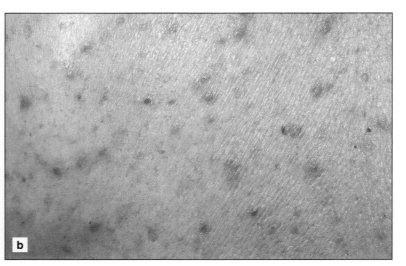

Figure 9.13 (**a**,**b**) Itchy red bump disease. These tiny red bumps of the trunk are very itchy. Often, their cause is unknown.

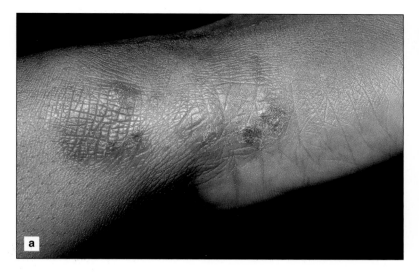

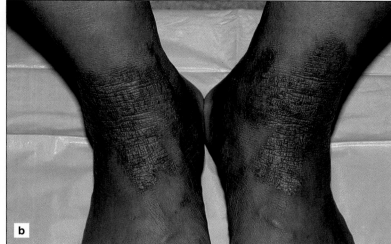

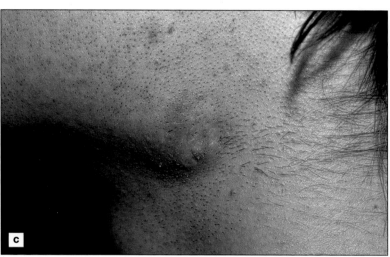

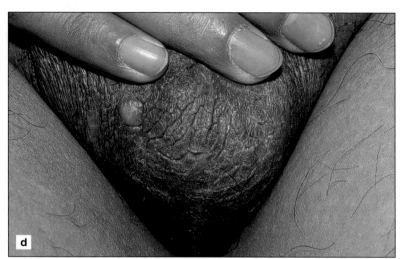

Figure 9.14 Lichen simplex chronicus (LSC). (**a**) Note the lichenification, excoriations, and accentuation of skin lines that have resulted from repeated scratching. (**b**) The skin of LSC may take on a lichenoid appearance, as shown here in a lesion on the leg. (**c**) Fiddler's neck. The chronic pressure and friction of a violin caused this indurated, thickened plaque. (**d**) LSC of the scrotum. Note the thickened, fissured skin. An epidermal inclusion cyst is seen in the skin on the right side of the scrotum.

margins. LSC may occur virtually anywhere, but common sites include the ankle, shin, scrotum, vulva, and nape and side of the neck. It is often less threatening and more helpful when trying to elicit a history of chronic scratching to ask the patient 'Does it itch?' rather than asking 'Do you scratch?'

In prurigo nodularis, 5–15-mm hyperkeratotic, verrucous nodules scattered on the extensor surfaces of the arms and legs are characteristic (Fig. 9.15). Onset is usually in middle age, and women are more commonly affected. Many patients have a family history of atopy.

A condition of prurigo nodularis lesions that develop in patients with bullous pemphigoid has been called pemphigoid nodularis.

In any condition where widespread scratching or rubbing occurs in the absence of an overt primary dermatosis, the area of the back where the patient is unable to reach to scratch may be spared (the butterfly sign, Fig. 9.16), but beware of missing the subtle causes of generalized pruritus discussed earlier, for example dermatographism (Fig. 9.17).

Differential diagnosis

Lichen simplex chronicus is usually fairly obvious by its morphology, the most notable differential diagnosis being chronic areas of lichen planus. Psoriasis may be diagnosed, but solitary lesions of psoriasis are uncommon, and LSC has neither the sharp margin nor the hard silvery scale that are typical of psoriasis.

Nodular prurigo is also usually characteristic but may need to be distinguished by biopsy from a range of other conditions, especially lichen planus (especially nodular lesions on the legs), granulomatous disorders, and neoplasms.

Treatment

Don't scratch! This single admonition is often left out by the doctor, leading to treatment failure. Tell the patient, 'No matter how strong a steroid I give you, this problem will continue if you continue to scratch'. Explore with the patient when they scratch: at night, when nervous, etc. Remember that scratching and rubbing occur at night even if the patient is asleep, and even if daytime itch is controlled.

Many factors may need to be combined for therapeutic success (Table 9.6).

PRACTICE POINTS

- In lichen simplex and nodular prurigo, remember that scratching and rubbing occur at night even if the patient is asleep, and even if daytime itch is controlled.
- Contact allergy may cause or complicate vulval lichen simplex chronicus.

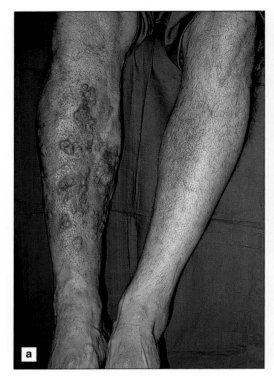

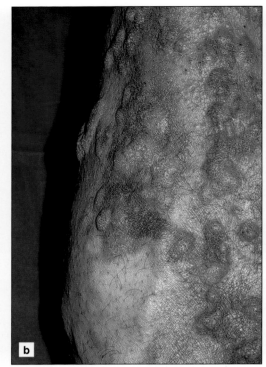

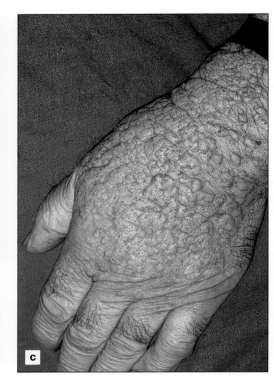

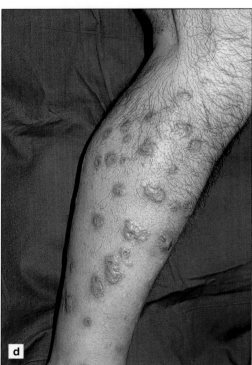

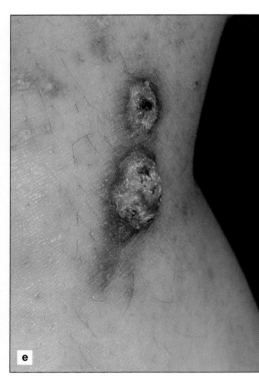

Figure 9.15 Prurigo nodularis. (**a**) Multiple hyperkeratotic nodules and plaques on the right leg, caused by daily scratching. (**b**) Close-up view. (**c**) Prurigo of the hand. (**d**) Multiple discrete indurated nodules on the legs. Some have an excoriated surface. In this case, the only causative factor identified was iron deficiency due to previous gastrointestinal bleeding. (**e**) Prurigo nodules showing the nodular lesions and the surface excoriation.

If the mid- and upper back is completely spared by an otherwise generalized itch rash (the butterfly sign), then the implication is that the rash is secondary to scratching, rather than representing a primary dermatosis.

Any form of chronic rubbing or excoriation is likely to be difficult to treat and may require the combination of several treatment modalities.

Dermatitis artefacta
Etiology and pathogenesis
The term dermatitis artefacta refers to skin lesions inflicted consciously with the intent of gaining sympathy, avoiding work, collecting insurance, or avoiding responsibility. Absolute proof of the diagnosis may be difficult to obtain.

Clinical
Irregularly shaped, bizarre skin lesions on easily accessible skin including the face (Figs 9.18 and 9.19) and arms (Fig. 9.20) are characteristic. The appearance depends on the mode of creation, which can include caustic substances, injection of foreign material, fingernails, or hot metal. Extensive scarring can result (Fig. 9.21).

Differential diagnosis
The range of differential diagnoses is immense, depending on the pattern of artifact. A useful clue, other than the often non-natural appearance of the rash, is the patient's apparent lack of concern ('la belle indifference'). Patients who use methamphetamines should be encouraged to enter a drug rehabilitation program.

Treatment
Referral for psychologic counseling may or may not be welcomed by the patient. If the patient is a child, there should be a tactful but open discussion with the parents about the suspected diagnosis.

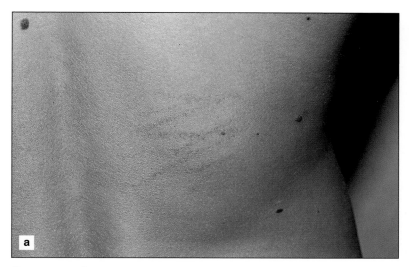

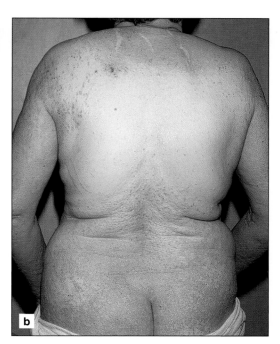

Figure 9.16 Some effects of scratching. (**a**) Linear purpura from scratching. (**b**) Butterfly sign. The mid- and upper back is relatively inaccessible to the hands. Some patients have a diffuse eruption, except for this area. The appearance has been likened to a butterfly. The implication is that any rash is secondary to scratching, rather than representing a primary dermatosis. Note that, with the use of a back scratcher or other instrument, even this area is accessible.

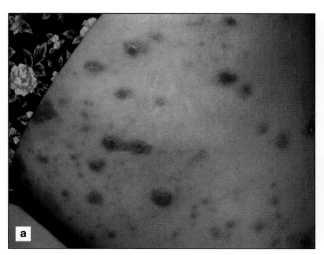

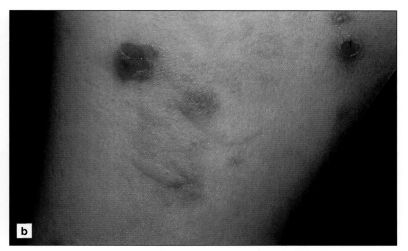

Figure 9.17 Prurigo nodularis and excoriations. (**a**) This woman presented with a diffuse pruritic rash that on initial inspection was thought to merely represent excoriations and prurigo nodularis. (**b**) Closer inspection showed the primary lesions of dermatographism.

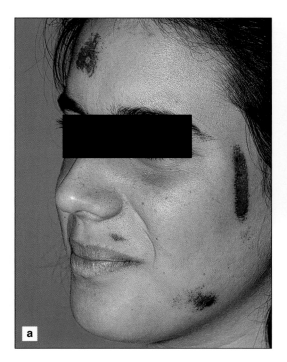

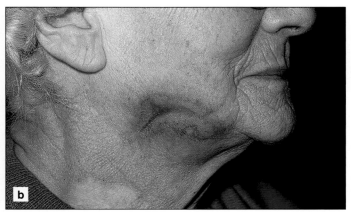

Figure 9.18 Dermatitis artefacta. (**a**) This teenaged girl said she woke up with these large facial lesions and has no idea how they got there. She has had approximately 10 episodes in 1 year and never seems to be very upset about them. (**b**) Dermatitis artefacta in an elderly woman who lives alone.

Table 9.6   MEASURES THAT MAY BE REQUIRED TO TREAT CHRONIC RUBBING OR SCRATCHING IN LICHEN SIMPLEX CHRONICUS OR NODULAR PRURIGO

Explanation of the role of scratching or rubbing in causation or at least in perpetuation of the lesion.

Short-term high-potency topical steroids are helpful to alleviate the itch. Use until the lesion is flat. Steroid-impregnated tape is helpful for small lesions. Intralesional steroids can be used.

Cover the lesion to prevent damage (e.g. use occlusive bandages for limbs with nodular prurigo), and ensure that the dressings are not removed until they are due to be replaced (remove the window of opportunity to scratch). Many dressings or bandages can be applied in conjunction with the topical steroid applied.

Decrease the potential to cause damage (e.g. cut the fingernails, get the patient to wear gloves).

Give sedating antihistamines, especially at night, or possibly a tricyclic antidepressant (which have both sedating and powerful antihistamine effects as well as their antidepressant function).

Avoid irritants, especially soaps for vulval lichen simplex chronicus (LSC), and replace with emollients.

Have family members encourage compliance.

Consider other topical agents, such as topical doxepin, topical local anesthetics, and topical capsaicin cream (although this was not helpful in LSC in one double-blind, placebo-controlled trial in which itching was described as worse at the active drug site).

Consider other options, such as phototherapy for nodular prurigo and excision for localized scrotal LSC.

Hypnosis or psychotherapy are less commonly used but have potential value.

Remember that there may be a systemic cause for itch in nodular prurigo, or a local cause in LSC, and investigate appropriately. For example, lichenification may conceal many primary dermatoses of the vulva, and contact dermatitis (e.g. to fragrances in hygiene wipes) may be either a cause or a secondary factor at this site.

Keep treating: remember that any excoriations noted on follow-up indicate continued scratching by the patient.

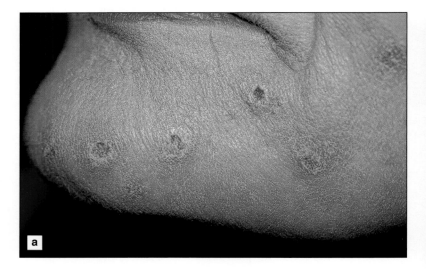

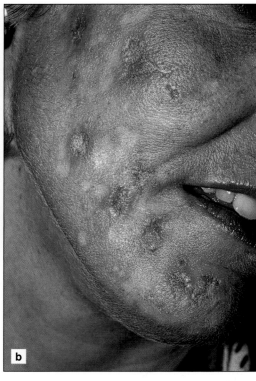

Figure 9.19   Acne excoriée. (**a**) Women often will excoriate their acne to such a degree that the acne is no longer visible. Significant scarring often results. (**b**) This patient has a severe case and has caused much scarring.

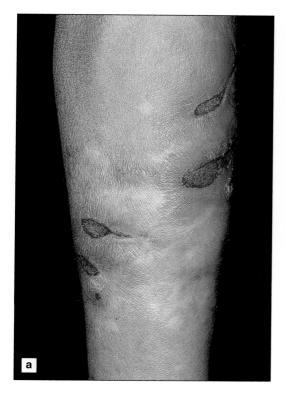

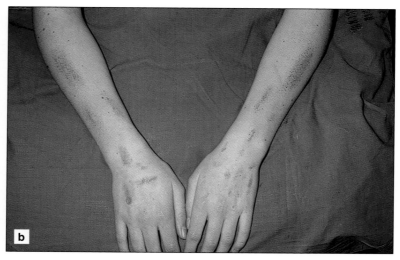

Figure 9.20 Dermatis artefacta. (**a**) This patient had injured herself on a thorn bush almost a year prior to the photograph. She was convinced that thorns were still embedded in the skin. Her constant digging prevented the skin from healing. Note the oval and linear pattern. (**b**) Dermatitis artefacta in a teenaged girl.

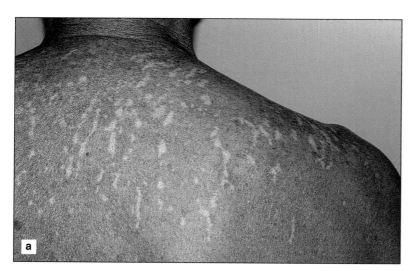

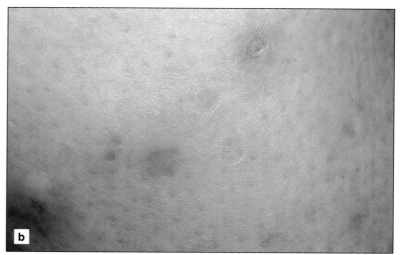

Figure 9.21 Scars. (**a**) This pattern of linear white scars on the upper back is a typical pattern that occurs as a result of years of scratching. (**b**) Shallow hypopigmented and/or pink circular scars are common on the legs, as shown here. Unfortunately, they are permanent. Acute excoriations are also seen.

FURTHER READING

Bernhard JD (ed) Itch: mechanisms and management of pruritus. New York: McGraw-Hill, 1994

Champion RH, Roberts SOB, Carpenter RG, et al. Urticaria and angio-oedema: a review of 554 patients. Br J Dermatol 1969; 81: 588–97

Denman ST. A review of pruritus. J Am Acad Dermatol 1986; 14: 375–92

Dreskin SC (ed) Urticaria. Immunol Allergy Clin North Am 2004; 24(2)

Goodkin R, Wingard E, Bernhard JD. Brachioradial pruritus: cervical spine disease and neurogenic/neuropathic (corrected) pruritus. J Am Acad Dermatol 2003; 48: 521–4

Grattan C, Powell S, Humphreys F. Management and diagnostic guidelines for urticaria and angio-oedema. Br J Dermatol 2001; 144: 708–14

Greaves MW. Chronic urticaria. N Engl J Med 1995; 332: 1767–72

Hellgren L. The prevalence of urticaria in the total population. Acta Allergol 1972; 27: 236–40

Holgate ST, Church MK (eds) Allergy. London: Mosby-Wolfe, 1993

Koo J. Psychodermatology: a practical manual for clinicians. Curr Probl Dermatol 1995; 7: 199–234

Sabroe RA, Seed PT, Stat C, et al. Chronic idiopathic urticaria: comparison of the clinical features of patients with and without anti-Fc or anti-IgE autoantibodies. J Am Acad Dermatol 1999; 40: 443–50

Volcheck GW, Li JT. Exercise-induced urticaria and anaphylaxis. Mayo Clin Proc 1997; 72: 140–7

10 Acne, Rosacea and Related Disorders

INTRODUCTION

Acne may be defined broadly as any condition that begins with the microcomedone. This therefore encompasses acne vulgaris, neonatal and infantile acne, and acne fulminans. However, rosacea and its variants do not fit this definition: even though rosacea superficially appears acneiform, having erythematous papules and pustules, and occurring mainly on the face, no comedones are seen. The follicular occlusion triad represents a group of diseases—hidradenitis suppurativa, acne conglobata, and dissecting cellulitis—that often occur together and that result from occlusion of the follicle.

ACNE AND RELATED CONDITIONS

Neonatal acne and neonatal cephalic pustulosis
Etiology and pathogenesis
There is a bit of controversy over neonatal acne and neonatal cephalic pustulosis. Neonatal acne has traditionally been thought to represent true comedonal and papulopustular acne induced by maternal hormones that cause excessive facial sebum production in the infant. Neonatal cephalic pustulosis is a newer entity, which describes a pustular condition of the head in neonates without comedones that is thought to be caused by overgrowth of various *Malassezia* species. Further studies are needed to identify features that help the clinician to differentiate between these two in the office setting.

Clinical
Papules and pustules on the face of an infant, usually in the first month of life, are characteristic (Fig. 10.1).

Differential diagnosis
Numerous conditions may cause pustules in the neonate; few, however, are confined to the face and none include a comedonal component. The main differentials to consider are as follows.
- Miliaria—papules and pustules occur, often on the head and neck, although other sites may be affected.
- Infections—especially due to *Staphylococcus aureus* or candida.
- Papular eruptions (some may have pseudopustular lesions) such as Langerhans cell histiocytosis and benign cephalic histiocytosis.

Treatment
Treatment in either case is rarely needed, as the condition resolves spontaneously in 1–2 months. If needed, topical erythromycin can be given, and low-strength benzoyl peroxide or tretinoin has been recommended for neonatal acne. If overgrowth of *Malassezia* species is suspected, ketoconazole (2% cream twice a day) can clear lesions within 1 week.

Infantile acne
Etiology and pathogenesis
The child with infantile acne is usually a male infant, 2–4 months of age, with inflammatory acne of the face. It has been suggested that infant boys are affected preferentially because they have near-pubertal levels of testosterone for the first 6–12 months of life. One study has suggested that these patients are more likely to develop more severe acne vulgaris as adolescents.

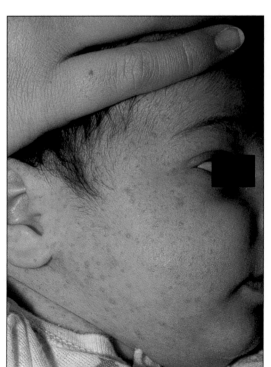

Figure 10.1 Neonatal acne. This condition, which is common in neonates, results from the mother's hormones, which increase facial oil production in utero, leading to acne. It typically resolves after 1–2 months of life without treatment, as the maternal hormones are no longer present.

Clinical

Clinically, one sees comedones, papules, pustules, and even larger inflammatory nodules on the face, especially the cheeks (Fig. 10.2).

Differential diagnosis

If the full spectrum of acne lesions is present, then diagnosis is straightforward. Diagnostic problems may arise if only one type of lesion is present, for example pustular lesions or a solitary nodule. Possible differentials include the following.

- Papular rash.
  Infection-related—molluscum contagiosum, plane warts, steroid-attenuated dermatophyte infections, viral exanthem, and Gianotti–Crosti syndrome.
  Inflammatory and others—irritant eczema due to dribbling saliva may be papular on the cheeks (often asymmetric); keratosis pilaris affecting the face; also, rarer conditions such as tuberous sclerosis, zinc deficiency (perioral, usually confluent eczematous appearance but can be papular), facial African-Caribbean childhood eruption (FACE), and histiocytoses (e.g. benign cephalic histiocytosis).
- Pustular rash—infections (staphylococcal and candidal) are the important issue to exclude in this age group.
- Solitary or few nodules—pilomatrixoma (see Ch. 23), insect bites, and idiopathic facial aseptic granuloma of childhood (usually on the cheek, usually solitary, mean age 5 years; resembles an inflamed acne cyst or nodule, and is usually self-limiting over many months).

Treatment

Congenital adrenal hyperplasia or a virilizing tumor should be excluded (e.g. by checking serum dehydroepiandrosterone sulfate, DHEAS, free testosterone, and 17-hydroxyprogesterone), although elevation of these hormones is uncommon. Oral erythromycin combined with tretinoin or benzoyl peroxide is usually sufficient. Other oral antibiotics appropriate for use in children (e.g. cephalexin and trimethoprim–sulfamethoxazole) may be tried. The disease tends to remit anywhere after 2 months to 4 years. Tetracyclines should be avoided in this age group. Rarely, isotretinoin may be needed.

Acne vulgaris

Etiology and pathogenesis

Acne is defined as any disease that begins with a microcomedo, and includes acne vulgaris, neonatal acne, infantile acne, and pomade acne. Rosacea, steroid folliculitis, and periorificial dermatitis are excluded.

Hormone surges in a child aged 7–10 years begin the changes that lead to acne. Adrenal maturation and gonadal development cause androgen production and subsequent sebaceous gland enlargement. Both the 'acne hormone' DHEAS and sebum production increase at this time. As the sebum levels increase, the follicular lining hypercornifies, leading to plugging of the follicle. Thus the comedo is formed. These pathophysiologic changes are typical of the young teen with an oily face and scattered centrofacial comedones.

Later, the bacterium *Propionibacterium acnes* proliferates in the oily milieu of the follicle. The patient's immune system reacts to this bacterium, and inflammation results. The clinical manifestation is the inflammatory papule or pustule. A plugged follicle in which *P. acnes* and the immune system do battle results in increased follicular pressure and a weakened follicular wall. Some of these follicles burst, resulting in an inflammatory nodule. Much damage is done by this process, and the skin may take many months to heal. The clinical manifestation of this healing process is the erythematous macule that remains after the inflammatory nodule has receded. Dermal scarring may be a permanent sequela.

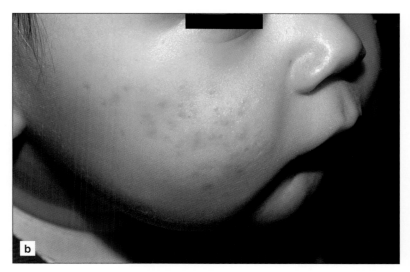

Figure 10.2 Infantile acne. (**a**,**b**) Infants, particularly boys, may develop the typical nodular lesions of acne. A hormonal profile should be obtained, although it is usually normal. In milder cases, more comedonal lesions are present. Standard acne therapy is used (but tetracyclines are avoided so as not to affect the teeth).

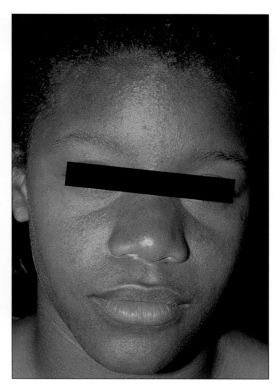

Figure 10.3 Prepubertal acne. One of the first signs of puberty is an oily face and centrofacial comedones.

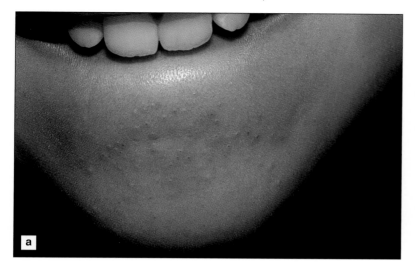

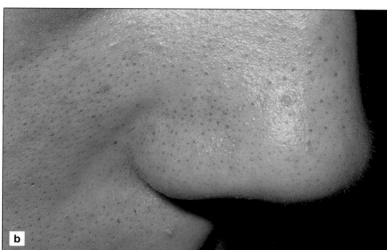

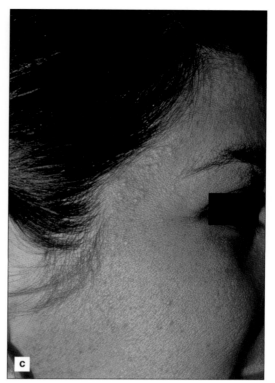

Figure 10.4 Comedonal acne. (**a**) Increased prepubertal hormones cause increased oiliness, clogging the pores. The black color is melanin, not dirt. (**b**) Topical retinoids are most effective for clearing the pores. (**c**) Acne along the hairline. Increased heat if covered by hair, natural oils from the scalp, and comedogenic substances from conditioners and shampoos may contribute.

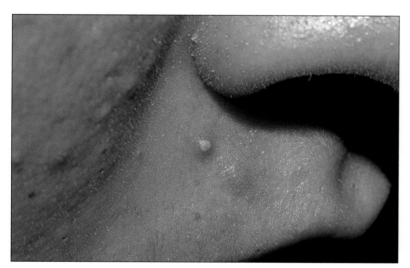

Figure 10.5 Inflammatory acne. The growth of *Propionibacterium acnes* and the body's immune response result in inflammatory lesions such as the pustule shown here.

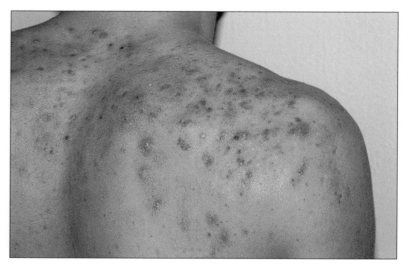

Figure 10.6 Acne on back and shoulders. This acne is typically inflammatory and usually needs oral antibiotics or possibly isotretinoin, but the patient may apply topical medication as well. Heat and sweat may aggravate.

Clinical

A clear indication that the pubertal hormones are beginning to surge is the development of an oily face and multiple comedones (Fig. 10.3). Open comedones (blackheads, Fig. 10.4) and closed comedones (whiteheads) are seen scattered across the central face. Later, inflammatory papules and pustules (Fig. 10.5) develop. They are more numerous and more deeply seated than simple comedones. Scarring may occur at this stage. If the acne becomes severe, deep, painful 'cysts' develop on the face, chest, and back (Fig. 10.6). Scarring is typical. Red macules are the common end result of inflamed lesions, and these will fade over time.

Scarring (Fig. 10.7) may be in the form of pits, smooth depressions, or keloidal nodules.

Differential diagnosis

It is uncommon that there is any real differential diagnostic problem for acne. However, on occasion the scenarios listed in Table 10.1 may cause problems.

Treatment

All acne treatment should involve the educational points as outlined in Table 10.2. A simple but effective therapeutic approach is presented in Table 10.3.

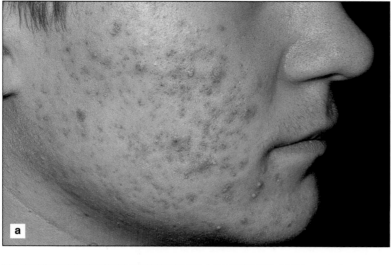

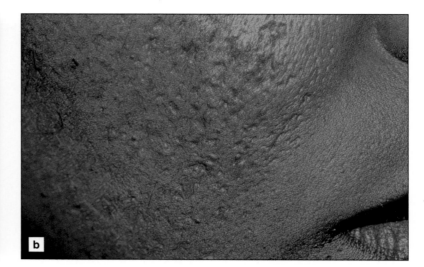

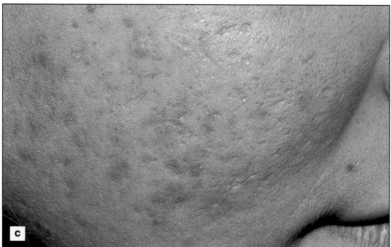

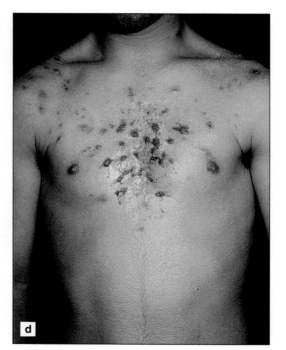

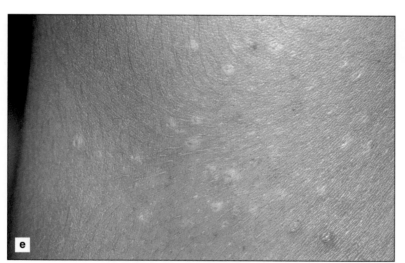

Figure 10.7 Acne scarring. (**a–c**) Acne with scarring on the cheeks. Acne lesions of any size may scar. When scarring is present, treatment with isotretinoin should be strongly considered. (**d**) Acne of the chest with early keloidal scarring. Acne commonly scars. When keloids form as well, the cosmetic consequences are even worse. Therapy is often difficult. (**e**) Papular acne scars on the back. These appear as white, dermal, perifollicular lesions. They are benign, and there is no good therapy other than preventing more acne.

Table 10.1   DIFFERENTIAL DIAGNOSIS OF ACNE VULGARIS (MAINLY APPLICABLE TO MID-CHILDHOOD TO YOUNG ADULT AGE GROUP)

Pattern of lesion	Type of process	Examples	Comments
Comedones or papules	Follicular lesions Infections Others	Simple milia Keratosis pilaris Plane warts, molluscum contagiosum Tuberous sclerosis (see Ch. 19) Facial African-Caribbean childhood eruption (FACE)	Often around eyes. Usually present on arms as well. Mainly central face; teenage diagnosis is not uncommon, especially in sporadic cases.
Pustules	Infections Other causes of pustules	Staphylococcal infection, gram-negative folliculitis, herpes folliculitis Pityrosporum folliculitis (see Ch. 26) Corticosteroid-induced acne Pseudofolliculitis barbae	Usually confined to the beard area, which helps to distinguish them; on the other hand, there is no reason why they cannot coexist with acne, and they may be an explanation for a sudden flare of 'acne'. Because of *Malassezia* yeasts; typically occurs on the trunk; usually in a slightly older age group than acne vulgaris, but the two conditions may overlap. May cause an acneiform rash that usually consists mainly of rather monomorphic papules or pustules. Discussed under *Rosacea* in this chapter. However, the full spectrum of acne lesions, including comedones, may occur. Common, but mainly on the neck and jaw area.
Nodules or cysts	Infections Follicle-related Others	Furuncle, carbuncle Epidermoid cyst, pilar cyst; pilomatrixoma Insect bites Lymphocytoma cutis Spitz nevus Idiopathic facial aseptic granuloma of childhood	See Chapter 24. See Chapters 23 and 30. Usually history of a bite. See Chapter 11. See Chapter 31. See discussion in section on differential diagnosis of infantile acne.
Varied, may be full acne spectrum	Drug-induced acne	Corticosteroids, anabolic steroids, lithium, isoniazid, anticonvulsants (see Ch. 18)	See also discussion of steroid rosacea in this chapter. Note that anabolic steroids are increasingly used by young men in the acne age group for bodybuilding purposes; they are a potent trigger for acne.

Table 10.2   TREATMENT OF ACNE: NOTES FOR THE PATIENT

Regular use of prescribed medications is critical.

Acne therapy is usually given in combination. Use all the medications prescribed.

Any regimen should be given at least 6–12 weeks to work.

Any moisturizer or make-up should be non-comedogenic or non-acnegenic.

Chocolate and french fries may not be good for the waistline but do not cause acne.

No picking, as this does not help and can lead to scarring.

Wash the face twice a day with a gentle cleanser. No scrubbing.

Do not spot treat acne. Spread the medication all over.

Table 10.3   STANDARD THERAPY FOR ACNE

Severity	Suggested therapy
Mild	Topical antimicrobial, particularly one that contains benzoyl peroxide, daily, plus a topical retinoid (e.g. adapalene or tretinoin) daily.
Moderate	Add to the above a tetracycline (e.g. tetracycline 500 mg or doxycycline 100 mg twice daily). If either of these fail, switch to minocycline (50–100 mg twice daily).
Treatment-resistant	Isotretinoin
Severe	Isotretinoin

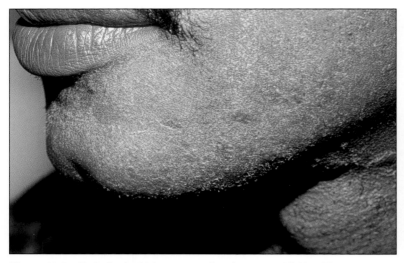

Figure 10.8   Topical retinoid therapy causing dryness and flaking. The term 'ashy' is often used by darker-skinned patients to describe this appearance. Non-comedogenic moisturizers should be recommended.

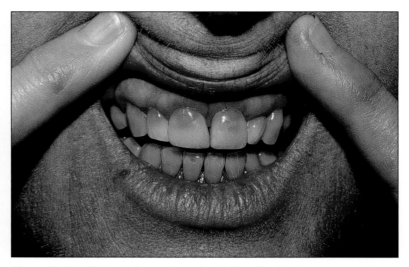

Figure 10.11   Blue teeth from minocycline. A blue discoloration may occur after many years of minocycline therapy, in this case 15 years for treatment of rosacea.

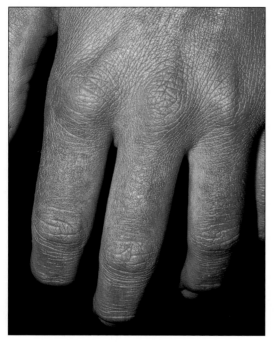

Figure 10.9
Photosensitivity with doxycycline. The dorsa of the hands and nose develop a characteristic erythema in patients on doxycycline exposed to significant sunlight.

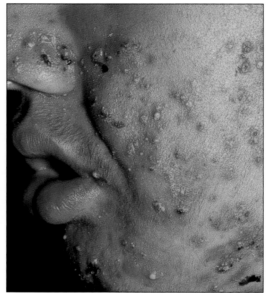

Figure 10.12   Severe acne. Acne this severe on presentation should prompt the consideration of early use of isotretinoin. The dose should be low initially to prevent a severe flare. An oral tetracycline or erythromycin may be helpful to calm the acne prior to isotretinoin.

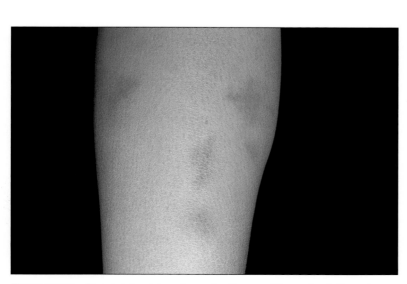

Figure 10.10   Blue patches from minocycline therapy. Minocycline is the only tetracycline that can cause blue patches on the skin. These probably start out as bruises, but never fade. Women are more commonly affected.

The foundation of any acne therapy is the combination of a topical retinoid (Fig. 10.8) and an antimicrobial. The retinoid opens up the pore and the antimicrobial kills *P. acnes*. Adapalene is one of the more versatile retinoids, as it is effective with a low level of irritation. Tretinoin packaged in a vehicle that reduces irritation is a good alternative. Any retinoid may be effectively combined with a topical benzoyl peroxide-containing product, although the combination may be more drying than either alone. For any patient with persistent comedonal disease, a salicylic acid cleanser could be considered, although these usually have only mild efficacy, and acne 'surgery' (extraction) may be a helpful adjunct.

For moderate to severe acne, a 3–6-month course of an oral antibiotic should be given in conjunction with the above topical regimen of a topical retinoid and benzoyl peroxide daily. The two standard first-line options are tetracycline or oxytetracycline (the dose used for either is the same: 500 mg twice a day) and doxycycline (100 mg twice a day). Doxycycline is more photosensitizing (Fig. 10.9) than the other tetracyclines, and thus may be less desirable in the summer. Most patients do fine on tetracycline in the summer months as long as a sunscreen is worn. The advantage of doxycycline is that it may be taken with food. Erythromycin (500 mg twice a day or 333 mg three times a day) is an alternative.

If the acne fails to respond after 6–8 weeks, minocycline (100 mg every day or twice a day) should be given along with the topical retinoid and benzoyl peroxide. Although minocycline is the most effective oral antibiotic against acne, it does carry the risk of several unpleasant side

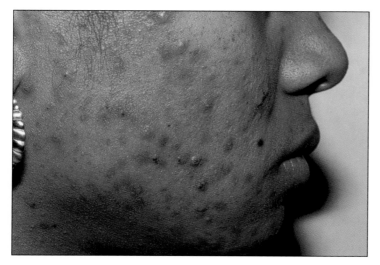

Figure 10.13 Inflammatory acne prior to beginning isotretinoin. Indications for isotretinoin are inflammatory acne that has failed to improve sufficiently on conventional therapy (as shown here), acne that relapses chronically after multiple courses of oral antibiotics, acne that scars, and acne in patients who have significant psychologic overtones to their acne.

effects. First of all, patients, particularly women, may develop nausea or dizziness with the first few doses. Second, it can cause bruises to persist, particularly on the legs of women (Fig. 10.10). Third, the teeth can develop a bluish color over time, especially if 100 mg twice daily is used over several years (Fig. 10.11). Finally, several systemic reactions have been noted, for example urticaria, rashes, hypersensitivity syndromes, hepatitis, arthralgias, and lupus-like syndrome. Thus every patient on minocycline should be asked at each visit if they have noticed any blue patches of the skin, blue teeth, or any unusual symptoms. It is also recommended that an antinuclear antibody test should be checked at 6–9-month intervals in those taking minocycline long term.

The alleged decrease in effectiveness of oral contraceptives by the above oral antibiotics has not yet been proved but should be discussed with the patient; it is prudent to recommend the use of additional barrier contraception during the first month of treatment in case there is disturbance of the enterohepatic circulation by the antibiotic, thus affecting absorption of the oral contraceptive agent.

For moderate or severe acne (Figs 10.12 and 10.13) that has failed conventional therapy, isotretinoin is the drug of choice. Additional indications for isotretinoin include any acne that is scarring and acne present for many years that quickly relapses off oral antibiotics. Isotretinoin is a potent teratogen and should be given only by someone trained in its use. Typically, one gives 40 mg/day for the first month until the patient acclimatizes to the side effects (Fig. 10.14, Tables 10.4 and 10.5). This also reduces the risk of an initial flare (Fig. 10.15). Then, a dose of 1 mg/kg per day is given and the patient's condition is followed until a total dose of 120 mg/kg is reached.

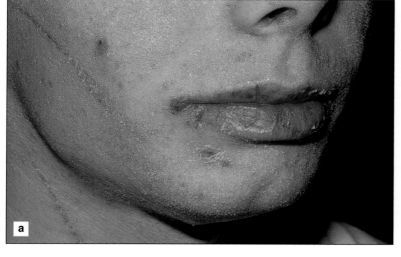

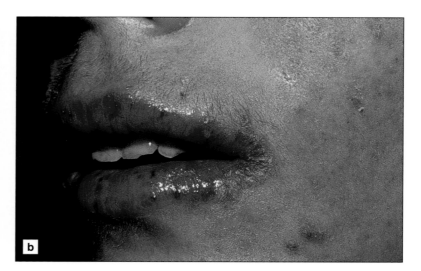

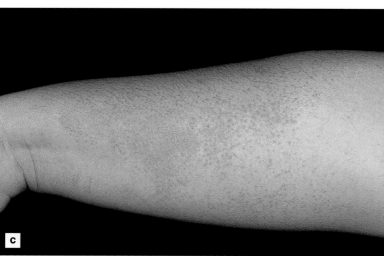

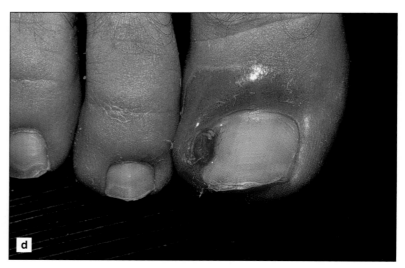

Figure 10.14 Side effects of isotretinoin. (**a**) The face during isotretinoin therapy. The skin is dry and peeling. The lips are inflamed, red, and scaly. Bacterial superinfection by staphylococci may occur. The corners of lips are often affected, as in perlèche. (**b**) Isotretinoin cheilitis. (**c**) Retinoid dermatitis of arms during therapy with isotretinoin. (**d**) Pyogenic granuloma and paronychia in a patient on isotretinoin therapy. The periungual skin may develop various complications during isotretinoin therapy, including ingrown nails, bacterial paronychia, and the formation of pyogenic granuloma.

Table 10.4 COMMON SIDE EFFECTS OF ISOTRETINOIN AND THEIR TREATMENT

Side effect	Suggested therapy
Dry, chapped lips	Lip balm many times per day
Dry facial skin	A non-comedogenic lotion several times a day
Dry skin of the body	A heavy cream applied immediately after the shower
Headache	Aspirin, ibuprofen, etc. (but stop isotretinoin if severe)
Nosebleed	Petrolatum applied in the nose three times per day
Reduce isotretinoin dose if frequent/severe
Backache	Aspirin, ibuprofen
Delayed menses	No treatment other than to confirm that the patient is not pregnant
Hypertriglyceridemia	Lower dose, lipid-lowering agent (e.g. gemfibrozil)
Paronychia	Antistaphylococcal antibiotic, may need partial nail avulsion
Impetigo	Antistaphylococcal antibiotic
Elevated liver enzymes	Stop isotretinoin, repeat test in 1–2 weeks. Ask about changes in general heath, alcohol intake.

Table 10.5 RARE BUT SERIOUS SIDE EFFECTS OF ISOTRETINOIN

Side effect or event	Intervention
Depression	Stop isotretinoin, refer for psychosocial evaluation
Decreased night vision	Stop isotretinoin, refer to ophthalmologist
Severe headache	Stop isotretinoin, refer to neurologist
Pregnancy	Stop isotretinoin, refer for genetic counseling and consideration of abortion

If the face is clear, the isotretinoin is stopped. Triglyceride levels and liver function should be monitored during therapy. For women, a baseline and then monthly pregnancy test is required, as isotretinoin is a serious teratogen. If a woman is of childbearing potential and still a virgin, abstinence is sufficient. Otherwise, two methods of birth control are mandatory in the USA. If some acne remains at the end of the course, treatment may be given for another month or two. If a predominance of macrocomedones emerges as therapy progresses, these lesions should be removed (Fig. 10.16). Multiple courses may be necessary in some patients, particularly women.

A small percentage of patients flare on isotretinoin therapy. These patients tend to be young, male, and with many macrocomedones (also known as sebaceous retention). Therapy for these patients is to lower the isotretinoin dose (or even stop it for a time), to give an oral corticosteroid (e.g. prednisone) for several weeks, and to use acne surgery to remove the macrocomedones.

Depression has been linked to isotretinoin therapy, but the incidence is rare. Each patient should be asked at every visit if their mood has changed. If depressive symptoms develop, the isotretinoin should be stopped and the patient referred to a psychiatrist.

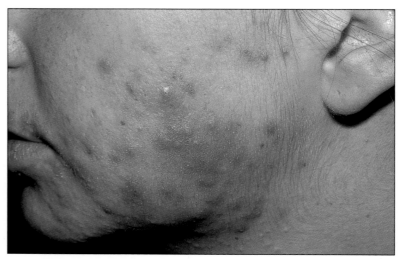

Figure 10.15 Flare of acne on isotretinoin. Acne may flare for several reasons during the first month of isotretinoin treatment. First, conventional therapy is usually stopped when isotretinoin is started, and isotretinoin needs several months to improve acne. Second, isotretinoin causes rapid death of *Propionibacterium acnes*, and the body's response to this antigenic load may be significant. Third, isotretinoin may thin the follicular wall, making it more susceptible to rupture.

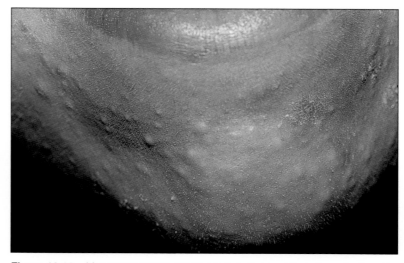

Figure 10.16 Macrocomedones. These small, 1–2-mm white balls under the skin do not clear easily with isotretinoin therapy and may prolong the course. Acne surgery clears them. They are often best seen when the skin is stretched.

For a severe flare of acne (Fig. 10.17), an oral corticosteroid may be given. For individual large lesions, intralesional triamcinolone (2.5 mg/mL) is helpful, but it must be documented that the patient accepts the risk of a permanent atrophic area. If the lesion is a cyst, the steroid injection should be placed within the cyst rather than into overlying skin, or it will be ineffective but may cause depigmentation. If a cyst is inflamed, this may be due to secondary infection or due to leakage into the skin; aspiration to exclude infection is prudent before considering steroid injection. Some patients complain of a lesion that recurs consistently in the same place. This may represent a persistent sinus tract that must be removed surgically. Sometimes the clinician may suspect a sinus tract or fistula by an oblong or linear acne 'cyst' (Fig. 10.18). Occasionally, a bacterial infection can mimic acne (Fig. 10.19).

Acne in adult women

Acne tends to remit in male patients by age 20 years. Unfortunately, this is not at all true for women, as persistence of acne through the twenties and thirties is common. The adult woman with acne usually does not have the degree of oiliness of the skin nor the visible comedones that are likely in a teenager. Instead, she mainly gets inflammatory papules and pustules scattered on the face. The cheeks and jawline are favored areas of the face to be affected (analogous to the beard area in men), which helps to distinguish acne from rosacea in this population. Microbiologic studies

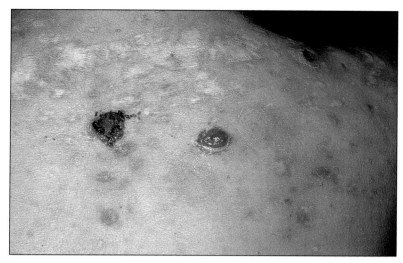

Figure 10.17 Pyogenic granuloma lesions during isotretinoin therapy. These crusted, bleeding lesions may form early in the course of isotretinoin therapy. They are most common in patients with severe disease prior to initiating isotretinoin. For these patients, the dose should be low initially and increased after 1–2 months to try to avoid this complication. Scarring almost always occurs.

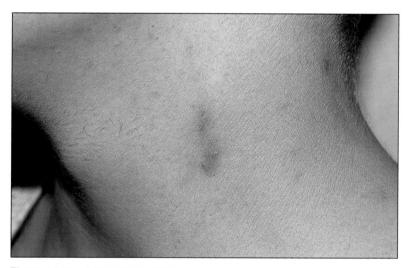

Figure 10.18 A sinus tract. Whenever an acne lesion is oval or linear (as shown here), the possibility of a sinus tract or fistula should be considered. These lesions do not clear with acne therapy and may require surgery. Note the opening at the superior end.

have failed to demonstrate differences in the bacterial milieu between adult women and teenagers with acne.

Treatment is usually similar to that for standard acne, except for increased use of hormonal approaches. Thus an oral antibiotic, for example tetracycline, combined with a topical retinoid and benzoyl peroxide, is appropriate. Some oral contraceptives have been shown in controlled trials to benefit acne, for example Ortho Tri-Cyclen and Yasmin. These agents are not usually used as monotherapy, but instead as an adjunct to conventional therapy. If standard approaches fail, isotretinoin is usually given. For women who relapse after multiple courses of isotretinoin, a hormonal evaluation (e.g. DHEAS and free testosterone) is recommended. If an abnormality is found, it is usually an elevation in testosterone, and referral to an endocrinologist is in order.

For women who relapse after isotretinoin, or who want to consider an alternative, the combination of spironolactone (75–100 mg/day), an oral antibiotic (e.g. minocycline, 100 mg/day), and an oral contraceptive is very effective. Side effects of spironolactone include decreased libido and breast tenderness but are unusual at this dose. The blood pressure should be monitored (spironolactone is an antihypertensive) and the potassium checked initially until it is stable. A topical retinoid (e.g. adapalene gel daily) and benzoyl peroxide (5% daily) may be given as well. In the UK, cyproterone (an antiandrogen) may be given, usually in a low-dose (2 mg daily) combination form with an oral contraceptive (Dianette). In hirsute patients, but not usually for acne in isolation, a higher dose may be given by adding cyproterone 50 mg on days 5–15 of the menstrual cycle, in conjunction with the same oral contraceptive combination.

Acne in the darker-skinned patient
Etiology and pathogenesis
Acne in the darker-skinned patient is caused by the same factors as acne in a pale-skinned patient. Indeed, recent studies have shown that the inflammation is just as common in black as in white patients: it is just more hidden by the patient's pigment. Some differences are seen clinically, however. For example, postinflammatory hyperpigmented macules abound and are often slow to fade. Lesions along the hairline may be more numerous if pomades are used in the hair.

Clinical
Acne in darker-skinned patients is characterized by the usual comedones, papules, pustules, and nodules. Unique to black patients, however, are the multiple brown or black spots at the site of prior acne (Fig. 10.20). Patients usually complain more of these lesions than of the acne.

Differential diagnosis
The differential is that of acne generally. However, the presence of hyperpigmented lesions and the decreased visibility of inflammation in

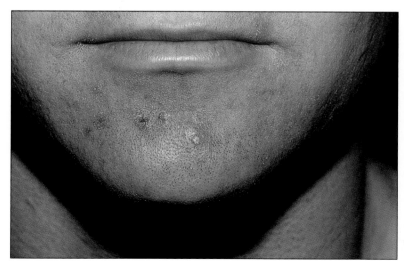

Figure 10.19 Staphylococcal infection mimicking acne. Both gram-positive and gram-negative bacteria can cause an eruption that mimics acne. Unusual cases should prompt a culture. The absence of comedones should elicit suspicion of this possibility.

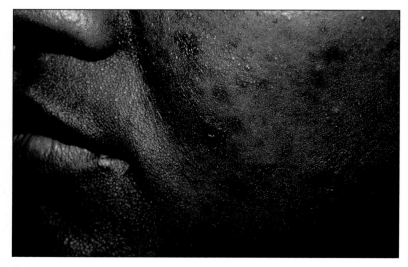

Figure 10.20 Postinflammatory hyperpigmentation. Dark-skinned patients frequently develop hyperpigmented macules at the sites of acne lesions. Much of the pigment is epidermal. Often, there is also significant residual inflammation.

darker skin may make the diagnosis more difficult. Additionally, there are differential diagnoses that may apply specifically to darker skin (such as FACE and pomade acne) and some conditions that are commoner in dark skin (such as papular sarcoidosis) that may widen the usual differential diagnosis.

Treatment

The treatment of acne in the darker-skinned patient is the same as that given to white patients, with a few exceptions. For example, controlling the acne with the standard therapy (e.g. a topical retinoid, topical benzoyl peroxide 5%, and an oral tetracycline) is very effective, as noted earlier. If many postinflammatory hyperpigmented macules are present, this is particularly important, as it is much easier to prevent the development of a brown spot than to remove it once it appears. Additionally, the individual black areas may be treated with azelaic acid, which has benefit both to treat acne and to lighten dark spots. Alternatively, 4% hydroquinone twice a day, applied only to the dark areas, may be given. (Histologic studies of these brown macules show most of the melanin to be epidermal, which makes them accessible to topical therapy.)

PRACTICE POINTS

- Acne is characterized by comedones (open and closed), papules, pustules, nodules, and cysts; comedones are essential for the diagnosis, but usually several of these lesion types coexist to leave little diagnostic doubt.
- A sudden flare of pustular acne on the face may be due to superimposed staphylococcal or gram-negative infection; always send microbiology samples from pustular eruptions if sudden or if the diagnosis is in doubt.
- In treating acne, it is essential to realize that antibiotics are not anticomedonal, and that results of treating inflammatory acne with antibiotics are improved if anticomedonal treatment is also used.
- Any treatment for acne needs to be used for long enough—typically at least 2 months—and any topical treatment should be applied to the whole zone of skin where the acne occurs, not just to individual lesions that are present at the time.

Acne excoriée
Etiology and pathogenesis

Many patients, particularly women, try to scratch away their acne. This practice is common and should be discouraged. In acne excoriée, however, this behavior is both obsessional and destructive.

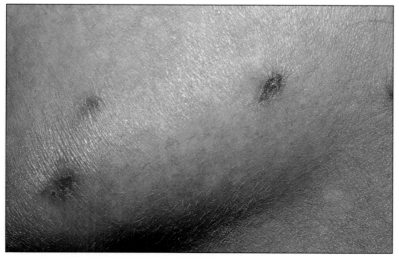

Figure 10.21 Excoriations in acne. Some patients with acne are unable to keep their hands away from their face. Multiple excoriations are the result. The physician can learn to recognize these patients by the large, red spots their fingernails leave. Patients with no underlying acne but who still scratch their face must be excluded.

Clinical

Often, no or only minimal acne is visible. Instead, the excoriations (Fig. 10.21), crusting, and scars from the patient's manipulation are evident. Patients who have no acne but still scratch should not really be considered under this term.

Differential diagnosis

Although the gouge marks of acne excoriée are usually very obvious to a dermatologist, the patient has often been treated unsuccessfully for infection previously. Commonly considered diagnoses for the scabbed or depressed areas of old ulceration include the following.
- Infection—staphylococcal and herpetic.
- 'Old spots' or cysts.
- Keratoses—although the lesions are generally around the mouth and jaw area.

Treatment

The patient should be encouraged not to touch the acne, as the manipulation itself usually causes more scarring than the acne alone. Often, however, this advice is not heeded, and the more successful course is simply to clear the acne. Thus aggressive treatment of the acne with oral antibiotics combined with topical medication is necessary. Isotretinoin may even be warranted. Topical antiitch preparations may be tried, but usually itch is not the culprit. Only a minority of patients will be amenable to psychiatric intervention, which may include psychotherapy and rarely antipsychotic medication (e.g. olanzapine).

Acne fulminans
Etiology and pathogenesis

Acne fulminans (AF) is a severe form of acne that tends to affect young males. In most patients, there is no obvious triggering event. The history is often of mild acne vulgaris, which then 'explodes' on the chest and back and which is accompanied by malaise, fever, arthralgias, myalgias, etc. In other patients, AF is precipitated by isotretinoin, usually in the first 7 weeks of therapy. However, this diagnosis should not be applied to a patient who is only experiencing a flare of acne without systemic symptoms. Finally, some teenage boys have developed AF in the setting of long-term testosterone therapy.

Clinical

White, male teenagers are most commonly affected, with the acute onset of inflammatory nodules on the chest and back, which may break down, leaving crusted ulcerations (Fig. 10.22). Virtually all patients complain of fever, arthralgias, and myalgias. Other reported findings include malaise, weight loss, erythema nodosum, and hepatosplenomegaly. Common laboratory abnormalities include an elevated erythrocyte sedimentation rate (ESR) and leukocytosis. Elevated liver function tests (LFTs), microscopic hematuria, and hypergammaglobulinemia have also been reported. Significant scarring usually occurs on healing.

Differential diagnosis

The most important differential diagnosis is to exclude secondary bacterial or (less likely) herpetic infection.

The skin lesions themselves often resemble pyogenic granulomas, but if explosive and crusted could suggest the possibility of a vasculitis.

Treatment

Antibiotics alone are ineffective. Prednisone or prednisolone at approximately 1 mg/kg per day should be instituted to quickly gain control of the outbreak. A course of isotretinoin (initially low dose to try to avoid pyogenic granuloma lesions) or high-dose tetracycline may then be instituted to try to prevent a flare or later recurrence. The prednisone should be tapered slowly over 2–4 months to avoid relapses. The musculo-skeletal symptoms respond well to oral corticosteroids and non-steroidal antiinflammatory drugs. Obviously, if isotretinoin precipitated the AF, it should be stopped. Minocycline or dapsone may be helpful for some patients.

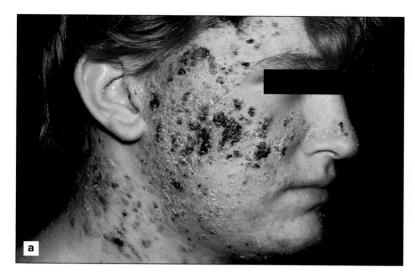

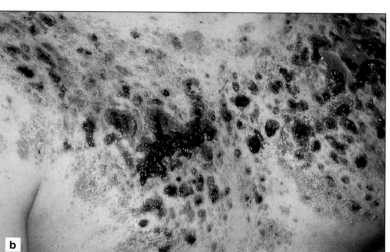

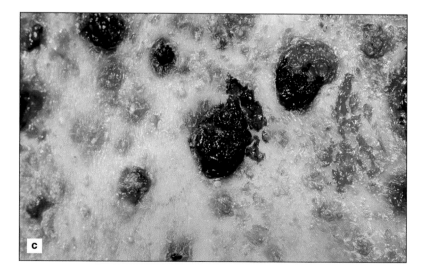

Figure 10.22 Acne fulminans. (**a**) This teenager developed severe hemorrhagic crusted 'acne' during the first month of therapy with isotretinoin. He also had fever and malaise. (**b**) Multiple crusted nodules on the back. Severe scarring invariably results. (**c**) Close-up view.

For any pyogenic granuloma-like lesions, a very potent topical steroid ointment is usually effective. Alternatively, pulsed dye laser has been reported to work rapidly.

ROSACEA AND RELATED CONDITIONS

Rosacea
Etiology and pathogenesis
Rosacea is characterized by papules and pustules on the cheeks and nose

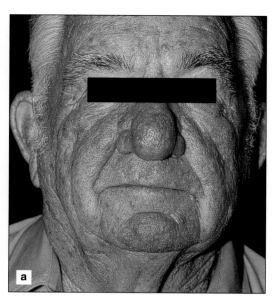

Figure 10.23 (**a,b**) Rosacea, the classic appearance. Multiple papules and a few pustules are scattered on the nose and cheeks. The nose shows almost confluent erythema.

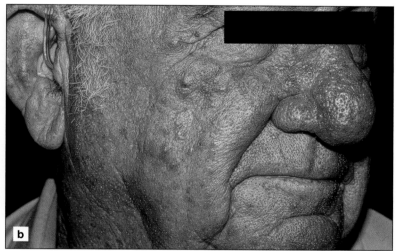

of an adult. Comedones are absent. Fair-skinned patients (particularly Celts) are prone to this disease. Black-skinned patients are rarely affected.

The exact cause of rosacea is unknown. *Demodex* mites (see later in this chapter) and gastrointestinal colonization with *Helicobacter pylori* have been proposed as the reason for rosacea, although never proved to have a true causal association. Recent evidence suggests that the warm milieu of the highly vascularized nose and cheeks causes resident bacteria to secrete a greater amount and a different composition of proteins as compared to with normal flora.

Clinical
Clinically, one sees inflammatory papules and pustules of the central face, especially the nose (Fig. 10.23). A Maltese cross distribution has been described in which the nose, each cheek, central forehead, and point of the chin are affected. The areas immediately around the mouth and the eyelids are characteristically spared, although, paradoxically, the eyelids may be affected in isolation in a variant of rosacea.

Erythematous papules usually outnumber pustules. The erythema may extend for 1–2 cm beyond the center. Comedones are absent. When severe, the redness may be confluent (Fig. 10.24).

Telangiectasias may accumulate over time, and ocular involvement (e.g. blepharitis, conjunctivitis, and ocular dryness) may occur as well. Facial telangiectasias, a reddish appearance of the face, and periodic flushing are often associated. Hot liquids and a hot environment may induce flushing. When this flush is the main component, diagnosis may be difficult. Unilateral rosacea may suggest demodicosis (Fig. 10.25). Enlargement of the nose (rhinophyma; Fig. 10.26) occurs in the minority, and patients

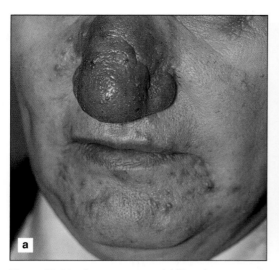
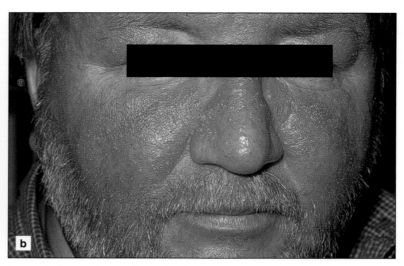

Figure 10.24 Severe rosacea. (**a**) Note the scattered papules on the face and the confluent involvement of the nose. Alcohol ingestion is not related to this appearance. (**b**) Note the severe inflammation with confluent redness and significant edema.

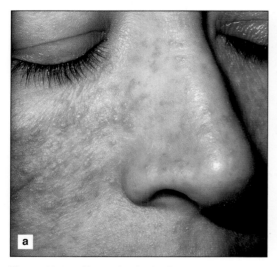
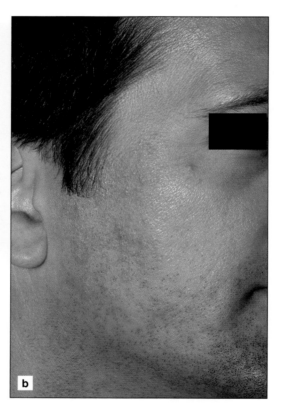

Figure 10.25 Demodicosis. (**a**) *Demodex* can appear exactly as rosacea. (**b**) The presence of unilateral rosacea should prompt the consideration of *Demodex* infection. Examination of a scraping of the lesions under the microscope is in order.

should be reassured that this is uncommon; it is more common in men, and the degree of rosacea present may be minimal. Tremendous edema may develop in rosacea (Fig. 10.27), sometimes without preceding erythema or other skin lesions.

Differential diagnosis

There are three common differential diagnoses that arise.

- Eczema—especially seborrheic dermatitis but also atopic and contact dermatitis affecting the face. Seborrheic dermatitis is a particular issue, as it affects the mid-face and is common. Distinction between rosacea and seborrheic dermatitis can usually be made on the basis of the features listed in Table 10.6. However, both are common conditions and may coexist, so diagnosis can be difficult.
- Systemic lupus erythematosus (SLE)—this may be suggested due to the presence of a butterfly rash on the cheeks. However, it would be very unusual for a patient with active SLE not to have additional features such as malaise, arthralgia, diffuse alopecia, raised ESR, or a positive antinuclear antibody. Additionally, although the butterfly rash

of SLE may consist of semiconfluent papules and plaques, the pustules that occur in rosacea are absent in SLE.
- Corticosteroid-induced skin changes—this situation is discussed later under the term perioral dermatitis. Redness and telangiectasia are typical on the cheeks, but papular lesions may occur around the mouth.
- Other conditions to consider—rosacea may have a prominent flushing component (for differential diagnosis of flushing, see Ch. 12). Acne, and disorders in the differential of acne, may also need to be considered (see previously in this chapter).

Treatment

Tetracycline or oxytetracycline (250–500 mg once or twice a day) is the mainstay of therapy for the papules and pustules of rosacea. In fact, these agents are more effective for rosacea than for acne, and a response is usually seen within 2–3 weeks. Patients can often maintain a clear face with a 500-mg capsule every day or every other day. It should be made clear to the patient that therapy may be lifelong. Control is the rule, not cure. It is also important to stress at the outset that papules and pustules may respond

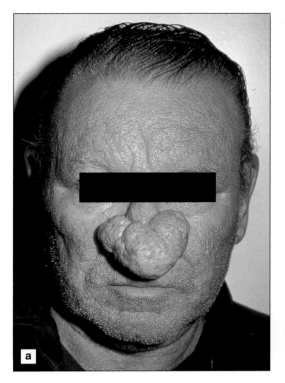
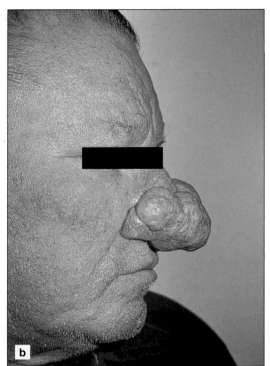

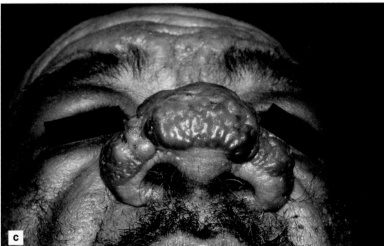

Figure 10.26 (**a,b**) Severe rhinophyma. (**c**) Severe rhinophyma in a black patient. (Panels a and b courtesy of Michael O. Murphy, M.D.)

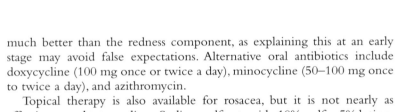

much better than the redness component, as explaining this at an early stage may avoid false expectations. Alternative oral antibiotics include doxycycline (100 mg once or twice a day), minocycline (50–100 mg once to twice a day), and azithromycin.

Topical therapy is also available for rosacea, but it is not nearly as effective as oral tetracyclines. Sodium sulfacetamide 10%–sulfur 5% lotion, or metronidazole 0.75% or 1% cream every day, are modestly effective topical agents. Clindamycin lotion or benzoyl peroxide are alternatives. Combining an oral tetracycline with one of these initially is a good approach for more severe cases. Alternatively, topical therapy may be used to prevent relapse when oral medications are stopped. Isotretinoin has been employed for severe cases, although it has no product license for this indication. A low dose (e.g. 20–40 mg/day) is usually given for 4–5 months.

Topical retinoids have little benefit. Any trigger factors of flushing (e.g. hot liquids) should be avoided.

It is important to help the patient understand that this therapy will not improve any telangiectasias. These so-called broken blood vessels do not respond to medical therapy. They can, however, be cleared nicely with the pulsed dye laser.

The excessive tissue of rhinophyma may be removed surgically to give excellent cosmetic results. Both cold steel and laser techniques may be employed.

It is vital to avoid use of topical steroids in rosacea. While they transiently reduce redness, their effect is of limited duration, and suddenly stopping them may cause a rebound flare. In either of these situations, a stronger agent may be applied to control the disease, thus worsening the situation and increasing the risk of local side effects (see Ch. 3 and perioral dermatitis, later in this chapter). It is all too easy for the unwary to become trapped in this vicious cycle.

Ocular rosacea

A chronic blepharitis, conjunctivitis, and ocular dryness are common in patients with rosacea (Fig. 10.28). Keratitis may occur.

Tetracycline or oxytetracycline is effective, as is doxycycline (100 mg twice a day) or minocycline (100 mg twice a day). Artificial tears are helpful for the dryness.

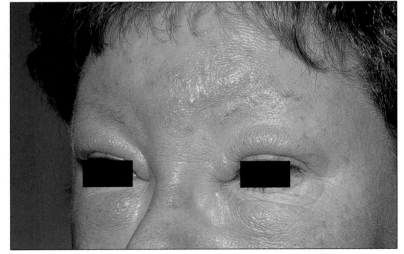

Figure 10.27 Edema of the forehead from rosacea. The inflammation of rosacea may cause significant edema. Edema about the eyes or of the entire face occurs.

Table 10.6   FEATURES THAT MAY HELP TO DISTINGUISH ROSACEA FROM SEBORRHEIC DERMATITIS

Feature	Rosacea	Seborrheic dermatitis
Color	Bright red	Brownish red
Scaling	No	Yes
Papules	Yes (but may be absent after antibiotic therapy, while redness may remain)	No
Pustules	Yes (but may be absent after antibiotic therapy, while redness may remain)	No
Telangiectasia	Yes, but may be absent early on	No, but telangiectases on sun-exposed cheeks are common, so may cause diagnostic problems
Flushing tendency	Frequent	No, but degree of rash may have some temperature or humidity variation
Specific localization	Nose, cheeks (usually confluent with nasal redness), central forehead, point of chin	Nasolabial folds and paranasal (not usually nasal dorsum or tip), scalp margin, ears, central chest, and back (mainly in male patients)
Associated skin features	Rhinophyma	Dandruff
Ocular features	Dry eye, red eye (conjunctivitis, keratitis), blepharitis	Seborrheic blepharitis

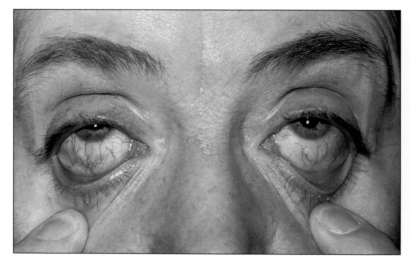

Figure 10.28   Ocular rosacea. Approximately half of patients with rosacea will have ocular rosacea as well. Dry eyes and irritation are common.

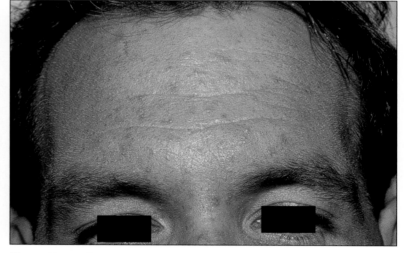

Figure 10.29   Steroid rosacea resulting from prolonged use of a high-potency topical steroid. Although the initial rash may be gone, the patient is continuing to use the medication, hoping that the new rash will improve.

Steroid rosacea

Etiology and pathogenesis

The chronic use of a high-potency or oral steroid can result in an acneiform eruption called steroid rosacea. The exact mechanism is unknown.

Clinical

Relatively monomorphic erythematous papules and follicular pustules are characteristic (Fig. 10.29). Comedones are absent.

Differential diagnosis

The diagnosis is generally apparent from the clinical setting. The most important differential, especially if the patient has had prolonged oral steroid therapy, is to ensure that the lesions (especially pustules) do not represent opportunistic infection.

The differential may include the following.

- Papules—see Table 10.1.
- Pustules—infection (bacterial, *Malassezia*, candidal, fungal, and herpetic) and eosinophilic folliculitis (HIV-associated).

Treatment

The offending steroid should be stopped, but the patient must be made aware that the disease may flare for the first 1–2 weeks. Tetracycline or oxytetracycline (e.g. 500 mg twice a day) or minocycline (e.g. 50–100 mg twice a day), with topical metronidazole (0.75% gel twice a day) or benzoyl peroxide daily, are effective therapies and will blunt this flare.

Demodicosis

Clinical

Although the human *Demodex folliculorum* mite is a normal component of the facial skin, some patients can develop a rosaceaform pustular rash of the face (Fig. 10.25) in the setting of excessive numbers of *Demodex* mites, as seen on KOH scraping. Often, the rash is 'unilateral'. Topical tacrolimus has precipitated this condition.

Treatment

Topical permethrin 5% cream and oral metronizadole have been used.

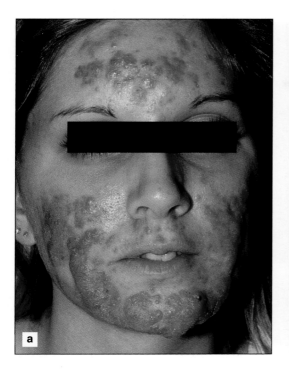
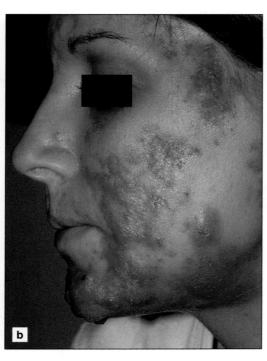

Figure 10.30 Rosacea fulminans. (**a**) The acute onset of large, deep, inflammatory nodules and abscesses on the face of a young adult woman is characteristic of rosacea fulminans, formerly called pyoderma faciale. (**b**) Close-up view.

Rosacea fulminans
Etiology and pathogenesis
The acute onset of large, deep, inflammatory nodules and abscesses on the face of a young adult woman is characteristic of rosacea fulminans, formerly called pyoderma faciale (Fig. 10.30). The cause is unknown. Bacterial cultures show the usual acne pathogens. Constitutional symptoms are generally absent (in contrast to AF). Comedones are absent, as are typical acne lesions on the chest and back. Increased facial oiliness prior to onset is typical.

Clinical
The chin, cheeks, and forehead are preferentially affected by inflammatory plaques with a variable amount of pustules. A localized form may occur, with a solitary lesion affecting the jaw, chin, or one cheek.

Differential diagnosis
The important differential is from infected lesions, such as staphylococcal abscesses. The main differentials are as follows.

- Infections—especially staphylococcal abscesses or infected cysts (including those of true acne); less commonly the disorder may be mimicked by other infections, such as a fungal kerion.
- Inflammatory diseases—Sweet disease (plaques with pseudopustules, rather than frank abscess formation), lupus erythematosus tumidus (solid plaque without pustules), Jessner lymphocytic infiltrate (plaques without pustules, more chronic evolution), pyoderma gangrenosum of the head and neck (rare, but may present with inflamed nodules), 'malignant pyoderma' (more ulcerative, probably actually a term that has historically included both pyoderma gangrenosum and Wegener granulomatosis).

Treatment
Prednisone or prednisolone at a dose of 0.5–1.0 mg/kg per day is given for the first 1–2 weeks to gain control of the outbreak. Then isotretinoin (e.g. 0.2–0.5 mg/kg per day) is begun. The oral corticosteroid may be tapered over 2–3 weeks and the isotretinoin continued until resolution occurs. Warm compresses and a high-potency topical steroid may be used during the first 1–2 weeks. If staphylococcal infection is a possibility when the patient is first seen, even though rosacea fulminans is the likeliest diagnosis, an antibiotic that might be useful for either condition (such as erythromycin 1–2 g daily) may be given while awaiting confirmation that bacterial cultures are negative and before starting a systemic corticosteroid that would be contraindicated in the presence of infection; the advantage of erythromycin over tetracyclines is that it can be given concurrently with isotretinoin if required, so the treatments can overlap. Note that pus for culture from a fluctuant lesion should be obtained by aspiration; formal incision and drainage should not be done, as it causes too much scarring. Dapsone has also been used as alternative therapy.

PRACTICE POINTS

- The commonest differential diagnosis of rosacea is seborrheic dermatitis, which is common and mid-facial; however, it is less red, has fine scaling, affects the nasolabial crease, and has no pustular or telangiectatic component, so should usually be easy to distinguish.
- Redness in rosacea (other than immediately around papules or pustules) responds poorly to antibiotics, even though the papulopustular component responds extremely well to tetracyclines; always warn the patient of this differential response in advance.
- It is vital to avoid use of topical steroids in rosacea to avoid escalating use of more potent agents and the associated rebound flare that may occur when they are stopped.
- Ocular involvement in rosacea is underestimated but can rarely be sight-threatening; if in doubt, and particularly if it does not respond quickly to oral tetracyclines, get an expert opinion.

Crusted folliculitis of the scalp
Etiology and pathogenesis
Some adult men complain of very itchy bumps on the scalp. They usually scratch away any primary lesion such that, at the time of the examination, only a crusted papule hidden in the hair is seen. On occasion, the true primary lesion, a pustule, is found (Fig. 10.31). Previous authors have called this condition acne necrotica, and others have opted for calling it *P. acnes* folliculitis, as they have found *P. acnes* in the follicles. Still others have found staphylococci, *Malassezia* spp., or gram-negative bacteria. Indeed, there may be several organisms that can cause crusted folliculitis of the scalp, some that are easily cultured and others that are not. Finally, some consider this to be a variant of rosacea or of seborrheic dermatitis.

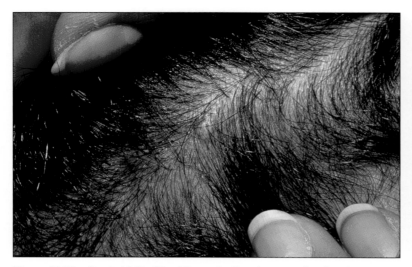

Figure 10.31 Crusted folliculitis of the scalp. Pustules occur first, but they are usually scratched away quickly.

Clinical

As documented earlier, the lesions may be a pustule, a crusted papule, or simply a mark from previous excoriation.

Differential diagnosis

The differential is usually between the following.

- Simple excoriation and excoriation due to neurosis.
- Infections, primary or secondary—some of the bacterial 'causes' discussed earlier might as easily be contaminants of primary excoriations.
- Rosacea of scalp—especially likely in those with rosacea of the face as well.

Treatment

Picking should be discouraged. A potent topical steroid may be prescribed if the itch is significant. The patient must be encouraged not to scratch. An oral antibiotic (e.g. tetracycline, 500–1000 mg/day) is often effective and should be tried. Other antibiotics (such as amoxicillin) may be used on the basis of bacteriology results, but culturing the causative organism (and knowing whether it is a cause, a relevant contributor, or simply a contaminant) may be difficult. Some have considered seborrheic dermatitis to be contributory, therefore this should be cleared with ketaconazole shampoo or a tar shampoo every day or every other day. A suggested regimen is ketoconazole shampoo daily combined with tetracycline 500 mg b.i.d. Finally, isotretinoin has been recommended for therapy-resistant cases.

Perioral dermatitis (periorificial dermatitis)
Etiology and pathogenesis

Perioral dermatitis is an inflammatory condition that occurs around the mouth. It has a strong female predilection, and most patients are young or early middle-aged adults. Its cause is unknown, although prolonged use of a potent topical steroid is one definite predisposing and aggravating factor. Some cases undoubtedly start out as seborrheic dermatitis, which the patient treats with a potent topical steroid. Still others seem to arise de novo. Histologically, perioral dermatitis resembles rosacea, and it is unfortunate that the 'dermatitis' part of its name has been used, as it encourages treatment with topical steroids as for eczema, rather than steroid avoidance (as discussed earlier for rosacea).

One recent study compared the follicular organisms in patients with perioral dermatitis versus those with seborrheic dermatitis. In all patients with perioral dermatitis and in two normal subjects, 20–70% of sample hairs were positive for fusiform bacteria. *Malassezia*-positive hairs were rarely seen in these cases. Seborrhoeic dermatitis showed the opposite results. Perioral dermatitis may tend to develop under fusiform bacteria-rich conditions, rather than *Malassezia*-rich conditions as in the case of seborrhoeic dermatitis.

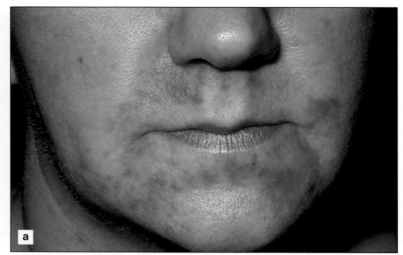

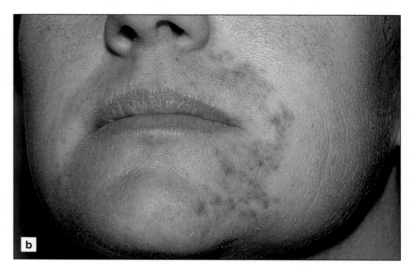

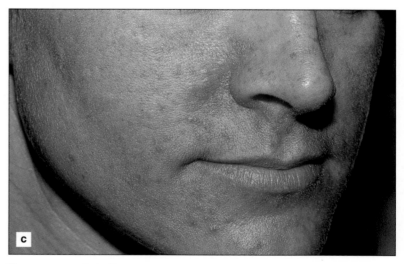

Figure 10.32 Periorificial dermatitis. (**a**) Periorificial papules are seen. Itching and burning are common in this disease of young women. (**b**) Tiny erythematous papules, pustules, and a small amount of scale occur about the mouth in periorificial dermatitis. (**c**) Confluent erythema of the nasolabial fold is a classic sign, and a narrow zone about the lips is typically spared. The use of a potent topical steroid may trigger or contribute to the eruption. Comedones are absent.

Clinical

Multiple red papules, and occasionally pustules, around the mouth in a woman aged 20–30 years, are characteristic (Fig. 10.32). Often there is a sensation of burning or itching. Confluent erythema of the nasolabial fold is characteristic. As a rule, perioral dermatitis is bright red and papular, whereas seborrheic dermatitis is red-brown and scaly. Rarely, children may be affected. Variants occur around the nostrils and eyes (Fig. 10.33),

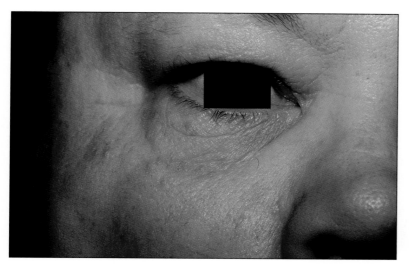

Figure 10.33 Periorificial dermatitis about the eyes. Usually, the outer, lower area is affected. This condition is a variant of perioral dermatitis. Oral tetracycline is effective.

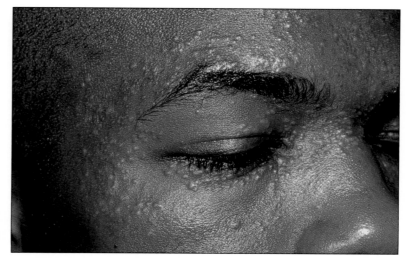

Figure 10.34 Papular periorificial dermatitis in an older teenaged boy. This condition is thought to represent a papular variant of periorificial dermatitis in the darker-skinned patient.

and are treated similarly. For this reason, the term periorificial dermatitis is preferred by some.

Differential diagnosis

The clinician should consider the following.

- True forms of dermatitis.
  Allergic contact dermatitis—for example, to a component of toothpaste (e.g. cinnamic aldehyde) or lipstick (e.g. propylene glycol or red dye no. 7).
  Seborrheic dermatitis—may cause redness in the same areas, but there is typically scale as opposed to papules.
  Lip lick dermatitis—usually in children, perioral but causes a confluent, sharply defined rash.
  Atopic dermatitis of face—usually more widely distributed, more likely to be in the differential of the periocular than of the perioral variant of perioral dermatitis.
- Other causes of inflammatory facial papules—including sarcoidosis, popular perioral dermatitis (Fig. 10.34), lupus miliaris disseminate faciei (discussed later), or granulomatous rosacea; these are all usually more widely distributed rather than being confined to the perioral region.
- Plane warts—browner color, and perioral distribution is common.

Treatment

Perioral dermatitis has many similarities to rosacea, one of them being its responsiveness to tetracycline. Indeed, tetracycline or oxytetracycline (250–500 mg twice daily) is the best current therapy. It will clear the condition within 4–8 weeks. Some patients may be able to stop the tetracycline then and remain clear, while others may need to keep it on hand for occasional flares, and finally some may need to take a low-maintenance dose (from one per day to one per week). Doxycycline or minocycline are effective oral alternatives. Topical therapy (e.g. metronidazole 0.75–1% or benzoyl peroxide) is significantly less effective, but may be preferred by some.

If any topical steroids are being used, they should be discontinued. Patients may be told that their skin has become 'addicted' to the steroid, so it may flare for several weeks on its discontinuation. If the patient had been on a high-potency topical steroid, one of low potency may be given for 10 days to blunt the flare.

For children aged 12 years or younger, tetracyclines must be avoided. Topical metronidazole gel or cream, 0.75–1%, twice daily is the preferred treatment. Alternatively, one can try topical clindamycin, topical erythromycin or benzoyl peroxide, or both.

Lupus miliaris disseminatus faciei ('acne agminata')
Etiology and pathogenesis

Lupus miliaris disseminatus faciei (LMDF) is a papular eruption of the face that histologically shows tuberculoid granulomas. No relation to

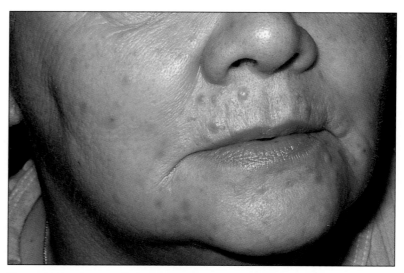

Figure 10.35 Lupus miliaris disseminatus faciei. Despite its name, no relationship to lupus is present. This condition is thought to represent a form of granulomatous rosacea.

tuberculosis has been found, however, and LMDF is thought to be a form of granulomatous rosacea.

Clinical

Multiple, symmetric, flesh-colored to brown papules are distributed on the forehead, temples, eyelids, chin, and cheeks (Fig. 10.35).

Differential diagnosis

This includes acne, plane warts, papular sarcoidosis, miliary forms of lymphocytoma cutis, and histiocytoses. The latter conditions do not normally enter the differential of other disorders discussed in this chapter, but do need to be considered in this condition due to its chronicity and therapeutic resistance.

Treatment

This condition is often difficult to treat. Tetracycline or erythromycin (1 g/day) can be tried. Isotretinoin and dapsone have been reported to be helpful. None of these options are consistently reliable.

FOLLICULAR OCCLUSION TRIAD

The follicular occlusion triad represents a group of diseases that commonly coexist, namely:

169

- hidradenitis suppurativa,
- acne conglobata, and
- dissecting cellulitis.

The first two will be discussed in turn here, and the latter in Ch. 28.

Hidradenitis suppurativa
Etiology and pathogenesis

This disease is often mistaken for a bacterial infection, as it presents with what looks like recurrent 'boils' in the groin and axilla. It actually seems to result from clogged pores, much like acne. Any bacterial infection is secondary. Although the disease affects areas inhabited by apocrine glands, it appears to be a process of poral occlusion of the pilosebaceous unit with secondary inflammation of the apocrine glands. Histology of early lesions shows an occluding spongiform infundibulofolliculitis. It is also more prevalent in hirsute women, and either more prevalent or more troublesome in obese individuals. Smoking and hidradenitis suppurativa may be linked.

Clinical

The patient presents with inflammatory nodules and sterile abscesses in the groin (Fig. 10.36a), the axilla (Fig. 10.36b,c), the inframammary area, or the perianal area. Later, with chronic inflammation, sinus tracts, fistulas, and hypertrophic scarring develop. Activity in the axilla is most common. One site only or all sites may be affected. Rarely, in severe cases, lesions may develop on the extremities (Fig. 10.36d). Women are more commonly affected, with onset from puberty to middle age.

This disease may occur with other diseases of the follicular occlusion triad (acne conglobata and perifolliculitis capitis abscedens et suffodiens). As noted earlier, initial lesions are sterile. Later, secondary infection occurs, most commonly with staphylococci, streptococci or *Escherichia coli*. Other organisms that may be found include *Bacillus proteus*, *Pseudomonas* spp., *Streptococcus milleri* and anaerobes (e.g. *Bacteroides* spp.). Squamous cell carcinoma may rarely be a complicating factor, most commonly in the anogenital region. Often there is a delay in diagnosis, and metastasis and death are common. Any chronic, non-healing areas should be biopsied.

Differential diagnosis

The usual diagnosis in patients with hidradenitis suppurativa, often over many years, is 'recurrent boils' or 'cysts'. The importance of applying the correct label, as outlined in the following *Treatment* section, is that the approach to antibiotic treatment, both in terms of duration and choice of agent, differ from the treatment of simple infected follicles that constitute a boil.

Treatment

Reduction of friction by weight loss and the avoidance of tight-fitting clothing should be recommended. Tight clothing and bras for women with inframammary disease should be avoided as much as possible. Any smokers should quit.

Once lesions have become chronic, and especially if drainage is present, antibiotics, both topical (e.g. clindamycin) and oral, are helpful. Typically recommended oral agents are tetracycline, oxytetracycline or erythro-

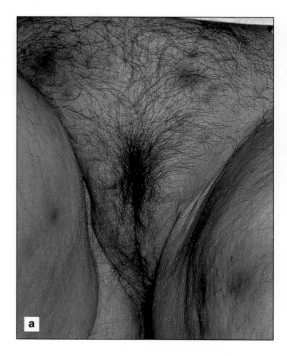

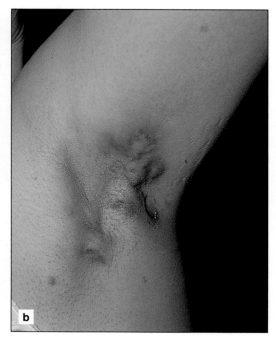

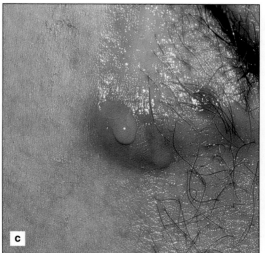

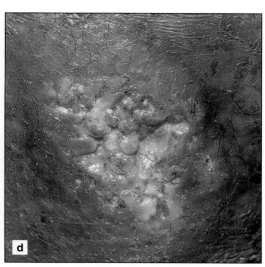

Figure 10.36 Hidradenitis suppurativa. (**a**) Multiple inflammatory lesions of the vulva. Intralesional triamcinolone is often helpful for early lesions that have not drained. (**b**) Hidradenitis suppurativa of the axilla. This is the classic appearance, with inflammatory nodules and scarred areas. This condition is commonly misdiagnosed as a bacterial infection. (**c**) Hidradenitis suppurativa of the axilla. A close-up view of the draining pus. When intact, the lesions represent sterile abscesses. Once open, they may become secondarily infected. (**d**) Acne conglobata of the leg. A rare variant seen in severe disease. Intralesional triamcinolone may be given for early lesions. More established lesions may be healed with curettage and desiccation, but scarring is significant.

mycin (all 1–2 g/day in divided doses), trimethoprim–sulfamethoxazole or minocycline (100 mg twice a day). Culture for both anaerobes and aerobes may direct therapy (e.g. clindamycin orally for *Bacteroides* spp.). Other than occasional short-term use if a specific infection has been identified, it is vital that antibiotic therapy is used for prolonged periods, sometimes indefinitely, as it is probably their antiinflammatory properties as well as antiinfection properties that are important; this is why the agents of choice and the stress on adequate duration of use are similar to those recommended for acne. Daily use of an antiseptic soap may be helpful.

Exteriorization of chronically draining sinuses, or incision and drainage of an acutely tender fluctuant lesion, may be necessary, but neither constitutes adequate long-term surgery, and such procedures may add to the scarring. Courses of isotretinoin and acitretin have met with some success, and it has been suggested that acitretin is more effective than isotretinoin; however, the requirement to abstain from pregnancy for 2 years after stopping the drug is a major disincentive. Prednisone or prednisolone 40–60 mg may be given for 1–2 weeks for acute, severe flares. Despite all these interventions, the patient often develops new lesions and is a frequent visitor to the doctor's office for intralesional injection of early lesions with triamcinolone (2.5–5.0 mg/mL).

Premenstrual exacerbation is common in female patients and, for them, antiandrogen therapy can be quite helpful. In the USA, spironolactone may be given. In the UK and elsewhere, cyproterone acetate (50–100 mg, days 5–15 of the menstrual cycle) with Dianette is recommended. Anecdotally, and probably logically, this approach seems to be more effective in those with a premenstrual flare than in those who do not report this, although it is worth trying in any female patient without contraindications to hormonal treatment.

For definitive cure, wide surgical excision with healing by secondary intention should be performed, preferably by someone with experience in this area. This intervention may seem excessive, but the patient may welcome this approach after suffering for years with many tender, draining lesions. Narrow excision of inflamed areas has a high recurrence rate.

Although surgery remains the treatment of choice for severe hidradenitis suppurativa, infusion of infliximab has proved beneficial in selected patients.

Acne conglobata
Etiology and pathogenesis
Acne conglobata is a specific variant of acne characterized by the large comedones with multiple openings. The face and back are typically affected, and the course is chronic. An inherited susceptibility to this disease is likely, and a positive family history is often elucidated. Some patients with acne conglobata may have chronic peripheral oligoarthritis, which is indistinguishable radiologically from the classic, seronegative spondyloarthropathies (e.g. Reiter syndrome and psoriatic arthritis).

Clinical
The patient is affected with multiple comedones, inflammatory nodules with pus, scarring, and sinus tracts of the back, buttocks, face and chest (Fig. 10.37a,b). The characteristic lesion of this disease is a large 'fistulated' or 'bridged' comedone with multiple openings (Fig. 10.37c). This disease most commonly affects young males, and may occur alone or in combination with other diseases of the follicular occlusion triad (hidradenitis suppurativa and perifolliculitis capitis abscedens et suffodiens). Acne conglobata and a generalized lichen spinulosa–like eruption have recently been reported in patients with HIV.

Treatment
Oral antibiotics, such as tetracycline (500 mg twice a day) or other antibiotics, as directed by culture, may be tried. A course of isotretinoin is recommended by many but is not as effective as in acne vulgaris. Incision and drainage of acutely inflamed or fluctuant areas may be necessary. Chronically draining sinus tracts may need to be externalized.

Dissecting cellulitis of the scalp
See Chapter 28.

MISCELLANEOUS

Acne keloidalis nuchae
Etiology and pathogenesis
Acne keloidalis nuchae (AKN) is a chronic, progressive, keloidal scarring process of the nape of the neck in dark-skinned men. Onset is usually after puberty, and most patients present in the second or third decade. Despite the name, acne vulgaris does not appear to be associated. Infection can contribute greatly to the inflammation and scarring but is thought to be a secondary event. The coexistence of pseudofolliculitis barbae has been noted in many patients, implying an underlying predisposition to both disorders, although there is no clinical or histologic evidence of recurving of superficial hairs into the skin in AKN.

Clinical
Clinically, the patient presents with a follicular pustular eruption on the nape of the neck (Fig. 10.38a–c). Comedones are not seen. Later, firm follicular papules develop. Large keloids with sinus tracts, pus, and scarring alopecia may form (Fig. 10.38d). Inside the keloidal nodules are crypts of trapped hairs. Often, these groups of hairs emanate from one opening (tufted hairs or polytrichia).

Pustules, crusting, and drainage are usually manifestations of a secondary infectious component, but at times, the inflammation is non-infectious and cultures are sterile. When a bacterium is found, it is usually *S. aureus*. The occipital posterior hairline is the overwhelmingly preferred location, but in one study, 3% had parietal lesions.

Differential diagnosis
Traumatic causes of keloid may need to be considered if there is a solitary confluent lesion without the semiconfluent follicular papules that are commonly seen. Simple ingrowing hairs (pili incurvatum) or follicular infection may be considered in early lesions. Generally, however, there is little diagnostic doubt.

Treatment
The hair should be allowed to grow long in the affected area. Some patients staunchly resist this advice, as they are fond of the shaved look. Mechanical irritation by a tight collar should be avoided if possible, although some patients find this difficult because of the professional attire required by their work. The patient should be encouraged not to pick or squeeze lesions. To control the infectious component, either topical antibiotics (e.g. clindamycin or erythromycin) or oral antibiotics (e.g. tetracycline or oxytetracycline 500 mg twice daily, doxycycline 100 mg twice daily, or minocycline 100 mg twice daily) should be given. If any pustules are present, bacterial culture should be done to assure that an appropriate antibiotic is being used. Hair oils should be avoided.

Sometimes the inflammatory or infectious component, or both, resist the above measures. It may be that previous scarring has created pockets of infection that are not fully exposed to therapy. Rotation of antibiotics, reculture, and even a course of isotretinoin may be needed. Once the inflammation has been controlled, as evidenced by the absence of pustules, crusting, or pain, the keloids may be treated by injection with triamcinolone (10–40 mg/mL every 4 weeks). If significant shrinkage of lesions is not obtained after three or four injections, a surgical approach

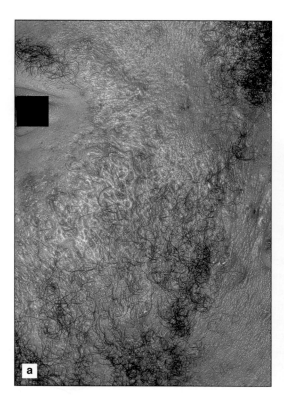

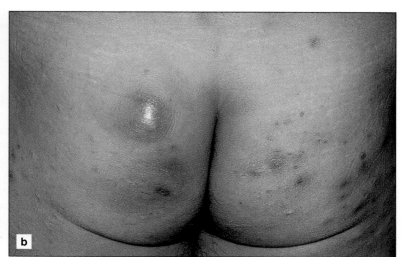

Figure 10.37 Acne conglobata. (**a**) Longstanding acne conglobata of the cheeks leads to this characteristic appearance of multiple pitted scars. (**b**) Large inflammatory nodules may occur. If fluctuant, they may be drained. If not, intralesional triamcinolone may be used. (**c**) The comedo with multiple openings (fistulated comedo) is characteristic of acne conglobata. It forms by multiple sebaceous follicles merging via an inflammatory process and represents a scar. The only effective treatment is unroofing of the cavity. (**d**) A wooden stick pushes through the lesion, illustrating the connection between the openings and the keratinous debris within.

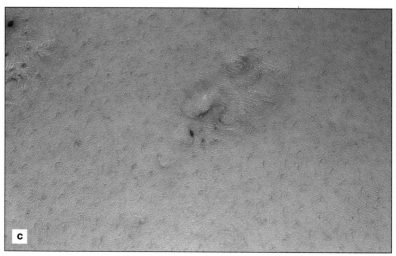

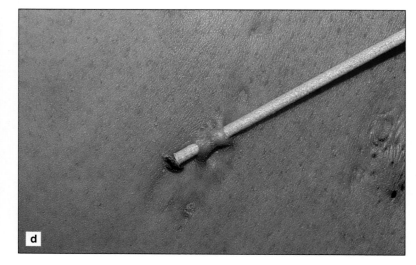

may be tried. Some success may be achieved with shaving lesions flat, followed by postoperative intralesional corticosteroid therapy (e.g. triamcinolone 20–40 mg/mL every 2-4 weeks) combined with a potent or very potent topical steroid (e.g. clobetasol propionate) and an oral antibiotic. However, this approach is not nearly as reliable as those that remove diseased tissue to the subfollicular level. In fact, larger keloids may result. Small, papular lesions may be removed via punch biopsy (e.g. using a hair transplant punch down to fibrous tissue). The CO_2 laser may be used effectively if removal is carried out to a subfollicular depth. Healing should be allowed to occur through secondary intention. In patients not responding to more conservative therapies and who don't mind permanent loss of hair, laser-assisted epilation should be considered.

Definitive therapy of severe disease with large keloids and sinus tracts is obtained by surgical debulking. The best results in one study were achieved with horizontal elliptic excision including the posterior hairline down to muscle fascia or the deep subcutaneous tissue (Fig. 10.39). The wound may be allowed to heal by secondary intention. Alternatively, primary closure after wide undermining for smaller lesions, and the use of a tissue expander inserted above the keloid for larger lesions, may be done. It cannot be overemphasized that any excision or destruction must be carried out to the subfollicular depth. If any portion of the hair follicle is left, recurrence is common and wound contraction is not as great.

The patient should be informed that the goal of such therapy is an asymptomatic but alopecic scar.

Chloracne
Etiology and pathogenesis
Chloracne results from poisoning by halogenated aromatic compounds. These agents are prevalent in agriculture.

Clinical
Multiple comedones are concentrated over the malar eminences and retroauricular areas in chloracne. In severe cases, comedones may appear on the trunk and extremities. Large cysts may develop. Central nervous system symptoms such as headache and fatigue are usually associated with acute exposure, whereas peripheral sensory neuropathy may represent a late complication. Xerosis, folliculitis, and cystic lesions may be seen.

Differential diagnosis
This diagnosis should be considered if there is acne predominantly around the ears, although ordinary acne may occasionally occur to a significant extent on the retroauricular skin. Comedones within the concha of the ear may occur in discoid lupus erythematosus, but other lesions in the acne spectrum are absent in this condition.

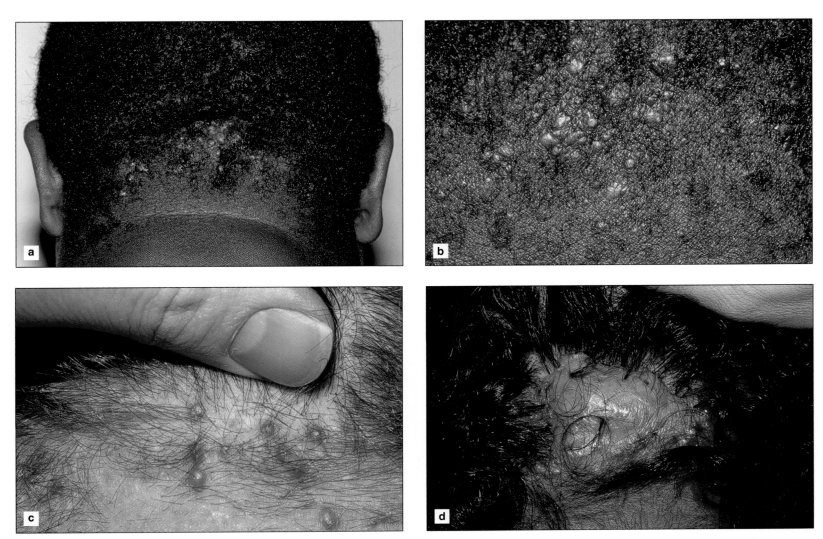

Figure 10.38 Acne keloidalis. (**a**) Acne keloidalis nuchae (AKN) in a dark-skinned man. The nape of the neck is the usual location for this papular condition of young, dark-skinned men. Short hair and trauma (e.g. football helmets and scratching) predispose. (**b**) Pustules and papules are characteristic of early lesions. (**c**) AKN in a pale-skinned man. White men may rarely be affected. (**d**) Large keloidal lesions may form. Tufts of hair may emanate from multiple openings. Surgical excision is needed here.

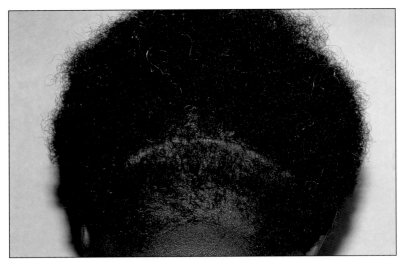

Figure 10.39 A horizontal elliptic excision of acne keloidalis nuchae down to the subfollicular depth may be done.

Treatment

Slow resolution often occurs after cessation of the exposure. All forms of conventional acne therapy may be tried. Light cautery after topical anesthesia (e.g. EMLA) has been used.

FURTHER READING

Bergfeld WF. The pathophysiology of acne vulgaris in children and adolescents, Part 1. Cutis 2004; 74: 292–7

Callender VD. Acne in ethnic skin: special considerations for therapy. Dermatol Ther 2004; 17: 184–95

Haider A, Shaw JC. Treatment of acne vulgaris. JAMA 2004; 292: 6726–35

Smolinski KN, Yan AC. Acne update: 2004. Curr Opin Pediatr 2004; 16: 4385–91

11 Cellular and Metabolic Cutaneous Infiltrates

INTRODUCTION

All inflammatory and papulosquamous disorders include a component of inflammatory infiltrate, but most can be allocated to either a more precise morphologic classification (such as eczema or psoriasis) or classified by cause (e.g. inflammation due to infection).

Some patterns of tissue reaction are usefully grouped together according to the major component of the cutaneous infiltrate. Examples include:

- neutrophilic infiltrates (see Ch. 14),
- eosinophilic tissue reactions,
- lymphocytic infiltrates,
- granulomatous infiltrates,
- mast cell infiltrates,
- histiocytic infiltrates,
- xanthomatous infiltrates,
- mucinous infiltrates,
- amyloid deposition, and
- other metabolic deposits (e.g. calcium deposition and gout).

These disorders are the subject of this chapter. However, as indicated, the neutrophilic infiltrates are discussed in Chapter 14, as their histologic pattern may overlap with that of the common neutrophilic vasculitides. There is also some degree of overlap with other chapters; for example, mucinosis associated with thyroid disease and calcinosis associated with renal failure are considered in Chapter 12 (*Cutaneous signs associated with disease of internal organ systems, and dermatoses of pregnancy*). A diverse group of benign lymphocytic infiltrates are considered here; cutaneous lymphoma and its precursors are discussed in Chapter 33.

EOSINOPHILIC TISSUE REACTIONS

A variety of eosinophilic syndromes may include skin involvement. Eosinophil proteins, such as eosinophil major basic protein and eosinophil cationic protein, are highly proinflammatory and contribute to, for example, blister formation in bullous pemphigoid and itch in atopic dermatitis. An eosinophilic component is common in the vasculitis associated with connective tissue diseases, and also in the cutaneous infiltrate in some drug eruptions, for example it may help to distinguish idiopathic from drug-induced lichen planus.

This section is restricted to dermatoses in which tissue eosinophilia is the predominant component (Table 11.1).

Eosinophilic cellulitis (Wells' syndrome)
Etiology and pathogenesis
The etiology is uncertain, although some cases are felt to follow insect bites.

Clinical features
Lesions usually affect distal limbs and resemble cellulitis (Fig. 11.1). They are urticated or infiltrated, and may be annular or bullous. They gradually enlarge then resolve over a few weeks, but may recur at intervals. Tissue eosinophilia is very marked, and there may be a granulomatous reaction around large clumps of eosinophilic material known as flame figures. Peripheral eosinophilia is less consistent.

Table 11.1   DERMATOSES IN WHICH TISSUE EOSINOPHILIA IS PROMINENT

Eosinophilia usually the predominant component	Eosinophilia often a significant feature
Eosinophilic cellulitis (Wells' syndrome) Hypereosinophilic syndrome Scleroderma-like syndromes: eosinophilic fasciitis, eosinophilia myalgia syndromes Eosinophilia with vasculitis: Churg–Strauss syndrome (Ch. 14) Angiolymphoid hyperplasia with eosinophilia and Kimura Eosinophilic folliculitis (see section on HIV, Ch. 12) Localized eosinophilic lesions: insect bites (early lesions), scabies (Ch. 27) Edematous syndromes: episodic angioedema with eosinophilia, solid facial edema with eosinophilia	Vasculitis associated with collagen vascular diseases (Ch. 13) Granuloma faciale (a vasculitis) Drug eruptions (Ch. 18) Immunobullous disorders: bullous pemphigoid (dermal and epidermal), pemphigus (epidermal: eosinophilic spongiosis) Eosinophilic granuloma (a variant of Langerhans cell histiocytosis; usually in bone, disease but can affect skin)

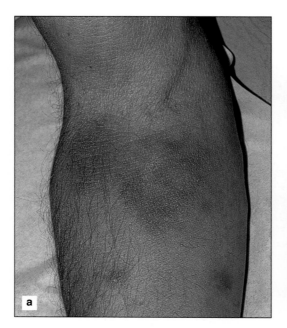

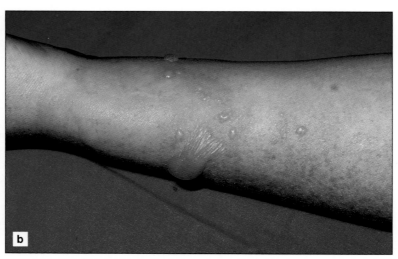

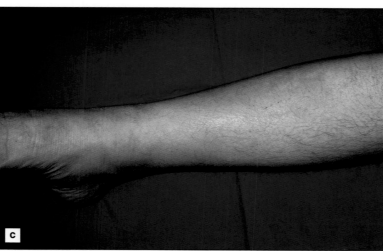

Figure 11.1   Eosinophilic cellulitis and fasciitis. Eosinophilic cellulitis (Wells' syndrome) causes inflammatory lesions that may resemble infective cellulitis (**a**) and may cause local blistering (**b**). Eosinophilic fasciitis (**c**) is a deeper and more diffuse process, typically affecting limbs; in this case, the skin appears tight and tethered on the lower legs.

Differential diagnosis

The main differential is infective erysipelas or cellulitis. Insect bite reactions, panniculitides, and sometimes blistering disorders may need to be considered.

Treatment

The condition usually responds well to systemic steroids (prednisolone, 40–60 mg daily, reduced over a few weeks).

Eosinophilic fasciitis (Schulman disease)

This condition presents as diffuse symmetric edema, usually most prominent on the lower leg (Fig. 11.2), with peau d'orange appearance of the skin and symptoms of myalgia and tightness. It is sometimes apparently provoked by exercise. Dermal and fatty inflammation is minimal, but there is a predominantly lymphocytic fasciitis with a disproportionate eosinophilic infiltrate. The disorder is often quite steroid-responsive, unlike acral scleroderma, but there may be progressive fibrotic changes and an association with morphea-like skin lesions. There is no specific serologic test, but typically there is an elevated eosinophil count, erythrocyte sedimentation rate, and gamma-globulin level.

Eosinophilia myalgia syndrome

This is a relatively recently described condition, which shares some features with eosinophilic fasciitis: myalgia is prominent, and some patients have sclerodermoid skin lesions. Muscle spasm and weakness occur, and neuropathies are also associated with this disorder. Outbreaks have been associated with various toxins (contaminated batches of L-tryptophan, and toxic oil syndrome).

Hypereosinophilic syndrome

Etiology and pathogenesis

This is a disorder of unknown etiology, which is probably reactive but in some cases behaves as an eosinophilic myeloproliferative state. It is defined by the presence of prolonged eosinophilia, for which other causes such as parasitic infections have been excluded, with internal organ involvement. Most patients are men, usually middle-aged or older.

Clinical features

Persistent eosinophilia for which no other cause can be found is required to consider the diagnosis. Skin lesions include an itchy eczematous or papular eruption (Fig. 11.2), which may become erythrodermic and occasionally develops blisters. Angioedema and dermographism may occur. Mucosal lesions affect the mouth and genitalia predominantly, and are usually erosive.

Internal organ involvement affects the heart (cardiomyopathy) and other organs (such as nephritis, pneumonitis, and thromboses).

Differential diagnosis

The skin lesions are non-specific and therefore have a wide differential diagnosis, including eczemas, cutaneous T-cell lymphomas, psoriasis and other papulosquamous diseases, and the differential diagnosis of erythroderma (Ch. 7).

Treatment

Symptomatic treatment with topical steroids and oral antihistamines are of value. Systemic therapy includes prednisolone, azathioprine, dapsone, hydroxyurea, cyclophosphamide, interferon-alpha, vincristine, etoposide, and others.

Angiolymphoid hyperplasia with eosinophilia, and Kimura disease

Etiology and pathogenesis

Angiolymphoid hyperplasia with eosinophilia (ALHE) is an uncommon condition in which there is a combination of angiomatous vessels, lymphoid infiltrate with germinal centers, and eosinophilic infiltrate. The cause is unknown, and interpretation is difficult due to overlapping features of rather different disorders reported from different geographic areas. Some parts of the spectrum behave as benign reactive processes, but others as invasive hemangiomatous processes.

Clinical features

Lesions usually occur on the head and neck in elderly patients, and are reddish-colored nodules or cobblestoned plaques (Fig. 11.3), which clinically may resemble malignant tumors such as basal cell carcinoma. Multiple lesions may occur. In Japanese patients, a more aggressive disorder known as Kimura disease occurs, usually in young men.

Differential diagnosis

This very much depends on the clinical pattern. Localized lesions may be confused with basal cell carcinoma or cysts. More extensive areas on the ear may resemble infective perichondritis, relapsing polychondritis, or pseudocyst of the auricle. Inflammatory conditions such as sarcoidosis or lymphocytomas may be considered, and even cutaneous lymphoma.

Treatment

Treatment is generally surgical excision or radiotherapy; local recurrences are common.

BENIGN LYMPHOCYTIC INFILTRATES

Several dermatologic disorders are characterized by a predominantly lymphocytic skin infiltrate. Some of these are generalized processes, such

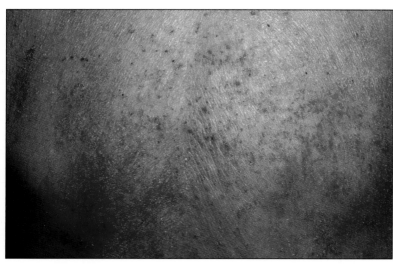

Figure 11.2 Hypereosinophilic syndrome. Non-specific eczematous lesions, as shown here, are a common presentation.

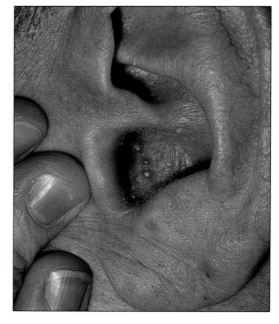

Figure 11.3 Angiolymphoid hyperplasia with eosinophilia.

as eczemas, psoriasis (which may have significant neutrophil infiltrate also), lichen planus, alopecia areata, and many others. These are not considered here, as they are not usually a source of problems for differential diagnosis. It is, however, worth being aware that many lesions alter over time; for example, most insect bites have a significant eosinophil component in their infiltrate, but more chronic bite reactions may be predominantly lymphocytic and thus enter the pathologic differential diagnosis of some of the disorders discussed in this section. The main disorders that are usually considered to fit into the category of cutaneous lymphocytic infiltrates are:

- Jessner lymphocytic infiltrate,
- lupus erythematosus (see Ch. 13),
- polymorphic light eruption (see Ch. 17),
- lymphocytoma cutis,
- erythema annulare centrifugum and other annular (figurate) erythemas,
- erythema multiforme, and
- cutaneous lymphoma (see Ch. 33).

Jessner lymphocytic infiltrate, Jessner–Kanof disease
Etiology and pathogenesis
This is a benign lymphocytic infiltrate that most closely resembles lupus erythematosus (LE), and is considered by some to be a variant of it. Like LE, provocation by sunlight is a common feature. There are, however, some immunopathologic differences from LE.

Clinical features
Lesions consist of (usually multiple) erythematous plaques and papules, which are most frequent on the head and upper trunk or upper arms (Figs 11.4 and 11.5). In some instances, they may be markedly annular. They do not have the follicular plugging or atrophic changes seen in discoid LE. Premenstrual exacerbation is prominent in some cases.

Differential diagnosis
This includes the following.
- Lupus erythematosis—the distinction from LE can be both clinically and histologically difficult, and may require passage of time for the situation to become clear (see also Fig. 13.5).
- Polymorphic light eruption—this is usually much more obviously related to sunlight, although some patients with Jessner lymphocytic infiltrate do report photoaggravation.
- Rosacea—occasionally very difficult to distinguish clinically, although pustules are usually present in rosacea (cutaneous demodicosis enters the same differential).
- Lymphocytoma cutis—usually a problem only if there are few and rather nodular lesions.
- Sweet syndrome—often affects the face, and usually more acute and pustular; histology will differentiate.
- Annular erythemas—may be histologically similar, but usually do not affect the face, which is a common site for Jessner lymphocytic infiltrate.

- Other annular eruptions that may affect the face—such as sarcoidosis, and annular lesions in Sjögren syndrome; these are usually distinguished by histology or by other clinical or laboratory features.
- Cutaneous lymphoma and potential lymphoma precursors such as follicular mucinosis.

Treatment
Response to treatment is unpredictable. Sunscreens may be useful prophylaxis. Topical steroids and systemic antimalarials or dapsone can be helpful.

Lymphocytoma cutis (Spiegler–Fendt sarcoid)
Etiology and pathogenesis
This term is used for a reactive B-lymphocyte proliferation that may resemble a cutaneous lymphoma (Ch. 33) but has benign behavior. Some cases may follow insect bites, scabies nodules, and inoculations or tattoos.

Clinical features
Lesions may be solitary or multiple, and consist of firm purplish-colored dermal nodules (Figs 11.6–11.8). The face and upper trunk are common sites; lesions may affect the nipple.

Differential diagnosis
The main differential diagnoses are insect bite reactions, cutaneous sarcoidosis, and cutaneous lymphoma. On the face in particular, skin tumors such as basal cell carcinoma are in the differential (as well as less

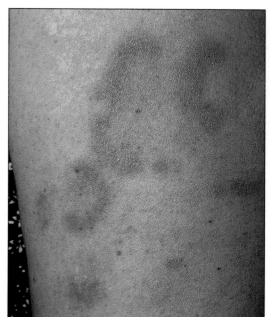

Figure 11.5 Multiple lesions of Jessner lymphocytic infiltrate. Annular and arciform lesions are common in this condition, and may be difficult to distinguish from the group of 'annular and figurate erythemas', such as erythema annulare centrifugum.

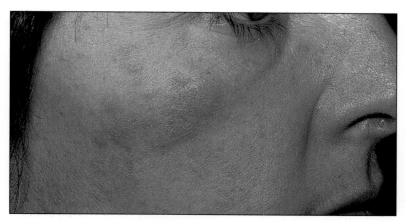

Figure 11.4 Jessner lymphocytic infiltrate. A slightly tumid plaque on the cheek, which clinically may resemble an early lesion of discoid lupus erythematosus (LE), but which lacks the epidermal component of LE.

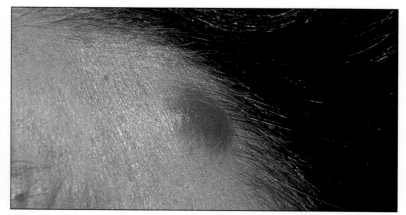

Figure 11.6 Solitary lesion of lymphocytoma cutis on the forehead. At this site, the differential diagnosis might include basal cell carcinoma, sarcoidosis, Jessner lymphocytic infiltrate, and LE.

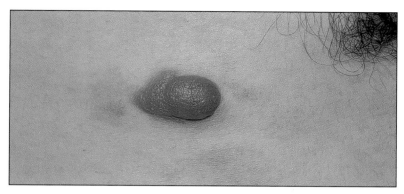

Figure 11.7 A lesion of lymphocytoma cutis on the trunk. This patient developed several similar lesions, and clinically was thought likely to have a B-cell lymphoma, although the histologic and immunocytochemical features strongly favored a benign process. Some such cases may be very difficult to characterize with confidence.

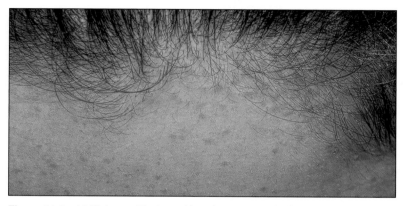

Figure 11.8 Multiple small lesions of lymphocytoma cutis, known as a miliary pattern.

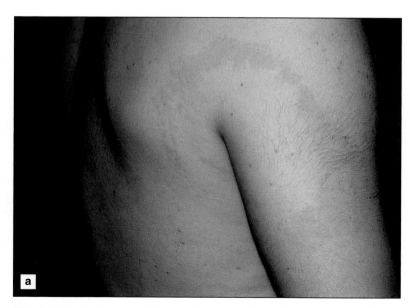

Figure 11.9 Erythema annulare centrifugum. Arciform lesions (**a**) and sometimes multiple concentric annular areas (**b**) are common. This type of eruption is commonly confused with fungal infections unless samples are taken for mycologic examination.

common but typically firm purple-colored tumors such as cylindromas; see Ch. 23). Cutaneous metastases occasionally need to be considered and, ←ED: Updated. especially in the case of more widespread lesions, the other lymphocytic infiltrates discussed in this section.

Treatment
Some lesions regress spontaneously. Intralesional steroid injection is a useful therapy.

Erythema annulare centrifugum and the 'annular (figurate) erythemas'
Etiology and pathogenesis
The annular or figurate erythemas are a poorly defined and poorly understood group of disorders, which are felt to be a reactive dermatosis. The most characteristic is erythema annulare centrifugum (EAC; Figs 11.9–11.11), which is usually idiopathic, although cases have occasionally

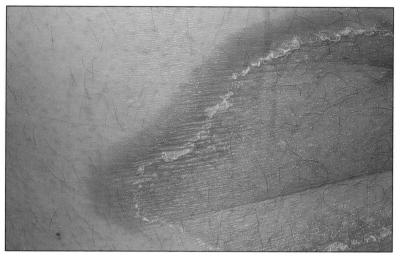

Figure 11.10 Some lesions of erythema annulare centrifugum have a well-developed scaling component. This is typically inward-pointing and proximal to the inflammatory advancing edge of the lesion, giving the impression that the scale is trailing the active lesion.

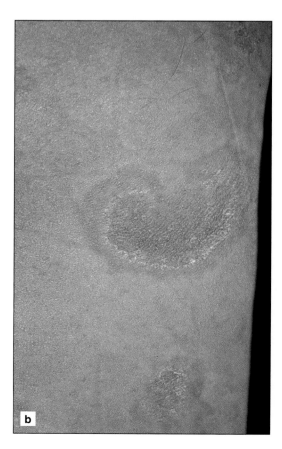

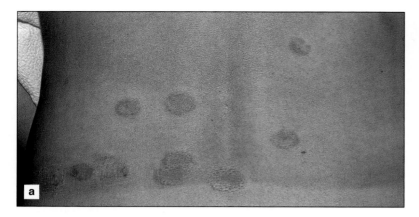

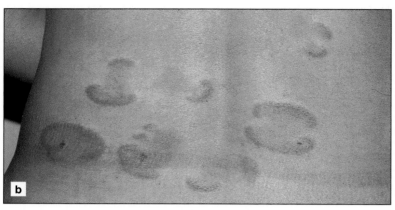

Figure 11.11 Erythema annulare centrifugum. (**a**,**b**) Evolution of lesions, which typically move and enlarge over a period of days or weeks. They do not have the day-to-day variability in size and site that occurs in urticaria, but enlarge more rapidly than most fungal infections.

Table 11.2	CAUSES OF ERYTHEMA MULTIFORME
Category	**Causes**
Infections	Herpes simplex, orf, mycoplasma, hepatitis, streptococcal, coxsackie, many others
Drugs	Sulfonamides, penicillins, anticonvulsants, non-steroidal antiinflammatory drugs, estrogens, gold, cytotoxics
Other	Lupus erythematosus, inflammatory bowel disease, neoplasia, idiopathic

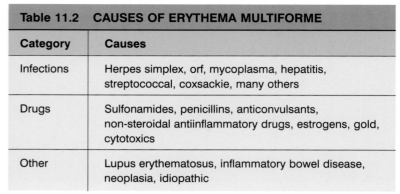

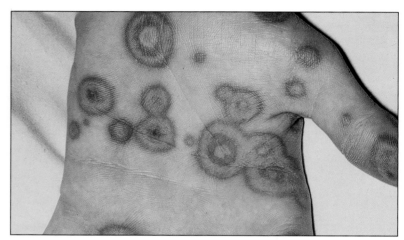

Figure 11.12 Target lesions of erythema multiforme. Although 'classical', neat concentric circles of this type are relatively uncommon; the trigger is almost always herpes simplex when the lesions are palmar and with this pattern.

been documented to be caused by a wide range of triggers, such as infections (dermatophytes and *Candida*), drugs (chloroquine and penicillin), foods (blue cheese), and tumors (Hodgkin disease). It may also rarely occur as a familial disorder.

Erythema chronicum migrans due to borreliosis (Ch. 24), erythema marginatum (a transient migratory rash in patients with rheumatic fever), and erythema gyratum repens due to gastrointestinal malignancy (Ch. 12) are usually included under the heading of annular erythemas. Neonatal LE is also often listed in this group but should probably be viewed as separate, as there is usually diagnostic serology (Ch. 13).

Clinical features

Erythema annulare centrifugum is an annular dermatosis with central clearing. It starts as a small macule with radial enlargement, occasionally over days but more typically over weeks or months. The edge is often urticated but with a trailing edge of scaling, and the central area clears, hence most lesions are erroneously diagnosed as ringworm dermatophyte infection (Ch. 26).

Differential diagnosis

This includes the following.
- Ringworm—a frequent and reasonable initial diagnosis, best excluded by mycology testing of skin scrapings.
- Lupus erythematosus—especially neonatal and subacute cutaneous forms, generally distinguished by positive serology for anti-SSA.
- Erythema multiforme—more acute, lesions expand but do not migrate or centrally clear, and different histology.
- Granuloma annulare—there is no scaling, the (slowly) expanding edge of the lesion has a cobblestoned feel, and often more acrally sited.
- Lyme borreliosis—usually larger, more rapidly spreading, and more inflammatory; serology may differentiate.
- Jessner lymphocytic infiltrate—usually on the face, and lesions do not tend to migrate.

- Sarcoidosis—annular lesions may occur but are more fixed; different histology.
- Cutaneous lymphoma—annular lesions may occur but are more fixed; histology will differentiate.
- Sjögren syndrome—annular lesions are usually on the face and are uncommon in non-Japanese.

Treatment

Most cases gradually subside, and response to treatment is variable. Topical steroids and oral antimalarials are used if required.

Erythema multiforme
Etiology and pathogenesis

Erythema multiforme (EM) is an abused term that is applied by non-dermatologists to many rashes with mixed morphology. It is best defined by the clinicopathologic correlation of appropriate skin lesions (described here) and consistent histologic features, which include an upper dermal lymphocytic infiltrate with (usually) exocytosis into the epidermis, upper dermal edema and erythrocyte extravasation, and epidermal cell death.

Causes of EM include drugs, infections, and others (Table 11.2). About a third of cases are clearly linked to herpes simplex infection, and the 30% of cases that are idiopathic probably include a large proportion in which herpes simplex is the trigger but has been clinically unapparent. The disease spectrum includes mucosal lesions (Stevens–Johnson syndrome), and features overlap with those of toxic epidermal necrolysis (Ch. 18).

Erythema multiforme is more common than the other conditions discussed in this section.

Clinical features

Onset is relatively acute and may be preceded or accompanied by fever, malaise, and arthralgia. The characteristic clinical lesion of EM is the target lesion (Figs 11.12–11.16), which is usually most typical on the palms, especially in EM secondary to herpes simplex infection. Lesions may

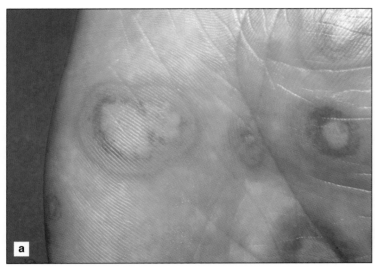

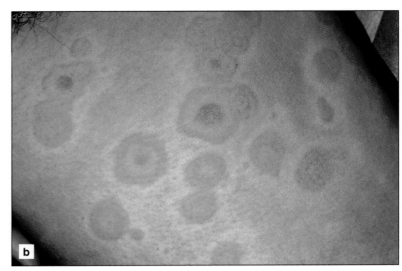

Figure 11.13 Target lesions of erythema multiforme. In (**a**) the cause was herpes simplex; in (**b**), with identical morphology, the lesions were drug-induced. The patient in (**a**) also had mucosal features of Stevens–Johnson syndrome.

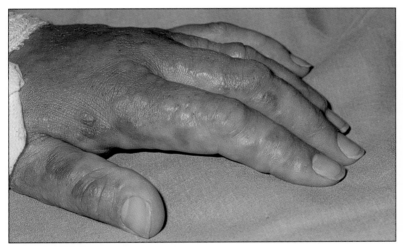

Figure 11.14 Nodular lesions of erythema multiforme (EM). This pattern, which usually affects the dorsal aspect of hands and forearms, is the typical morphology of EM related to orf infection. There is often associated swelling of the hands and general malaise.

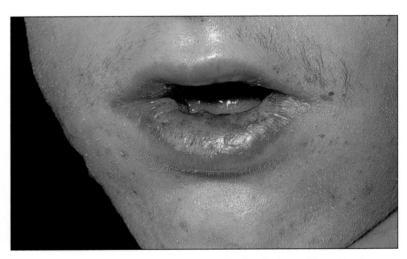

Figure 11.15 Stevens–Johnson syndrome affecting the lips, with confluent erosion. Occasionally, it can be difficult to distinguish between lip lesions of herpes simplex and those of Stevens–Johnson syndrome, but this may be important therapeutically.

Figure 11.16 (**a**) Ocular involvement in Stevens–Johnson syndrome. Note that there is a lesion of erythema multiforme (EM) on the nose in (**b**). Conjunctivitis can occur in cases of EM without other mucous membrane involvement.

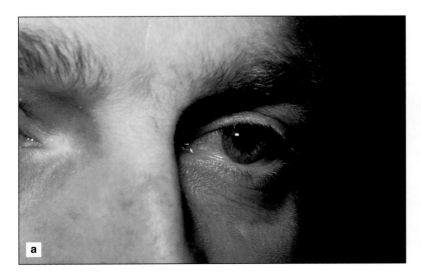

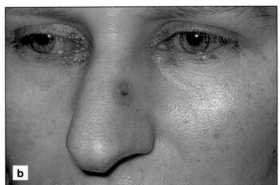

expand initially, classically producing concentric rings of pallor, erythema, or duskiness, and there may be central necrosis or blistering. They do not migrate or centrally clear in the manner seen in EAC. Often the eruption consists of papules and plaques with grayish central epidermal necrosis, rather than the multiple concentric circles of 'classic' target lesions. Crops of lesions may occur over a week or two.

Mucous membranes may be affected, including erosions of the lips (Fig. 11.15), oral vesicles, conjunctivitis (Fig. 11.16), and genital lesions. These may also occur in isolation, particularly in EM due to mycoplasma infection. In severe cases, esophageal or bronchial mucosae may be involved.

Differential diagnosis

Erythema multiforme is usually readily differentiated from the other lymphocytic infiltrates by its rapid onset, multiplicity and predominantly acral distribution of lesions, morphologic appearance, strong association with herpes simplex, and tendency to spontaneous resolution.

Vasculitis does, however, need to be considered in the differential in some patients, especially if lesions are purpuric.

It may be difficult clinically to decide whether oral lesions are those of EM or those of a causative herpes simplex infection.

Some patients get frequent premenstrual episodes of EM (probably caused by herpes simplex reactivation in most cases); this may be difficult to distinguish from progesterone dermatitis (Ch. 12).

Treatment

The skin lesions cause few symptoms and may need no treatment. A topical steroid is generally sufficient for symptomatic areas. Systemic steroids are useful if there is significant malaise or swelling of the hands (as often occurs in EM due to orf virus), but should be used with caution in patients with underlying infective causes of EM. Mouth and eye care is important where these are involved, and oral steroids are usually administered in such cases.

PRACTICE POINTS

- Annular erythemas are not common but should be considered if annular scaling lesions migrate and have negative mycology results or do not respond to antifungal agents.
- Mixed clinical morphology of a rash does not mean it is erythema multiforme (EM); this is a specific clinicopathologic diagnosis.
- Recurrent EM is almost always due to herpes simplex infection, even though this may be clinically occult.
- In patients with predominantly mucosal EM, mycoplasma infection may be the trigger.

GRANULOMATOUS REACTIONS

The granulomatous reaction

Granulomatous disorders (Table 11.3) are a difficult diagnostic and therapeutic problem. Many granulomatous lesions are clinically non-specific and pathologically similar. Additionally, some disorders that may cause granulomas in some patients more commonly occur in a non-granulomatous form (e.g. rosacea). A useful clinical clue to a granulomatous process is the brownish 'apple jelly' color that can be seen when blood is compressed out of the skin by diascopy.

Granulomas are formed due to chronic antigen exposure, either due to slow release of antigen or slow degradation of poorly soluble antigens. The reaction is characterized by the presence of tissue macrophages (histiocytes) and multinucleated giant cells, which usually group together as intradermal nodules. Depending on the causative process, there may be associated vasculitis (e.g. Wegener granulomatosis), suppuration (e.g. deep fungal infections), necrosis (e.g. tuberculosis), collagen damage known as necrobiosis (e.g. granuloma annulare), or none of these (e.g. sarcoidosis,

---

Table 11.3   CAUSES OF GRANULOMATOUS TISSUE REACTIONS

Process	Comments
Sarcoidosis	See text, this chapter
Granuloma annulare	See text, this chapter and Chapter 12
Necrobiosis lipoidica	See Chapter 12
Annular elastolytic giant cell granuloma (Miescher granuloma)	See text, this chapter
Granulomas associated with rheumatologic and collagen vascular disease	Rheumatoid nodules, multicentric reticulohistiocytosis, interstitial granulomatous dermatitis (see Ch. 13)
Granulomas associated with vasculitis	Wegener granulomatosis, Churg–Strauss disease, granuloma faciale (see Ch. 14)
Granulomas due to infections	Mycobacterial infection (tuberculosis, atypical mycobacteria such as fish tank granuloma, leprosy), deep fungal infections (includes candidal granuloma, Majocchi granuloma, sporotrichosis, blastomycosis, coccidiodomycosis, others), secondary syphilis, granuloma inguinale (donovanosis), leishmaniasis, histoplasmosis, protothecosis
Crohn disease, orofacial granulomatosis	See Chapter 12
Granulomas due to foreign material or keratin	Foreign body granuloma, ruptured epidermoid cyst or follicular rupture (see text, this chapter)
Neoplastic and histiocytoses	Granulomatous slack skin (mycosis fungoides variant), lymphomatoid granulomatosis, necrobiotic xanthogranuloma, eosinophilic granuloma
Miscellaneous	Granulomatous rosacea, tuberculides (see text, this chapter), chronic granulomatous disease, focal Miescher granulomas in erythema nodosum, granuloma gluteale infantum

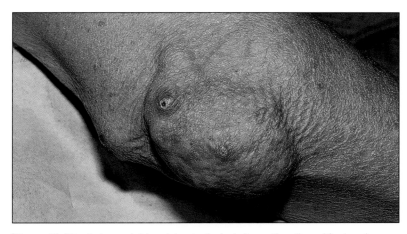

Figure 11.17 A rheumatoid nodule at a typical site on the elbow. Most such lesions occur in patients with well-documented rheumatoid disease, but smaller nodules or those at unusual sites may cause diagnostic problems. Multiple tiny rheumatoid nodules sometimes occur in association with vasculitis.

Crohn disease, and foreign body granuloma). Some disorders may have variable histologic features; for example, some foreign body reactions are necrobiotic, vasculitis has been reported in granulomas of Crohn disease, and so on.

Some of these granulomas are illustrated without further discussion, for example rheumatoid nodules (Fig. 11.17), which rarely present to dermatologists unless they occur at unusual sites. Granulomatous vasculitis is discussed in Chapter 14, and Crohn disease and necrobiosis lipoidica are described in Chapter 12; otherwise the more important medical causes of cutaneous granulomas are discussed further here.

Note that the term *granuloma* is also applied to some lesions that do not have typical granulomatous histology, such as pyogenic granuloma (a benign vascular proliferation) and lethal midline granuloma (now termed nasal NK/T-cell lymphoma), or in which a granulomatous component is either minor or inconsistent, such as granuloma fissuratum (due to friction on the ear from spectacles) or granuloma faciale (a low-grade chronic vasculitis). These are not discussed here.

Granuloma annulare
Etiology and pathogenesis
Granuloma annulare (GA) is a relatively common disorder that has several morphologic variants. Some of these have an association with diabetes mellitus and are discussed in Chapter 12, but this is not now felt to apply to ordinary lesions of GA. Trauma may be involved in the pathogenesis, as lesions are often over bony prominences. Rarely, GA is recurrent on a seasonal basis (spring or summer). Pathologically, GA lesions occur in the mid-dermis and demonstrate necrobiosis (literally, death and life) of collagen, with mucin deposits between the damaged collagen and a surrounding infiltrate of lymphocytes and histiocytes.

Clinical
Lesions are most common over bony prominences such as knuckles, elbows, and the dorsum of fingers. The initial lesion is a firm, pink, yellowish, or skin-colored plaque, which gradually expands radially, and has the appearance of coalesced papules producing a cobblestoned morphology (Figs 11.18–11.24). About 50% of GA lesions resolve within 2 years, gradually flattening with some residual purplish staining. In the generalized form, the papules are usually much smaller, but more extensive sheets of superficial GA occur.

The perforating variety is discussed in Chapter 12. Deep GA presents as a non-specific firm subcutaneous nodule or plaque.

Differential diagnosis
This varies according to the site and pattern.
- Lesions on fingers or knuckles may be confused with warts, knuckle pads or callosities, or ringworm infection.
- Lesions on the trunk or limbs are usually annular and are most commonly confused with ringworm, although they can be differentiated by the lack of scaling in GA. Other granulomatous lesions with annular morphology discussed in this section, such as annular sarcoidosis, may be difficult to differentiate, especially in small early lesions. Other eruptions with annular morphology, such as some lichen planus, or erythema chronicum migrans, may also need to be considered.
- Perforating GA causes non-specific crusted lesions with a wide differential diagnosis; other perforating disorders are an important consideration and are discussed later in this chapter.
- Diffuse papular GA should be distinguishable from disorders such as diffuse mucinoses or histiocytoses on pathologic grounds, but may be difficult to distinguish with certainty from micropapular sarcoidosis.

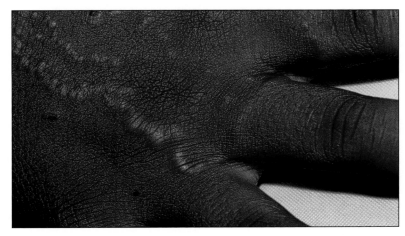

Figure 11.19 Granuloma annulare on the dorsum of the hand, also a common site (in this case in a child). The morphology of the border of the lesion is characteristic.

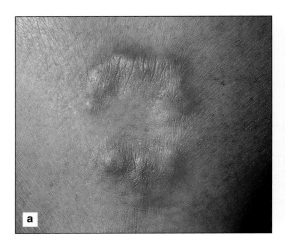

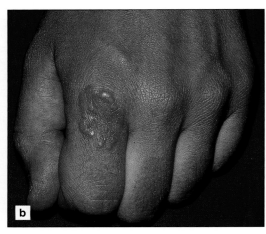

Figure 11.18 Typical annular lesions of granuloma annulare, the appearance being that of multiple semiconfluent papules forming the annular border. Both lesions were also typical in being situated near bony prominences, (**a**) over the ulna at the elbow and (**b**) over the knuckles.

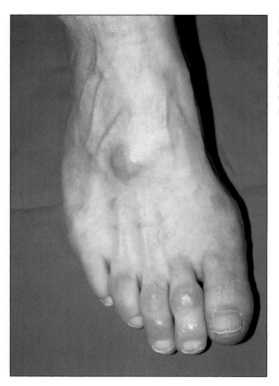

Figure 11.20
Granuloma annulare on the foot, again being situated over a bony prominence but showing a more nodular (and less easily diagnosed) morphology.

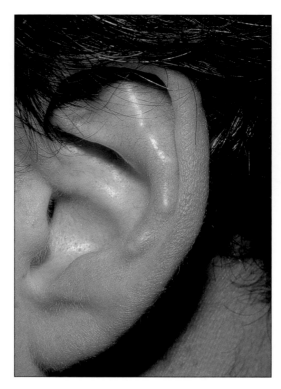

Figure 11.23 A characteristic, but often unrecognized, site for granuloma annulare is the antihelix of the ear, as shown here. This variant may occur in isolation, or there may be lesions at other sites. There are usually multiple lesions, and both ears are usually affected (although not necessarily to the same extent).

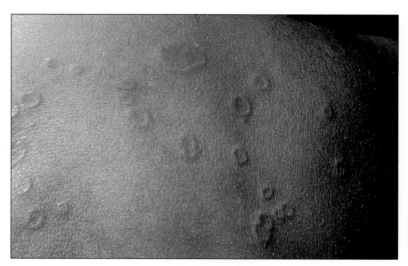

Figure 11.21 Multiple small lesions of granuloma annulare is an uncommon pattern.

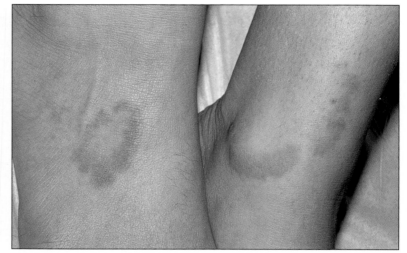

Figure 11.24 Resolving lesions of granuloma annulare are often brown or violaceous, and have a flatter border. These seem to cause undue diagnostic confusion, and are often erroneously treated as ringworm infection.

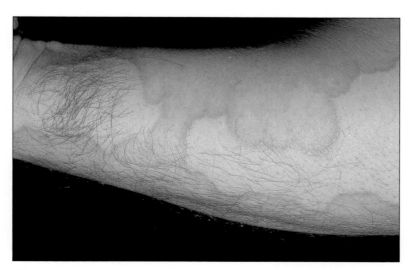

Figure 11.22 A small proportion of patients with granuloma annulare describe photoaggravation, as in this case. The lesions are a more extensive sheet of granulomatous appearance.

- The deep form of GA is clinically similar to deep morphea, subcutaneous sarcoidosis, or interstitial granulomatous dermatitis.

Treatment
Often, no treatment is required. During the early expanding phase, there may be erythema and itch, in which case topical corticosteroids can be useful. Photochemotherapy (PUVA) can be used, usually for those with more extensive lesions.

Annular elastolytic giant cell granuloma
Annular elastolytic giant cell granuloma (AEGCG) may be a granulomatous reaction to damaged elastic fibers (Fig. 11.25). It occurs in sun-damaged skin and, using appropriate histologic stains, fragments of elastic tissue can be seen within macrophages and giant cells. Like those of GA, lesions are typically annular, but often more serpiginous and without the cobblestoned character of GA. The two disorders are very similar histologically.

Sarcoidosis

Etiology and pathogenesis

The etiology is uncertain. Some evidence suggests an infective cause, combined with an abnormal degree of humoral and cell-mediated immune response. Polyclonal hypergammaglobulinemia is common in chronic sarcoidosis, and there is an association with a variety of autoimmune disorders and with Sjögren syndrome.

Clinical features and variants

Sarcoid skin lesions are extremely varied (Figs 11.26–11.37). They include erythematous or purplish plaques and nodules, papules (which may be widespread and very numerous in micropapular sarcoid), hypopigmented patches, atrophic lesions, and scar sarcoid. Lesions may mimic psoriasis or morphea, or may be subcutaneous. Atrophic, alopecic, pustular, and ulcerative lesions may occur. Massive granulomatous nodules are uncommon but may resemble lymphedema if a limb is affected. Nails may be affected (usually with underlying osteolysis), as may mucous membranes. Diffuse erythrodermic or ichthyotic presentation causes particular diagnostic difficulty.

Additionally, non-specific lesions such as erythema nodosum (Ch. 22) occur in acute sarcoidosis, usually with hilar lymphadenopathy.

Other organs that are affected are listed in Table 11.4.

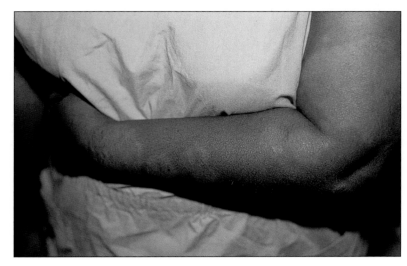

Figure 11.27 Hypopigmented sarcoid is most frequent in black skin, although this may reflect the difficulty of identifying such lesions in white skin.

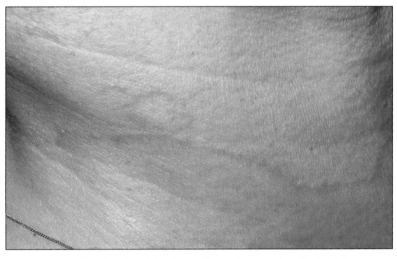

Figure 11.25 Annular elastolytic giant cell granuloma. This entity is felt by some authors to be a variant of granuloma annulare (both have some elastic tissue damage and elastin within tissue macrophages), and by others to be a type of solar damage (lesions occur in sun-exposed skin and resemble O'Brien actinic granuloma). Annular and arciform lesions are typical.

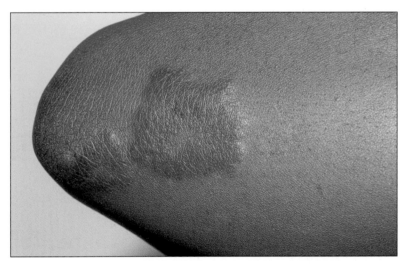

Figure 11.28 An individual plaque of sarcoidosis. Patients with chronic cutaneous sarcoid often also show involvement of the lungs and bones.

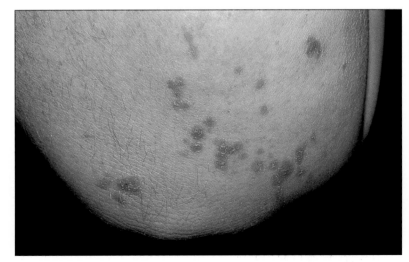

Figure 11.26 Sarcoidosis, showing multiple, small, papular lesions. The rather purple color is quite frequent, although a range of browns and flesh tones may occur.

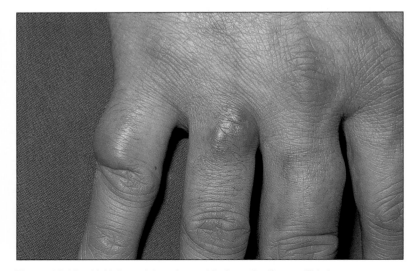

Figure 11.29 Multiple nodules of sarcoidosis on the fingers. This is an uncommon pattern resembling multicentric reticulohistiocytosis, which may also be similar histologically.

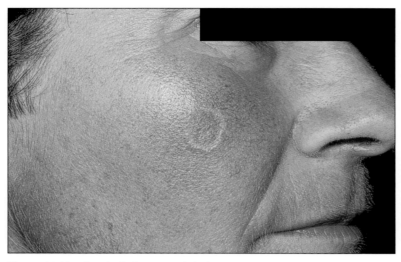

Figure 11.30 Annular lesions are relatively common in sarcoidosis, in this case affecting the cheek. This lesion was very atrophic centrally, and responded poorly to a variety of topical and systemic therapies.

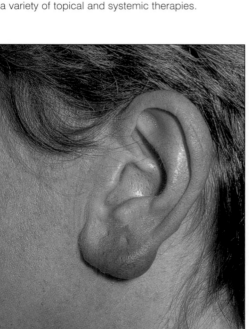

Figure 11.31 Sarcoidosis affecting the earlobe, with a prominent purple color. Lymphomas can produce very similar lesions at this site.

Figure 11.33 Micropapular sarcoidosis is a relatively uncommon variant. It may be difficult to distinguish, both clinically and histologically, from the diffuse form of granuloma annulare.

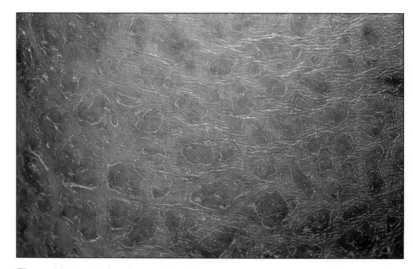

Figure 11.34 Ichthyotic sarcoidosis is another uncommon variant that may cause diagnostic difficulty. The combination of acquired ichthyosis and systemic symptoms is also suggestive of lymphoma or other internal malignancy.

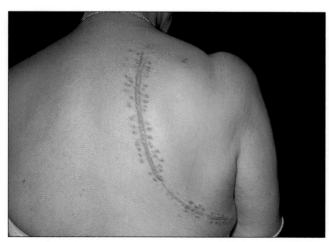

Figure 11.32 Scar sarcoid is a common phenomenon. It differs from a Koebner reaction in that old scars are commonly affected as a gradual process. In this case, a large proportion of an old thoracotomy scar was affected.

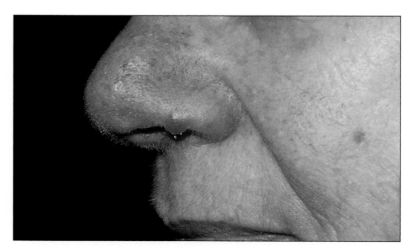

Figure 11.35 Lupus pernio of the nose. This is a chronic variant of sarcoidosis that typically affects the nose and central face, is usually very purple, and may be destructive locally. This type of lesion may also become verrucous, but can respond well to low-dose methotrexate.

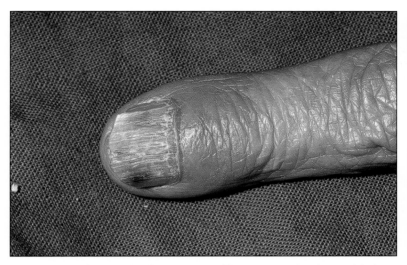

Figure 11.36 Sarcoidosis affecting the nail. This occurs in chronic sarcoidosis, and is a marker of bony involvement of the underlying terminal phalanx (see Fig. 11.37).

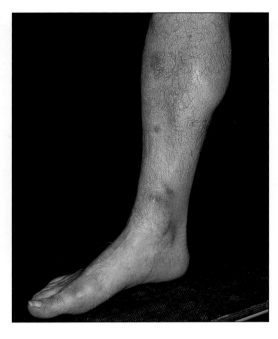

Figure 11.38 Erythema induratum (Bazin disease). This disorder is poorly defined, and is best considered as a type of nodular vasculitis in which the proof of a tuberculid process is unconvincing. Most cases occur in relatively stout female lower legs as a recurrent problem in winter or spring, and probably have a vascular etiology.

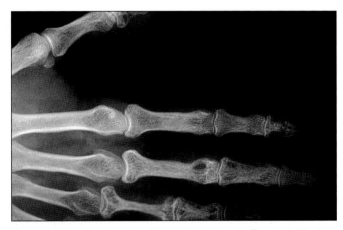

Figure 11.37 Radiograph of the patient shown in Figure 11.36, demonstrating bone cysts in the terminal phalanges.

Lupus pernio

This is a form of chronic cutaneous sarcoidosis that affects predominantly the central face and ears (Fig. 11.35). It is typically purple, but the site on the face may lead to it being confused with LE. It is commonly associated with other features of chronic sarcoidosis, such as restrictive pulmonary disease or bone cysts.

Differential diagnosis

This varies hugely depending on the clinical pattern (Table 11.5).

Treatment

Treatment options for sarcoidosis include strong topical or intralesional corticosteroids, systemic steroids, antimalarials, and methotrexate, depending on the pattern and severity of both the skin disease and other organ involvement. In lupus pernio, physical modalities such as laser, electrocautery, or surgery may be useful. Methotrexate seems to be of particular benefit in verrucous lesions. Allopurinol appears to be beneficial, for uncertain reasons. PUVA may have a role, as does infliximab for severe disease.

Erythema induratum and tuberculides
Etiology and pathogenesis

Direct infection with *Mycobacterium tuberculosis* (scrofuloderma and lupus vulgaris) and with atypical mycobacteria (e.g. fish tank granuloma) are discussed in Chapter 24.

The precise pathogenesis of tuberculides is more controversial. Some are felt to represent delayed hypersensitivity to tuberculosis, whereas some evidence favors local reaction to disseminated mycobacteria, or parts of them. Polymerase chain reaction technology has demonstrated mycobacterial DNA sequences in some tuberculide lesions, but also in some cases of sarcoidosis. Lichen scrofulosum and papulonecrotic tuberculid are most convincingly associated with tuberculosis.

Clinical features

Erythema induratum (Bazin disease, Fig. 11.38) is a nodular granulomatous panniculitis that occurs on the lower leg. Clinically, it may be difficult to differentiate from nodular vasculitis, which may occur due to polyarteritis or following phlebitis or chronic perniosis.

Lupus miliaris disseminatus faciei (Fig. 11.39) is a facial eruption consisting of numerous small papules. Some authorities feel that it is probably a form of granulomatous acne, but it is very refractory to treatment that would normally be used for acne.

Tuberculin skin tests are positive in many of this group of disorders, but the variable strength of reaction is a reason to suppose that many cases may

Table 11.4 ORGAN SYSTEMS THAT MAY BE INVOLVED IN SARCOIDOSIS	
Organ system	**Comments**
Skin	See text, this chapter
Eyes	Especially anterior uveitis
Chest	Hilar lymphadenopathy in acute-onset sarcoidosis, pulmonary fibrosis in chronic disease
Bones	Arthralgia in acute sarcoidosis, cysts (mainly digital)
Visceral organs	Splenomegaly, hepatomegaly
Heart	Commonly asymptomatic, but conduction defects and heart failure occur
Neurologic	Especially facial palsy (may occur with uveitis and parotid enlargement)
Lymph nodes	Especially hilar, peripheral in about 25%

Table 11.5   DIFFERENTIAL DIAGNOSIS OF SOME PATTERNS OF CUTANEOUS SARCOIDOSIS

Pattern of cutaneous sarcoidosis	Differential diagnosis or comments
Chronic plaques (discoid or annular)	Psoriasis, discoid eczema, lichen simplex, morphea, lymphocytoma cutis, cutaneous lymphomas, foreign body and chronic insect bite reactions, atypical mycobacterial infection; causes of annular lesions (see Table 1.2); other granulomatous disorders, as discussed in this section
Micropapular	Micropapular variants of granuloma annulare, lichen planus; other eruptions with scattered small lesions, for example folliculitis, scabies, some histiocytoses
Lupus pernio	Rosacea, lupus erythematosus
Scalp	Causes of scarring alopecia (usually with inflammation); see Chapter 28
Hypopigmented	Vitiligo, pityriasis versicolor, hypopigmented mycosis fungoides
Scar	Usually late event in patients with known sarcoidosis (therefore not consistent with simple hypertrophic or keloid scar); foreign body granuloma is the main differential (either traumatic with foreign material in the wound, or application of talc to a scar); rarely, nodular scleroderma or cutaneous metastasis to a scar may appear similar
Nail	Usually only in patients with known chronic sarcoidosis; may need to exclude fungal disease or subungual tumor if single nail affected; may mimic many forms of nail dystrophy, or finger clubbing
Ichthyotic	Other causes of acquired ichthyosis: hypothyroidism, lymphoma, late-onset atopy, malnutrition
Subcutaneous (Darier–Roussy disease)	Subcutaneous variants of granuloma annulare, morphea; interstitial granulomatous dermatitis; various causes of panniculitis (Ch. 22), cutaneous metastases, rare lymphoma variants
Erythema nodosum	A reaction to sarcoidosis, not actually cutaneous involvement by sarcoidal granulomas; may occur with fever, hilar lymphadenopathy, and arthritis (Löfgren syndrome); see also Chapter 14

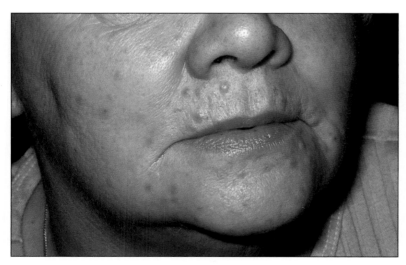

Figure 11.39 Lupus miliaris disseminatus faciei: multiple papular lesions on the face are typical (see also Ch. 10).

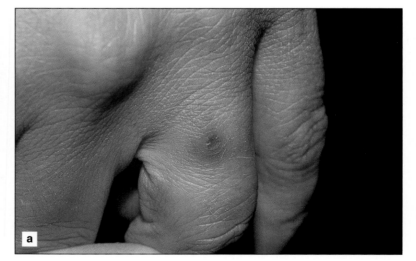

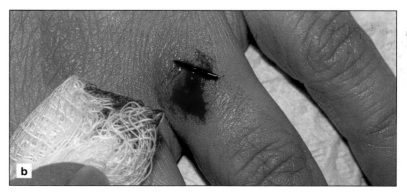

Figure 11.40 Foreign body granuloma. (**a**) A nodule at the site of injury from a thorn (from a yucca bush) over 4 years previously. (**b**) The thorn that caused the damage, after removal from the skin.

not be related to tuberculosis. In the true tuberculides, a strong positive skin test reaction is usual.

Differential diagnosis

This varies according to the tuberculide being considered.

Erythema induratum may resemble ordinary chilblains, venous stasis disease, other types of vasculitis, or panniculitis.

Lupus miliaris disseminatus faciei is usually diagnosed clinically as acne or rosacea, less commonly as demodecosis. It may resemble the miliary form of lymphocytoma cutis, which also tends to affect the face.

Treatment

Cases in which there is evidence to support a true tuberculid should be treated with full antituberculous therapy. Some of the acne- or rosacea-like tuberculides may respond to tetracyclines or to isotretinoin. Nodular vasculitis may respond to steroids, to dapsone, or to vasodilating drugs if there is a perniotic component.

Foreign body reaction

Etiology and pathogenesis

Foreign body granulomas (FBGs) may occur due to numerous agents (Figs 11.40–11.43), and the granulomas may be sarcoidal or necrobiotic in type. Examples include the following.

- Keratin from ruptured epidermoid cysts, folliculitis with disruption of hair shafts, and ingrowing hairs.
- Plant materials—thorns, cactus spines, wood splinters, etc.
- Animal derived—arthropod bites (e.g. tick mouth parts), sea urchin spines, and jellyfish stings.
- Metabolic causes—calcinosis and gout (discussed later in this chapter).
- Iatrogenic and other inoculations—suture material, talc, aluminum in vaccines, foreign collagen or silicone, paraffin (sclerosing lipogranuloma), and tattoo pigments.
- Other essentially inert materials—silica, zirconium, and beryllium.

Clinical features

Most foreign body reactions present either as a non-specific inflammatory nodule or in obvious relation to a preceding scar. The features may also vary according to the causative agent and type of injury; for example,

granuloma formation due to illicit injection of paraffin for tissue augmentation may produce a broad area of abnormality, whereas a thorn injury is usually very localized. Pathologically, many foreign bodies will be visible by polarized light microscopy, thus confirming the diagnosis.

Differential diagnosis

Lesions in relation to a preceding scar are usually suspected to be due to foreign material, although keloid scarring and transepidermal elimination of subcutaneous sutures (both early events), and recurrent neoplasms or scar sarcoid (both later events), may be in the differential. In the case of ruptured cysts or follicles, or foreign material in a penetrating wound, the usual differential is from infection or from localized skin nodules such as dermatofibroma. On the sole of the foot, warts or callosities may be suspected.

Treatment

In some cases, it may be possible to extrude a foreign body (e.g. thorns and splinters), or it may be extruded by the skin as a form of transepidermal elimination. In some cases, there may be a good response to intralesional corticosteroids. Some FBGs, such as vaccination granulomas, appear to resolve slowly or to just leave an asymptomatic, deep nodule. Persistently symptomatic localized FBGs may need to be excised.

Multicentric reticulohistiocytosis

Etiology and pathogenesis

This is a granulomatous disorder, usually of unknown etiology but associated with internal malignancy in about 25% of cases.

Clinical

Lesions typically affect skin, bones, and joints, less commonly heart, lungs, eyes, and nervous system. Arthritis is usually manifest in the fingers and knees. The skin lesions usually consist of multiple reddish brown or purple nodules, usually affecting the dorsa of the hands and fingers, and the head and neck (especially around the ears) (Fig. 11.44).

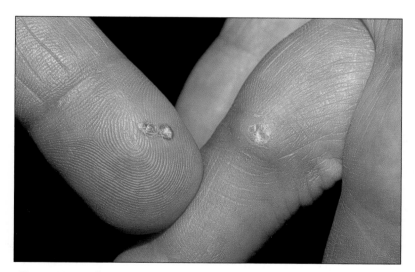

Figure 11.41 Granulomatous lesions on the fingers due to spines from a sea urchin.

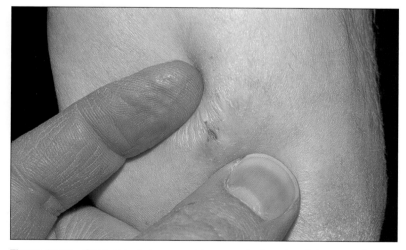

Figure 11.43 Silica granuloma caused by a penetrating glass injury more than 10 years prior.

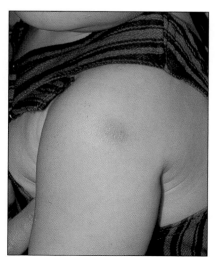

Figure 11.42 Vaccination granuloma at a typical site on the upper arm. This is due to aluminum, which is used to absorb the vaccine antigen and improve the production of an immune response. Such individuals usually have positive patch tests to aluminum salts, and the reactions may last for many years. Symptoms, if any, generally settle with intralesional corticosteroid injection. Any further vaccinations should use non-adsorbed agents where these are available, and should use the buttock injection site, where any nodule is less apparent.

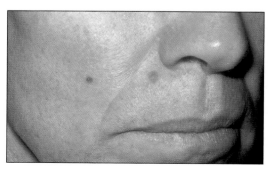

Figure 11.44 Multicentric reticulohistiocytosis: small lesions on the face in a patient with associated malignancy (myelofibrosis).

Differential diagnosis

There is a wide differential, as lesions can be varied. Small papular lesions may suggest sarcoidosis, lymphocytomas, or lupus miliaris disseminata faciei. Larger lesions may resemble rheumatoid nodules.

Treatment

Underlying disorders should be treated. The arthritis may respond to non-steroidal antiinflammatory drugs (NSAIDs). Systemic steroids are of variable benefit, as are antimalarials, cyclophosphamide, and chlorambucil. In some patients, the active disease gradually remits.

PRACTICE POINTS
- Sarcoidosis is one of the great mimics in medicine: the cutaneous patterns are extremely diverse.
- Previously ruptured cysts or hair follicles are the commonest cause of a localized granulomatous reaction.
- The historical link between granuloma annulare and diabetes is largely disproved for most patterns; more complex investigations than a simple urinalysis for glucose are unnecessary.
- In an immunosuppressed patent with a skin lesion that has granulomatous histology, always consider the possibility that it may be due to fungal infection.

MASTOCYTOSIS

Etiology and pathogenesis

Mastocytoses are the deposition of abnormal numbers of mast cells in skin or other organs. Most cases are sporadic, a few are familial, and some are associated with other myeloproliferative disease. It is now known that adults, and a small proportion of children, with sporadic mastocytosis have mutations in the protooncogene *c-kit*. The product of this gene, KIT, is expressed on mast cell surface membranes and is normally activated by stem cell factor, leading to cell growth and increased survival. Mutations in *c-kit* lead to constitutive activation of KIT.

In addition to the well-known histamine content of mast cells, numerous other chemicals from mast cell granules play a part in producing the symptoms of mastocytosis. These include proteases, carboxypeptidase A, heparin, leukotrienes, prostaglandins (leukotriene B4, leukotriene C4, prostaglandin D_2, and platelet-activating factor), and cytokines (interleukin [IL]-1, IL-3, IL-4, IL-5, IL-6, granulocyte–monocyte colony-stimulating factor, and tumor necrosis factor). Release of IL-5 leads to eosinophilia, which may be prominent in some cases.

Mastocytosis is divided on clinical grounds into the following types.
- Type Ia: indolent mastocytosis, no systemic disease.
- Type Ib: indolent mastocytosis, with systemic disease.
- Type II: mastocytosis associated with a myeloproliferative (IIa) or myelodysplastic (IIb) disorder (skin lesions may or may not be present; urticaria, dermographism, or flushing usually occur).
- Type III: lymphadenopathic mastocytosis with eosinophilia (also termed aggressive mastocytosis; rare, usually no skin lesions).
- Type IV: mast cell leukemia (rare, usually no skin lesions).

This text will concentrate on the skin lesions.

Clinical

Cutaneous mastocytosis presents with several different morphologies (Table 11.6 and described later), each of which has a different age group of predilection (Figs 11.45–11.50). Lesions in children contain many more mast cells than those in adults, hence the greater tendency for lesional urtication or blistering in the younger age group. Clinical features of the lesions include itch, urtication when rubbed (Darier sign), blistering in some cases, and pigmentation. Dermographism and urticarial lesions may occur more widely. Systemic symptoms include flushing (Ch. 12), alcohol intolerance, headache (especially in adults), and peptic ulceration (Table 11.7).

Table 11.6   CLINICAL VARIANTS OF CUTANEOUS MASTOCYTOSIS

Pattern	Description	Differential diagnosis
Solitary mastocytoma	Yellow-brown plaque (may be macular or papular morphology). Urticates or blisters easily. Virtually always in children.	Early macular lesions may resemble a café-au-lait patch or congenital nevus. Congenital or early-onset lesions are often confused with a variety of birthmarks, or with some form of intrauterine or perinatal trauma. Juvenile xanthogranuloma may have a similar yellowish color. Bullous lesions may be confused with impetigo, burns, or child abuse.
Urticaria pigmentosa: childhood pattern	Variable number of yellow-brown macules, plaques; usually fewer if later age of onset. Usually urticate easily; blistering is a feature, especially if extensive and young age. Larger lesions (may be 1–2 cm) compared with the adult pattern.	Includes café-au-lait patches, bite reactions, pseudolymphomas, ordinary and Spitz nevi, impetigo, other pediatric bullous disorders (all rare), burns, child abuse.
Urticaria pigmentosa: adult pattern	Numerous red-brown macules or papules, usually each < 0.5 cm, mainly on trunk. May be difficult to urticate.	Lichen planus, freckles, nevi.
Diffuse cutaneous mastocytosis	Semiconfluent yellow–pale brown plaques, skin may be wrinkled and doughy. Rare; usually children.	May be confused with immunobullous disorders, impetigo, erythema multiforme if there is extensive blistering. Flushing episodes may suggest carcinoid syndrome.
Telangiectasia macularis eruptive perstans	Telangiectatic macules; may be discrete or semiconfluent. Urtication is often subtle. Usually adults.	Usually non-specific description of telangiectasia or red patches; may be assumed to represent aging or solar damage.
Xanthelasmoid pattern	Yellowish plaques; may urticate. Rare.	Xanthomatoses, pseudoxanthoma elasticum.
No skin lesions	Systemic disease may occur without skin lesions	Depends on organ(s) involved and symptoms; see Table 11.7.

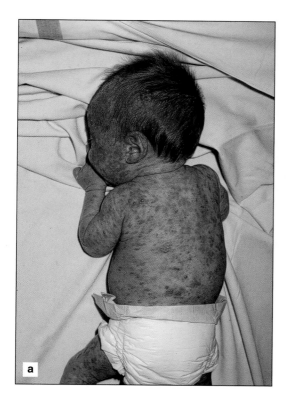

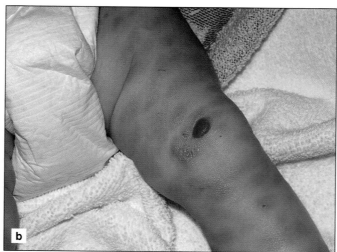

Figure 11.45 Examples of extensive neonatal mastocytosis. (**a**) This infant had diffuse cutaneous involvement; splenomegaly was a feature when he was a few years older. (**b**) This child had scattered red patches present at birth, but blisters, as shown here, and generalized flushing were the prominent problems during her early childhood.

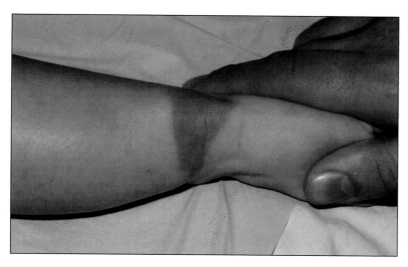

Figure 11.46 Solitary lesions (mastocytoma) are a pattern of mastocytosis that occurs in infants and young children, and often affects the distal part of a limb. In this case, blistering at the ankle was blamed on a name band used in the neonatal unit, but the characteristic brown color of mastocytosis made the diagnosis apparent.

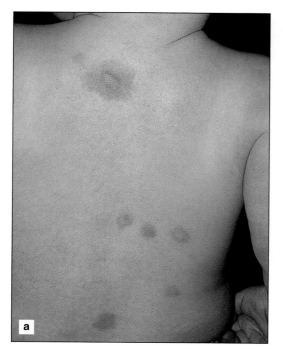

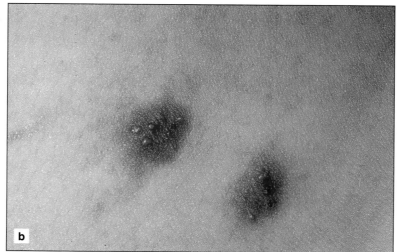

Figure 11.47 (**a**) Urticaria pigmentosa is the most frequent type of mastocytosis in the second half of the first decade of life. The lesions typically urticate when rubbed, swelling up and developing a flare around them (Darier sign), as shown here. (**b**) Blistering may occur as a more extreme response to release of inflammatory mediators from mast cells, particularly in infants and young children with widespread lesions.

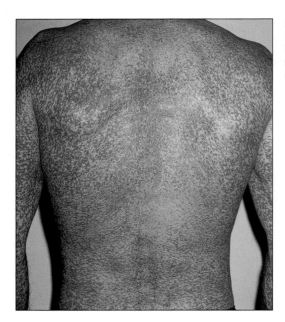

Figure 11.48
Mastocytosis in an adult. Pigmentation of lesions may be prominent, as shown here.

Mastocytoma

These lesions are generally solitary or few in number, and usually present within the first few months of life. They often cause blistering, and may be a diagnostic challenge until the typical brown pigmentation develops. Most resolve spontaneously.

Urticaria pigmentosa

This is the commonest childhood form of mastocytosis, presenting as scattered (predominantly truncal) reddish brown or yellow-brown plaques that become red and raised, with a surrounding erythematous flare after rubbing. Most of those with early age of onset remit or just leave faint staining by teenage years. Those with onset in the second half of childhood, or in adult years, usually have more, but smaller, lesions, which are more persistent.

Other cutaneous mastocytoses
Telangiectasia macularis eruptiva perstans

Telangiectasia macularis eruptiva perstans (TMEP) is an essentially asymptomatic variant of mastocytosis that usually occurs in middle-aged women and is characterized by prominent telangiectasia. Symptomatic urtication is usually mild, but the telangiectasia or variable redness of lesions causes cosmetic concern (Fig. 11.50).

Figure 11.49 Extensive adult mastocytosis lesions. Some such patients have minor symptoms, but in this case there was considerable itch due to the dermographic tendency illustrated.

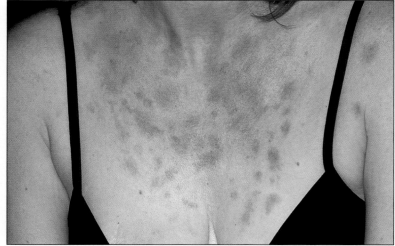

Figure 11.50 Telangiectasia macularis eruptiva perstans. Unfortunately, the upper trunk is a common site in female patients, although urtication and symptoms are usually minor.

Table 11.7 SYMPTOMS AND ORGAN-SPECIFIC FEATURES THAT MAY OCCUR IN MASTOCYTOSIS

Organ system	Symptom or feature	Comments
Skin	Itch (mediated by prostaglandin D_2), wheals (leukotrienes), flushing (chymase), blisters (histamine)	Wheals in localized disease (mastocytoma, limited urticaria pigmentosa) are at the site of lesions, but they may occur elsewhere in more extensive disease. Blisters are most commonly a feature of extensive mastocytosis in infants and young children, improving with time.
General	General malaise or tiredness, fever	Constitutional symptoms suggest significant systemic involvement.
Cardiac	Palpitations, dizziness, fainting, chest pain	Different mediators involved in the different symptoms.
Respiratory	Dyspnea	Uncommon.
Gastrointestinal and abdominal	Nausea or vomiting, diarrhea, cramps, dyspepsia; splenomegaly, hepatomegaly	Epigastric pain suggests peptic ulcer and systemic disease. Splenomegaly probably occurs in about 50% with systemic disease.
Bone and bone marrow	Osteoporosis, bone pain	Focal radiolucent or radiopaque bone lesions are fairly common. Subclinical bone marrow involvement (increased bone marrow mast cells) occurs in most adults with mastocytosis but is rare in children. Bone pain may occur in systemic disease.
Neurologic	Headache	Cognitive impairment may occur in systemic disease.

Diffuse cutaneous mastocytosis

This rare pattern usually presents in the first few years of life, typically in infancy. The skin may exhibit thickening, with a doughy peau d'orange texture, but in the earliest stages there may be blistering with little else visibly abnormal. Flushing and diarrhea are common, but improvement within a few years is anticipated.

Xanthelasmoid pattern

Rare, and may be confused with xanthomatoses or with pseudoxanthoma elasticum.

Systemic mastocytosis and investigations

About 20% of adults with urticaria pigmentosa will have some involvement of bone marrow or gastrointestinal tract, causing systemic features such as headache, diarrhea, or flushing. A small proportion, probably less than 2%, develop more aggressive disease associated with myeloproliferative features, lymphoma, neutropenia, lymphadenopathy and eosinophilia, or even mast cell leukemia. Such developments may be accompanied by an apparently paradoxical improvement in skin symptoms, which presumably reflects development of a less well-differentiated mast cell population.

Measurement of mast cell tryptase or of urinary histamine or its metabolites (N-methyl histamine, 1,4-methylimidazole acetic acid, MeImAA) may be useful in assessment of systemic symptoms. A radiologic or isotope skeletal assessment is recommended in adults with mastocytosis, even in the absence of overt systemic disease, and a bone marrow biopsy is also recommended if there is either an abnormal complete blood count or evidence of bone lesions.

Differential diagnosis

This is discussed for each pattern of skin lesions in Table 11.6. Biopsy of skin lesions will usually confirm the diagnosis, but additional investigations as described earlier for systemic disease may also be useful.

Treatment

This falls into three main categories for cutaneous disease.

- Avoid triggers of mast cell degranulation. This is especially important if there are significant systemic features due to widespread skin lesions. Friction is an important factor in causing urtication or blistering of lesions in children. More important is the potential for significant mediator release due to drugs such as opiates, aspirin, NSAIDs, alcohol, and many anesthetics (propofol, vecuronium, and fentanyl appear to be safe).
- Local treatments. These include topical corticosteroids, PUVA, and UVA1 (the last is not widely available). If using topical corticosteroids, potent agents are required, so there is a risk of atrophy with prolonged use. Short-term use under occlusion may be worthwhile, or intra-lesional depot steroid (usually for localized mastocytomas). Rarely, troublesome mastocytomas may be treated by excision.
- Systemic treatments. In patients with more widespread urticaria pigmentosa, or with systemic symptoms, symptomatic treatment with oral H_1 antihistamines is usually required. H_2 antagonists are also useful, especially if there is associated peptic ulcer disease. Mast cell stabilizing agents, such as ketotifen and sodium cromoglycate, are also useful in some cases, as is doxepin (which has powerful antihistaminic activity).

PRACTICE POINTS

- In childhood mastocytosis (and less reliably in adult forms), lesions are usually brown but become edematous, itchy, and with a surrounding red flare when rubbed.
- Patients with systemic symptoms such as flushing or urticaria associated with cutaneous mastocytosis should avoid drugs that cause mast cell degranulation; opiates and anesthetic agents are of particular importance.
- In adults with mastocytosis, any abnormality of blood counts is an indication that a bone marrow biopsy should be performed.

MUCINOSES

The classification of cutaneous mucinoses, and the rationale for each different version, is a constant source of debate and is beyond the scope of this text. A tentative but clinically relevant approach is given in Table 11.8 (Figs 11.51–11.58).

Some disorders in which mucin deposition occurs are discussed elsewhere; most of the remainder are rare (with the exception of digital myxoid cyst, which is common) but are briefly discussed here.

Reticulate erythematous mucinosis
Etiology and pathogenesis

This is an uncommon dermatosis, affecting women more often than men, usually in young adults. There are many similarities to LE, particularly the photosensitivity that is frequently reported; indeed, the two disorders may be associated, and some patients have other autoimmune diseases. However, internal involvement as seen in LE does not occur, and immunofluorescence of skin biopsies is negative. The degree of mucin deposition is greater than the small amounts seen in some cases of LE.

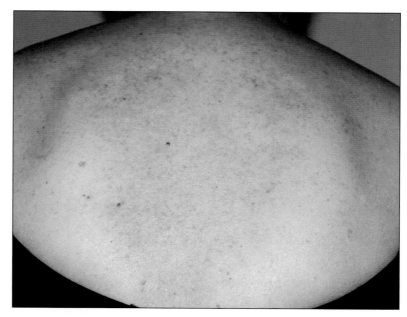

Figure 11.51 Reticulate erythematous mucinosis. The upper back and V of the neck areas are the typical sites for lesions, which are typically rather non-specific erythematous papules or reticulate plaques. Most patients are female.

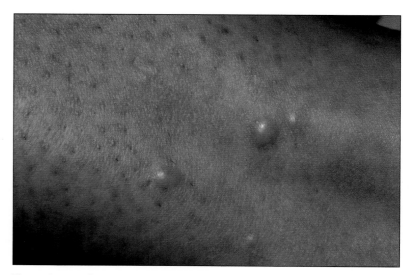

Figure 11.52 Small, scattered lesions with the typical gray color, which can occur in small lesions of mucinosis; the patient also had deep granuloma annulare but no evidence of autoimmune endocrine or metabolic diseases (especially diabetes or thyroid disease), and no paraproteinemia, and did not wish further investigations. (Courtesy of Dr. L. Barco.)

Table 11.8   A CLINICALLY RELEVANT CLASSIFICATION OF CUTANEOUS MUCINOSES

Pattern	Mucinosis	Comments
Extensive or generalized	Scleromyxedema (generalized lichen myxedematosus) Scleredema Generalized myxedema	Papular and sclerodermoid components See text, this chapter See Chapter 12
Diffuse but localized site	Pretibial myxedema Reticular erythematous mucinosis	See Chapter 12 See text, this chapter
Focal	Lichen myxedematosus, papular form (Digital) myxoid (mucinous) cyst Other focal myxomas	Divided into five types: discrete papules, any site; acral persistent papular mucinosis; self-healing papular mucinosis (adult and juvenile variants); papular mucinosis of infancy; and nodular form See text, this chapter For example subcutaneous myxomas (usually facial, periauricular) in the LAMB[a] syndrome
Follicular	Follicular mucinosis Secondary follicular mucinosis	See Chapter 33; may be associated with mycosis fungoides Mucin may be present in follicles in dermatitis, lupus erythematosus, lichen planus, insect bites, and others
Associated with inflammatory dermatosis	Mucinosis in lupus erythematosus and others	Usually microscopic only, but occasionally massive deposition in lupus erythematosus; epithelial deposition may occur in dermatitis, and dermal deposition in dermatomyositis, sclerodermoid graft-versus-host disease, granuloma annulare, Degos disease, some scars, and others
Within localized skin lesion	Mucinous nevus (Angio)myxoma Secondary deposition	Hamartoma Neoplastic Mucin may be found in basal cell or squamous cell carcinoma, keratoacanthoma, viral warts, and others

[a]LAMB: lentigines, atrial myxomas, mucocutaneous myxomas, blue nevi.

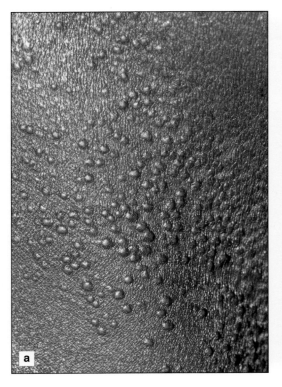

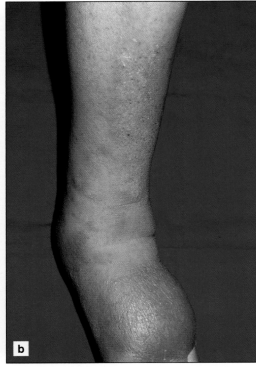

Figure 11.53   Lichen myxedematosus. (**a**) The typical form, having a sheet of discrete, small, skin-colored papules. (**b**) Nodular form. This is an unusual variant, not well served by the term *lichen*; it may be confused with simple edema or lymphedema, or with a soft nodule such as a lipoma, although this would be an unusual site. Some rather more cobblestoned lesions, more typical of this disease, are apparent further up the shin.

Figure 11.54 Scleredema typically affects the upper trunk and causes a marked peau d'orange appearance; the dermis is expanded by mucin, but the follicles are tethered.

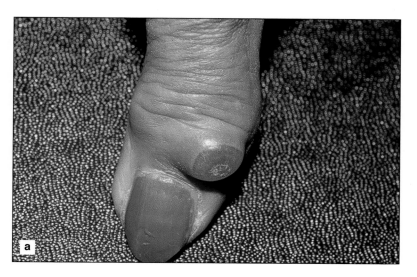

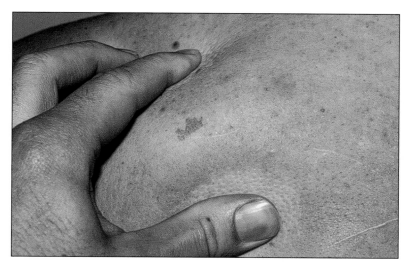

Figure 11.55 Scleredema diabeticorum. The peau d'orange appearance can be exaggerated by pinching the skin, which also demonstrates a massive increase in dermal thickness. (See also Fig. 12.18.)

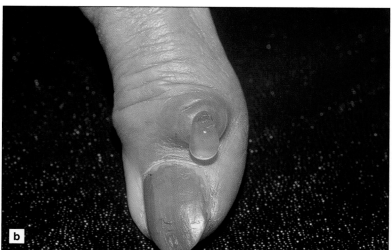

Figure 11.57 (**a**) Digital myxoid (mucinous) cyst at a typical site on the dorsal aspect of the terminal phalanx of a finger. (**b**) Puncture of the cyst demonstrates extrusion of sticky, jelly-like, mucinous fluid.

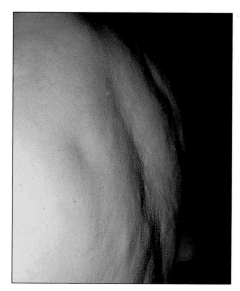

Figure 11.56 A side view of the upper back in a patient with scleredema demonstrates the pitting of the skin that occurs after pressure (or squeezing, as in Fig. 11.55). This is typically very slow to regain a normal contour, presumably due to the high viscosity of the mucinous infiltrate.

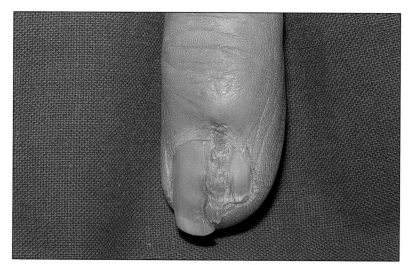

Figure 11.58 Digital myxoid cyst demonstrating the associated nail dystrophy that is a common feature. This is due to compression of the nail matrix within the proximal nail fold, therefore causing a groove that runs along the length of the nail.

Clinical features

The disorder usually occurs on the chest and V region of the neck, and consists of patchy or reticulate-patterned lesions, which are often just palpable (Fig. 11.51). Exacerbation due to sunlight, and occurrence confined to the summer months, are common findings, but routine phototests and provocation tests are negative.

Differential diagnosis

The main differential is from LE or polymorphic light eruption.

Treatment

There is usually a dramatic response to oral hydroxychloroquine or mepacrine.

Generalized lichen myxedematosus (scleromyxedema)
Etiology and pathogenesis

Lichen myxedematosus (Fig. 11.53a) is a rare disorder that consists of extensive papular lesions, or a more diffuse sclerodermoid pattern. It is usually associated with benign monoclonal gammopathy, usually IgG λ type, although the titer does not appear to correlate with disease severity. Histologically, there is extensive deposition of mucin throughout the dermis.

Clinical features

Lesions are papular and waxy in appearance, but merge into confluent, firm, shiny, infiltrated plaques that may become generalized and resemble scleroderma. Facial features become coarsened, and inability to open the mouth adequately may be a significant problem. Sclerodactyly and inability to extend the fingers are frequent, but the telangiectasia of systemic sclerosis is not seen, and there is always some degree of a papular

component in scleromyxedema. The Koebner phenomenon has been reported in scleromyxedema.

Differential diagnosis

The main differential diagnoses in established cases are systemic sclerosis (Ch. 13) and scleredema (discussed later). The papular lesions may suggest micropapular sarcoidosis or the diffuse form of GA, but these generally affect the trunk predominantly. Some histiocytoses, or rare disorders such as lipoid proteinosis, may also need to be considered on clinical grounds.

Treatment

The localized versions may regress spontaneously, and even generalized scleromyxedema may improve without any intervention. In more severe cases, treatment of the underlying gammopathy, usually with melphalan, may lead to improvement in the cutaneous features. A dramatic response to intravenous immunoglobulin has recently been reported.

Localized forms of lichen myxedematosus

All forms (Fig. 11.53b, Table 11.8) are uncommon or rare. Lesions are off-white or grayish colored, often translucent, papules, sometimes with a lichenoid appearance. Some forms are defined by the specific site affected, as is apparent from the nomenclature. Biopsy confirms mucin deposition.

Scleredema
Etiology and pathogenesis

This disorder may occur after streptococcal or viral upper respiratory infections (scleredema of Buschke), and also occurs in association with chronic diabetes mellitus, especially in those patients with insulin resistance. It may also occur in association with myeloma or monoclonal

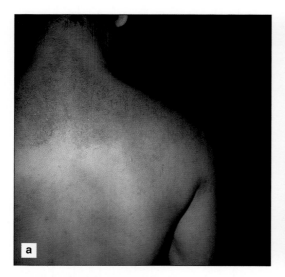
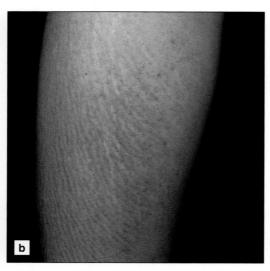
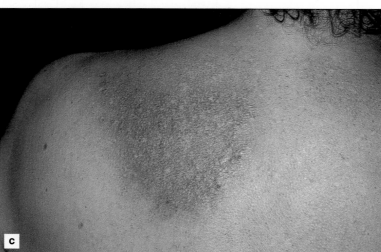

Figure 11.59 Macular amyloid typically occurs as a pigmented region with a rather rippled appearance, as shown on the upper back (**a**) and arm (**b**). It seems to be disproportionately common in Asian skin, when it may be very extensive. (**c**) In at least some individuals, it is probably just a response to chronic rubbing, as was almost certainly the case in this patient with a very localized area corresponding to the position achieved by rubbing the left upper back with the (dominant) right hand.

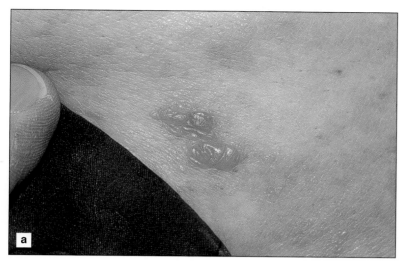

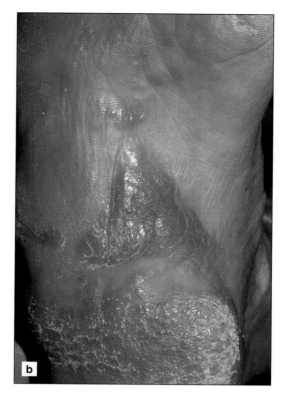

Figure 11.60 Nodular amyloid usually presents as one or a few brownish nodules (**a**), which may resemble granulomatous nodules such as sarcoidosis or granuloma faciale (really a type of vasculitis; discussed in Ch. 14). Some lesions become quite large (**b**). Note that some localized skin tumors may also generate large amounts of amyloid material, usually detected only when they are examined histologically.

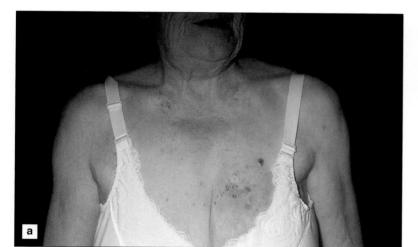

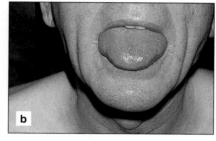

Figure 11.61 Systemic amyloidosis. (**a**) Fragility of cutaneous vasculature is typical, and extravasation of erythrocytes may occur in poorly supported skin after coughing or a Valsalva maneuver. In this case, the linear purpura was probably due to pressure from clothing or minor scratches. Extensive eyelid bruising may also occur. (**b**) Macroglossia is a useful diagnostic feature in systemic amyloidosis.

gammopathy. By contrast with scleromyxedema, there is less mucin deposition and abnormal thickening of collagen.

Clinical features

The clinical appearance is striking, especially in the postinfective patients in whom onset is often quite rapid. The skin of the upper back and nape of neck becomes indurated and tethered, with a peau d'orange appearance and erythema (Fig 11.54–11.56). It may extend to other areas, such as the face and proximal limbs.

Differential diagnosis

This includes systemic sclerosis and scleromyxedema.

Treatment

Treatments such as antibiotics in the infective cases, corticosteroids, immunosuppressive agents, and penicillamine all appear to be equally ineffective.

Digital myxoid cyst

This is a common disorder, which is most commonly seen on fingers but can occur on toes. Some cases appear to occur following local injury, but most are probably caused by extrusion of fluid from the adjacent distal interphalangeal joint (which often has changes of osteoarthritis). The fluid

tracks distally beneath the skin of the dorsum of the finger toward the proximal nail fold, where it may intermittently discharge or may compress the nail matrix, thereby causing distortion of the nail plate (Figs 11.57 and 11.58; see also Ch. 29). Treatment is by surgery, cryotherapy, or intralesional steroid, but recurrence is frequent unless the proximal source of fluid can be obliterated.

This lesion is generally readily diagnosed if the practitioner has seen a case previously. The referral diagnosis may include warts, various tumors and cysts, foreign body reactions, and traumatic or non-specific nail dystrophies.

AMYLOIDOSES

General aspects, etiology, and pathogenesis

Amyloid is a group of disorders characterized by deposition of abnormal tissue proteins in a fibrillar form with β-pleated sheet configuration. The deposits also contain serum amyloid P, which is a globulin similar to C-reactive protein. The clinical pattern varies depending on the type of fibrillar protein and its localization (Figs 11.59–11.64).

The main types of amyloid proteins of dermatologic relevance are as follows.

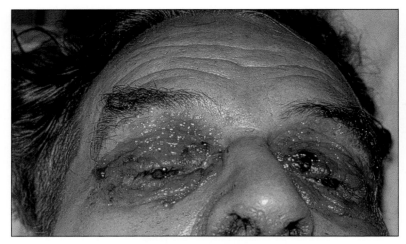

Figure 11.62 Systemic amyloid with massive periorbital deposits. (Courtesy of the Department of Dermatology, University of California, San Diego.)

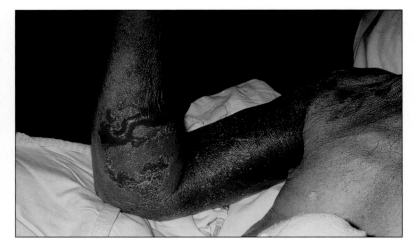

Figure 11.64 Diffuse cutaneous involvement by amyloid, with extensive bruising and bullae.

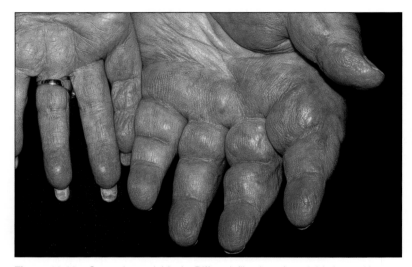

Figure 11.63 Systemic amyloidosis. Diffuse infiltration of amyloid along with lymphedema may lead to massive enlargement of tissue. In this case, the hand and fingers on the left are massively enlarged compared with the normal hand on the right.

- Amyloid fibrils derived from immunoglobulin light chains (mainly of λ type), known as amyloid L (AL). This occurs in primary systemic amyloid or in systemic myeloma-associated amyloid. Less commonly, immunoglobulin heavy chains (AH) constitute the amyloid protein in these types of amyloid. Nodular amyloid (of the skin or at other internal sites) also contains AL.
- Amyloid derived from serum amyloid A precursor protein, this type being termed amyloid A (AA). AA occurs secondary to a wide variety of chronic inflammatory disorders, such as tuberculosis, rheumatoid and other chronic arthritis, bronchiectasis, some lymphomas, and chronic venous ulceration. Of particular dermatologic relevance, as there are cutaneous as well as systemic features, AA occurs in familial Mediterranean fever and other periodic fevers, as well as in familial cold urticaria and Muckle–Wells' syndrome (a familial disorder with urticaria and deafness).
- Amyloid derived from altered keratin—this occurs in several skin tumors, such as basal cell carcinoma and Bowen disease, and in benign lesions, such as seborrheic keratoses and porokeratosis, but is rarely prominent clinically. It is probably also the amyloid type in macular amyloid and lichen amyloidosis, in which scratching may play a part in disrupting keratinocytes.

About 20 other proteins are implicated in amyloidosis of various internal organs.

Clinical features

Cutaneous involvement in different types of amyloidosis is listed in Table 11.9.

Systemic amyloid may present as malaise, edema (with proteinuria), arthritis, neuropathy, cardiomyopathy, and many other symptoms. The cutaneous presentation is typically as purpura, due to amyloid infiltration of walls of small blood vessels in the skin. Linear purpura after scratches, pinch purpura (especially at thin skin areas), and periorbital purpura are most typical, but widespread purpura, bullae, and waxy plaques may also occur. Macroglossia is a frequent feature.

Localized cutaneous amyloid occurs as several distinct forms.

- Nodular amyloid occurs mainly in older patients, and consists of one or several reddish brown nodules that appear mainly on the face and extremities. Most nodular amyloid is probably due to a polyclonal reactive process of AL fibrils, but some patients have a monoclonal gammopathy or urinary Bence Jones protein.
- Lichen amyloidosis occurs mainly in patients of Chinese origin, and causes small, brown, keratotic papules on the shins.
- Macular amyloidosis is most common in Asian and South American populations, but also occurs in white ones. It usually affects the upper back and presents as rippled brown lines. It may be associated with chronic itch and scratching or rubbing, for example in notalgia paresthetica (Ch. 9).

Differential diagnosis

This depends on the pattern.

- Purpura in systemic disease—may resemble many causes of purpura or coagulopathy. Lesions around eyes may be felt to resemble simple bruising.
- Waxy plaques in systemic disease—may resemble syringomas (eyelids) or multiple trichofolliculomas (paranasal and eyelids) in early stages; differential later might include histiocytoses, mucinoses, xanthomatoses, necrobiotic xanthogranuloma, and cutaneous metastases.
- Nodular amyloidosis—differential includes primary skin tumors, such as basal cell carcinoma; granulomatous diseases, such as GA or sarcoidosis; xanthomas; granuloma faciale (a vasculitis); and skin lymphoma.
- Lichen amyloidosis—most likely to be confused with simple lichenification; lichen planus and lichen myxedematosus (papular lesions) are possible differentials.
- Macular amyloidosis—other causes of rippled hyperpigmentation include lichenification, nostalgia paresthetica, and the so-called atopic dirty neck. The last in particular has the same rippled pigmented appearance as in macular amyloidosis. Although it is not routinely detectable, amyloid has been observed in such lesions by electron microscopy, so it may be a similar process. Notalgia paresthetica may be a form of entrapment neuropathy but is often felt to overlap with macular amyloid.

Treatment

Systemic amyloidosis is treated with a variety of chemotherapeutic agents, particularly melphalan, to control the underlying plasma cell dyscrasia,

Table 11.9 CUTANEOUS INVOLVEMENT IN AMYLOIDOSIS

Clinical type	Amyloid protein	Skin findings
Primary cutaneous amyloidosis Macular amyloidosis Lichen amyloidosis Nodular amyloidosis	?Keratin ?Keratin Amyloid L (AL)	Rippled pigmentation, usually trunk. Lichenoid papules, usually legs. Usually solitary, yellowish brown, sometimes rather translucent nodule.
Secondary cutaneous amyloidosis Related to localized lesions	Keratin	Amyloid may be present in numerous lesions, including basal cell carcinoma, nevi, seborrheic keratosis, porokeratosis.
Systemic amyloidosis Primary systemic (AL) amyloidosis and myeloma-associated amyloidosis	Mainly AL	Skin findings in about 30–40%. Also macroglossia. Skin features are as follows. Purpura: due to vascular wall infiltration, especially at areas of minor trauma (includes 'pinch purpura'), or periorbital (raccoon sign) if increased vascular pressure by coughing etc. Plaques: due to skin infiltration; waxy yellowish or purpuric, often papular or cobblestoned plaque morphology. Others: bullae, sclerodermoid plaques, paronychia or nail dystrophy.
Reactive amyloidosis (amyloid A, AA)	AA	Skin findings are rare, although the diagnosis may often be made by subcutaneous fat aspirate for histologic examination. There may be features of a chronic skin disorder that has led to reactive amyloidosis, for example psoriasis, scleroderma, lupus erythematosus, hidradenitis suppurativa.
Hereditary forms	AA	Familial Mediterranean fever may cause urticaria-like skin lesions; Muckle–Wells' syndrome is familial urticaria and deafness (note: there are many other hereditary amyloidoses in which other amyloid proteins are involved).

together with symptomatic treatment of complications such as cardiac failure.

Localized nodular amyloid is generally treated surgically by excision, curettage, or laser.

Macular amyloid is generally treated with antipruritic measures.

XANTHOMAS

General aspects, etiology, and pathogenesis

This group of disorders is characterized by deposition of abnormal lipid in the skin. At some sites, such as the eyelids (xanthelasma), this is often in the context of normal serum lipid levels. However, xanthomas at other sites are usually a manifestation of systemic hyperlipidemia (Table 11.10).

In many cases, xanthomas occur in patients with a hereditary predisposition (primary), although there may be environmental interaction (diet, alcohol, etc.). The primary hyperlipidemias were classified types I–V (World Health Organization classification, Fredericksen classification) but are now classified as follows (World Health Organization classification in square brackets):

- hypercholesterolemia (familial and polygenic types) [IIa, IIb],
- combined hypercholesterolemia [IIa, IIb],
- remnant particle disease (dysbetalipidemia) [III],
- hypertriglyceridemia (familial hypertriglyceridemia [IV] and familial combined hypertriglyceridemia [V]),
- chylomicronemia [I], and
- unclassified high-density lipoprotein abnormalities.

Secondary hyperlipidemias may be due to cholestasis, hypothyroidism, diabetes, nephrotic syndrome, renal failure, monoclonal gammopathy, or drugs. Most drug-induced hyperlipidemia does not cause dermatologic features, but olanzapine has been implicated as a cause of eruptive xanthomas due to hypertriglyceridemia; dermatologists also need to be aware of hyperlipidemia due to use of oral retinoids. Cholesterol and triglyceride are the most relevant lipids, but abnormal levels of other sterols may also be dermatologically relevant, for example elevated cholestanol in cerebrotendinous xanthomatosis.

Note that some lesions that carry the name xanthoma are actually correctly classified as histiocytoses (e.g. xanthoma disseminatum or necrobiotic xanthogranuloma) and are discussed briefly later.

Clinical features

Xanthomas are usually clinically apparent from their yellow color (Figs 11.65–11.70). The main patterns are summarized in Table 11.10.

Differential diagnosis

This varies according to the pattern (see Table 11.10). Note that juvenile xanthogranuloma, a type of histiocytosis that occurs in children, may produce yellow-orange lesions that resemble xanthomas; however, these are usually on the scalp and face, whereas this would be an uncommon distribution for most xanthomas. Nodular lesions may superficially resemble cysts, but the latter are more white in color and are spherical rather than having the lobulated feel of xanthomatous nodules.

Treatment

In the majority of cases, in which there is an underlying hyperlipidemia, treatment is by dietary correction, drugs such as statins, and correction of other cardiac risk factors such as smoking and hypertension. Some xanthomas, especially eruptive lesions, will regress as serum lipid levels are corrected. Local treatment, such as excision, is occasionally required for xanthomas at difficult sites.

Xanthelasmas may be treated with a variety of destructive modalities, such as trichloroacetic acid, electrocautery, excision, and laser.

PRACTICE POINTS

- Always check a lipid profile in patients with xanthelasma; a significant minority will have a treatable hyperlipoproteinemia.
- Most xanthomas can be suspected from their yellowish color.
- Eruptive xanthomas are important to recognize, as they are usually a consequence of very high serum triglyceride levels.
- Extensive cutaneous mucinosis is rare, but is important, as it has a significant association with myeloma and monoclonal gammopathy.

Table 11.10   THE MAIN PATTERNS OF XANTHOMAS AND THEIR DIFFERENTIAL DIAGNOSIS

Pattern	Lipid abnormality	Clinical features	Differential diagnosis
Tendon xanthomas	Mainly in type II or III hyperlipoproteinemia. Associated with diabetes mellitus, hypothyroidism, obstructive liver disease. Tendon xanthomas also occur, with neurologic deficit, in cerebrotendinous xanthomatosis.	Usually most apparent on hands and ankles over the extensor tendons	Usually distinctive but may be confused with rheumatoid nodules or giant cell tumor of tendon sheath, less often with lipomas.
Tuberous xanthomas	Occur in type III or type II hyperlipoproteinemia.	Often occur on elbows or knees	May be confused with localized neurofibromas (but tuberous xanthomas are usually symmetric) or with uncommon conditions such as erythema elevatum diutinum (a chronic vasculitis that causes fibrotic nodules, often on elbows or knees)
Plane xanthomas	Depends on site. Antecubital and finger web plane xanthomas occur in type II hyperlipoproteinemia. Hand and foot involvement occurs in cholestasis. See also specific types discussed below (palmar crease, xanthelasma, normolipemic type).	Antecubital and finger webs; hands and feet, becoming generalized	Antecubital pattern might be confused with lichenification, erythrasma, tinea. Broader areas of plane xanthoma on the neck or larger flexures, or more widespread lesions, may resemble pseudoxanthoma elasticum or the rare xanthelasmoid variant of mastocytosis.
Palmar crease xanthomas (xanthoma striatum palmare)	Almost diagnostic of type III hyperlipoproteinemia.	Occur in the palmar creases	Occasionally confused with carotenemia, but this does not localize to the creases.
Eruptive xanthomas	Occur due to marked elevation of triglyceride levels (occurs in type I, IV, and V hyperlipoproteinemia). Associated with diabetes mellitus, hypothyroidism, and pancreatitis.	Tiny spots, eruptive pattern; typically occur on the buttocks but may be generalized	May be confused with folliculitis, diffuse pattern granuloma annulare, or with some histiocytoses.
Xanthelasma	A significant minority (about 25%) of patients have hyperlipidemia, usually type II.	Occur on the eyelids	Nodular elastoidosis, a disorder of elderly sun-damaged skin that occurs predominantly on the cheeks and in the vicinity of the eyes (but which is also characterized by comedones). Sebaceous hyperplasia lesions are more circular, usually not on eyelids. Syringomas occur on eyelids but are more discrete small skin-colored lesions. Necrobiotic xanthogranuloma (a histiocytosis associated with paraproteinemia) often produces lesions around the eyes (Fig. 11.73) but is usually more destructive.
Normolipemic plane xanthomatosis	None	Sheets of small yellowish papules; strongly associated with paraproteinemia or myeloma; also linked with acquired type of C1 esterase inhibitor deficiency	Differential includes several of the histiocytoses, but the diagnosis is usually apparent from the yellow color of the xanthomatosis lesions. Plane xanthomas associated with hyperlipoproteinemia are usually much more localized.

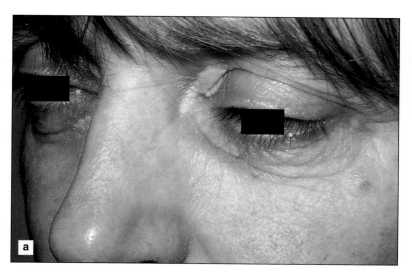
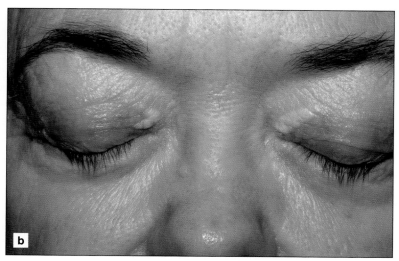

Figure 11.65 (**a**,**b**) Xanthelasma. This is a common lesion, which may be associated with hyperlipidemia in about 25% of cases. It is typically bilateral and fairly symmetric, as shown in (b), and usually involves the medial part of the eyelids. Extensive involvement of the eyelids with large lesions is indicative of a likely abnormality of lipid levels.

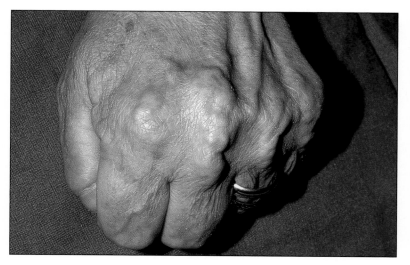

Figure 11.66 Tendon xanthomas are often associated with endocrine disorders causing hyperlipidemia, such as hypothyroidism or diabetes mellitus.

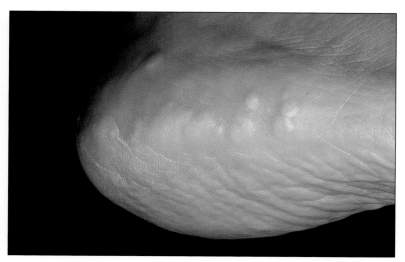

Figure 11.68 Eruptive xanthomas typically affect the buttocks and limbs but may present at any site. When they occur on the weight-bearing area of the feet, our experience suggests that they may be relatively large lesions (compare with the eruptive xanthomas shown in Fig. 11.67), sometimes being painful as a result of their size and site.

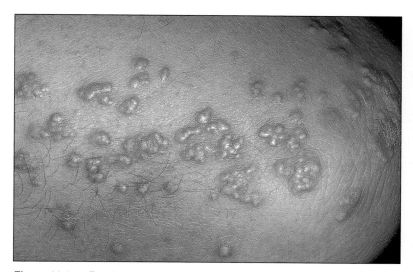

Figure 11.67 Eruptive xanthomas may be misdiagnosed as pustules due to their yellow color. They are due to an underlying hypertriglyceridemia.

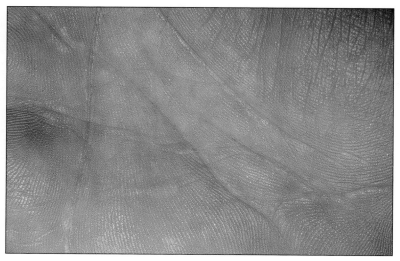

Figure 11.69 Palmar crease xanthomas (xanthoma striatum palmare) are a feature of type III hyperlipidemia, and often resolve when the associated lipid abnormality is treated. Carotenemia (Fig. 1.17) may be confused with these lesions. (Courtesy of Stephen H. Ducatman, M.D.)

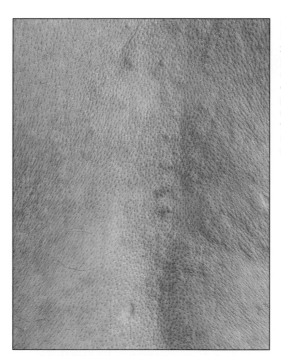

Figure 11.70
Normolipemic plane xanthomatosis with paraproteinemia. The skin lesions are sheets of confluent yellowish papules, which are usually most apparent on the trunk and proximal limbs. (Courtesy of Dr. Mary M. Carr.)

LANGERHANS CELL HISTIOCYTOSIS AND OTHER HISTIOCYTOSES

Langerhans cell histiocytosis (histiocytosis X)

This histiocytic disorder (Ch. 19) is most frequent in children. It causes a rash that resembles a severe seborrheic rash, with crusted papular lesions, erosions, granulomatous areas, and purpuric areas. The rash may present on the nappy area, trunk, or scalp. Internal involvement may occur, especially diabetes insipidus (in 25–50% with systemic disease), and treatment is usually with radiotherapy or chemotherapy, or both.

Occasionally, solitary nodular skin lesions known as eosinophilic granuloma of the skin may occur as a rare variant of Langerhans cell histiocytosis (LCH), which may be cured by excision, radiotherapy, or intralesional steroid injection.

Juvenile xanthogranuloma

Juvenile xanthogranuloma (JXG) is much the commonest of the histiocytic disorders. It occurs in children, usually as one or a few yellowish orange papules or nodules, most commonly on the scalp or face (Fig. 11.71). As discussed earlier, its yellow color is most likely to be interpreted as a xanthoma, but it also enters the differential diagnosis of mastocytosis. It does not have any significance in most cases, and lesions generally resolve without treatment. However, involvement of the eyes may occur, and there is a rare association between JXG, neurofibromatosis type 1 (NF1), and juvenile myelomonocytic leukemia (although JXG and NF1 can coexist without leukemia also).

Other histiocytoses

Most other histiocytoses are rare. They include types that are the following.

- Familial—familial sky blue histiocytosis and hereditary progressive mucinous histiocytosis.
- Eruptive or disseminated—benign cephalic histiocytosis (usually in children), generalized eruptive histiocytosis (mainly in adults), and xanthoma disseminatum (Fig. 11.72).
- Paraneoplastic—diffuse plane xanthomatosis and necrobiotic xanthogranuloma (with paraproteinemia) (Fig. 11.73).
- Usually systemic but occasionally confined to skin—massive sinus histiocytosis (Rosai–Dorfman disease, Fig. 11.74).

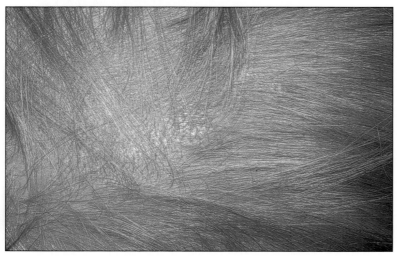

Figure 11.71 Juvenile xanthogranuloma. This child had a few very orange-colored lesions in the scalp. Although usually yellowish in color, and usually solitary or few in number, this diagnosis can be difficult in cases with many lesions or those with a more brown color.

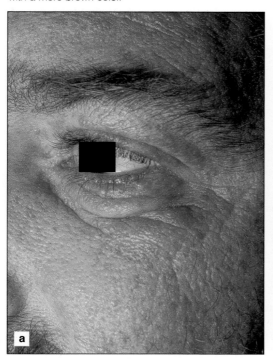

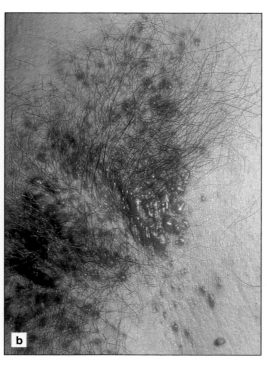

Figure 11.72 Xanthoma disseminatum (**a,b**). A rare histiocytic disorder in which lesions are typically brownish and grouped together in the axillae and other flexures. The perioral skin and buccal mucosa may be affected, and systemic symptoms arise from involvement of respiratory epithelium and meninges. (Courtesy of the Department of Dermatology, University of California, Irvine.)

a

b

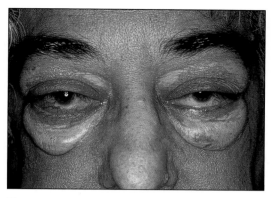

Figure 11.73 Necrobiotic xanthogranuloma is a rare disease, associated with paraproteinemia (usually of IgG type). Lesions are nodules and plaques that may be annular and, due to their yellowish color, may resemble necrobiosis lipoidica. Periorbital involvement is typical, and the lesions may be locally destructive. Early periorbital lesions may be confused with xanthelasma. (Courtesy of Theodore Sebastian, M.D.)

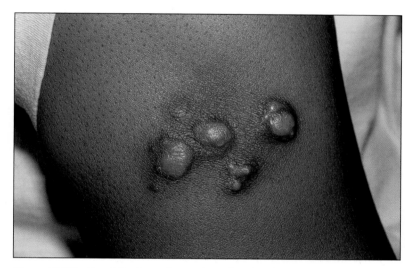

Figure 11.74 Rosai–Dorfman disease (massive sinus histiocytosis). The skin is involved in a minority of cases, but it may be the dominant or the presenting feature on some occasions. Pigmented plaques and nodules are the typical skin lesion in this rare disorder.

OTHER METABOLIC INFILTRATES AND DEPOSITS

Perforating disorders

This is a group of disorders in which dermal tissue is extruded through the epidermis or into the follicles (perforating folliculitis), a process known as transepidermal elimination (Fig. 11.75). This is an important group of disorders, as they are associated with systemic disease, notably diabetes and chronic renal failure, and are discussed further in Chapter 12. However, the same process of transepidermal elimination may occur sporadically and also occurs as isolated lesions in several other situations, which are usually more obvious. For example, subcutaneous suture material ('spitting' sutures), fragmented hair shafts (e.g. after simple folliculitis), or insect mouthparts may all be eliminated through the skin surface.

Calcinosis

Cutaneous calcinosis (Fig. 11.76) occurs by various mechanisms, the clinical features being very varied and depending on the disease entity. The major mechanisms are as follows (and are listed, with examples, in Table 11.11).

- Dystrophic calcification. In this mechanism, calcium is deposited in previously abnormal tissue or is related to specific local factors. This occurs, for example, in some connective tissue disorders (widespread in juvenile dermatomyositis, locally in CREST [calcinosis, Raynaud phenomenon, esophageal dysfunction, sclerodactyly, and telangiectasia] syndrome; see Ch. 13), occasionally in longstanding venous stasis or

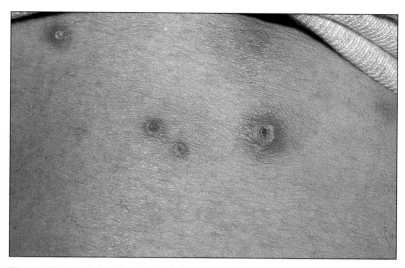

Figure 11.75 Perforating folliculitis in a renal transplant recipient. These lesions are often quite pruritic, and relatively difficult to treat. In this instance, they responded to prompt application of a potent topical corticosteroid ointment.

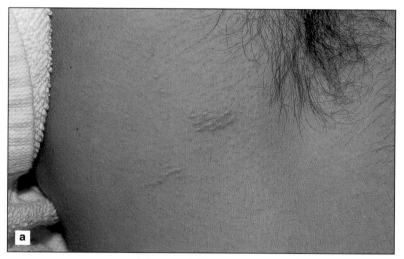

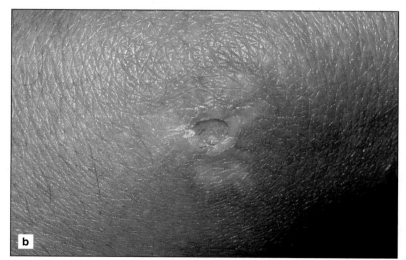

Figure 11.76 Calcinosis cutis: (**a**) showing small striate plaques that are firm to touch, (**b**) showing an ulcerated lesion with typical white color of the calcified plaque.

Ehlers–Danlos syndrome (Ch. 22), and after various injuries. Calcification of the ear occurs most commonly after cold injury but also in some endocrine disorders. There are also some specific entities in which calcification occurs, such as pilomatricoma (a benign tumor of hair follicle origin, Ch. 23).

- Metastatic calcification. This occurs due to either elevated calcium or phosphate levels, or both. Most cases occur in renal failure with

Table 11.11   SOME EXAMPLES OF CUTANEOUS CALCINOSIS

Mechanism of calcinosis	Examples
Dystrophic	Post-traumatic: scars, hematomas, fat injury Localized lesions: cysts, angiomas, lipomas Neoplastic: pilomatricoma, some sarcomas Inflammatory diseases: sclerodermas, dermatomyositis, acne Other skin conditions: venous stasis disease, pseudoxanthoma elasticum, Ehlers–Danlos syndrome
Metastatic	Hyperparathyroidism, pseudohypoparathyroidism, chronic renal failure, milk-alkali syndrome Sarcoidosis Malignant disease with hypercalcemia
Idiopathic	Calcinosis universalis, calcinosis circumscripta Solitary nodular calcinosis (cutaneous calculus) Idiopathic calcinosis of the scrotum

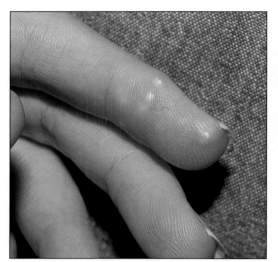

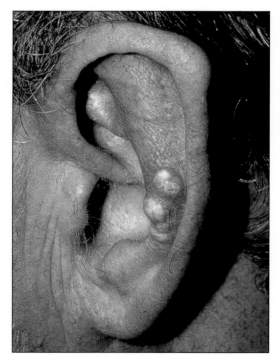

Figure 11.77   Gouty tophi on the finger. The lesions are hard, and white or yellowish. Large lesions may need to be treated surgically (Fig. 2.29a), but smaller lesions may resolve when prophylactic treatment is established, as in this case.

Figure 11.78   Gouty tophi on the ear. The antihelix is the typical site. Multiple yellowish nodules at this site on the ear in a patient without joint disease are unlikely to be due to gout, and granuloma annulare should be considered (Fig. 11.23).

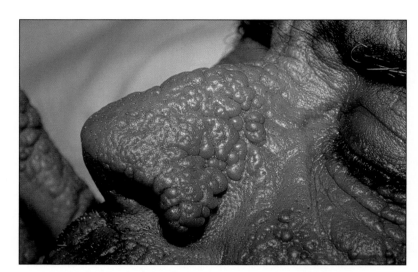

Figure 11.79   Waxy yellowish deposits in the skin in chronic erythropoietic protoporphyria. This disorder is apparent as severe and immediate photosensitivity in early childhood, but it may be relatively asymptomatic in later years. The liver may also be affected in some cases. (Courtesy of Gary W. Cole, M.D.)

Gout

Etiology and pathogenesis

Gout is a disorder in which excessive urate is deposited in the tissues. This may occur for a variety of reasons, including a familial tendency, failure of excretion (e.g. chronic renal failure), or excessive purine load (e.g. from breakdown of damaged cells during chemotherapy).

Clinical features

Gout primarily affects the joints, causing severe acute pain. However, in chronic gout there may be development of cutaneous nodules known as tophi (Figs 11.77 and 11.78). These affect primarily the fingers and the ears. They are hard, yellowish white subcutaneous nodules.

Differential diagnosis

On the fingers, the differential diagnosis includes bony abnormalities, such as Heberden nodes; other abnormal tissue deposits, such as calcinosis; and some firm cutaneous nodules, such as foreign body reactions. On the ears, the most common mimic of gouty tophi is GA, which may also present as multiple nodules over the antihelix (see Fig. 11.23). Solitary nodules on the ear may be confused with chondrodermatitis nodularis (Ch. 30) or pilomatricoma (Ch. 23).

Treatment

Individual tophi may be excised if required. Prophylactic treatment of the underlying metabolic disorder should be instituted with allopurinol.

secondary hyperparathyroidism. Rarely, this may cause deposits of calcium in the skin; the more significant disorder that occurs is calcific uremic arteriolopathy, which is discussed in Chapter 12.

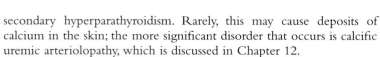

- Idiopathic calcification. At least some examples of apparent idiopathic calcification are probably due to unrecognized injury and are really dystrophic in type.

Porphyrias

Porphyrias are discussed in Chapter 17. However, the yellowish waxy scars that may occur in erythropoietic protoporphyria (Fig. 11.79) may be confused with other tissue infiltrates such as xanthomas or mucinoses, especially in older patients in whom the photosensitive symptoms may have abated considerably compared with childhood years. The main differential diagnosis of these lesions if they occur in younger patients is a rare inherited condition known as lipoid proteinosis.

Lipoid proteinosis

Also termed hyalinosis cutis et mucosae or Urbach–Wiethe disease, this is an autosomal recessive disorder in which hyaline material is deposited in various organs. In the skin, waxy papules develop mainly around eyelid margins, nose, and lips. The skin is generally thickened and may appear verrucous over extremities or bony prominences. Hoarseness due to laryngeal involvement is an early feature that may suggest the diagnosis. Dental abnormalities and sickle-shaped calcification of the temporal lobes occur.

The main differential diagnoses are other deposition disorders such as porpyhria (discussed earlier), amyloidosis, mucinoses, or histiocytoses.

FURTHER READING

Braverman IM. Skin Signs of Systemic Disease, 3rd edn. Philadelphia: Saunders, 1998

Breathnach SM. Amyloid and amyloidoses. J Am Acad Dermatol 1988; 18: 1–16

Caputo R. Text Atlas of Histiocytic Syndromes. London: Martin Dunitz, 1998

Dauod MS, Lust JA, Kyle RA, et al. Monoclonal gammopathies and associated skin disorders. J Am Acad Dermatol 1999; 40: 507–35

Hartmann K, Henz BM. Mastocytosis: recent advances in defining the disease. Br J Dermatol 2001; 144: 682–95

Metcalfe DD (ed) Clinical advances in mastocytosis: an interdisciplinary roundtable discussion. J Invest Dermatol 1991; 96: 1S–65S

Rongioletti F, Rebora A. Updated classification of papular mucinosis, lichen myxedematosus, and scleromyxedema. J Am Acad Dermatol 2001; 44: 273–81

Stephens CJM, McKee PH, Black MM. The dermal mucinoses. Adv Dermatol 1993; 8: 201–26

Tharp MD, Chan IJ. Mastocytosis. Adv Dermatol 2003; 19: 207–36

Touart DM, Sau P. Cutaneous deposition diseases. Part 1. J Am Acad Dermatol 1998; 39: 149–71

Touart DM, Sau P. Cutaneous deposition diseases. Part 2. J Am Acad Dermatol 1998; 39: 527–44

INTRODUCTION

The cutaneous signs of internal disease are a fascinating and varied series of eruptions, some of which are disease-specific and therefore of critical diagnostic importance as an early indicator of systemic disease. In some internal diseases, the cutaneous features may be non-specific (such as pruritus or pigmentation), but recognition that these features may have a systemic cause is important for a logical approach to investigation.

The majority of sections in this chapter are 'organ-oriented', and some multiorgan systemic diseases are discussed in other chapters. In particular, most multisystem inflammatory and granulomatous skin eruptions (several of which may be due to disorders with internal involvement) are covered in Chapter 11, collagen vascular diseases in Chapter 13, and vasculitis and neutrophilic dermatoses in Chapter 14. Non-epidermal neoplastic conditions that may have a systemic component but that also affect the skin (such as cutaneous T-cell lymphomas) are discussed in Chapter 33.

SKIN SIGNS OF THYROID DISEASE

There are several mechanisms by which cutaneous features may be linked with thyroid disease.

- Features due to high (thyrotoxicosis) or low (hypothyroidism) thyroid hormone levels.
- Immunologically mediated cutaneous features (e.g. pretibial myxedema).
- Features of associated autoimmune diseases (e.g. vitiligo and urticaria).

Thyrotoxicosis
Etiology

Thyrotoxicosis may occur due to several causes, of which the most frequent is a diffuse overactive goiter (Graves disease), which occurs as an autoimmune condition. In addition to the elevated levels of thyroxine (T_4), and sometimes of triiodothyronine (T_3) in this condition, there are immunologic abnormalities. From a dermatologic viewpoint, the most important are the thyroid-stimulating immunoglobulins, or long-acting thyroid stimulator (LATS), which are typically demonstrated in Graves disease, but also in 10–20% of patients with Hashimoto thyroiditis.

There are associations between autoimmune thyroid disease and other organ-specific autoimmune diseases such as vitiligo, myasthenia gravis, adrenalitis, insulin resistance, and others. Other disorders of dermatologic relevance that are more frequently linked with thyroid disease, or with the presence of thyroid autoantibodies, than expected by chance include atopic dermatitis, chronic urticaria, psoriasis and palmoplantar pustulosis,

Sweet syndrome, granuloma annulare, bullous pemphigoid, Sjögren syndrome and other collagen vascular diseases, and sarcoidosis. These associations may cluster in some individuals, giving rise to acronyms such as TASS (thyroiditis, adrenalitis, Sjögren syndrome, and sarcoidosis) or TOASSUC (thyroiditis, other autoantibodies, Sjögren syndrome, sarcoidosis, and ulcerative colitis). Cutaneous features of these conditions are discussed elsewhere but may coexist with features of thyroid disease.

Cutaneous features due to elevated thyroid hormone levels

Some features occur in any situation in which thyroxin levels are elevated (such as Graves disease, early thyroiditis, isolated 'hot' nodules, or exogenous administration of thyroxin). These include hot or sweaty skin, fine hair and increased hair loss (Fig. 12.1), and palmar erythema (Table 12.1).

Immunologically mediated cutaneous signs of thyrotoxicosis
Pretibial myxedema

This cutaneous mucinous infiltrate is strongly associated with the presence of circulating LATS, which is identifiable in over 90% of patients. Pretibial myxedema can also occur in Hashimoto thyroiditis, in which some patients have LATS in serum. However, the degree of the disorder does

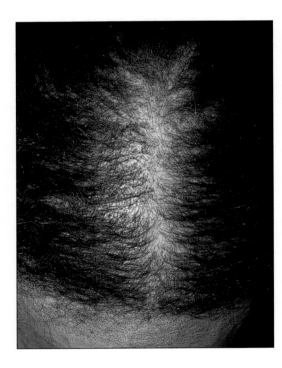

Figure 12.1 Diffuse alopecia due to thyrotoxicosis. The hair is often fine in texture as well, but these are all rather subjective symptoms.

not correlate with LATS titer in serum, and LATS is not identified immunologically in lesional skin. The process typically affects the pretibial skin, as implied by the name, but the toes (especially the dorsal aspect of the hallux) are also frequently involved. Erythema and slight edema are the early signs, with subsequent peau d'orange appearance as the degree of infiltration increases (Figs 12.2 and 12.3). Treatment is difficult, as control of the thyroid disease does not alter the immunologic situation. Topical or intralesional corticosteroids may reduce the inflammation and mucinous infiltrate; in some individuals with large masses on digits, surgery is required.

A similar pattern of pretibial mucin deposition in euthyroid patients has been associated with venous stasis and may respond to compression therapies, as discussed in Chapter 15.

Thyroid acropachy

Clubbing of digits with increased nail curvature may cause concern, as it has a number of other causes, including bronchial neoplasia (see Ch. 29). However, it is a recognized, although usually not severe, feature of Graves disease (Fig. 12.4).

Hypothyroidism

A wide spectrum of skin changes occur in hypothyroidism (Table 12.1), and these contribute to a typical 'myxedema facies'. Lethargy and stiffness may also contribute to the rather expressionless appearance. Histologically, there is a mucinous infiltrate in the skin. The cutaneous features (Figs 12.5–12.8) include dry, coarse skin, which may appear ichthyotic; diffuse alopecia with coarse hair; loss of lateral eyebrows (also seen due to aging); puffiness of the face and hands; periorbital edema; excoriations due to itch; and palmar hyperkeratosis, which may rarely be the presenting feature. Carotenemia may be prominent. Hyperlipidemia is frequent, but uncommonly at a level sufficient to cause skin lesions. Carpal tunnel syndrome may occur. Treatment is by administration of thyroxine to achieve normal serum levels.

SKIN SIGNS OF DIABETES

Numerous skin lesions may be associated with diabetes or its treatment (Table 12.2). Many of these are not specific and are discussed elsewhere, such as cutaneous xanthomas (Ch. 11), scleredema (Ch. 11), arterial disease (Ch. 15), lipodystrophies (Ch. 22), and drug reactions (Ch. 18). Vitiligo is increased in frequency but is discussed in detail in Chapter 21. Perforating disorders are discussed in the section on renal disease in this chapter.

Table 12.1	**CUTANEOUS FEATURES RELATED TO ABNORMALITIES OF THYROID HORMONE LEVELS**	
Feature	**Thyrotoxicosis**	**Hypothyroidism**
Skin	Soft, smooth, velvety, warm Palmar erythema, facial flushing Pruritus Hyperpigmentation Pretibial myxedema[a] (May also be features of associated autoimmune diseases, e.g. vitiligo, urticaria)	Pale, cold, scaly, wrinkled Puffy edema of hands, face, and eyelids Pruritus (due to xerosis or asteatotic eczema) Ivory-yellow color (in part due to carotenemia) Purpura and ecchymoses Xanthomatosis (secondary to hyperlipidemia)
Sweating	Increased	Decreased
Nails	Fast growth Soft nails, koilonychia, distal onycholysis Thyroid acropachy[a]	Slow nail growth Brittle and striated nails
Hair	Fine thin hair, diffuse alopecia Loss of pubic, axillary, and facial hair Loss of lateral eyebrows	Coarse hair, diffuse alopecia

[a]Resulting from autoimmune thyrotoxicosis; not a feature of other reasons for elevated thyroid hormone levels.

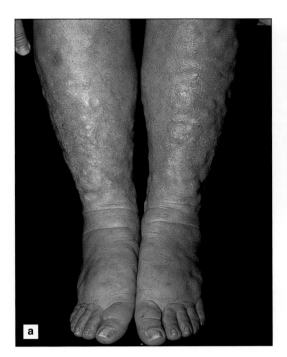

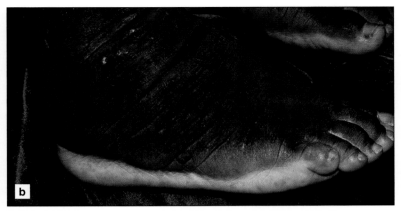

Figure 12.2 Pretibial myxedema in thyrotoxicosis. Deposition of mucin in this condition is often variable in degree, leading to a cobblestoned appearance of the lower legs. Toes are also often affected. The patient shown in (**b**) shows an interesting cut-off at the Wallace line, an area that may be a junction between areas of lymphatic drainage. This pattern may also occur in patients who have idiopathic pretibial myxedema.

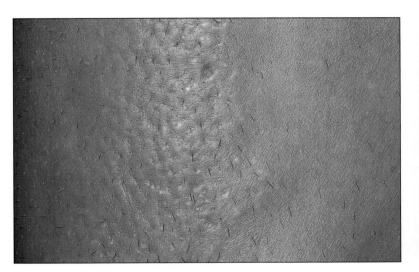

Figure 12.3 Pretibial myxedema demonstrating the peau d'orange appearance that is typical of diffuse cutaneous mucin deposition (see also scleredema, Fig. 11.54).

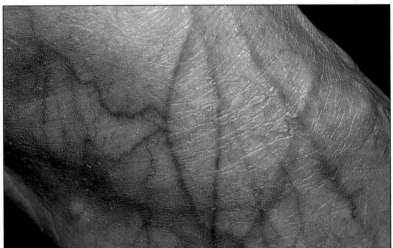

Figure 12.5 Acquired ichthyosis or dry skin occurs in numerous conditions, but thyroid function should always be tested in such cases, as ichthyosis may occur in both hyper- and (as shown here) hypothyroidism.

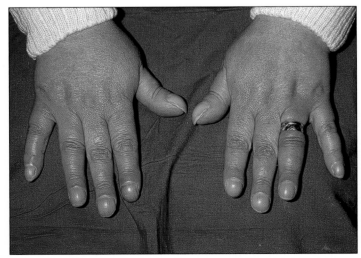

Figure 12.4 Mild clubbing of the nails in thyrotoxicosis, a condition known as thyroid acropachy. The combination of acropachy with exophthalmos and pretibial myxedema is known as the Diamond triad.

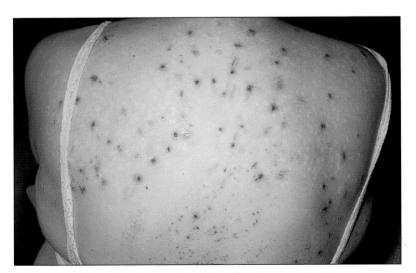

Figure 12.6 Excoriations in a patient with previously unrecognized hypothyroidism. Note the relative sparing over the lower scapulae where the patient cannot reach; this is known as the butterfly sign (more dramatically illustrated in Fig. 12.60) and proves that the eroded areas are secondary to scratching.

209

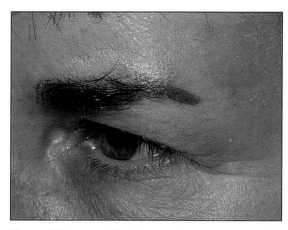

Figure 12.7 Loss of the lateral eyebrow may occur in the elderly, without pathologic significance. This loss in a young patient, who has tried to conceal it with cosmetics, is likely to be relevant. This patient also had excoriations similar to those of the patient in Fig. 12.6, with borderline low thyroxine level and elevated thyroid-stimulating hormone ('compensated hypothyroidism'), and her itch resolved after starting thyroxine treatment.

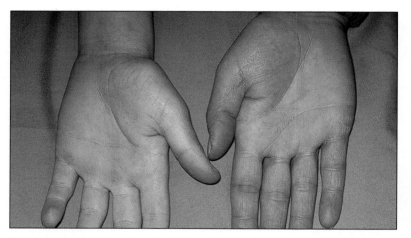

Figure 12.8 Hypothyroidism in a teenaged boy (left) who was referred due to eyelid edema but also had dramatic palmar carotenemia (shown with a normal hand for comparison).

Infections

Infections of various types may occur, several of which are probably not increased in frequency but are more resistant to standard therapy compared with the situation in healthy individuals.

- Bacterial—checking a urinalysis for glucose is prudent in patients with episodic staphylococcal furunculosis (see Fig. 24.10). Infection of foot ulceration is particularly important (discussed later). Malignant otitis externa, a severe invasive *Pseudomonas* infection of the ear, is rare but is strongly linked with diabetes (see Fig. 24.38).
- *Candida*—recurrent vulval candidiasis should always raise the suspicion of diabetes; it is the usual cause of vulval itch in diabetes. Flexures may also be affected (intertrigo).
- Other fungi—dermatophyte infections may possibly be increased in frequency, and may occasionally be extensive; more important is the fact that tinea pedis may predispose to cellulitis of the lower leg, and may be unrecognized if chronic or if it occurs in the neuropathic foot. Some

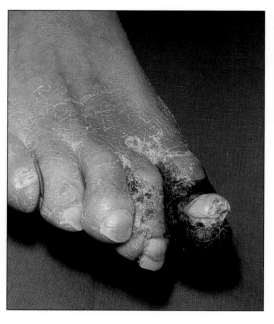

Figure 12.9 Gangrene of the hallux in a diabetic patient. This patient also had well-marked red streaks up the leg, and impaired glycemic control, due to secondary infection with lymphangitis.

Table 12.2 CUTANEOUS FEATURES ASSOCIATED WITH DIABETES

Feature	Comments
Infections	Mainly bacterial (furunculosis) and candidiasis; pseudomonal otitis externa is rare but more specifically diabetes-related, and rare fungal infections such as mucormycosis are more common
Peripheral vascular and small-vessel disease	See Chapter 15 for details of skin features of vascular disease
Neuropathy	Usually presents on the sole of the foot with punched-out ulceration over a bony prominence or area of trauma from footwear
Itch	Often said to be a feature of diabetes but actually uncommon, other than indirectly (e.g. vulval candidiasis)
Necrobiosis lipoidica	Uncommon, but about two-thirds of individuals with this have diabetes (see text for details)
Granuloma annulare variants	A link with diabetes probably exists only for deep, systemic, perforating, and possibly generalized variants
Perforating disorders	Perforating folliculitis, reactive perforating collagenosis
Xanthomas	Related to associated hyperlipidemia
Scleredema	A rare complication; see cutaneous mucinoses, Chapter 11
Drug-related	For example insulin injection site reactions, dry skin due to hydroxymethylglutaryl-CoA reductase inhibitors (statins), several patterns of rash due to sulfonylureas (see Ch. 18)
Features of associated autoimmune disease	For example vitiligo, features of thyroid disease

rare infections, such as mucormycosis and other zygomycoses, probably do occur with increased frequency in diabetic patients.

Neurovascular changes and the diabetic foot

Diabetes predisposes to atheroma of large vessels, and also to micro-angiopathy. The most frequent site at which these changes are of dermatologic importance is the foot, where three factors may combine to cause severe morbidity (Figs 12.9–12.11).

- Neuropathy—leads to lack of awareness of pain, for example from poorly fitting footwear, and also to shape changes that will alter weight-bearing pressure points; both of these contribute to risk of ulceration.
- Vasculopathy—both large- and small-vessel disease predispose to poor healing, ulceration, and gangrene; cholesterol emboli from proximal atheroma may also occur.
- Infection—bacterial infection of ulcerated or gangrenous areas (Fig. 12.9) adds to the problems of healing; tinea pedis may be less apparent in the context of impaired sensation.

Ulceration is the most important complication, which is usually associated with reduced sensation and variably with signs of vascular compromise. Impaired skin sensation increases the risk of penetrating injury, but the ulcers often arise under areas of callosity that are due to the combination of rigid keratin (because of glycosylation) and altered weight-bearing (due to foot deformity caused by neuropathy affecting the intrinsic foot muscles). Regular foot examination is important in diabetic patients, with particular attention to treatment of tinea pedis, checking sensation, and checking that there are no irregular areas within the sole of footwear. Special footwear may need to be made to avoid pressure, or lightweight casts designed to remove pressure from areas of neuropathic ulceration.

Necrobiosis lipoidica

Two-thirds of individuals with necrobiosis lipoidica have diabetes, and a further 20% develop it later or have a positive family history of diabetes; conversely, 0.3% of diabetic patients will develop this complication. In such cases, it is known as necrobiosis lipoidica diabeticorum (NLD); however, most discussion of NLD is equally applicable to non-diabetic necrobiosis lipoidica. The lesions are most frequent on the shin, with a female predominance, and bilateral disease in 10–20%. Active lesions have a yellowish-colored atrophic center with visible cutaneous blood vessels, and an erythematous inflammatory border (Figs 12.12–12.14).

Topical corticosteroids may have a role in reducing this inflammatory component, but they should be used with care in view of the central atrophy, which can be worsened by excessive topical steroid administration. A variety of agents with antiplatelet effects have been used thera-

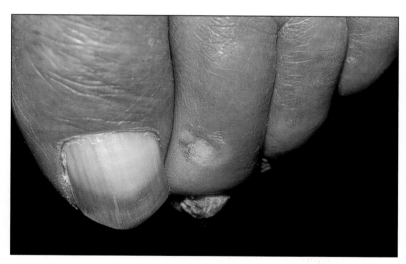

Figure 12.10 Smooth, shiny, red skin, with a small digital ulcer, and a 'Terry nail' (pale, with a distal band of reddish brown color) due to chronic renal failure. This combination is highly suspicious of diabetic complications.

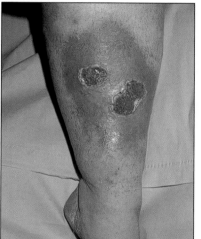

Figure 12.12 Ulceration is a feature in a minority of cases of necrobiosis lipoidica, usually in larger lesions at areas prone to injury (the shin is the most common site for this disorder). Secondary infection of ulcerated areas should be treated promptly, especially in diabetic patients, and adherent dressings should be avoided, as they may cause further damage when removed from the fragile atrophic skin around the ulcers.

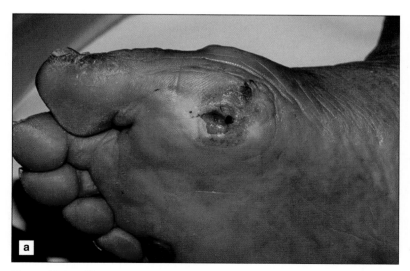

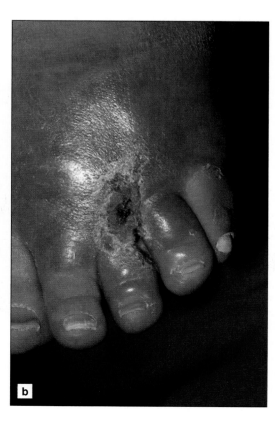

Figure 12.11 Neuropathic ulceration of the foot. (**a**) Neuropathy in a diabetic patient. This patient requires careful attention to his footwear, and regular review to exclude secondary infection (which may be asymptomatic due to the neuropathy). (**b**) An example in which infection has occurred; this patient has a toe web sinus due to spina bifida and has developed local cellulitis, which would normally be painful at this site even before development of redness.

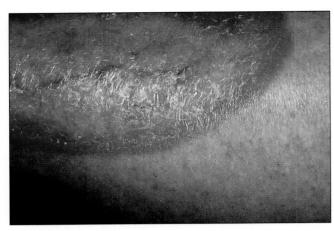

Figure 12.13 A typical lesion of necrobiosis lipoidica in which there is cutaneous atrophy, telangiectasia (easily visible dermal vessels), and a background yellowish color. (From Lawrence CM, Cox NH. Physical Signs in Dermatology, 2nd edn. London: Mosby, 2002.)

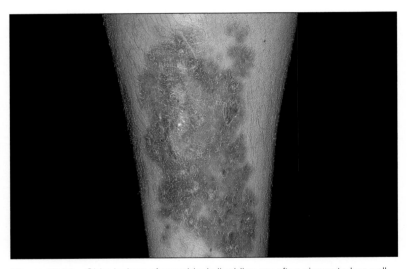

Figure 12.14 Older lesions of necrobiosis lipoidica are often pigmented as well as obviously atrophic, but often lose the more inflamed appearance of more recent lesions.

peutically, with mixed results, based on the fact that there are changes in the vessel wall intima in diabetes and also increased platelet aggregation. Photochemotherapy (PUVA) has been used with success in several recent reports. Excision and grafting can be effective, but there is potential for poor healing and graft failure, so this procedure is usually reserved for patients with recurrent or severe ulceration of the atrophic lesions, in whom the balance of risks and benefit is most favorable. Cultured tissue grafts may be useful for ulceration but are expensive.

Other cutaneous features of diabetes
Granuloma annulare
The association between granuloma annulare (GA) and diabetes has been the subject of debate for some time. This disorder is clinically distinct from NLD but has many similar histologic features, in particular the presence of necrobiotic collagen. The typical clinical appearance is of a small plaque that gradually expands; the border is raised and thickened, often with a cobblestoned morphology, whereas the central skin may be slightly pigmented or purplish in color. Lesions tend to occur over bony prominences of the knuckles, elbows, knees, or dorsum of the foot. Large studies of this disorder do not confirm a significant association between this 'ordinary' pattern of GA and diabetes, and investigation is not usually performed in the typical young and otherwise well patient who develops this disorder. There is greater uncertainty about patients with some rare forms of GA, in whom it appears prudent to perform urinalysis.

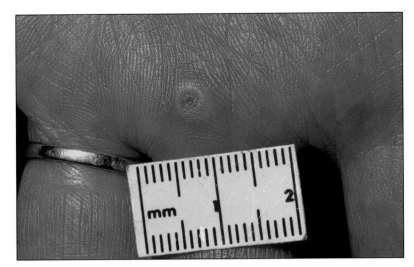

Figure 12.15 Perforating granuloma annulare (GA). The palm is an uncommon site for GA, and perforating disorders generally are associated with diabetes; both the atypical site and variant of GA therefore suggest this possibility.

Diffuse GA is an uncommon variant that presents as myriad tiny papules, which usually show some degree of grouping and sometimes a vaguely annular patterning. This usually affects older individuals, and the suspicion of an increased frequency of diabetes may simply reflect the predominant age group.

Perforating GA is a rare variant in which the necrobiotic collagen is expelled through the surface of the skin (Fig. 12.15). The lesions are often acral, and are scabbed or discharging papules. About 30% of patients have diabetes.

Deep and systemic variants of GA are rare but appear to be associated with higher risk of diabetes.

Treatment of GA can be difficult. Topical corticosteroids may reduce inflammation in the border of active lesions, but many lesions are seen at a static and asymptomatic phase, in which case active treatment is often not required: about 50% resolve spontaneously within 2 years. As with NLD, photochemotherapy can be quite useful (usually for disseminated or extensive plaque forms of GA).

Diabetic dermopathy
This disorder is common in diabetes but is found fairly commonly in other endocrine disorders, and occasionally in healthy individuals. It consists of small, red papules that subside to leave small, brown, atrophic patches (Fig. 12.16). Within the skin in these areas, there is evidence of thick-walled blood vessels, but this is seen to some extent in the skin of the lower leg in all individuals. One theory is that the disorder is due to minor trauma, in which case the inherently abnormal vasculature in diabetic patients may lead to a more obvious residual defect compared with non-diabetic skin.

Stiff skin, cheirarthropathy, and similar disorders
An interesting phenomenon in diabetes is the development of stiff, thick skin that resembles the changes in scleroderma but without the vascular and other features of this disorder (Figs 12.17 and 12.18). This is most apparent at acral sites, and may be associated with limited joint mobility (also known as cheirarthropathy) due to the abnormal collagen. The physical sign that demonstrates this entity is known as the prayer sign. When the two palms are pressed together at 90° to the forearms, affected patients cannot oppose the fingers and palms fully. The condition is particularly prominent in patients with poor glycemic control over many years. The proposed mechanism is an increased cross-linking of collagen, known as non-enzymatic glycosylation (NEG), which produces stiffer collagen. In support of this concept, it has been demonstrated that NEG of skin collagen is related to duration of diabetes and to other features of poor glycemic control.

Diabetic finger pebbles (Fig. 12.19) are another interesting skin texture change in diabetic patients.

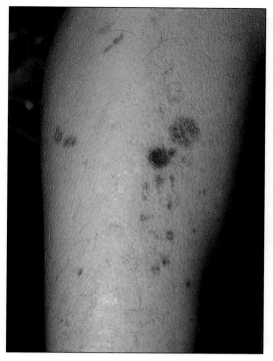

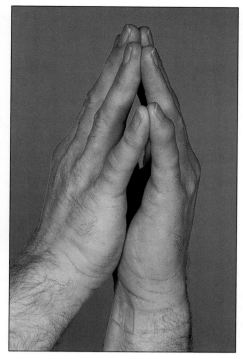

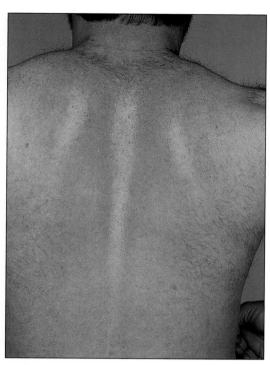

Figure 12.16 Diabetic dermopathy (skin spots). These small, brown lesions are relatively non-specific; the extent of lesions in this case is uncommon (except in diabetes). They probably represent microvascular damage and tend to occur at sites of minor trauma.

Figure 12.17 Cheirarthropathy prayer sign. (Courtesy of Dr. S. Russell.)

Figure 12.18 Sclerederma in a patient with cheirarthropathy. (Courtesy of Dr. S. Russell.)

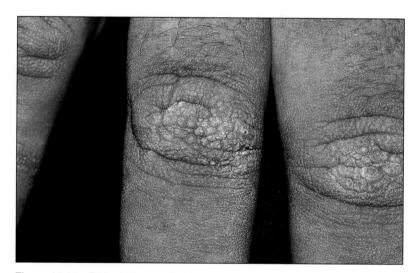

Figure 12.19 Diabetic finger pebbles are an exaggeration of the skin markings over the knuckles and on the dorsal aspect of the terminal phalanges. They are more cobblestoned than knuckle pads (Ch. 22), with which they may be confused.

Diabetic bullosis

This is a poorly defined entity (or entities, as various intraepidermal and subepidermal sites of blistering have been described). Blisters are usually acral, vary in size but are usually of diameter one to a few centimeters, arise on a non-inflamed background, and may be induced by trauma or by sunlight in some individuals. Diagnosis is largely by exclusion of some common blistering conditions (pompholyx eczema and friction blisters), mechanobullous disorders (inherited types of epidermolysis bullosa), porphyrias (especially if photosensitive), and immunobullous disorders (especially epidermolysis bullosa acquisita).

PRACTICE POINTS

- In patients with recurrent furunculosis, test the urine for glucose.
- Particular attention must be paid to the feet of patients with diabetes: to treat any infection, to detect any sensory loss or vascular compromise, and to ensure that footwear is well fitting.
- Itch, other than due to localized vulval candidiasis or due to statin-induced skin dryness, is not a common feature of diabetes and requires consideration of other causes.
- Painful otitis externa in a diabetic patient may be due to potentially highly invasive *Pseudomonas* infection and requires urgent attention.

DISORDERS OF PITUITARY AND ADRENAL FUNCTION

Hypopituitarism

The effects of hypopituitarism depend on the cause, which may include infarction (Sheehan syndrome, Fig. 12.20), infiltrations such as sarcoidosis or tumors, and iatrogenic (surgery) and idiopathic causes. In general, thyroid-stimulating hormone (TSH) is relatively well maintained compared with, for example, the sex stimulating hormones. Thus the skin in patients with hypopituitarism is usually fine, smooth, and 'infantile', but may be more ichthyotic and scaly if there is significant thyroid under-activity (Fig. 12.20). Loss or absence of secondary sexual hair is typical, due to reduced gonadal stimulation. Pallor is characteristic, due to the reduced levels of proopiomelanocortin, a pituitary protein that is cleaved to form hormones that would normally stimulate pigmentation; these are adrenocorticotropic hormone (ACTH), α-melanocyte-stimulating hormone (α-MSH), and β-lipotropin.

Cushing syndrome

This may occur due to adrenal hyperplasia, adrenal carcinoma or benign adenoma, a pituitary tumor secreting ACTH, or other neoplasm (usually of lung) secreting ACTH. The adrenal causes usually give a mixed picture

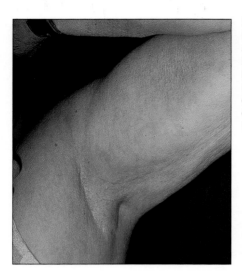

Figure 12.20 Hypopituitarism. Loss of secondary sexual hair and soft, fine skin produce an infantile appearance. This patient had a history of severe blood loss in pregnancy, a situation in which diagnosis of pituitary failure is often delayed for several years (Sheehan syndrome).

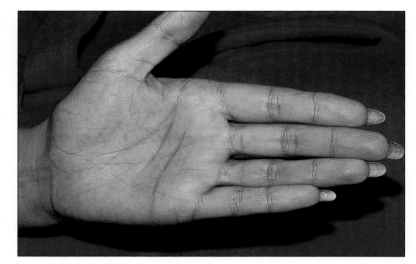

Figure 12.21 Addison disease causing increased pigmentation of palmar creases. This patient had a history of previous tuberculosis, which caused initial concern about the possibility of tuberculous adrenal disease, but also had positive autoantibodies and subsequently became thyrotoxic.

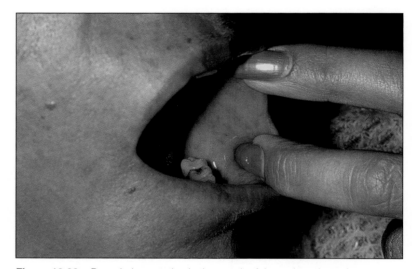

Figure 12.22 Buccal pigmentation in the mouth of the patient shown in Fig. 12.21.

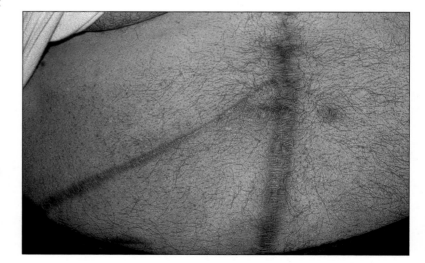

Figure 12.23 Pigmentation of scars is a particular feature of Addison disease due to adrenal failure or surgery.

of increased glucocorticoid, mineralocorticoid, and androgenic hormones. Iatrogenic Cushing syndrome is due to administration of glucocorticoids or, rarely, to excessive use of topical steroids on skin or by inhalation.

The characteristic clinical picture is of truncal obesity and a 'moon' face. Hypertrichosis and telangiectasia of the face are typical, and other features of virilization may occur with the primary adrenal causes. Striae of the skin are frequent, and a monomorphic pustular pattern of acne may occur, especially when exogenous topical steroids are implicated.

Addison disease

Adrenal failure may be due to infarction (e.g. in Henoch–Schönlein purpura) or infiltration (tumor and tuberculosis), or be iatrogenic (surgery), but most instances are of idiopathic autoimmune etiology. There is an association with vitiligo in 15% of the autoimmune cases.

The resulting cutaneous feature is excessive pigmentation, due to a compensatory increase in ACTH and the other pigmenting pituitary hormones discussed earlier. Pigmentation is most apparent in skin creases, scars, friction sites, and genital and areolar skin, but diffuse pigmentation and increased pigmentation of hair may be prominent in some individuals (Figs 12.21–12.23). Spotty intraoral pigmentation of the buccal and gingival mucosa is characteristic. The same, but particularly prominent, pigmentation may be seen after adrenalectomy for Cushing syndrome in the small proportion of patients who develop an ACTH-producing pituitary adenoma (Nelson syndrome).

Acromegaly

This is usually due to increased secretion of growth hormone and insulin-like growth factor-1 from pituitary adenoma. In children, this causes gigantism, but in adults the typical feature is slowly increasing coarseness of the facial features and enlargement of extremities. The skin becomes thickened with increased furrowing, especially of the brow (cutis verticis gyrata, Ch. 22). Increased pigmentation and hypertrichosis also occur.

OTHER DISORDERS OF THE ENDOCRINE SYSTEM

Acanthosis nigricans

Acanthosis nigricans (AN) is best known as a paraneoplastic phenomenon (see later), but this is very rare; much more commonly, AN occurs in relation to endocrine disease. It can also occur as an idiopathic or hereditary disorder.

The endocrine associations have been grouped together under the term HAIR-AN (hyperandrogenism, insulin resistance, AN). Insulin resistance leads to chronic hyperinsulinemia, which in turn stimulates increased ovarian production of testosterone and also has growth-promoting effects on fibroblasts and keratinocytes to produce the clinical features.

Insulin resistance may occur as primary and secondary forms; it is common in obesity, which explains AN in this context. The primary types

have been divided into type A (young patients with severe AN and hyperandrogenism, who have decreased numbers or function of insulin receptors) and type B (older women with less severe AN, who have blocking autoantibodies that bind to the insulin receptors).

Other causes of hyperandrogenism, such as polycystic ovary, ovarian dermoid, and other ovarian lesions, may also cause this syndrome, as may

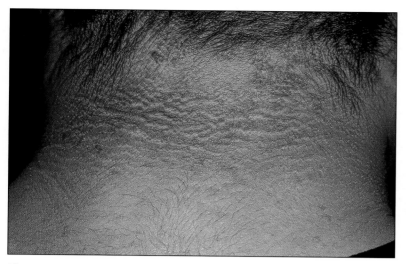

Figure 12.24   Brownish-colored warty hyperkeratosis on the nape of the neck, in a patient with acanthosis nigricans and insulin resistance.

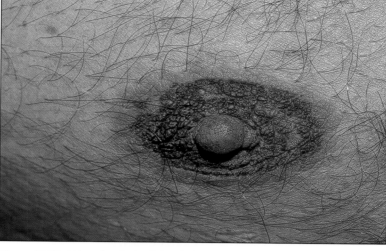

Figure 12.26   Hyperkeratosis of the nipple is not uncommon in elderly men, but is usually a pale brown, greasy color. This dark-brown pigmentation is clearly abnormal, and was associated with other features of acanthosis nigricans.

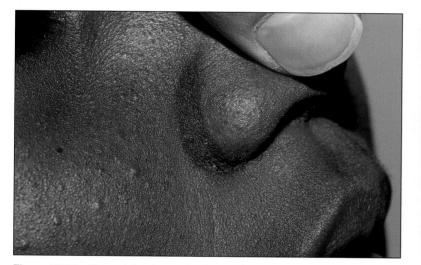

Figure 12.25   Pigmentation in acanthosis nigricans is most marked at flexural sites. This pattern of well-demarcated pigmentation in the skin crease around the alae nasi is unusual and striking, and led to a diagnosis of hyperinsulinemia in this child.

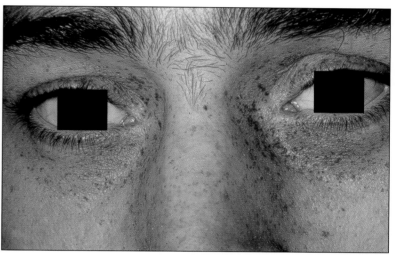

Figure 12.27   Peutz–Jeghers syndrome. Dark-brown lentigines around the mouth and eyes are typical. This patient had a history of intussusception in childhood.

other causes of insulin resistance, such as lipoatrophic diabetes and pineal lesions. Drugs such as estrogens, corticosteroids, nicotinic acid, and recently somatotropin have been documented as causes of AN.

The clinical features are coffee-colored or gray-brown velvety and papillomatous thickening of the skin around the nape of the neck, axillae, antecubital fossae, and groin (Figs 12.24–12.26). In the malignant type, palms, soles, and oral and ocular mucosae are also often involved; this should be suspected in older patients with weight loss, whereas the insulin-resistant patients are most often either young or the obese elderly.

Treatment is that of the underlying disorder where possible, weight loss, and topical agents such as emollients or keratolytics. Metformin may help to normalize the background endocrine abnormalities.

Multiple endocrine neoplasia syndromes

Three syndromes of multiple endocrine neoplasia (MEN) may have features of dermatologic relevance over and above the features of the individual endocrinopathies. These are known as MEN 1 (multiple endocrine adenomatosis), MEN 2a (Sipple syndrome), and MEN 2b (multiple mucosal neuromas syndrome). Mucosal neuromas and marfanoid habitus are particular features of MEN 2b, with medullary carcinoma of thyroid and pheochromocytomas. Notalgia paresthetica (see Ch. 9) has been reported in association with MEN 2a. Facial angio-fibromas and collagenomas similar to those of tuberous sclerosis have also been reported in MEN 1.

PRACTICE POINTS

- Loss of secondary sexual hair is very suggestive of hypopituitarism.
- Addison disease may have a very gradual onset; if suspected from palmar crease pigmentation, inspect the buccal mucosa and any old scars for supportive features.
- Most acanthosis nigricans is not due to malignant disease; suspect endocrine abnormality in young overweight patients, and malignancy in old patients with sudden weight loss.

DERMATOSES ASSOCIATED WITH GASTROINTESTINAL, HEPATOBILIARY, AND NUTRITIONAL DISEASE

Disorders associated with polyposis or adenocarcinomas
Peutz–Jeghers syndrome

Peutz–Jeghers syndrome (see also Ch. 19, and Figs 19.50 and 19.51) is manifest dermatologically by lentigines (dark, freckle-like lesions) of lips and mouth, eyelids, and extremities (Figs 12.27 and 12.28). Intestinal polyps may occur at any location except the esophagus, and usually present because of pain or bleeding; intussusception occurs in almost half

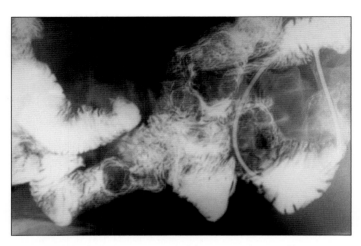

Figure 12.28 Small bowel enema of the patient shown in Fig. 12.27, demonstrating numerous filling defects due to intestinal polyps.

the affected patients. Malignancy has been estimated to occur in 2%, but prophylactic bowel resections are not advised, as the polyps are scattered widely throughout the gastrointestinal tract. There is also a five- to tenfold increased risk of testicular and ovarian neoplasia. An important differential diagnosis is Laugier–Hunziker syndrome (Ch. 29), a cause of multiple lentigines on the lip that occurs mainly in older patients; nail pigmentation is also apparent, and bowel investigations are not required.

Gardner syndrome
This consists of epidermoid cysts, fibrous tumors and desmoids, and dental and jaw lesions (osteomas in 75%, dental cysts, and abnormal teeth), associated with colonic polyps and carcinomas. Pigmentation of the ocular fundus is found in 90% of cases but is asymptomatic. The polyps occur in a pattern similar to familial polyposis, but are preceded by the cutaneous cysts, which are first apparent in early childhood.

Cowden syndrome
Cowden syndrome (see Fig. 23.27) consists of multiple hamartomas, and is associated with tumors of breast (30–50% of female patients) and thyroid (10% of female patients), as well as colonic carcinoma. The main dermatologic features are facial trichilemmomas, fibromas, and oral mucosal papillomatosis; keratoses may also be present on the dorsum or palms of the hands, and lipomas are also frequent.

Neurofibromatosis
Neurofibromatosis (see Ch. 9) is a common genodermatosis, which is autosomal dominant but with about 50% of cases being sporadic new mutations (all dermatologists occasionally see new referred cases because of multiple 'moles' that are actually neurofibromas). Associated skin pigmentary abnormalities are diagnostically useful, and include multiple café au lait patches and axillary freckling (Crowe sign). Neurofibromas may occur in the gastrointestinal tract but are usually asymptomatic.

Canada–Cronkhite syndrome
This is a rare disorder that is associated with generalized gastrointestinal polyposis. The cutaneous features are a triad of pigmented patches (mainly on hands and arms), diffuse alopecia, and nail plate shedding and splitting.

Muir–Torre syndrome
This is discussed in Chapter 23.

Disorders associated with vascular lesions
Hereditary hemorrhagic telangiectasia
This is a moderately common, autosomal dominant disorder in which typical punctate and mat-like cutaneous telangiectases usually develop in early adult life (Fig. 15.34). The face and digits are the most commonly

affected sites, including lips, tongue, and conjunctivae. Epistaxis is the most frequent symptom and may occur earlier in childhood; significant gastrointestinal bleeding is unusual before the fourth decade. Large internal vascular malformations may cause shunting, with anemia and high-output cardiac failure; they can be a focus for chronic infection, which is similar to infective endocarditis.

Blue rubber bleb nevus syndrome
This is less common, but gastrointestinal bleeding is the most frequent internal manifestation. The skin lesions are larger, blue-colored, compressible, cavernous angiomas, which are typically tender on direct pressure. Similar lesions occur throughout the gastrointestinal tract, especially the small bowel. From a dermatologic point of view, it is impossible to distinguish the skin lesions from multiple glomangiomas; in the absence of any history of gastrointestinal bleeding, the presence of oral mucosal lesions may be a useful indicator of which patients to investigate.

Pseudoxanthoma elasticum
This is the term used for a group of disorders that are characterized by yellowish, cobblestoned patches of skin in flexures and sides of the neck, likened to a plucked chicken appearance (Ch. 22). Some forms have a marked tendency to gastrointestinal hemorrhage, which is caused by a generalized blood vessel defect in which abnormal elastic fibers and subsequent calcification reduce contractility of arterial walls.

Ehlers–Danlos syndromes
These are a group of inherited defects of collagen (Ch. 22). Some, particularly type IV, have a strong predisposition to hemorrhage in various organs, including the gastrointestinal tract. Other gastrointestinal complications include diverticula, dilatation, and even rupture of the bowel, and diaphragmatic disease causing hiatus hernia and eventration.

Disorders associated with inflammatory bowel disease
Disorders associated with inflammatory bowel disease (IBD) can be categorized as shown in Table 12.3.

Reactive lesions
Most of the indirect reactive associations between IBD and the skin are more frequently linked with ulcerative colitis than with Crohn disease. Pyoderma gangrenosum is the most striking; it occurs in 1–2% of patients with ulcerative colitis, and is five times as common in ulcerative colitis compared with Crohn disease. Others include erythema nodosum, Sweet disease, pustular dermatoses, and vasculitis. As with pyoderma gangrenosum, all these have other non-gastrointestinal causes, which may need to be considered. However, each of them occurs mainly during periods of exacerbation of IBD, so the link with underlying bowel disease is usually readily apparent.

Erythema nodosum and Sweet disease are discussed in Chapter 22 and Chapter 14, respectively.

Pustular eruptions in association with IBD may be a variant of pyoderma gangrenosum. Histology shows neutrophilic abscesses in the epidermis. Vasculitis may occur in association with IBD, and may be pustular (Fig. 12.29). In patients with ulcerative colitis, this is usually of leukocytoclastic type, presenting as palpable purpura due to immune complex deposition, whereas patients with Crohn disease may develop polyarteritis nodosa.

Crohn disease
Patients with Crohn disease may have direct cutaneous involvement or indirect associations that also occur in other IBDs, such as pyoderma gangrenosum.

Cutaneous lesions of Crohn disease (Figs 12.30–12.33) include those in direct continuity with the gastrointestinal tract (oral or perineal lesions); more rarely, 'metastatic' Crohn disease develops, in which skin lesions occur in skin without apparent direct connection with the gut, usually occurring in the region of the umbilicus or groin. Those at the umbilicus may in fact be in continuity with the bowel by virtue of residual embryologic connections. All these have a granulomatous histology (see Ch. 11).

Table 12.3   DISORDERS ASSOCIATED WITH INFLAMMATORY BOWEL DISEASE

Feature	Comments
Reactive lesions	These include pyoderma gangrenosum, Sweet disease, pustules, vasculitis, and erythema nodosum. They are most commonly associated with ulcerative colitis rather than Crohn disease, and most (especially erythema nodosum and pustular vasculitis) occur in association with exacerbation of the associated bowel disease. Most examples have a neutrophilic infiltrate histologically (Ch. 14); a granulomatous histology, as occurs in Crohn disease itself, is not a feature.
Lesions occurring as direct extension from the bowel	This occurs mainly in Crohn disease, typically as fissures and fistula in the perianal area; oral lesions include ulceration, fissures, and cobblestoned thickening.
Cutaneous lesions of the associated bowel disorder	Crohn disease may occur at skin sites other than those in direct continuity with the bowel, known sometimes as 'metastatic' Crohn disease (see text of this chapter).
Skin lesions related to malabsorption	Discussed in the text of this chapter.
Skin lesions related to treatment	These include drug reactions (such as urticaria with sulfasalazine, side effects of systemic steroids), plus problems such as stoma dermatoses (e.g. irritant or allergic contact dermatitis).
Other associated dermatoses	Psoriasis has been demonstrated to be more common in patients with Crohn disease. Some blistering disorders (Ch. 16) have been linked with inflammatory bowel disease (IBD), for example epidermolysis bullosa acquisita with Crohn disease and linear IgA disease with ulcerative colitis. Ulcerative colitis is linked with several immunologic disorders, some of which may be expressed in the skin (e.g. sarcoidosis).
Associated oral lesions	In addition to the oral lesions of Crohn disease (above), non-specific aphthous ulceration occurs in association with (usually active) IBD; however, it also occurs in other bowel disorders, such as celiac disease, as well as in many other situations.

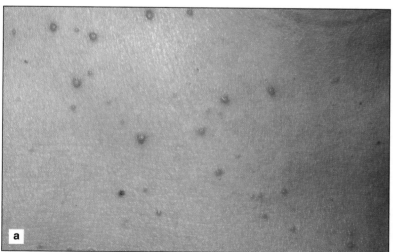

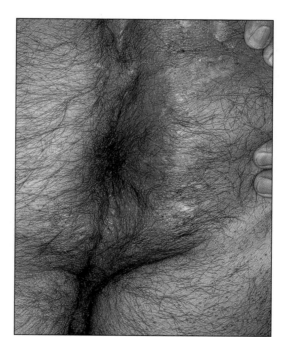

Figure 12.30   Crohn disease affecting the skin of the buttocks, with multiple sinuses and scarring. This patient had a lesion of pyoderma gangrenosum when first seen, and developed inflammatory plaques with the appearance of Sweet disease on the trunk (with the novel feature of a Koebner reaction into recent scars).

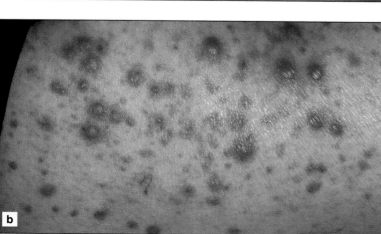

Figure 12.29   Pustular eruptions in patients with an acute exacerbation of inflammatory bowel disease. This type of lesion may be clinically bland (**a**) or much more inflammatory (**b**), in which case it is best regarded as a type of pyoderma gangrenosum or pustular vasculitis.

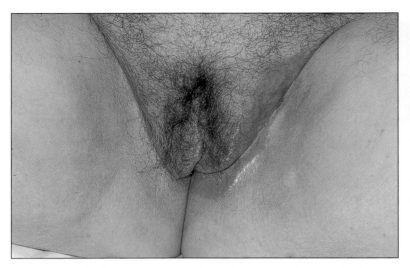

Figure 12.31 Crohn disease affecting the groin flexures. Inflamed and indurated granulomatous areas, often with discharge and sinuses, are typical of Crohn disease in the perineum and groin.

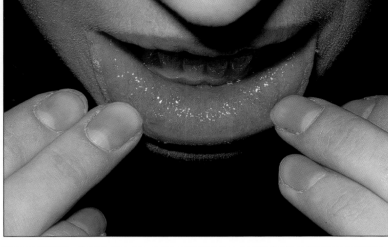

Figure 12.33 Crohn disease of the oral mucosa. In this fairly quiescent example, there is a granular cobblestoned appearance. Some patients have more aggressive fissured and ulcerated plaque lesions.

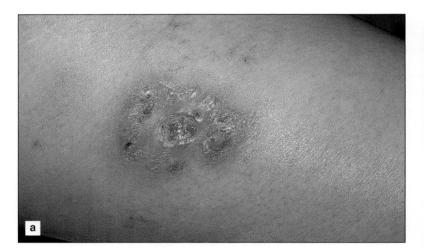

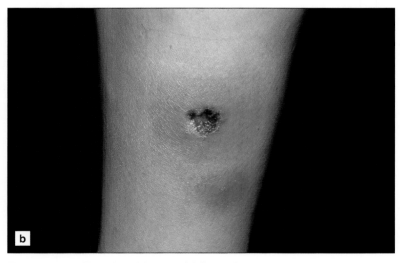

Figure 12.32 Examples of 'metastatic' Crohn disease on the thigh (**a**) and lower leg (**b**). These areas are not contiguous with any gastrointestinal lesions. Biopsy is often required to distinguish between the granulomatous infiltrate of Crohn disease (as in these cases), compared with the neutrophilic infiltrate of pyoderma gangrenosum that may occur as a consequence of inflammatory bowel disease (see Figs 12.29 and 14.57–14.64).

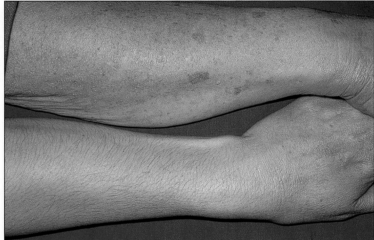

Figure 12.34 A patient with malignancy of the biliary tract causing obstructive jaundice. The yellow color of her arm is clearly apparent by comparison with the arm of her nurse.

This may be difficult to distinguish from a disorder known as orofacial granulomatosis, in which food allergies can sometimes be demonstrated (e.g. to potato, chocolate, and other specific foods). This may actually be a localized form of Crohn disease, and some patients who appear to have localized oral lesions do develop intestinal Crohn disease at a later stage.

Treatment of cutaneous Crohn disease is primarily aimed at the underlying disease; in severe cases, this may include infliximab, azathioprine, or methotrexate. Topical or intralesional corticosteroids may also be useful for localized granulomatous areas.

Cutaneous signs of hepatobiliary disease

Jaundice is the cardinal sign of biliary disease (Figs 12.34 and 12.35) however, there are other reasons for a yellow color in the skin (see Fig. 1.17). Itch is prominent in patients with obstructive causes of jaundice, and is a particular feature of primary biliary cirrhosis. The combination of xanthelasma and jaundice is highly suggestive of primary biliary cirrhosis.

Chronic hepatocellular disease, particularly cirrhosis, is associated with numerous skin changes. Vascular changes include spider nevi (Fig. 12.36) and palmar erythema; purpura may occur due to clotting factor deficiency. Loss of secondary sexual hair is common in men. Pale nail beds may occur due to hypoalbuminemia.

Hyperpigmentation occurs in several forms of cirrhosis but is particularly prominent in primary biliary cirrhosis (Fig. 12.37) and in hemochromatosis.

Perineal lesions are usually fissures or fistulae, which may be multiple. There is associated abscess formation, induration, and scarring, with large fleshy perianal tags.

The oral features include chronic swelling of the lips, and cobblestoned thickening of the mucosa, with granulomatous features on biopsy.

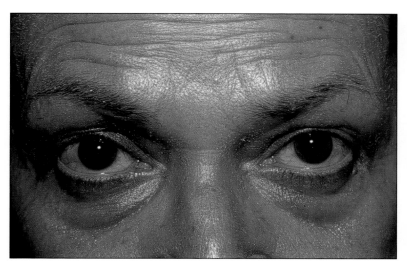

Figure 12.35 Jaundice also causes yellow sclerae of the eye, and this is often the most readily visible abnormality in mild jaundice, as there is no background melanin or vascular pigment to distract the examiner.

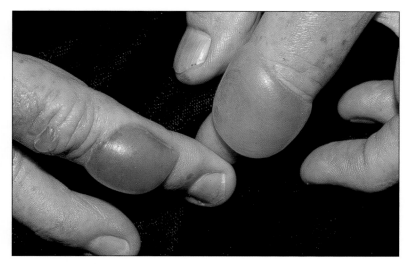

Figure 12.38 Porphyria cutanea tarda, demonstrating unilocular blisters that are usually most prominent on the dorsum of the hands. They leave pigmentation, scarring, and milia as they resolve. The most common trigger for this disorder, which is discussed in more detail in Chapter 17, is excessive alcohol intake.

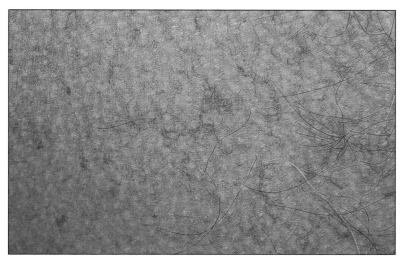

Figure 12.36 Telangiectasia on the chest in a man with alcoholic cirrhosis of the liver.

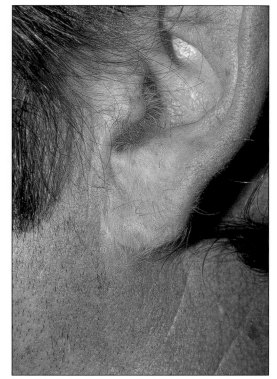

Figure 12.39 A less frequent feature of porphyria cutanea tarda is hypertrichosis; if present, it is usually apparent on the cheeks and lateral forehead area, but in this case was prominent on the earlobe.

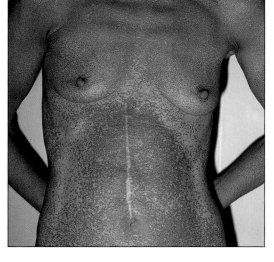

Figure 12.37 Marked pigmentation is a feature of some cirrhotic disorders, such as primary biliary cirrhosis. Jaundice and xanthelasma also occur in this disorder.

Hepatitis B infection may be associated with an urticarial or exanthematous rash, but this is non-specific in morphology, and other viral infections may cause both elevated transaminase levels and urticarial rash.

Hepatitis C virus (HCV) has been the subject of recent interest dermatologically, as it is associated with essential mixed cryoglobulinemia. This disorder causes cold-induced precipitation of serum cryoglobulin and causes vasculitis, which is manifest clinically as palpable purpura (Ch. 14), livedo lesions, urticaria, Raynaud phenomenon, and skin ulceration. Palpable purpura in particular appears to be a stronger feature of HCV-positive compared with HCV-negative cryoglobulinemia. There is also evidence linking HCV with non-familial porphyria cutanea tarda and with lichen planus.

Porphyria cutanea tarda presents as blistering and skin fragility, which is most apparent on the dorsum of the hands, with scarring and pigment disturbance (Figs 12.38 and 12.39). Hepatic iron overload is a feature of all such patients, and elevated liver enzyme and ferritin levels are a frequent feature. This is discussed in more detail in Chapter 17.

Lichen planus (Ch. 8) is associated with liver disease, predominantly with chronic active hepatitis; the strength of this association varies widely between studies from different geographic areas, which may reflect differences in hepatitis C prevalence.

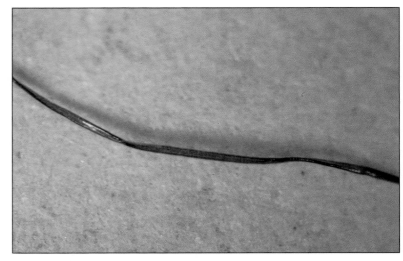

Figure 12.41 Microscopy of a 'corkscrew' hair from a patient with scurvy demonstrates that the hairs are actually multiply kinked rather than forming a neat spiral or corkscrew shape.

Nutritional disorders

Many bowel disorders may lead to malabsorption, resulting in multiple deficiencies of nutrients and vitamins. Additionally, some specific forms of malabsorption occur, such as that of zinc (hereditary acrodermatitis enteropathica, discussed later), and some specific dietary deficiencies (such as ascorbic acid deficiency, leading to scurvy) are also important. Some examples of disorders leading to deficiency, and of specific deficiencies, are provided here.

Celiac disease

This causes malabsorption of many nutrients, and may therefore have several cutaneous findings, such as those of fatty acid deficiency (acquired ichthyosis), iron deficiency anemia (pallor), and zinc deficiency (discussed later). It is also associated with aphthous ulceration.

Scurvy

Ascorbic acid (vitamin C) is essential for synthesis of collagen. Deficiency occurs most commonly in elderly patients with poor diet, especially with low fruit intake, and is probably underestimated. It causes abnormalities of collagen, which are particularly apparent in blood vessels, small peri-follicular hemorrhages being a typical feature (Figs 12.40–12.43). In more advanced scurvy, bleeding from gums and larger sheets of hemorrhage in the skin, which resolve with woody induration, may occur. Teeth may become loose due to defective supporting collagen. Hairs are flattened and irregularly kinked (known as corkscrew hairs), and arise from keratotic follicles. These must be distinguished from rolled or coiled hairs, which occur around friction areas such as the waist (Ch. 28).

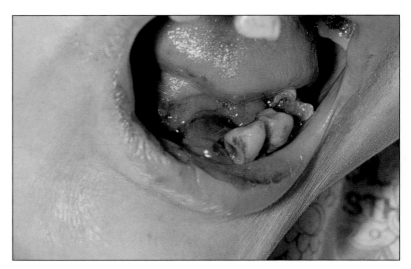

Figure 12.42 Scurvy in a patient with marked self-neglect and anemia. She had loose teeth and bleeding from the gums.

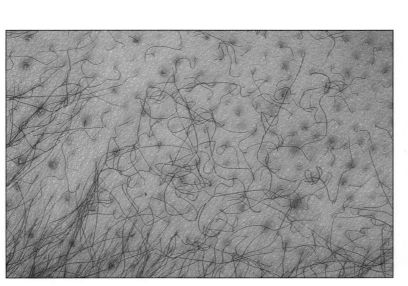

Figure 12.40 Scurvy in a patient with esophageal stricture, with a very limited and mainly fluid diet. Perifollicular papules and keratoses are associated with kinked hairs. This disorder is underestimated in elderly individuals.

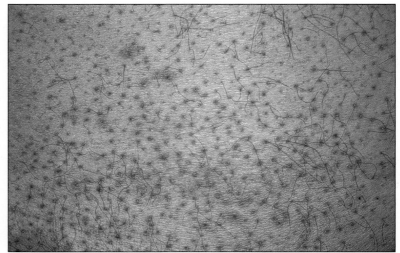

Figure 12.43 Scurvy, demonstrating rather more hemorrhagic follicular lesions. This pattern is often seen on the legs, where gravitational stresses encourage leakage through the abnormal blood-vessel walls.

Zinc deficiency and acrodermatitis enteropathica

Zinc deficiency may occur for dietary reasons in alcoholism, malabsorption, enteral nutrition without supplementation, and protein malnutrition (such as marasmus). The typical eruption is of rather eczematous or erosive appearance but with a strong predilection for the extremities, and perioral and perineal regions.

Acrodermatitis enteropathica is an autosomal recessive disorder of zinc absorption. The rash is the same as in acquired zinc deficiency, and is associated with diarrhea, offensive stools, and eventual growth retardation.

Other nutritional deficiencies

Fatty acid deficiency causes dryness of the skin. It may occur in patients with malabsorption, in whom the combination of acquired ichthyosis and weight loss may suggest lymphoma in the differential diagnosis.

Pernicious anemia (vitamin B_{12} deficiency) is an autoimmune disease that is associated with vitiligo.

Vitamin B complex deficiency usually involves several vitamins rather than isolated deficiencies. Angular cheilitis and sore tongue are typical features, although both have more common causes, such as candidiasis. Nicotinic acid (vitamin B_3) and dietary tryptophan deficiency cause pellagra, in which there is diarrhea, dermatitis (in a photosensitivity distribution), and dementia; this condition is most frequent in chronic alcoholism but may also occur secondary to isoniazid therapy.

Vitamin K deficiency causes easy bruising, which may occasionally resemble actinic purpura.

Protein energy malnutrition is important worldwide but uncommon in developed countries. It may cause kwashiorkor (in which there is relative carbohydrate excess) or marasmus. In both conditions, there is dry cracked skin, pigmentary disturbance, and poor hair.

Iron deficiency is discussed in the section on hematologic disorders (later in this chapter).

SKIN SIGNS OF RENAL DISEASE AND OF ORGAN TRANSPLANTATION

A number of dermatologic disorders have associations with renal disease, which fall into several broad categories.

- Skin lesions that are a sign of uremia or are related to chronic renal failure.
- Skin lesions that are associated with renal transplantation (essentially, those due to chronic therapeutic immunosuppression).
- Skin disorders that are associated with specific types of renal disease, such as partial lipodystrophy (Ch. 22).
- Skin lesions of multisystem disorders that may also affect the kidney, such as systemic lupus erythematosus, systemic sclerosis, vasculitides, amyloidosis, and Fabry disease (all discussed elsewhere).

Features of uremia

Typical changes include:

- dry skin and itch,
- pigmentary change (usually increased),
- nail changes, and
- indirect changes related to uremia (e.g. drug-related).

Dry skin and itch are common in uremia, occurring to some degree in most patients and disabling in intensity in some. The etiology of renal itch is uncertain, but is probably not simply due to the urea level. Parathormone may be involved, as parathyroidectomy improves symptoms in some individuals. Other contributory factors include the fact that many patients are elderly with consequent skin dryness, and control of hyperlipidemia with statins may contribute to dryness as a direct pharmacologic side effect. Scratching may also cause purpura, as platelet function is impaired.

Treatment of itch can be difficult, and the response to dialysis is variable: some patients slowly improve, but others get increased symptoms after dialysis. Emollients are important, and sedating antihistamines may reduce the severity of itch. Phototherapy with UVA or UVB helps some patients, and cholestyramine, charcoal, and evening primrose oil have all

been used with benefit. Recently, naltrexone (an opiate antagonist) has shown promising results, presumably by a central effect on central nervous system opiate receptors.

Pigmentary changes in uremic patients are multifactorial, due to a combination of anemia (pallor), carotenemia (yellow), and increased levels of β-MSH in the tissues (causing increased melanin pigmentation).

'Half and half' nails (pale proximally, reddish brown distally) occur in about 25% of uremic patients, and total leukonychia may also occur.

Indirect changes include drug eruptions due to the multiplicity of drugs taken by many patients with renal failure, as well as rarer conditions related to dialysis. Blisters may occur in patients having hemodialysis, and resemble porphyria cutanea tarda (which may also occur in this group of patients, see Ch. 17).

Perforating disorders
Etiology and pathogenesis

This is a group of disorders in which dermal tissue is extruded through the epidermis or into the follicles (perforating folliculitis), a process known as transepidermal elimination. The term is usually applied to extrusion of collagen (reactive perforating collagenosis) or elastic fibers, but it requires histologic examination and special stains to determine the nature of the extruded material.

This is an important group of disorders, as they are associated with systemic disease, notably diabetes and chronic renal failure (or both together). Perforating granuloma annulare (GA) is discussed in Chapter 11.

The same process of transepidermal elimination occurs as isolated lesions in several other situations, which are usually more obvious. For example, subcutaneous suture material ('spitting' sutures), fragmented hair shafts (e.g. after simple folliculitis), or insect mouthparts may all be eliminated through the skin surface.

Clinical features

Clinically, the lesions are fairly non-specific. They are usually multiple, scattered, small crusted or umbilicated papules with variable degree of itch (Fig. 12.44; see also Fig. 11.75), which may discharge and regress. Crops of new lesions develop at intervals.

Differential diagnosis

This includes infections, folliculitis, abscesses, foreign body granulomas, and simple excoriations. Suture elimination from a scar may be felt to represent wound infection, and cases are often referred as recurrent tumor even though most suture elimination occurs within a month or so after surgery, far earlier than most tumor recurrence would be likely.

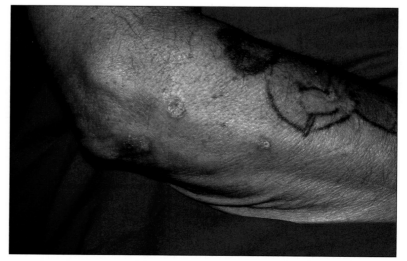

Figure 12.44 Perforating collagenosis, a disorder that is especially associated with diabetes and/or chronic renal failure. The inflammatory nodules often have a crusted or umbilicated center, as shown here, although this is not always clinically apparent. These lesions are often quite pruritic, and relatively difficult to treat.

Treatment

These disorders are difficult to treat. Strong topical corticosteroids may provide symptomatic relief from itch. Treatment of an associated systemic disease is clearly important.

Calcific uremic arteriolopathy ('calciphylaxis')

This is a severe disorder that presents as acute painful livedo and scattered large, deep, painful ulcers, usually on the limbs (Figs 12.45–12.47; see also Ch. 14 for discussion of the differential diagnosis of livedo, and Ch. 22 for discussion of other panniculitides). It occurs in patients with chronic renal failure, usually with renal osteodystrophy; calcium deposition in vessels is the initial pathologic event. Radiography may demonstrate pepper pot calcification of the skull and vascular calcification. Blood results show elevated creatinine and parathormone, and most patients have a calcium × phosphate product > 6.5 mmol^2/L^2. Protein C functional activity may be reduced. The disorder may be fatal, but the situation may be reversed by parathyroidectomy in patients who are sufficiently fit for this intervention. Response to a low-calcium dialysis regimen has also been described. A clinically identical picture occurs in primary hyperoxaluria, and can also occur in homocystinuria.

Nephrogenic fibrosing dermopathy

This is a newly described disorder that occurs almost exclusively in patients with chronic renal failure on dialysis. It may be preceded by thrombotic events or vascular surgery, and patients may have a thrombophilic tendency. Clinically, it consists of a symmetric scleroderma-like thickening of the skin, mainly affecting the limbs and often with rapid progression. Histologically, there is mucin deposition resembling scleromyxedema. The process may involve transforming growth factor-β, which is profibrotic.

The differential diagnosis includes sclerodermas, eosinophilic fasciitis, cellulites, scleredema, and scleromyxedema. Treatments that have had some success include systemic corticosteroids, plasmapheresis, and restricting use of erythropoietin, but response is generally slow or poor.

Immunosuppression and transplants

Cutaneous features that occur in transplant patients are mainly related to long-term immunosuppressive therapy. They are therefore not unique to renal transplantation, but this constitutes much the largest group of individuals, so the topic is discussed here. Potential dermatologic problems of the transplant patient are listed in Table 12.4.

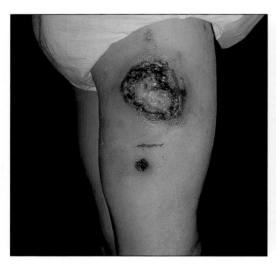

Figure 12.45 A large necrotic ulcer due to calciphylaxis in a patient with chronic renal failure and hyperparathyroidism. There were similar lesions on the buttocks and contralateral thigh.

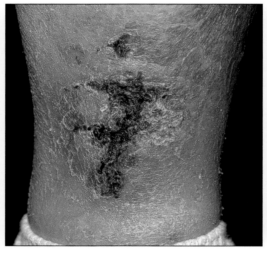

Figure 12.46 Irregular necrotic ulceration on the ankle due to calciphylaxis. This ulcer is clearly not typical of venous disease, as it has a rather stellate shape, suggesting a livedo pattern. This morphology of ulcer also occurs due to cholesterol emboli from proximal arteries.

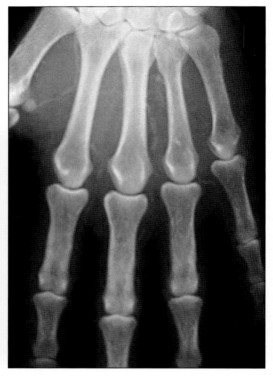

Figure 12.47 Radiographic evidence of vascular calcification is a frequent feature in patients with calciphylaxis, shown here in the arteries of the palm and digits.

Table 12.4 DERMATOLOGIC PROBLEMS OF RENAL TRANSPLANTATION

Feature	Example(s) and comments
Related to background renal disease	Features due to renal failure usually improve after transplantation: some, for example pigmentation, may persist
Drug side effects	For example striae due to steroids, rash due to azathioprine, hypertrichosis and gum hypertrophy due to ciclosporin, acneiform rash due to mycophenolate mofetil
Infections	Viral: warts, molluscum contagiosum, herpes simplex and herpes zoster (may be atypical), cytomegalovirus Bacterial: impetigo, cellulitis, ecthyma gangrenosum (*Pseudomonas*), *Nocardia*, atypical mycobacteria Fungal: candidiasis, *Pityrosporum*, dermatophytes, *Cryptococcus*, aspergillosis, mucormycosis Protozoal: *Pneumocystis*
Neoplasms and precursors	Especially increased risk of squamous cell carcinoma or Merkel cell carcinoma, but also increased risk of actinic keratosis, basal cell carcinoma, malignant melanoma, Kaposi sarcoma, anal carcinoma
Other lesions	Sebaceous hyperplasia (Ch. 23) may be prominent; porokeratosis (Ch. 32) may be more common. Graft-versus-host disease occurs rarely in solid organ transplants (see hematology section of this chapter)

It is important to recognize that immunosuppression not only makes unusual infections more likely, but they may also occur in atypical or masked forms. Warts (which are present in the majority of patients after 5 years) or molluscum contagiosum may be extensive and therapy-resistant; note that molluscum may resemble cryptococcal lesions in the immunosuppressed patient. Chronic herpes simplex may be difficult to diagnose, and disseminated herpes zoster (a life-threatening eruption in immunosuppressed patients) may occur. Unusual fungal variants include unusual patterns, such as proximal subungual onychomycosis (Ch. 26), or unusual organisms, such as *Mucor*. Any undiagnosed lesion should be biopsied, with samples for culture and histologic staining for fungi and other organisms.

The great concern in long-term transplant survivors is a variety of tumors, both cutaneous (Table 12.4) and systemic (e.g. non-Hodgkin lymphoma). The cutaneous lesions are felt to be related to long-term sun exposure, and the increased number may represent tumors of which at least a proportion would normally have been rejected by an intact immunologic system. There are several problems relating to the cutaneous tumors.

- There are significant increases in incidence of squamous cell carcinoma and Merkel cell carcinoma.
- Differential diagnosis of squamous cell carcinoma from viral warts, seborrheic keratosis, or actinic keratosis may be more difficult than normal (at least in part, because long-term transplant survivors usually have multiple lesions of all these types).
- The triggering sunlight exposure has generally been long term prior to immunosuppression, so 'the die has been cast'.
- Multiple primary lesions over time are common.
- Metastatic disease is more common and responds poorly to therapy in immunosuppressed individuals.
- There is usually no scope to reduce the immunosuppressive therapy.

Prevention is therefore important, and although the relevant sunlight exposure may have preceded renal failure and immunosuppression, it is prudent that all patients in whom a likelihood of transplant can be predicted should be advised about sun avoidance.

PRACTICE POINTS

- Itch is a particularly prominent cutaneous feature of chronic renal failure and may be very difficult to treat adequately.
- Patients who have long-term immunosuppression following renal transplantation almost all develop viral warts that are resistant to therapy.
- Always consider the possibility of rare infections in any undiagnosed skin lesion in an immunosuppressed patient.
- Sun avoidance is essential for patients on long-term immunosuppression; there is a markedly increased incidence of cutaneous squamous cell carcinoma and other sun-induced neoplasia in this group.

SKIN SIGNS OF HEMATOLOGIC DISEASE

Anemias and erythrocyte abnormalities
Iron deficiency

This causes itch, koilonychia, smooth tongue, angular cheilitis, and diffuse alopecia. It is important to be aware that itch due to iron deficiency may occur even when the hemoglobin level is within the normal range (e.g. in an anemic patient who receives transfusion but in whom underlying iron deficiency is not addressed).

Pernicious anemia

This is associated with vitiligo and other autoimmune disorders, and may be associated with premature graying of hair. The skin in patients with this type of anemia may be yellowish colored.

Polycythemia rubra vera

Polycythemia rubra vera (PRV) causes plethora, and itch that occurs typically after a hot bath or shower. PRV is also associated with erythro-melalgia, which presents as an episodic erythematous swelling of the feet with burning pain; it also occurs as an idiopathic disorder and is associated with other myeloproliferative states such as thrombocythemia. The hematologically related adult-onset types may respond to treatment with aspirin, but the idiopathic type responds better to serotonin reuptake inhibitors.

Hemoglobinopathies

Hemoglobinopathies such as sickle cell anemia may cause cutaneous ulceration with residual pigmentation.

Leukemias and myeloproliferative disease

Leukemia and myeloproliferative disease may affect the skin in numerous direct and indirect ways (see also polycythemia, discussed earlier). Many of these are discussed in other chapters, but some of the cutaneous associations are listed here for convenience. Possible manifestations and cutaneous associations include the following.

- Non-specific features—such as purpura due to thrombocytopenia.
- Direct cutaneous involvement—leukemia cutis (Ch. 33).
- Paraneoplastic neutrophilic dermatoses—pyoderma gangrenosum and Sweet disease (Ch. 14).
- Infections—due to the disease or treatment; includes severe herpetic infections, and unusual organisms such as zygomycosis or mucormycosis.
- Drug reactions—see Chapter 18.
- Other skin eruptions related to therapy—such as post–marrow transplantation graft-versus-host disease (discussed later).

Lymphomas

Many of the effects of leukemia just described also apply to lymphoma, such as infections, drug reactions, and effects of pancytopenia. Cutaneous involvement with lymphoma is much more common than with leukemia, and is discussed in Chapter 33. Lymphomas may also present with itch, sweating, erythroderma, or acquired ichthyosis (Fig. 12.48).

Purpura and coagulation defects
Platelet defects and clotting factor deficiencies

Clotting factor abnormalities tend to cause deep bruising, compared with platelet defects, which usually cause smaller purpuric lesions; neither commonly presents to dermatologists, as they are usually diagnosed by

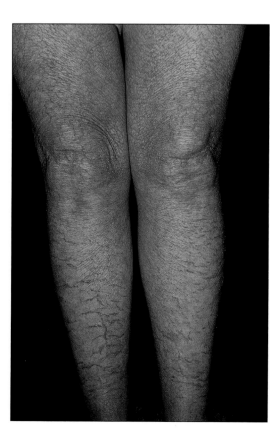

Figure 12.48 Acquired ichthyosis, with an asteatotic eczema pattern on the legs, in a patient with Hodgkin disease. Recurrence of this skin change was an early feature in a relapse over a year after an initial good response to chemotherapy.

Table 12.5	CAUSES OF PURPURA AND BRUISING
Category	**Causes**
Platelet disorders	Thrombocytopenia Abnormal platelet function Thrombocytosis
Coagulation disorders[a]	Hemophilias Anticoagulant drugs, vitamin K deficiency Disseminated intravascular coagulopathy
Intravascular occlusion	Dysproteinemias, cryoproteinemias Emboli, for example cholesterol from atheroma
Abnormal vessels, vascular support, or intravascular pressure	Actinic ('senile') purpura, corticosteroid purpura, scurvy, Ehlers–Danlos syndrome Severe coughing or vomiting, stasis dermatitis
Vasculitis and inflammatory disorders[b]	Vasculitis, for example Henoch–Schönlein purpura (see Ch. 14 for causes of vasculitis) Capillaritis (pigmented purpuric dermatoses) Purpura is common in any inflammatory dermatosis, especially on lower legs
Other causes of purpura or ecchymosis	Physical and artefactual causes, for example paroxysmal finger hematoma (Achenbach syndrome), painful bruising (autoerythrocyte sensitization, Gardner–Diamond) syndrome

[a]Usually cause larger bruises.
[b]Cause *palpable* purpura, other than capillary lesions.

blood tests. There are, however, many causes of purpura other than those due to platelet defects (Table 12.5), many of which are in the province of the dermatologist. Platelet abnormalities, including use of antiplatelet drugs such as aspirin, may also present to dermatologists as unexpected capillary oozing during operative procedures. It is of particular importance to distinguish between flat spots of purpura and 'palpable purpura', which is due to the combination of inflammation and vascular leakage, and which is the hallmark of vasculitis (discussed in Ch. 14). As some causes of intravascular occlusion lead to secondary inflammatory changes, by comparison with vasculitis, in which vessel wall inflammation is the primary event, assessment should always be directed at fresh purpuric lesions.

Causes of thrombocytopenia are not addressed here, but the association of thrombocytopenia with two more obviously dermatologic conditions is worth noting. It is a feature of Wiskott–Aldrich syndrome, a rare sex-linked disorder, with atopic dermatitis and severe infections. Thrombocytopenia also occurs with disseminated intravascular coagulation in a small proportion of large, congenital angiomas (Kasabach–Merritt syndrome).

Thrombophilia, protein C
Thrombophilias are of some importance in dermatology, particularly in relation to a livedo pattern of rash. Antiphospholipid syndrome, anticardiolipin antibodies, and lupus anticoagulant are discussed in Chapter 14 along with other causes of microvascular occlusion. The other important thrombophilic states are antithrombin III deficiency, protein C deficiency, activated protein C resistance (factor V Leiden), and protein S deficiency. Acquired functional protein C or protein S deficiency may occur in antiphospholipid syndrome.

Of this group, the most frequent is activated protein C resistance, which is due to a mutation in clotting factor V, rendering it relatively insensitive to the anticoagulant effect of activated protein C. Abnormalities of this anticoagulant system have been implicated as a cause of leg ulceration (especially in young individuals), neonatal purpura fulminans, disseminated intravascular coagulopathy, and coumarin-induced skin necrosis (see also Chs 14 and 18), as well as in thrombotic disorders of less direct dermatologic relevance.

Dysproteinemias and myeloma
Hypergammaglobulinemia
This is a feature of sarcoidosis (Ch. 11), various collagen vascular disorders (Ch. 13), and other disorders. In those patients in whom it causes skin lesions, this is typically a purpuric rash. Waldenström hypergammaglobulinemic purpura and other occlusive vasculitides are discussed in Chapter 14.

Cryoglobulins and cryofibrinogens
Cold-precipitating proteins such as cryoglobulins and cryofibrinogens are also discussed in Chapter 14. Mixed cryoglobulinemia is often secondary to hepatitis C infection, discussed earlier in this chapter.

Myeloma and monoclonal gammopathy
A wide range of cutaneous disorders are associated with either myeloma or monoclonal gammopathy, including the following.
- Non-specific signs due to pancytopenia or treatments (similar to those listed earlier for leukemias).
- Plasmacytoma—a localized, cutaneous, plasma cell tumor (Fig. 33.30).
- Hyperviscosity syndrome—similar to that of Waldenström macroglobulinemia.
- Amyloidosis—Chapter 11.
- Neutrophilic dermatoses (as for leukemias, but less common; see also Ch. 14) and normolipemic plane xanthomatosis (Fig. 11.70).
- Scleromyxedema—lichen myxedematosus (Ch. 11).
- POEMS (polyneuropathy, organomegaly, endocrine disorder, M protein, skin changes) syndrome—these patients have cutaneous features of pigmentation, hypertrichosis, tight edematous skin resembling scleroderma, capillary angiomas, hyperhidrosis, and clubbing. The M protein is usually of IgG-λ or IgA-λ type, and is associated with sclerotic bone lesions representing plasmacytomas. Hepatosplenomegaly, lymphadenopathy, and peripheral edema are common.

Graft-versus-host disease
Graft-versus-host disease (GVHD) is a skin eruption that occurs in recipients of allogeneic tissues, in which donor immune cells attack host tissues due to histoincompatibility. It can occur after any transplant operation, but is discussed here as it is most common after bone marrow transplantation. It may affect the gut, liver, lungs, marrow, and blood vessels as well as the skin. The cutaneous features evolve through a sequence of stages (Fig. 12.49).

In acute GVHD (within 100 days of transplant, usually within 7–21 days), the rash is of non-specific maculopapular appearance, mainly on palms, soles, and upper trunk, and is accompanied by malaise, diarrhea, and hepatitis. Occasionally, there may be hyperacute changes similar to

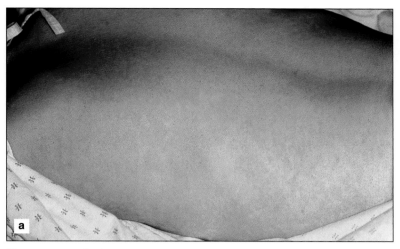 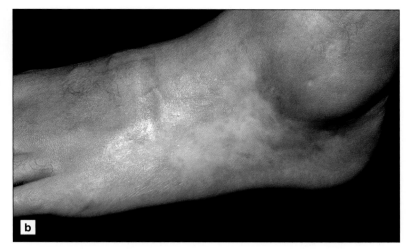

Figure 12.49 Graft-versus-host disease. The early rash (**a**) is non-specific, but a more lichenoid or sclerodermoid pattern, as shown here on the foot (**b**), develops in the chronic phase. (Figure 12.49a courtesy of Robert Sigafoes M.D.)

toxic epidermal necrolysis with extensive desquamation. The most important differential diagnoses at this stage, as they are common during the phase of marked immunosuppression and use of multiple drugs, are exanthems related to viral infection, cutaneous drug eruptions, and the eruption of lymphocyte recovery.

Chronic GVHD may develop from about 30 days after transplant, and persists (or occasionally appears de novo) more than 100 days after transplantation. It has chronic dermatitic, or rather lichenoid, features, and may include blotchy pigment disturbance, nail dystrophy, and alopecia. The differential diagnosis includes ordinary lichen planus or lichenoid drug eruptions, lupus erythematosus, and dermatomyositis. Mucosal manifestations may resemble lichen planus, or may cause xerostomia similar to that of Sjögren disease. In the later stages, a poikilodermatous or sclerodermatous pattern may develop. These two main patterns have been termed lichenoid chronic GVHD and sclerodermatous chronic GVHD, respectively.

Histologic examination of the skin can be helpful in identifying GVHD, as infections and drug eruptions are both common in this group of immunosuppressed patients. The features are lichenoid, with hydropic degeneration of the basal layer, and necrotic keratinocytes are surrounded by lymphocytes (a picture known as satellite cell necrosis). This is due to donor T lymphocytes attacking 'foreign' host histocompatibility antigens.

Treatment is by immunosuppressive drugs such as corticosteroids, azathioprine, methotrexate, or ciclosporin. Irradiation and cell depletion techniques are applied to donor blood to prevent GVHD.

PRACTICE POINTS

- Iron deficiency is an important cause of itch, and may occur in patients with a normal hemoglobin level.
- Itch specifically after a warm bath is suggestive of polycythemia rubra vera, but may also occur due to commoner disorders such as dermographism (from toweling or shower jets) or cholinergic urticaria (due to heat).
- It is of particular importance to distinguish between flat spots of purpura and 'palpable purpura', which is due to the combination of inflammation and vascular leakage, and which is the hallmark of vasculitis.
- Patients with a neutrophilic dermatosis such as pyoderma gangrenosum or Sweet syndrome may have an underlying myeloproliferative disorder; a complete blood count is essential.
- A livedo pattern of purpura or dusky discoloration may be due to intravascular occlusion; always include a biopsy and thrombophilia screen in the work-up.

FLUSHING

Causes and triggers for flushing

Flushing is a common symptom but very subjective, and most patients who complain of flushing have either a normal physiologic response or an exaggeration by several common triggers. There is also a racial predisposition (mainly east Asian), especially for flushing after alcohol. This is due to racial variations in levels of alcohol dehydrogenase: deficiency causes high blood levels of acetaldehyde after ingesting alcohol. Causes of flushing and common triggers are listed in Table 12.6; most can be identified from the history, without need for investigations. Some flushing due to occupational solvents resolve at weekends (Fig. 12.50). Features that suggest a systemic cause, and appropriate investigations, are discussed in the section on carcinoid syndrome below.

Table 12.6 CAUSES OF FLUSHING

Physiologic factors, such as the response to emotional stimuli or hot drinks

Endocrine causes, such as the menopause or oophorectomy

Idiopathic flushing

Alcohol, either alone or with:
- solvents, such as dimethylformamide (Fig. 12.50), thiuram chemicals
- medications, classically chlorpropamide (known as the chlorpropamide alcohol flush) and other hypoglycemics, also disulfiram (a thiuram used therapeutically in alcoholism), and antibiotics such as griseofulvin or metronidazole
- tumors (carcinoid [see below], lymphoma, medullary carcinoma of thyroid)

Autonomic epilepsy

Chemicals: nitrates and nitrites, monosodium glutamate (typically occurs after Chinese meals), nicotine, mithramycin, histamine

Neoplastic causes:
- Carcinoid (see text; Fig. 12.51)
- Other APUD tumors, such as medullary carcinoma of thyroid, pheochromocytoma, islet cell adenoma, oat cell tumor
- Systemic mastocytosis
- Renal carcinoma

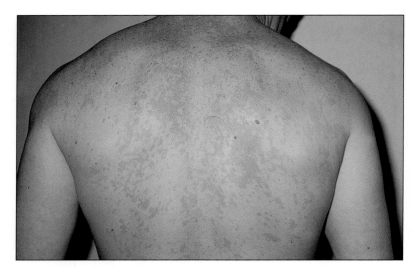

Figure 12.50 Flushing is a transient vasodilatation on the face and upper trunk. In this case, the flushing was induced by small amounts of alcohol in a patient who worked using a dimethylformamide solvent, but the morphology of the eruption is the same as in physiologic flushing.

Carcinoid syndrome

Etiology

Carcinoid syndrome is a rare but important cause of flushing, which must be differentiated from other neoplastic causes and the other etiologies listed earlier. The tumor may be intestinal (mainly appendix and distal ileum), bronchial, or ovarian; features vary according to the site, as the liver metabolizes mediators released into the portal venous system by a purely intestinal carcinoid tumor, and symptoms do not occur unless there is access to the systemic circulation.

Clinical features

Flushing is initially episodic but becomes more fixed, with development of erythema and telangiectases on the face and upper chest, and a pellagra-like photosensitivity rash (Fig. 12.51). Associated symptoms and signs include hypotension, tachycardia, diarrhea (all of which may occur in idiopathic flushing), bronchospasm, abdominal pain, right heart valve fibrosis, and hepatomegaly. The diagnosis is confirmed by demonstration of increased urinary 24-h excretion of hydroxyindole acetic acid (5HIAA), but this does not detect all cases; serotonin levels and vasoactive intestinal peptide levels may need to be measured as well. Extensive radiology and other localizing investigations (such as use of indium-labeled octreotide) may be required.

Differential diagnosis

The following features help to distinguish other neoplastic lesions that may resemble carcinoid.

- Systemic mastocytosis (Ch. 11) may have similar flushing and telangiectasia, but the latter is usually more generalized; bronchospasm is not a feature and heart valves are unaffected.
- Pheochromocytoma is associated with hyperhidrosis, hypertension, and headache; urinary metanephrines are increased but 5HIAA is normal.
- Islet cell tumors may cause increased 5HIAA levels, but hypoglycemia also occurs.
- Renal carcinoma causes increased prostaglandin levels but normal 5HIAA.
- Multiple endocrine neoplasia—other symptoms, especially diarrhea, may be prominent.

Treatment

Flushing in carcinoid responds to somatostatin analogs such as octreotide, and surgery to the primary tumor and metastases should be performed if feasible. Radioisotope-labeled octreotide or analogs (e.g. indium-labeled octreotide or yttrium-labeled DOTATOC) are also of value in disease control.

SIGNS OF INTERNAL MALIGNANCY, AND PARANEOPLASTIC SYNDROMES

A number of dermatoses are linked with internal neoplasia (Table 12.7). Some are rather non-specific and may have many other non-neoplastic causes (e.g. acquired ichthyosis), some have a sufficiently frequent link with malignancy generally that screening is appropriate (e.g. adult dermatomyositis), while others have such a close link that the site of associated malignancy can almost be assumed (e.g. acrokeratosis paraneoplastica). Selected examples are discussed here; direct metastases to the skin are covered in Chapter 33. Superior vena cava obstruction (Fig. 12.52) is a mechanical problem rather than paraneoplastic but is conveniently illustrated here.

Acanthosis nigricans

The benign endocrine-associated form of AN, the most common type, was discussed earlier in this chapter. AN also occurs as a paraneoplastic phenomenon, usually in elderly patients, and is most frequently associated with adenocarcinoma of stomach. By contrast to the insulin-resistant type of AN, patients with paraneoplastic AN are usually older, losing weight, and have more florid AN (often involving oral and conjunctival mucosae, and the palms) of recent onset (Figs 12.53–12.55; compare with Figs 12.24–12.26).

Dermatomyositis

About 25% of patients with dermatomyositis have an underlying malignancy, with approximately equal proportions diagnosed before, after, and at the time of the skin eruption. This disorder and the approach to diagnosis and evaluation are discussed in more detail in Chapter 13, but

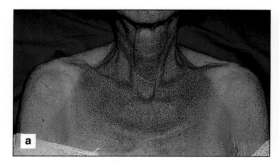

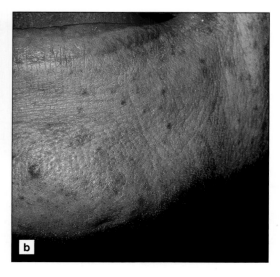

Figure 12.51 Carcinoid syndrome. There is a fixed erythematous area in the V of neck distribution (**a**). Telangiectasia becomes fixed in the distribution of flushing, as shown on the chin of the same patient (**b**).

Table 12.7   SOME SKIN ERUPTIONS THAT MAY BE PARANEOPLASTIC

Condition	Associated main tumor type	Description
Pruritus	Several	Itch, no primary rash
Acquired ichthyosis	Several, especially lymphoma	Diffuse dryness or asteatotic eczema pattern
Acanthosis nigricans	Adenocarcinoma of stomach	Warty brownish flexural rash, 'tripe palms'
Dermatomyositis	Common tumor types	Violaceous rash, periorbital involvement (Ch. 13)
Sign of Leser–Trélat	Gastrointestinal adenocarcinomas	Multiple, small, eruptive, itchy, seborrheic keratoses
Acrokeratosis paraneoplastica (Bazex syndrome)	Squamous carcinoma of upper aerodigestive tract	Psoriasiform scaling with acral pattern: fingers, toes, ears, nose
Palmar keratoderma (tylosis)	Carcinoma of esophagus (few families; investigate only if positive family history)	Diffuse keratoderma of palms (see also Ch. 7)
Acquired hypertrichosis lanuginosa	Several	Fine downy hair growth acquired in an overtly ill cachectic adult (also occurs as a benign congenital disorder)
Glucagonoma syndrome	Pancreatic α cells, sometimes other gastrointestinal sites	Necrolytic migratory erythema (see text), cheilitis, glossitis
Lobular panniculitis	Pancreatic carcinoma (and chronic pancreatitis)	Inflammatory nodules on legs, with lobular panniculitis histologic pattern and ghost fat cells
Malignancy-associated fasciitis–panniculitis	Several	Scleroderma-like, often acral pattern, progressive
Migratory thrombophlebitis (Trousseau sign)	Several; classically pancreatic, although bronchial carcinoma is more common	Tender, migrating, may be cord-like thrombotic areas
Erythema gyratum repens	Gastric carcinoma	Very rare; migratory rash with parallel erythematous scaling bands of wood grain appearance

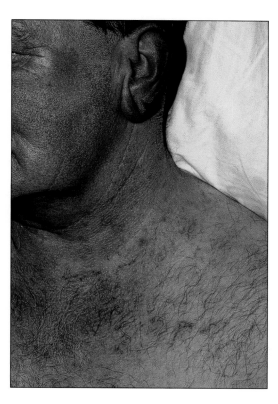

Figure 12.52   Superior vena cava obstruction causing dilated veins and plethora of the upper trunk and neck in a patient with bronchial carcinoma. Patients with superior vena cava obstruction are occasionally referred to dermatologists with suspected contact allergy (eyelid swelling) or angioedema (facial or hand swelling).

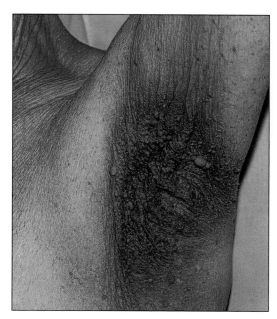

Figure 12.53
Malignant acanthosis nigricans in the axilla. The lesions are much more warty than those occurring in the hyperandrogenic or insulin-resistant types, and occurrence in a thin, elderly patient is highly suspicious of gastrointestinal carcinoma.

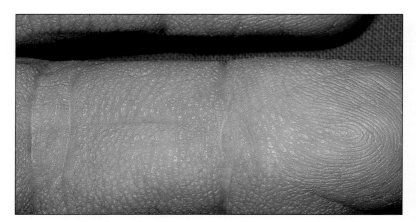

Figure 12.54 Palmar markings and fingerprints are exaggerated in malignant acanthosis nigricans, and are known as tripe palms. This is the fingertip of the patient shown in Fig. 12.53.

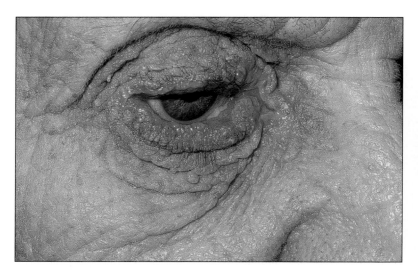

Figure 12.55 Warty lesions on the eyelids of the same patient as in Fig. 12.53. She also had warty areas of the oral mucosa.

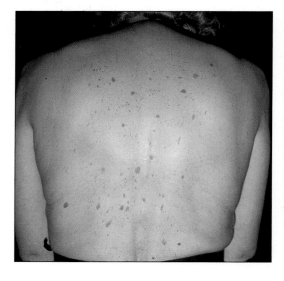

Figure 12.56 The sign of Leser–Trélat. This is sometimes overestimated, as multiple seborrheic keratoses are common in elderly patients, and this is the age group with the highest cancer risk. The important aspect is that the keratoses are eruptive and itchy. In this case, they occurred over a few months in a young adult who was found to have an ovarian carcinoma.

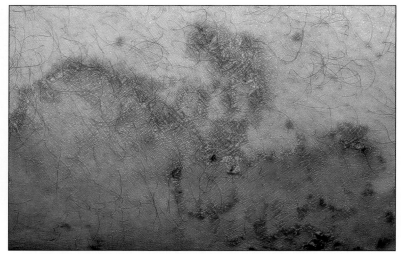

Figure 12.57 Necrolytic migratory erythema is the typical eruption of glucagonoma syndrome, and is typically crusted and rather annular, as shown here.

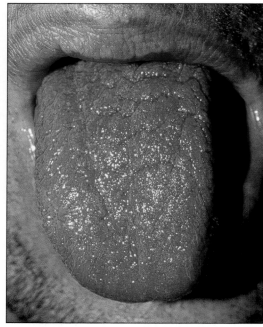

Figure 12.58 Examination of the tongue is useful in glucagonoma syndrome. Glossitis is a common and often severe feature, producing a beefy, red tongue.

all patients with multiple or itchy seborrheic keratoses is unlikely to be cost-effective, but suspicion is reasonable if the keratoses are multiple, small, itchy, and of concurrent recent onset (Fig. 12.56). They must not be confused with the small, eruptive acanthomas that occur during the resolution of erythrodermic disorders.

Glucagonoma syndrome

This is due to glucagon-producing tumors, usually arising in the pancreatic α cells but occasionally at other sites in the gastrointestinal tract. It occurs mainly in middle-aged or older women. The rash it produces is known as necrolytic migratory erythema (Figs 12.57 and 12.58). It typically affects the perineum and other flexures, causing expanding macular lesions with erosions and crusting, which may resemble pemphigoid. Postinflammatory pigmentation may occur. Angular cheilitis and glossitis are common, and weight loss, diarrhea, glucose intolerance, and anemia are typical. The rash may precede the other symptoms by many years, and suspicion is required for any biopsy of a rash that shows histologic evidence of necrolysis in the superficial epidermis.

A significantly elevated plasma glucagon level confirms the diagnosis, and amino acid levels are often low, as gluconeogenesis is impaired (low valine, leucine, and isoleucine). Zinc levels may be low; the rash of zinc deficiency is similar (Fig. 12.59). Extensive radiology may be required to determine the tumor site; radioisotope localization (indium-labeled

dermatomyositis is included here as it is one of the more characteristic paraneoplastic eruptions. Bronchial, colonic, breast, and genitourinary carcinomas are the most frequent associations with dermatomyositis.

Sign of Leser–Trélat

This sign is the sudden appearance of seborrheic keratoses in association with an internal malignancy (usually a gastrointestinal adenocarcinoma). It is somewhat subjective, as older patients (in whom most cancers occur) tend to have multiple seborrheic keratoses. In some cases, regression of keratoses after treating the malignancy supports the diagnosis. Screening

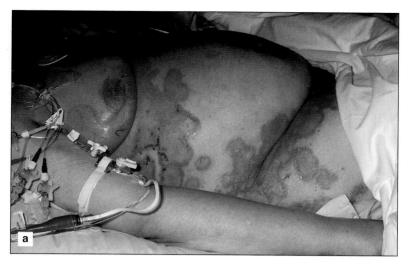

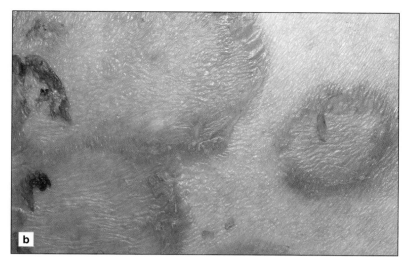

Figure 12.59 (**a**,**b**) Acquired zinc deficiency: the skin eruption is similar to that of glucagonoma syndrome, although periorificial rash may be the only feature.

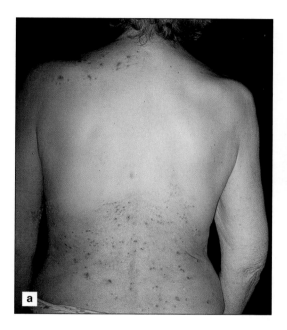

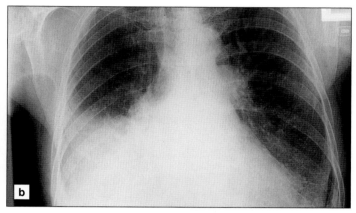

Figure 12.60 Itch is a symptom that may be due to underlying malignancy. This patient has the butterfly sign of scratch marks confined to the areas she can reach (**a**). The lack of rash in the spared central back demonstrates that the visible skin lesions are secondary to the scratching rather than due to a specific rash. A chest radiograph (**b**) demonstrated a pleural effusion that was due to underlying malignancy.

octreotide) is a recent development. Non-malignant causes of necrolytic migratory erythema with hyperglucagonemia should be excluded; these include administration of glucagon (to treat insulin-producing tumors), malabsorption (especially due to celiac disease), pancreatitis, and hepatitis.

Treatment is by resection of the tumor if possible. Drug treatment includes somatostatin, octreotide, radioisotopes (indium-labeled octreotide), and chemotherapy (streptozocin); dietary supplementation with zinc and amino acids may also improve the rash.

Other paraneoplastic eruptions and clinical approach

Numerous eruptions, some rather non-specific, may on occasion be paraneoplastic. The clinical problem is often that of deciding which patients require investigation. Most tumors are commoner in older patients but, conversely, older patients generally have more reasons for some skin eruptions, and over-investigation may be detrimental. For example, itch is a feature of some malignancies, especially lymphomas, although there are numerous other causes of generalized pruritus, such as dry skin in the elderly (see Ch. 6). Itch may present as 'eczema' or even as bruising due to scratching (Figs 12.60 and 12.61). Likewise, there are many causes of acquired ichthyosis; the clue that it is significant may be the degree, as it is sometimes dramatic, presenting as extensive asteatotic eczema (Fig. 12.62), especially in patients with lymphoma (Fig. 12.48).

In general, the more uncommon the pattern of eruption, then the greater the chance that it is significant (e.g. erythema gyratum repens). Other examples are given in Table 12.7.

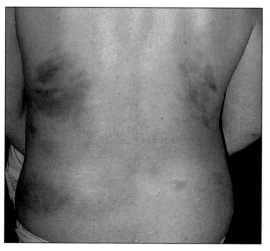

Figure 12.61
Occasionally, itch may be sufficiently severe that patients whose response is to rub the skin rather than to scratch it may get prominent bruising. This patient had a carcinoma of the ovary.

Questions that may help to direct the approach to the patient include the following.

- Type of eruption and known likelihood of malignancy—for example patients with necrolytic migratory erythema almost always have a glucagonoma, whereas generalized pruritus is only rarely a marker of malignancy.
- Age—is the patient the right age for the eruption? (For example, acquired ichthyosis due to aging, use of statins, etc. is common in the elderly but would be unusual in a 40-year-old).

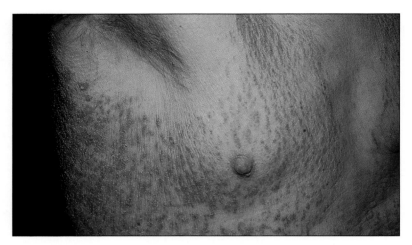

Figure 12.62 A rather poikilodermatous asteatotic eruption on the trunk. This was too prominent to be considered as an ordinary asteatotic eruption in an elderly man, especially on the trunk, and investigations revealed a carcinoma of the prostate.

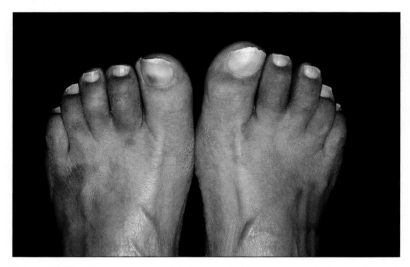

Figure 12.63 Bazex syndrome: this is a psoriasiform paraneoplastic eruption that typically includes involvement of the nose, ears, and distal digits. It is associated with upper aerodigestive tract neoplasms.

- Pattern and degree—is the pattern unusual? (Such as the distribution of the psoriasiform eruption in Bazex syndrome, Fig. 12.63.) Or is the degree of the eruption out of proportion to that normally seen? (For example severe asteatotic change in acquired ichthyosis or bruising due to generalized pruritus; Figs 12.48, 12.60–12.62.)
- Other features that cause concern—such as weight loss, anemia, nocturnal sweating, organ-specific symptoms, and strong family history of cancer.
- Response to treatment and results of previous investigation—a patient with ongoing symptoms despite simple therapies (such as emollients for ichthyosis), or with negative results of simpler tests, may require more detailed evaluation.

PRACTICE POINT

Consider an underlying systemic malignancy in any patient, especially the elderly and especially if non-specifically unwell or losing weight for unexplained reasons, and who has a rash that is:
- 'wrong' for the age-group,
- exaggerated in degree,
- morphologically bizarre,
- atypical for the clinical diagnosis,
- unresponsive to apparently appropriate therapies,
- known to have a link with internal malignancy, or
- associated with abnormal systemic clinical findings or blood results.

CUTANEOUS SIGNS OF HIV INFECTION

Infection with human immunodeficiency virus (HIV, a small RNA retrovirus) was initially associated with homosexual transmission, but in less than 20 years has become increasingly commonly transmitted by heterosexual contact, materno–fetal transmission, and infection from contaminated blood products (iatrogenic, shared needles in drug abusers, or by accidental occupational needle-stick injury). It causes an acquired defect of cell-mediated immunity, and is associated with a vast number of patterns of cutaneous, genital, and other organ involvement, including a wide range of infections. Some of these may vary according to the route of transmission of HIV, for example Kaposi sarcoma (KS) is most frequent in homosexual transmission.

HIV infection follows a variable course, with three main phases. After an initial asymptomatic period, there is a phase of rapidly increasing viremia, in which about half of infected individuals will have 'viral symptoms' and a transient non-specific rash, which is usually macular and which may be associated with oral and palmoplantar lesions. In this phase, infected patients are antibody-negative on enzyme-linked immunosorbent assay (ELISA) tests. Following this, there is a phase that lasts months or years without symptoms; in this phase there is a low level of viremia, mild reduction of CD4 lymphocyte count, and antibodies are present. In the final phase, there is increasing viremia, decreasing CD4 count, and increasing symptoms with increasing tendency to infections and neoplasia such as lymphomas and KS (known as the acquired immune deficiency syndrome, AIDS).

Kaposi sarcoma

Kaposi sarcoma is one of the most specific cutaneous signs of AIDS (Fig. 12.64), although a sporadic form known as classic KS also occurs unrelated to HIV infection. Classic KS usually occurs on the feet and lower legs (see Chapter 33). KS is strongly associated with human herpesvirus type 8 (HHV8) infection, and AIDS-related KS is seen predominantly in homosexual patients.

The skin lesions are typically purplish-colored patches and plaques that may occur at any site and are often subtle initially. Initial involvement of the head and neck is common, and lesions of the palate and other parts of the oral cavity are a notable and useful diagnostic feature. Most lesions occur in patients with known HIV infection, but biopsy for histologic confirmation may be necessary to exclude other diagnoses, such as infections (discussed later). Lesions progress from patches and plaques to become nodules, and may ulcerate or cause secondary lymphedema. Other organs, such as lungs and gastrointestinal tract, may be affected.

Other neoplastic skin lesions in AIDS include lymphomas, squamous cell carcinoma (which may occur at unusual sites, Fig. 12.65), and other papillomavirus-related cancers.

Oral lesions, oral hairy leukoplakia

The oral cavity, especially the palate, is a common site for KS. Oral candidiasis is a common, but not very specific, feature in HIV infection. The combination of median rhomboid glossitis (a candidal infection discussed in Ch. 26) together with a corresponding lesion on the hard palate may signify the presence of immunosuppression; it has been termed the thumbprint of AIDS, or the CIT-NIP syndrome (candidal infection of the tongue with non-specific inflammation of the palate).

Oral hairy leukoplakia is found mainly in homosexual persons, and is probably due to Epstein–Barr virus infection. The lesions are verrucous or reticulate streaky plaques on the sides of the tongue or buccal mucosa, which may resemble lichen planus, candidiasis (which may also be present), or leukoplakia.

Cutaneous infections

Numerous infections occur with increased frequency or severity in HIV infection, especially yeast and viral infections (Figs 12.66–12.72). Sexually transmitted infections are common, and genital ulcer diseases appear to increase the risk of HIV transmission. Oral candidiasis is a relatively early sign, which should arouse suspicion in adults without other predisposing causes such as frequent antibiotic use. Herpes simplex virus (HSV)

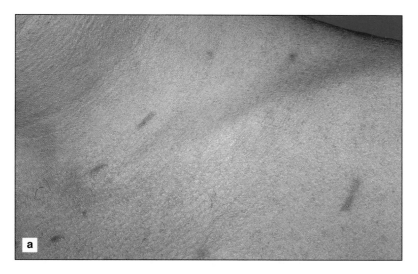

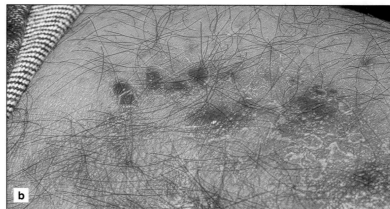

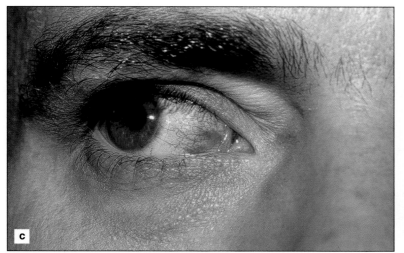

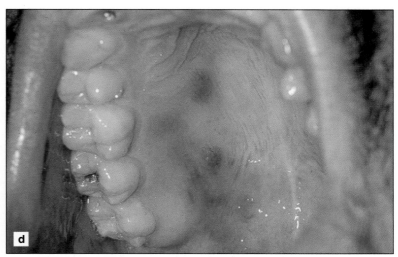

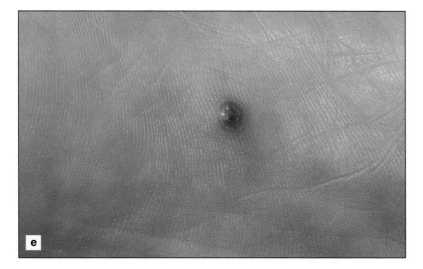

Figure 12.64   (**a–e**) Examples of AIDS-related Kaposi sarcoma. Lesions are usually purplish-colored patches and plaques or nodules, but may just resemble bruises or may resemble pyogenic granulomas (**e**). The palate (a common site) and conjunctivae may be affected as well as the skin.

infections may be chronic, severe, and atypical in morphology; chronic perineal HSV is particularly suspicious, although similar atypical patterns of HSV infection also occur in patients with hematologic malignancies. Perineal ulceration may be due to HSV or cytomegalovirus (CMV) infection, although most CMV infection in AIDS is inferred from positive serology; it also affects eyes and central nervous system, or causes disseminated disease. Extensive, often facial, viral warts or molluscum contagiosum may occur; the latter may be difficult to distinguish from cryptococcosis in patients with AIDS. Extensive impetigo or dermato-phytosis may occur in some patients, as well as less ordinary infections such as nocardiosis, histoplasmosis, blastomycosis, and coccidiomycosis.

An important infection that occurs mainly in immunocompromised patients, especially those with AIDS, is bacillary angiomatosis. This is

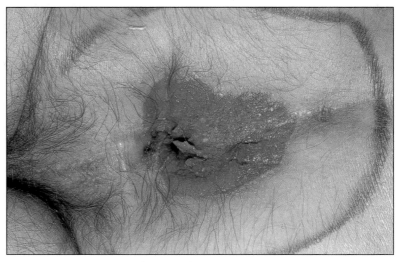

Figure 12.65   Squamous cell carcinoma in the perianal area of an HIV-positive patient. The marker outlines the radiation port for radiation therapy.

231

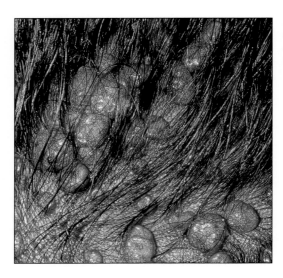

Figure 12.66 Giant molluscum contagiosum of the scalp in a patient infected with HIV.

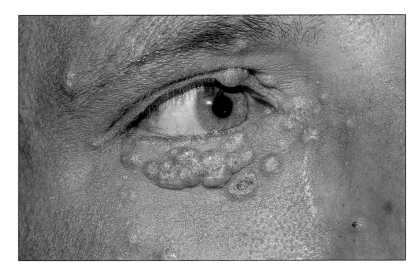

Figure 12.67 Molluscum contagiosum in a patient infected with HIV.

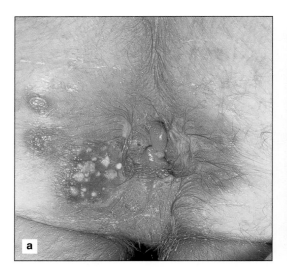

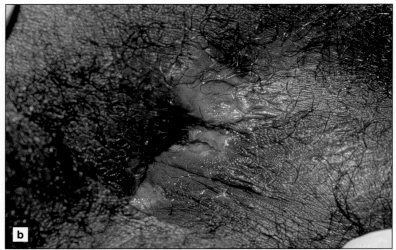

Figure 12.68 (**a**,**b**) Perianal herpes simplex infection in patients infected with HIV.

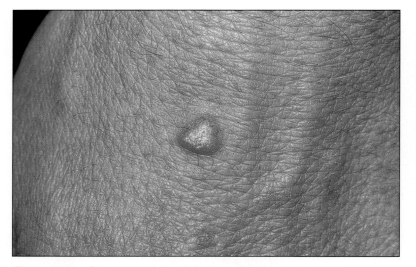

Figure 12.69 Cytomegalovirus infection in a patient infected with HIV.

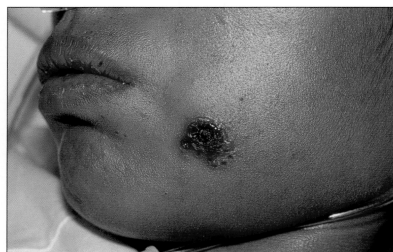

Figure 12.70 Herpes zoster in a woman with AIDS. Although this looks like localized herpes simplex, the patient had several scattered lesions and zoster was confirmed by virologic testing.

mainly due to *Bartonella henselae*, the cause of cat scratch disease. Its importance, apart from the close association with AIDS, is that it causes skin nodules that may resemble KS. It may also cause fever, weight loss, malaise, lymphadenopathy, and lesions of lung, brain, heart, and bone marrow in disseminated infection. Thus it may be confused with advanced-stage AIDS unless a biopsy is taken. The distinction is critical, as

bacillary angiomatosis usually responds to treatment with erythromycin or azalide antibiotics.

Severe and extensive seborrheic dermatitis is a particular feature of HIV infection. This is due to *Pityrosporum* yeasts, although there is some argument about whether this is quite the same as seborrheic dermatitis in HIV-negative individuals. Extensive pityriasis versicolor is also frequent.

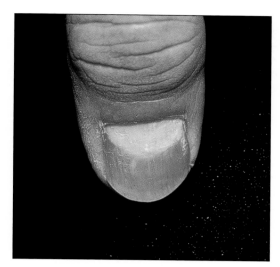

Figure 12.71 Proximal white onychomycosis is a fungal infection that occurs by invasion into the proximal nail fold and growth under the nail plate. It is strongly associated with HIV infection.

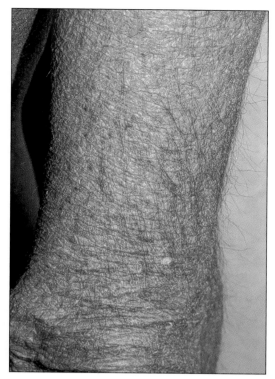

Figure 12.73 Ichthyosis may occur due to HIV infection. Clinically, it resembles a rather severe version of the relatively common and benign autosomal dominant type of ichthyosis.

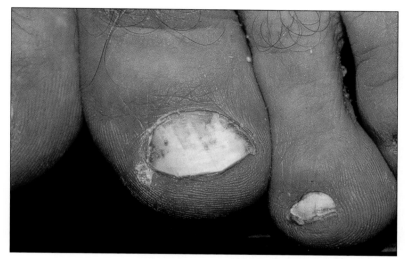

Figure 12.72 Superficial white onychomycosis affects the surface of the nail plate. It is a relatively uncommon pattern of fungal nail disease in immunocompetent individuals.

Miscellaneous

Acquired ichthyosis in young adults is suspicious of HIV infection (Fig. 12.73), but other diagnoses such as lymphoma must be considered. Psoriasis in HIV-positive patients may be severe and therapy-resistant, and there is an increased frequency of Reiter syndrome (discussed in Ch. 33). Severe acne may occur, but infection must be excluded as a cause of acneiform eruption.

Folliculitis is common in HIV infection. It may be due to infections (bacteria, *Pityrosporum*, or other yeasts), but a particularly itchy, sterile folliculitis may also occur. In some such cases, there is marked tissue eosinophilia (HIV-associated eosinophilic folliculitis, Figs 12.74 and 12.75). The papular pruritic eruption of HIV is probably part of this spectrum of follicular lesions. This is relatively resistant to all therapies, but may respond to UVB radiation, isotretinoin, or pentoxifylline. Scabies should be excluded, especially if eosinophilia is a feature.

Drug reactions are particularly common and severe in HIV infection, especially to co-trimoxazole (trimethoprim–sulfamethoxazole). Some drugs used primarily for HIV also cause reactions, such as nail pigmentation due to zidovudine, and penile ulcers due to foscarnet.

Elongated eyelashes have been described in several reports as a feature of AIDS. Elevated porphyrin levels, and less commonly porphyria cutanea tarda, occur with increased frequency in HIV infection.

Treatment

Treatment of HIV and AIDS is a constantly changing field. It incorporates components of antiretroviral treatment, prophylaxis and treatment of infections, treatment of complications such as KS, and general supportive measures. Antiretroviral treatment regimens are complex and have serious

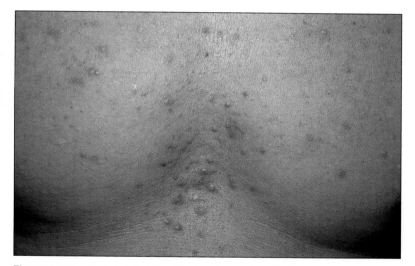

Figure 12.74 Eosinophilic folliculitis showing scattered lesions on the trunk.

Figure 12.75 Eosinophilic folliculitis, the non-specific, close-up morphology showing a tiny pustule with much surrounding erythema.

233

side effects, so need to be carefully considered. Current guidelines suggest that treatment should be offered to all those with symptoms due to HIV infection, and usually to those with a CD4 T-cell count below 0.35×10^9/L or with viral load, measured as the HIV RNA concentration, of more than 55 000 copies/mL. Viral load is a predictor of prognosis, and also (as the half-life is short) is a useful indicator of therapeutic response to antiretroviral infection. It is expected that viral load will be < 50 copies/mL at 4–6 months after starting treatment. It is now common to use highly active antiretroviral therapy (HAART), which consists of triple therapy with two nucleoside reverse transcriptase inhibitors (NRTIs) and a protease inhibitor (PI) for asymptomatic disease, or with two NRTIs and a non-nucleoside reverse transcriptase inhibitor (NNRTI), or two NRTIs and one or two PIs (depending on the agent) for established disease. Side effects of HAART include lactic acidosis, hyperglycemia, lipodystrophy, hyperlipidemia, osteopenia, and rashes including severe Stevens–Johnson syndrome and toxic epidermal necrolysis.

Treatments for KS include systemic antiviral therapy for the underlying HIV infection; local treatments such as radiotherapy, cryotherapy, or laser treatment; and systemic treatments with interferon or chemotherapeutic agents such as doxorubicin.

Infections are treated with appropriate antimicrobials, but courses of treatment may require high doses and prolonged therapy. Resistant organisms may also be a feature, for example aciclovir-resistant HSV is relatively common in patients with HIV but rare in other situations.

PRACTICE POINTS

- Common conditions and infections, such as oral candidiasis, viral warts, or seborrheic dermatitis may all be more extensive than usual or may occur concurrently in HIV infection.
- If you suspect a skin lesion may be Kaposi sarcoma, always examine the mouth: you may find Kaposi sarcoma (especially of the palate), oral candidiasis, or oral hairy leukoplakia.
- Extensive molluscum contagiosum is uncommon in immunocompetent adults; in the context of HIV infection, lesions may be at unusual sites or unusually large and may mimic cutaneous cryptococcosis.

CUTANEOUS ERUPTIONS OF PREGNANCY OR MENSTRUATION

Skin changes in pregnancy

A number of physiologic changes occur during pregnancy, including the following.

- Pigmentation is increased due to the action of estrogens. This is apparent at the areolae, genital skin, and sometimes the axillae. Facial melasma (chloasma) is frequent during pregnancy (see Ch. 21), and pigmented lines become more apparent (Figs 12.76 and 12.77). A linea nigra (a midline pigmented line on the abdomen, especially below the umbilicus, is particularly common).
- Striae develop on the central abdomen and upper thighs due to the enlarging fetus, weight gain, and increased adrenocorticoid levels (Fig. 12.78).
- Vascular changes occur, such as palmar erythema (Fig. 12.79) and spider nevi. The increased pressure of abdominal contents predisposes to hemorrhoids and varicose veins. Pyogenic granulomas (Fig. 12.80), especially of the gingiva, are relatively uncommon, but this site is rarely affected at any other time.
- Scalp hair often becomes thicker as hairs are maintained in anagen phase. This effect is often not appreciated until 2 or 3 months after the pregnancy is concluded, when the normal hair cycle returns and causes a synchronized loss of hair (telogen effluvium).

Polymorphic eruption of pregnancy

Polymorphic eruption of pregnancy (PEP), also known as pruritic urticarial papules and plaques of pregnancy (PUPPP), is the most common of the symptomatic pregnancy-specific dermatoses (Figs 12.81 and 12.82). It

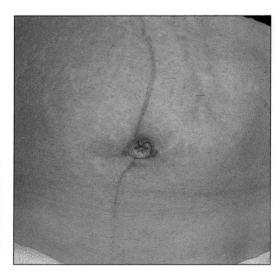

Figure 12.77 A pigmented line that runs down the abdomen (linea nigra) is very common in pregnancy.

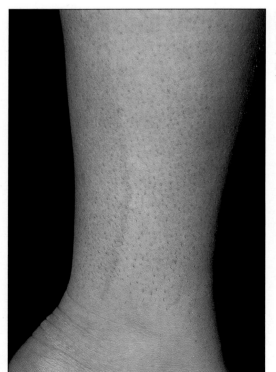

Figure 12.76 Pigmentary demarcation lines may become more apparent during pregnancy (in this case, type B lines on the leg).

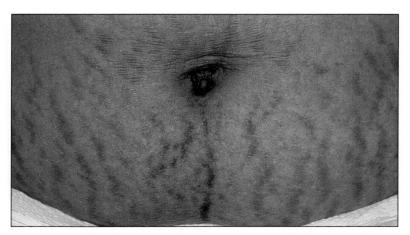

Figure 12.78 Stretch marks or striae are very common and often very red in color during pregnancy, but fade to a silvery white color subsequently.

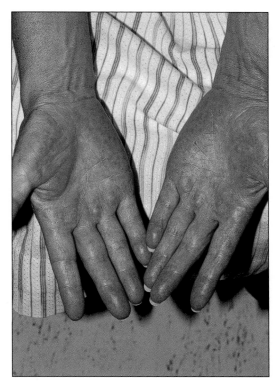

Figure 12.79 Erythema of the palms is a feature of several disorders, such as liver cirrhosis, but is also very common in pregnancy.

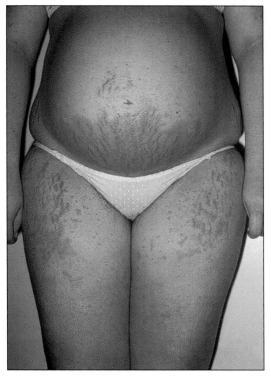

Figure 12.81 Polymorphic eruption of pregnancy on the abdomen and upper thighs.

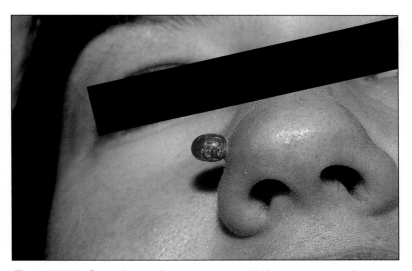

Figure 12.80 Pyogenic granulomas may appear during pregnancy, and may affect otherwise relatively uncommon sites, such as the gums or the nose, as shown here. If they are not removed, they may spontaneously regress after the pregnancy has been completed.

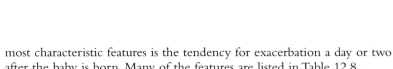

Figure 12.82 Polymorphic eruption of pregnancy on the abdomen.

is relatively common and resolves within a few days of childbirth. The important differential diagnosis is from pemphigoid gestationis, which is a rarer and more significant disorder. The clinical features and a comparison of these two dermatoses are given in Table 12.8.

Treatment is usually with topical corticosteroids and chlorpheniramine; however, corticosteroids may add to the tendency for striae, and sedating antihistamines may be best avoided prior to delivery to avoid fetal sleepiness manifesting as poor fetal movement.

Pemphigoid gestationis

This disorder, which was once confusingly named herpes gestationis, is a potentially severe eruption that has the tendency to present earlier and more floridly in subsequent pregnancies, and is therefore of diagnostic importance (Figs 12.83 and 12.84). It is an autoimmune disorder mediated by complement-fixing IgG1 antibodies, which bind to a 180-kDa bullous pemphigoid antigen, known as BP antigen 2, at the basement membrane zone. This probably occurs due to 'foreign' paternal histocompatibility molecules on the placenta; even in patients with several episodes, it may not recur if a subsequent pregnancy is to a different partner. One of the

most characteristic features is the tendency for exacerbation a day or two after the baby is born. Many of the features are listed in Table 12.8.

Treatment of typical cases is with systemic corticosteroids, which may need to be continued for several months after completion of the pregnancy. Even when most activity has settled, premenstrual exacerbations may occur. If blisters occur in the baby, these are transient, as they are due to passively transferred immunoglobulin across the placenta. However, it is important to recognize that milder versions do occur and may be amenable to control with topical corticosteroids alone, although proof of the disorder by biopsy for immunofluorescence is worthwhile in view of the risks of recurrence.

Other pregnancy eruptions

- Recurrent cholestasis of pregnancy is relatively uncommon, and occurs late in pregnancy. It is probably due to increased levels of bile acids. Clinically, it is characterized by itch, initially at night, and subsequently jaundice, although this is not apparent in all affected individuals. There is no rash as such, but excoriations may be a feature. There may be a familial tendency or a history of cholestasis due to oral contraceptives.

235

Table 12.8 COMPARATIVE FEATURES OF POLYMORPHIC ERUPTION OF PREGNANCY AND PEMPHIGOID GESTATIONIS

Feature	Polymorphic eruption of pregnancy (PEP)	Pemphigoid gestationis
Age and sex	Pregnant female patient, typically first pregnancy	Pregnant female patient, any pregnancy
Family history	Non-specific	Non-specific
Sites	Affects abdomen, thighs, and occasionally distal limbs. The rash usually starts in striae in the last month of pregnancy. The umbilical area is spared in 90%.	Starts on abdomen, initial lesions are periumbilical in 90%, but the rash may affect any body site at any stage of pregnancy (including the postpartum period).
Symptoms	Severe itch	Severe itch
Signs common to both	Erythematous urticated papules and plaques, vesicles	Erythematous urticated papules and plaques, vesicles
Discriminatory signs	Localization to striae. Vesicles are present in 40% of cases but remain small. The rash and itch rapidly regress after delivery.	Periumbilical involvement is typical, and annular lesions are more frequent than in PEP. Vesicles progress rapidly to larger bullae. Exacerbation at the time of delivery is common.
Associated features	None; in particular, the baby is unaffected.	Neonatal involvement may occur due to transplacental transfer of immunoglobulin, and causes urticarial lesions and sometimes bullae. These are usually mild and resolve spontaneously.
Important tests	Biopsy with direct immunofluorescence will distinguish between these two disorders if required. A very recent study has shown ELISA against BP180 NC16a is almost always positive in higher titer in pemphigoid gestationis but not in PEP.	Biopsy with direct immunofluorescence will distinguish between these two disorders if required. A very recent study has shown ELISA against BP180 NC16a is almost always positive in higher titer in pemphigoid gestationis but not in PEP.
Prognosis and recurrence	Common (1 in 250 pregnancies). PEP is typically a disorder of first or multiple pregnancies, especially if there is large weight gain. It resolves rapidly and usually does not recur in subsequent pregnancies.	Rare (1 in 25 000 pregnancies). This disorder may be severe and require systemic therapy; since introduction of systemic steroids, most studies have not reported increased fetal mortality or morbidity, apart from transient rash and some degree of placental insufficiency (slight increase in prematurity and small-for-dates babies). The eruption typically recurs in subsequent pregnancies with the same partner.

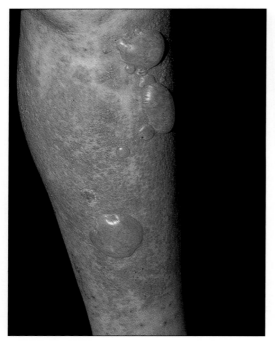

Figure 12.83 Frank blisters on the leg in a patient with pemphigoid gestationis. The lower leg would be an unusual site for polymorphic eruption of pregnancy, and would therefore raise suspicion about the possibility of pemphigoid gestationis.

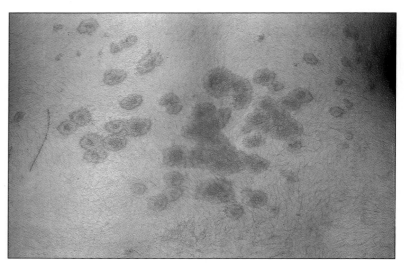

Figure 12.84 Erythema multiforme–like pattern of lesions in a patient with pemphigoid gestationis. The morphology of this eruption is quite variable, and some cases may be quite mild, but deterioration after the pregnancy is a useful feature to suggest the diagnosis.

- Pruritic folliculitis is a rare but possibly underdiagnosed condition that presents as multiple tiny follicular papules and pustules, which appear at any time in the second half of pregnancy and resolve in the few weeks after delivery.
- Impetigo herpetiformis is a rare disorder, which is essentially a form of generalized pustular psoriasis. Treatment is usually limited to systemic steroids and UV therapy, due to the potential for adverse effects on the fetus of the immunosuppressive agents and retinoids that would normally be used for this entity.
- A variety of other conditions, such as papular dermatitis of pregnancy, prurigo of pregnancy, and erythema multiforme gestationis, may all be morphologic variants of PEP.

- Various vascular lesions are either provoked by or more apparent during pregnancy. Effects of increased circulating estrogens, plus an increased circulating volume and hyperdynamic circulation, may all play a part. Unilateral nevoid telangiectasia is often first apparent during a pregnancy and usually fades (but may not fully disappear) afterward. Pyogenic granulomas may occur, with a particular predilection for oral mucosa compared with sporadic lesions outside pregnancy (which can affect oral mucosa, but much less commonly; Fig. 12.85).

Autoimmune progesterone dermatitis

This is not actually a pregnancy eruption but is specifically a female problem and is conveniently discussed here, although it is discussed in more detail in Chapter 9. Patients develop rash, which may have very mixed morphology (it may be eczematous as the name suggests, but may be more erythema multiforme-like or occasionally urticarial), and is confined to the high-progesterone phase of the menstrual cycle. It may be provoked by progestogen-based oral contraceptives, and conversely may respond to estrogen-based regimens. An estrogen-induced equivalent has been reported but is even rarer. Progesterone dermatitis must not be confused with exacerbations of atopic or contact dermatitis that occur in some women in the premenstrual phase of the cycle. Both proving the diagnosis and treating it are difficult.

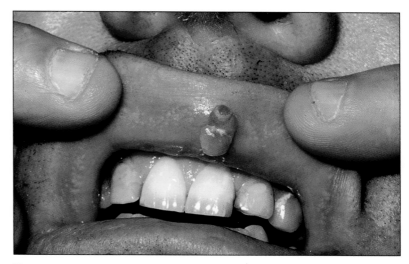

Figure 12.85   Pyogenic granuloma of the oral mucosa. This case is unusual, being in a male patient; most oral pyogenic granulomas are in pregnant women.

FURTHER READING

Aronson IK, Bond S, Fiedler VC, et al. Pruritic urticarial papules and plaques of pregnancy: clinical and immunopathologic observations in 57 patients. J Am Acad Dermatol 1998; 39: 933–9

Berg D, Otley CC. Skin cancer in organ transplant recipients. J Am Acad Dermatol 2002; 47: 1–17

Black MM, McKay M, Braude P. Obstetric and Gynecologic Dermatology. London: Mosby-Wolfe, 1995

Braverman IM. Skin Signs of Systemic Disease, 3rd edn. Philadelphia: Saunders, 1998

Callen JP (ed) Skin signs of systemic disease. Dermatol Clin 2002; 20: 373–560

Callen JP, Jorizzo JL, Bolognia JL, et al (eds) Dermatological Signs of Internal Disease, 3rd edn. Philadelphia: Saunders, 2003

Cox NH, Graham RM. Systemic disease and the skin. In: Burns DA, Breathnach SM, Cox NH, et al (eds) Rook's Textbook of Dermatology, 7th edn. Oxford: Blackwell Publishing, 2004: 59.1–75

Dybul M, Fauci AS, Bartlett JG, et al. Guidelines for using antiretroviral agents among HIV-infected adults and adolescents. Ann Intern Med 2002; 137: 381–433

English JC, Patel PJ, Greer KE. Sarcoidosis. J Am Acad Dermatol 2001; 44: 725–43

Fimiani M, De Aloe G, Cuccia A. Chronic graft versus host disease and skin. J Eur Acad Dermatol Venereol 2003; 17: 512–7

Gregory B, Ho VC. Cutaneous manifestations of gastrointestinal disorders. J Am Acad Dermatol 1992; 26: 153–66, 371–83

Harris P, Sag MS. Dermatologic manifestations of human immunodeficiency virus infection. Curr Probl Dermatol 1997; 9: 213–42

Heymann WR. Cutaneous manifestations of thyroid disease. J Am Acad Dermatol 1992; 26: 885–902

Miller SJ. Nutritional deficiency and the skin. J Am Acad Dermatol 1989; 21: 1–30

Penneys NS. Skin manifestations of AIDS, 2nd edn. London: Martin Dunitz, 1995

Perez MI, Kohn SR. Cutaneous manifestations of diabetes mellitus. J Am Acad Dermatol 1994; 30: 519–31

Poole S, Fenske NA. Cutaneous markers of internal malignancy. J Am Acad Dermatol 1993; 28: 1–13, 147–64

Stingl G (ed) Treatment of AIDS-related disorders. Dermatol Clin 1999; 12: 1–130

Wilkin JK. The red face: flushing disorders. Clin Dermatol 1993; 11: 211–23

INTRODUCTION

The collagen vascular diseases comprise lupus erythematosus, the scleroderma spectrum of diseases, mixed connective tissue disease (MCTD), dermatomyositis (and polymyositis), and various other rarer autoimmune disorders. They are also termed 'connective tissue diseases', but technically this term includes structural disorders of collagen, elastic, etc. (Ch. 22) and

may therefore be confusing. All the collagen vascular diseases are potentially of general medical importance, having both cutaneous and systemic manifestations, and all may have vasculitic manifestations (vasculitis is discussed more fully in Ch. 14).

Raynaud phenomenon may occur in several of these disorders, and is therefore discussed initially.

RAYNAUD PHENOMENON

Etiology and pathogenesis

Causes of Raynaud phenomenon are listed in Table 13.1. It is a vasospastic disorder that is relatively common as an isolated phenomenon, usually in women and mainly the young adult age group (2% of the overall population, but about 10–20% of young women). It may be familial, usually with a young age of onset (most below 30 years). Symptoms may vary with pregnancy, menopause, and menstrual cycle.

Five to ten percent of affected individuals will develop a collagen vascular disease, especially sclerodermas; this should be suspected especially in men who develop Raynaud phenomenon, as they less commonly suffer from idiopathic Raynaud disease. It is a feature in about 25% of patients with systemic lupus erythematosus (SLE) or Sjögren syndrome, and 95% of those with systemic sclerosis.

Within the microvasculature, the abnormal vasoconstriction appears to involve an imbalance between endothelium-derived constricting factors (endothelins) and relaxing factors (nitric oxide).

Clinical features

The characteristic lesion of Raynaud phenomenon is a sharply demarcated pallor of the digit (Fig. 13.1), usually with a cut-off in the region of the proximal interphalangeal joint, which is of sudden onset and may be triggered by a cold environment or by handling cold objects. This is followed by a dusky cyanosed phase, and a red hyperemic phase. The most common site is the fingers, but toes are also affected. Usually one or a few digits are affected at any one time, but affecting both hands and most digits on different occasions; if confined to one hand, a local cause of proximal vascular obstruction is likely. Rarely, the tongue may be affected, causing dysarthria.

Features that suggest an underlying collagen vascular disorder include elongated cuticles or nail fold telangiectasia, pulp atrophy of fingertips producing pitted scars, and positive antinuclear antibody (ANA) tests.

Differential diagnosis

The classic sharp cut-off and color change sequence is diagnostic, in which case the issue is to determine whether the disorder is idiopathic or has an underlying cause. Disorders that may be confused with Raynaud phenomenon include the following.
- 'Poor circulation'—all fingers and the hands generally are cold, and may variably appear pale.
- Acrocyanosis—the hands and all fingers are dusky blue or purplish, and prone to perniosis.
- Perniosis (chilblains)—individual lesions are painful, inflamed, and last days or weeks.
- Achenbach syndrome—affects a solitary digit, which becomes painful and then swollen and blue; this is due to venous rupture, often after a

Table 13.1 CAUSES OF RAYNAUD PHENOMENON

Mechanism	Examples
Idiopathic	(= Raynaud disease)
Arterial: mechanical obstruction	Extravascular causes (thoracic outlet, trauma), intravascular causes (thrombi, arteriosclerosis, stenosis, etc.)
Connective tissue disorders	Systemic sclerosis or scleroderma, polyarteritis nodosa, lupus erythematosus, vasculitis
Hematologic	Cold-precipitable proteins, other causes of hyperviscosity
Neurologic	Nerve compression, chronic disuse disorders (e.g. hemiplegia), reflex vasoconstriction
Trauma	Vibration white finger
Drugs	Beta-blockers, nicotine, ergot, bleomycin, vinyl chloride, methysergide

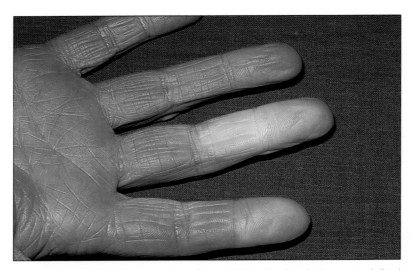

Figure 13.1 Raynaud phenomenon, demonstrating the sharply demarcated distal whiteness of affected digits. The affected fingers typically vary between episodes, although several may be affected at any one time.

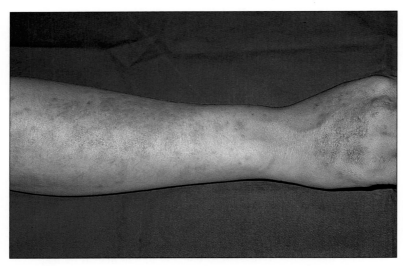

Figure 13.2 Lesions induced by sunlight in a patient with lupus erythematosus. This pattern of transient rash on the exposed forearm skin is very similar to polymorphic light eruption (see Ch. 28).

Treatment

Mild cases require no treatment other than gentle rewarming and sensible measures such as gloves and warm clothing to reduce the frequency of episodes. More complex clothing includes electrically heated gloves and socks.

A variety of vasodilator drugs may be helpful, especially calcium channel antagonists and pentoxifylline.

In the more severe cases with severe symptoms, ulceration, or vascular compromise (usually those with a collagen vascular disorder), additional treatments such as steroids, immunosuppressive agents, plasmapheresis, prostacyclin infusions, upper limb sympathectomy, and more recently digital sympathectomy may be applicable. Novel vasodilators such as calcitonin gene-related peptide (CGRP) have also been used.

PRACTICE POINTS

- Raynaud phenomenon in a male patient is strongly suggestive that there may be an associated collagen vascular disease.
- If all fingers are cold at the same time, the diagnosis is probably not Raynaud phenomenon.
- A painful and dusky finger without a preceding pale vasoconstrictive phase is probably not due to Raynaud phenomenon.
- Suggested screening tests in a patient with Raynaud phenomenon and no other clinical clues would be complete blood count, viscosity and autoantibody screen (to include antinuclear antibody, ribonucleoprotein, Scl-70, and anticentromere; see Table 13.4).

LUPUS ERYTHEMATOSUS

General aspects, diagnosis, and investigations

Lupus erythematosus (LE) is a multisystem disorder, which commonly affects the skin (sometimes in isolation). Possible effects on internal organs include renal, neurologic, cardiovascular, and lung disease. Some of the non-specific skin diseases that may occur is discussed more broadly elsewhere (e.g. vasculitis and diffuse alopecia). Aggravation by sunlight is frequent and may produce lesions resembling polymorphic light eruption (Fig. 13.2); expression of autoantigens by keratinocytes may be induced by sunlight. The specific patterns of skin involvement may differ according to the category of LE (Table 13.2) and are discussed below; the most important patterns numerically are discoid (DLE), subacute cutaneous (SCLE) and systemic (SLE).

In all types of LE (except the neonatal form), there is a female predominance, which is most marked in SLE. About 5–10% of patients meet criteria for SLE (Table 13.3).

Investigations

Investigations in LE are to establish the diagnosis, and to determine the presence and degree of internal organ involvement; the following may all be pertinent.

degree of trauma (e.g. twisting off a tight jar lid) and does not have the vasoconstrictive phase of Raynaud phenomenon.

- Buerger disease—a smoking-associated severe form of peripheral vascular disease characterized by digital necrosis.

TABLE 13.2 TYPES OF LUPUS ERYTHEMATOSUS AND THEIR DIFFERENTIAL DIAGNOSIS

Pattern of lupus erythematosus (LE)	Typical lesion pattern	Main differential diagnoses and comments
Discoid lupus erythematosus (DLE)	Discoid lesions, typically facial	Dermatitis, psoriasis, Bowen disease, telangiectatic actinic keratosis, reticulate erythematosus mucinosis (V of neck, see Ch. 11), polymorphic light eruption (more variable than typical DLE), tinea faciei, lupus vulgaris. Jessner lymphocytic infiltrate may be particularly difficult to distinguish. Scalp: consider lichen planus, folliculitis decalvans.
Subacute cutaneous lupus erythematosus (SCLE)	Lesions may be psoriasiform or annular; photosensitivity is also common	Psoriasis, dermatitis (especially seborrheic on trunk), tinea corporis, mycosis fungoides or lymphomas, polymorphic light eruption, reticulate erythematosus mucinosis, dermatomyositis, drug-induced photosensitivity.
Systemic lupus erythematosus (SLE)	Malar butterfly rash (for other lesions, the differential diagnosis is that of DLE or SCLE)	Especially rosacea, seborrheic dermatitis. Also contact dermatitis, polymorphic light eruption and other photosensitivity.
Lupus profundus	Inflammatory nodules affecting fat	Other panniculitides can usually be excluded by the tendency for lupus profundus to affect the face, upper arm, or upper trunk (unusual in other panniculitis); plus patients often have known LE or positive antibody tests. In acute inflammatory stage, soft tissue injuries, infections, or neoplasia may be in the differential.
Chilblain LE	DLE-like lesions of distal digits	Dermatitis, perniosis.
Neonatal LE	SCLE-like lesions, often facial	Dermatitis, skin infection, cutis marmorata.
LE tumidus	Tumid facial lesions	Polymorphic light eruption, Jessner lymphocytic infiltrate, pseudolymphomas, mucinosis.
Mucosal LE	Lip or buccal involvement	Lip: dermatitis, lichen planus. Buccal: lichen planus, candidiasis, leukoplakia.

Table 13.3 CRITERIA FOR DIAGNOSIS OF SYSTEMIC LUPUS ERYTHEMATOSUS[a]

Malar rash
Discoid rash
Photosensitivity
Oral ulcers
Arthritis
Serositis (pleuritis or pericarditis)
Renal disorder (proteinuria or casts)
Neurologic disorder (seizures or psychosis)
Hematologic disorder (hemolytic anemia, leukopenia, lymphopenia, or thrombocytopenia)
Immunologic disorder (positive lupus erythematosus cells, anti-DNA, or anti-Sm antibodies: false positive syphilis serology)
Antinuclear antibody

[a]Summarized from the 1982 American Rheumatism Association criteria (see *Further reading* list). Note that this list was designed for use in clinical studies rather than for clinical diagnostic purposes (see text for discussion).

Biopsy of skin lesions

This may show characteristic features, including a rather lichenoid dermo–epidermal junction infiltrate with basal keratinocyte vacuolation, which extends down the hair follicles. There is keratotic plugging of the follicles, most marked in chronic DLE. Rarely, the basal vacuolation may be sufficiently severe to cause clinically apparent blisters, usually in patients with acute cutaneous or subacute cutaneous LE.

Direct immunofluorescence studies on a skin biopsy (see Ch. 16 for details of the technique and further reading) may show deposits of IgG, complement C3, IgM, or IgA in the basement membrane zone in lesional skin, less commonly in sun-exposed non-lesional skin, and least commonly (the lupus band test) in non-exposed skin.

Tests for autoantibodies

Antinuclear antibody is often positive in patients with collagen vascular disorders, and is therefore useful as a screening test, but it has varying degrees of sensitivity and specificity between diseases. Various patterns of nuclear staining may occur.

- Homogeneous—anti-DNA antibodies and antihistone antibodies.
- Speckled—antibodies to SSA (Ro), SSB (La), Sm, and ribonucleoprotein (RNP).
- Centromere—anticentromere (typical of CREST [calcinosis, Raynaud phenomenon, esophageal involvement, sclerodactyly, and telangiectasia], less often found in systemic sclerosis).
- Nucleolar—typical of scleroderma, also occur in LE.

The ANA and other relevant antibodies, and their approximate frequency in different diseases, are listed in Table 13.4. Some antibodies are very specific to a particular disease or subset, even though they may occur only in a minority of patients (e.g. Sm in SLE). Others may be demonstrated in several disorders but have a particularly strong link with a particular disease, such as anticentromere antibodies with CREST, anti-RNP antibodies with MCTD, or antihistone antibodies with drug-induced LE.

Anti-SSA (anti-Ro) and anti-SSB (anti-La) are extractable nuclear antigens, which may be present in photosensitive, subacute cutaneous, neonatal, and late-onset LE, and in Sjögren syndrome (from which the 'SS' is derived), dermatomyositis (uncommonly), and others. SSA may produce positive tests in patients with ANA-negative LE, the combination of negative ANA and positive SSA being found particularly in SCLE and neonatal LE.

Table 13.4 SOME AUTOANTIBODIES IN COLLAGEN VASCULAR DISEASE AND THEIR SIGNIFICANCE[a]

Antibody	Approximate frequency of positive results in collagen vascular diseases			
	Positive in 90–100% with:	Positive in 50–90% with:	Positive in 20–50% with:	Positive in < 20% with:
Antinuclear antibody (ANA)	SLE, MCTD, CREST	SCLE, PSS	DLE, NLE, LEP	
ssDNA		SLE		MCTD, PSS, SCLE, DLE
dsDNA		SLE		
Sm			SLE	
U1RNP	MCTD		SLE, PSS	
SSA	NLE	SCLE	SLE	DLE, PSS, LEP
SSB			SLE, NLE	SCLE, DLE
Histone			SLE (mainly drug-induced)	
Scl-70			PSS	
Centromere	CREST			PSS

[a]Antiphospholipid and anticardiolipin antibodies and antibodies in dermatomyositis are discussed in the text.
CREST, calcinosis, Raynaud phenomenon, esophagus, sclerodactyly, telangiectasia; DLE, discoid lupus erythematosus; LEP, lupus erythematosus profundus; MCTD, mixed connective tissue disease; NLE, neonatal lupus erythematosus; PSS, progressive systemic sclerosis; SCLE, subacute cutaneous lupus erythematosus; SLE, systemic lupus erythematosus.

Antiphospholipid antibodies (anticardiolipin antibodies and lupus anticoagulant) may be linked with LE but are discussed in the section on antiphospholipid syndrome (Ch. 14), as they also occur without background LE. A skin lesion that can rarely occur in patients with LE, anetoderma, may be more common in patients with antiphospholipid antibodies.

Complement levels

These should be tested in patients with active LE. Complement C4 levels are often subnormal in patients with active systemic disease. Low levels are particularly linked with renal involvement. Occasional patients have familial LE due to inherited complement deficiency (usually C2 or C4), and there is an association with C1 esterase inhibitor deficiency, which causes hereditary angioedema.

Tests for involvement of internal organs

Tests for internal organ involvement may include urinalysis (proteinuria and casts), electrolytes, full blood count, liver function tests, erythrocyte sedimentation rate (ESR), and others, as determined by symptoms.

Drug-induced lupus

A wide range of drugs may provoke LE or LE-like eruption (Fig. 13.3). In some cases, patients may have a positive ANA test but no clinical symptoms (such as the majority of cases due to procainamide); even in symptomatic patients, anti–dsDNA and hypocomplementemia are rare in drug-induced LE. Sometimes, it may be difficult to be certain whether LE in a patient taking a relevant drug is actually drug-induced or idiopathic; the presence of antihistone antibodies suggests the possibility of drug-induced LE but is not specific. Patients with drug-induced LE typically have a photosensitive rash. Relevant drugs include the following.

- Cardiology—hydralazine, procainamide, captopril, methyldopa, quinidine, and spironolactone (also thiazides and beta-blockers, which are linked mainly with the SCLE pattern).
- Neurology—phenytoin, carbamazepine, levodopa, and lamotrigine.
- Psychiatry—lithium.
- Endocrinology—thiouracils and oral contraceptives.
- Infections—isoniazid and sulfonamides.
- Rheumatology—penicillamine, etanercept, and leflunomide.
- Gastroenterology—cimetidine.

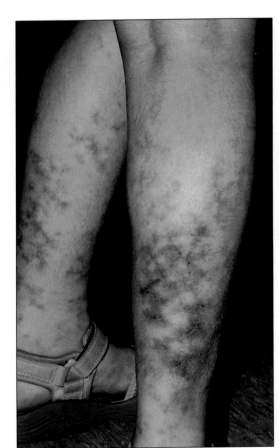

Figure 13.3 Lupus erythematosus: it was uncertain whether the disease was drug-induced, due to anticonvulsant therapy, or idiopathic. The clinical appearances are those of livedo (see Ch. 14), histologically with vasculitis. Serology was positive for antinuclear antibody, antihistone antibodies (a feature consistent with a drug etiology), and anti-dsDNA antibodies. (Courtesy of Dr. L. Barco.)

- Dermatology—griseofulvin and terbinafine.
- Other—COL-3 (a tetracycline used in oncology).

Discoid lupus erythematosus

Discoid lupus erythematosus is the most common form of LE (Figs 13.4–13.14). It may occur as one of several features leading to a diagnosis of SLE, but commonly DLE lesions occur in the absence of

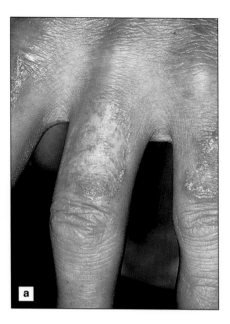

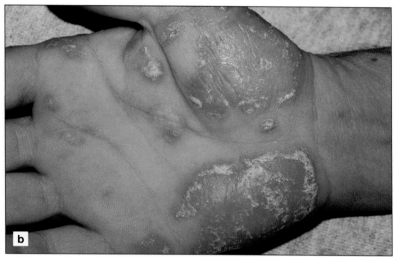

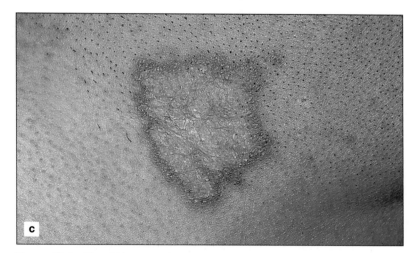

Figure 13.4 Discoid lupus erythematosus on the finger (**a**), palm (**b**) (an uncommon site), and beard area (**c**). A grayish color centrally is a common feature, due to the combination of disruption of pigment, which is caused by inflammation at the dermo–epidermal junction, and the subsequent atrophy. Note the scaling, follicular scarring, and follicular plugging shown in these pictures. (Panel a from Lawrence CM, Cox NH. Physical Signs in Dermatology, 2nd edn. London: Mosby, 2002.)

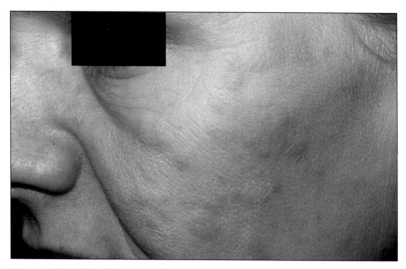

Figure 13.5 Discoid lupus erythematosus: early lesions on the face. This may be difficult to distinguish from Jessner lymphocytic infiltrate or from systemic lupus erythematosus.

other evidence of LE. Discoid lesions are erythematous, thickened plaques with scaling and plugging of follicles. They later become atrophic, scarred (including permanent loss of hair), telangiectatic, and variably pigmented. Most occur at sun-exposed facial sites, including the scalp (Figs 13.9–13.11). Ears are often affected (Fig. 13.12), as is the nasal tip (Fig. 13.13) and the lips more rarely (Fig. 13.14). Less commonly, annular (erythema multiforme-like) lesions may occur.

About 20–30% of patients with DLE have positive ANAs, but fewer than 10% progress to develop SLE.

Systemic lupus erythematosus

Classification as SLE is made by fulfilling four of a series of diagnostic criteria proposed by the American Rheumatism Association (Table 13.3), although these criteria were proposed for use in clinical studies and do not preclude the diagnosis being made on the basis of fewer criteria in clinical practice (especially as there is no requirement for four criteria to be simultaneous). Additionally, some less specific criteria are not included (such as malaise, alopecia, or nail fold telangiectasia), some clinical patterns that strongly suggest LE are not included (e.g. hypocomplementemic urticarial vasculitis), and some supportive antibody tests (e.g. anti-SSA and antiphospholipid antibody) were not included at the time the criteria were proposed. The dermatologic manifestations included in the SLE diagnostic criteria are a 'butterfly' malar rash (Figs 13.15 and 13.16), DLE, and photosensitivity; other cutaneous features that were not specific enough to form part of the diagnostic criteria include diffuse alopecia (Fig. 13.17), nail fold telangiectasia (Fig. 13.18), urticarial lesions (Fig. 13.19), and vasculitis (Fig. 13.20).

By contrast with DLE, the acute malar rash of SLE often parallels disease in other organ systems. This is of diagnostic benefit, as it is very unlikely that malar rash in an otherwise completely well patient is due to SLE; in such patients, other diagnoses, such as rosacea (Fig. 13.21), seborrheic dermatitis, contact dermatitis, and polymorphic light eruption should be considered. ANA tests are also more useful than in DLE, as they are positive in almost all patients with SLE, and over 50% with acute SLE also have anti-dsDNA antibodies, especially if there is active nephritis.

Subacute cutaneous lupus erythematosus

This variant of LE (Figs 13.22–13.27) is characterized by psoriasiform or annular skin lesions, photosensitivity, and mild systemic disease (usually arthritis). There is some overlap with SLE at the more severe end of the spectrum, and with DLE in other cases. A common feature is the demonstration of a negative ANA test but a positive anti-SSA (anti-Ro) antibody

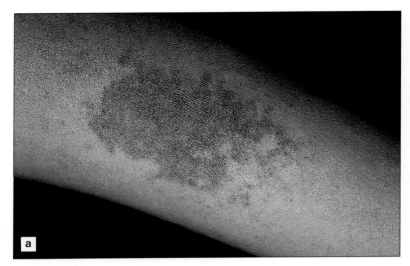

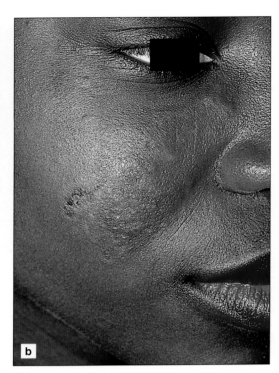

Figure 13.6 Discoid lupus erythematosus in colored skin on the arm (**a**) and face (**b**). Lupus erythematosus is more common in African-Caribbean patients, and needs prompt treatment due to the potential for pigmentary disturbance (a) and scarring (b). This is especially important on the face, a site at which the risks of atrophy due to treatment are outweighed by the potential benefits of potent topical steroids.

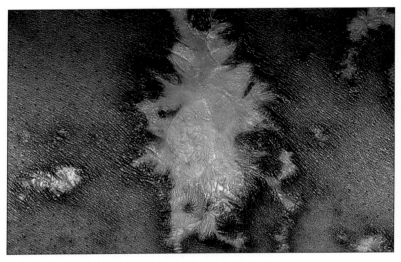

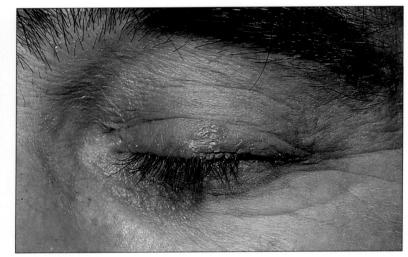

Figure 13.7 Discoid lupus erythematosus, demonstrating marked scarring and hypopigmentation.

Figure 13.8 Discoid lupus erythematosus (DLE) of the eyelid margin. This may be difficult to distinguish from neoplastic lesions if it occurs in isolation, but the upper eyelid margin is a rare site for skin tumors. Note the loss of eyelashes, which is typical of DLE at this site.

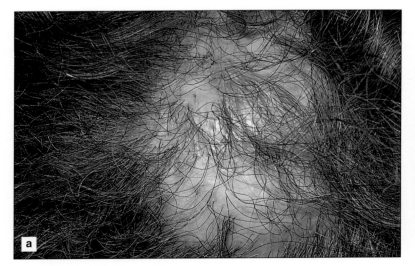

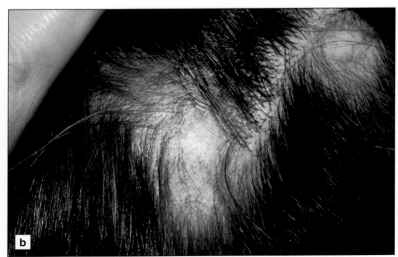

Figure 13.9 Discoid lupus erythematosus of the scalp usually presents as a scarring alopecia. In (**a**), there is patchy sparing of some hairs, and potent topical steroid treatment may halt the progression of alopecia, although this is more likely when an inflammatory component or intact follicles are visible (see Fig. 13.10). (**b**) A pattern resembling pseudopelade (an end point of several scarring dermatoses, see Ch. 28) in a patient with systemic lupus erythematosus.

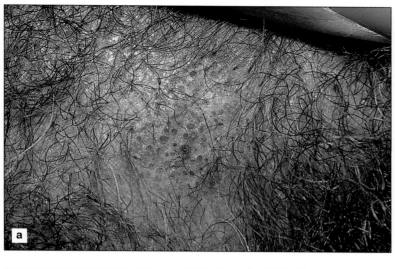

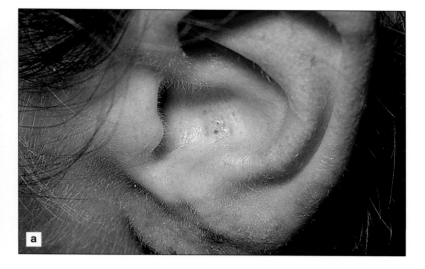

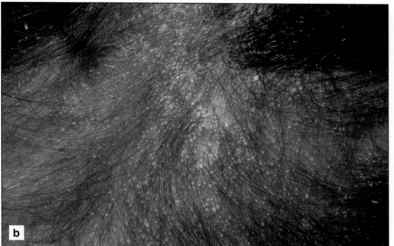

Figure 13.10 (**a**,**b**) Discoid lupus erythematosus of the scalp: two cases with inflammation and the characteristic plugging of follicles, particularly prominent in (**b**).

Figure 13.11 Discoid lupus erythematosus of scalp, demonstrating marked scarring and pigment change. This situation is irreversible. (Courtesy of Michael O. Murphy, M.D.)

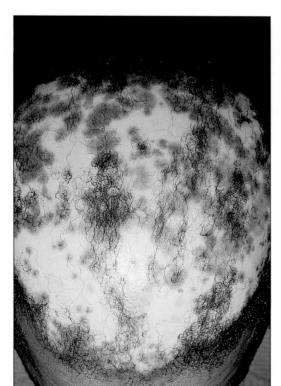

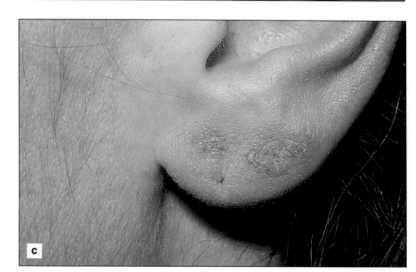

Figure 13.12 Discoid lupus erythematosus (DLE) of the ear. (**a**) Comedo-like follicular plugging may occur in the concha of the ear in some patients with acne. When it occurs in the absence of acne, as in this case, it should be considered as suspicious of lupus erythematosus (LE). This patient had a DLE lesion on the helix of the ear as well. (**b**) More typical LE also occurs at this site, and may be confused with other causes of otitis externa such as seborrheic dermatitis or psoriasis. (**c**) The earlobe is also a common site for DLE. It may be confused with nickel dermatitis from earrings, but the usual area affected is the lower part of the helix, just above the lobe, rather than at the typical site of piercing the ear (which is clearly spared in this illustration).

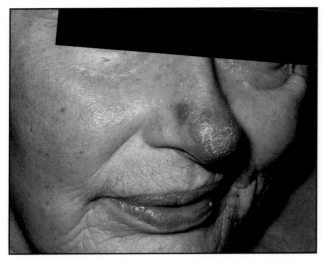

Figure 13.13 Discoid lupus erythematosus of the nasal tip; this is sometimes the only site affected.

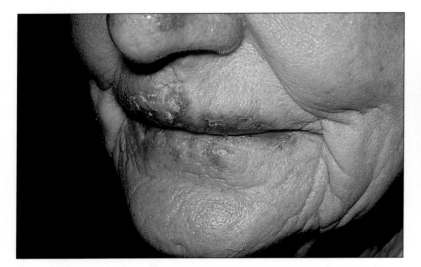

Figure 13.14 Discoid lupus erythematosus of the lip (note a small area on the nose as well). This patient had been told 30 years previously that there was no treatment, and presented due to weight loss, as she could not eat solid food; topical treatment with clobetasol propionate resolved the symptoms, and her weight increased by 7 lb in the following month.

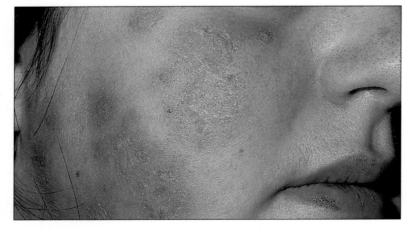

Figure 13.15 Acute facial lupus erythematosus. This shows rather tumid lesions, and was associated with a discoid area of lupus erythematosus in the scalp (which was treated before irreversible scarring occurred), general malaise, and mild leukopenia.

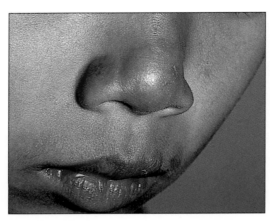

Figure 13.16 Systemic lupus erythematosus (SLE) rash on the nose in a child. In adults, most new-onset lupus erythematosus is of discoid type, but children seem more likely to have SLE.

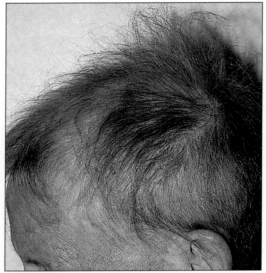

Figure 13.17 Diffuse alopecia in LE. Diffuse hair thinning is common in acute episodes of systemic lupus erythematosus (SLE), but would be an uncommon presentation in the absence of other symptoms. It also occurs for numerous other reasons (Ch. 24), and is too non-specific to be used as a formal diagnostic criterion for SLE.

in serum; additionally, particulate intraepidermal IgG positivity on direct immunofluorescence testing of skin biopsies may reflect binding of anti-SSA antibodies to keratinocytes.

Subacute cutaneous lupus erythematosus may be provoked by drugs, especially thiazides, and may occur in families with inherited complement deficiency or hereditary angioedema.

Chilblain lupus erythematosus

Chilblain (perniotic) LE is felt to be rare in the USA but more common in the UK (Figs 13.28 and 13.29). Patients have lesions around the nail folds of fingers and toes, often duskiness and hyperkeratosis of fingers and feet, and sometimes annular lesions of the limbs. Histologically, they have features of DLE. They are very refractory to treatment, but may respond to vasodilators as used for the treatment of Raynaud phenomenon.

Lupus erythematosus tumidus

It is unclear whether this should be treated as a separate variant of LE, but it does have some features that are different from more typical DLE. These include an acute and seasonal (summer) presentation, localized tumid lesions, marked photosensitivity, and good response to systemic antimalarials.

Lupus panniculitis

This is also known as lupus profundus (Figs 13.30 and 13.31). It is most common in women with LE, presenting as firm, inflamed nodules that may form a contracted scar with depression of the overlying skin surface.

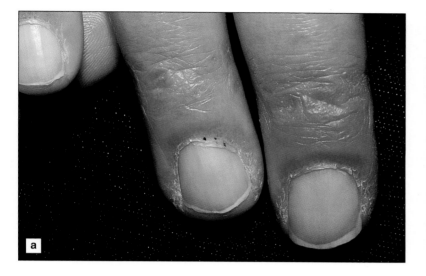

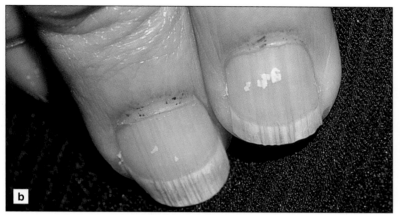

Figure 13.18 (**a,b**) Nail fold telangiectasia and dilated capillary loops, with ragged, elongated cuticles, are features of lupus erythematosus, scleroderma, and dermatomyositis.

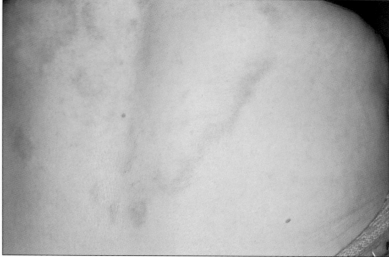

Figure 13.19 Large arcuate lesions in lupus erythematosus. These appear rather urticarial in morphology, but migrate more gradually than true urticaria.

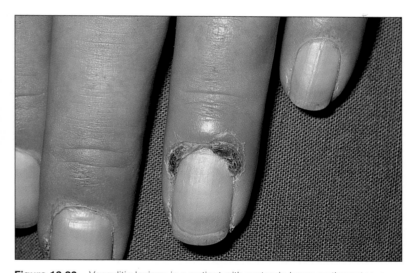

Figure 13.20 Vasculitic lesions in a patient with systemic lupus erythematosus, presenting as digital infarcts and splinter hemorrhages.

Mucosal lupus erythematosus

Mucosal lesions are probably underestimated. Lips are not uncommonly affected in patients with DLE. Palatal lesions (Fig. 13.32) and rather lichenoid-appearing buccal and gingival lesions (Fig. 13.33) may all be present.

Neonatal lupus erythematosus

This disorder is due to transplacental transfer of antibodies, most commonly anti-SSA but less commonly anti-SSB alone or anti-U1RNP. The mother may be asymptomatic, have Sjögren syndrome, or have SCLE, but will have positive antibodies (the diagnosis is usually confirmed by testing maternal blood). Skin lesions in the neonate are typically mild, usually annular, erythematous plaques, which resemble mild SCLE. They occur especially on the face and scalp (Fig. 13.34), typically involving the periorbital area ('owl eye' appearance), although limbs and trunk can also be affected. Crusting may be prominent, and photosensitivity is common, although not always clinically apparent. Telangiectasia, cutis marmorata, or angiomatous lesions may occur in the absence of more typical rash.

The important systemic feature that may occur is neonatal heart block, which may be detected from about the 20th week of pregnancy. By contrast to the skin lesions, which resolve spontaneously in the first 6 months postpartum, the heart block does not resolve. However, even in women with known SLE and anti-SSA antibodies, the risk is only about 10–20%. Other systemic involvement is uncommon, apart from thrombocytopenia. Systemic involvement may have a male predominance.

Differential diagnosis

This is indicated, by clinical pattern, in Table 13.2.

PRACTICE POINTS

- Always consider discoid lupus erythematosus (DLE) in any patient with scarring alopecia and evidence of inflammation (perifollicular erythema at the margin of scarred areas).
- The risks of atrophy due to treatment are outweighed by the potential ability of potent topical steroids to prevent permanent scarring in DLE.
- A butterfly rash without malaise or other systemic symptoms is unlikely to represent active systemic lupus erythematosus (SLE).
- If you suspect SLE in a patient with photosensitivity and DLE-like lesions, but the ANA test is negative, check for anti-SSA antibodies: the patient may have subacute cutaneous lupus erythematosus (SCLE).
- In a pregnant woman with SCLE or known anti-SSA antibodies, remember the possibility of neonatal congenital heart block.
- Patients on antimalarials for lupus erythematosus *must* stop smoking to get good benefit.

Treatment

Sunscreens are important therapeutically in all types of LE, especially SCLE and tumid LE. UVB-blocking ability is usually felt to be the most important factor, although there are cases of LE provoked by UVA tanning

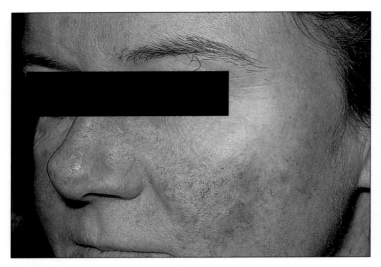

Figure 13.21 Rosacea is in the differential diagnosis of systemic lupus erythematosus on the face. It often involves the forehead and chin as well, and usually has a more prominent background erythematous component with some fixed telangiectasia, as well as pustular lesions and whiteheads, which are not a feature of lupus erythematosus.

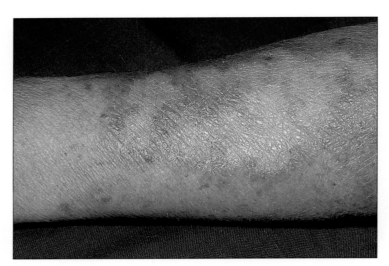

Figure 13.24 Subacute cutaneous lupus erythematosus. As with some discoid lupus erythematosus (DLE) lesions, a central grayish color is common. There is less central atrophy compared with DLE.

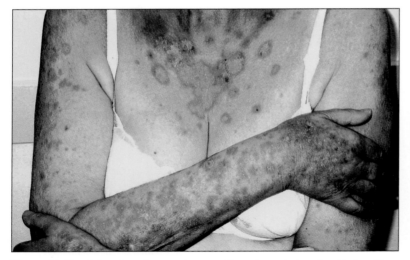

Figure 13.22 Subacute cutaneous lupus erythematosus lesions tend to be either annular or psoriasiform. In this patient, both types are present; those on the trunk are annular, but the arm lesions are more psoriasiform. Most patients, as in this case, have a positive test for Ro (SSA) antibody. (Courtesy of Dr. G. Dawn.)

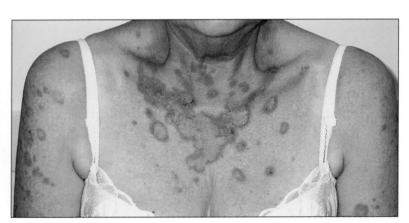

Figure 13.25 Subacute cutaneous lupus erythematosus demonstrating the ring of peripheral scaling that may lead to it being confused with dermatophyte 'ringworm' infections (same patient as in Fig. 13.22). (Courtesy of Dr. G. Dawn.)

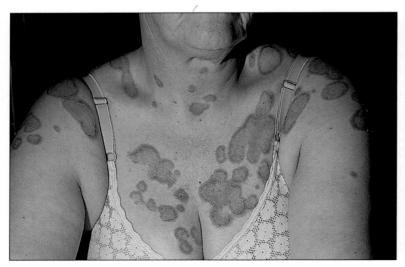

Figure 13.23 An example of subacute cutaneous lupus erythematosus with more strikingly annular lesions. When the trunk is involved, the rash often affects the upper torso predominantly.

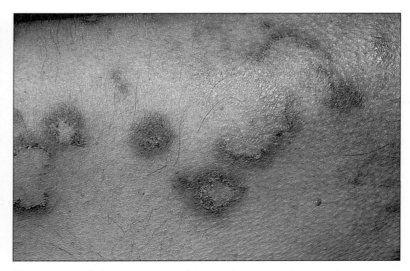

Figure 13.26 Subacute cutaneous lupus erythematosus demonstrating annular and arciform lesions.

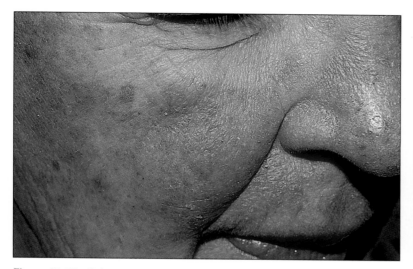

Figure 13.27   Subacute cutaneous lupus erythematosus affecting the face. In many patients, this type of lupus erythematosus is quite photosensitive, affecting the face, V of neck, and exposed areas of the forearms.

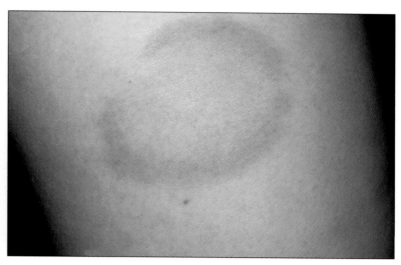

Figure 13.30   An early lesion of lupus profundus, at the initial inflammatory stage prior to atrophy and fibrosis of the subcutaneous fat. This lesion responded well to hydroxychloroquine.

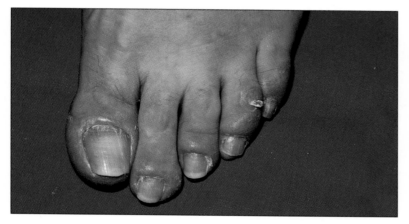

Figure 13.28   Dusky cold toes in a patient with the 'chilblain' pattern of lupus erythematosus. Most patients with this presentation have other systemic features, and it is often a very refractory condition with prominent symptoms of discomfort or pain.

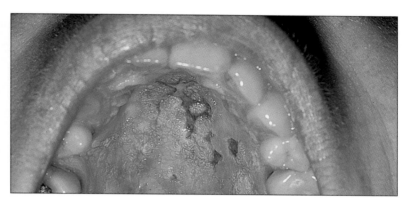

Figure 13.31   Lupus erythematosus of the palate in a patient with systemic lupus erythematosus and associated hereditary angioedema. This degree of oral involvement is uncommon.

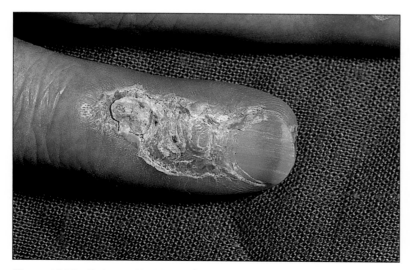

Figure 13.29   Patients with chilblain lupus erythematosus (LE) may develop discoid pattern LE lesions in the periungual region, as shown here.

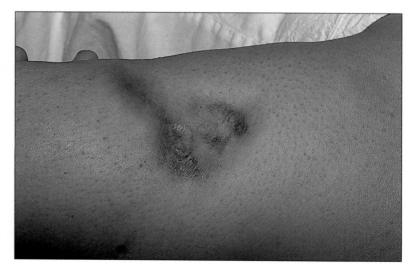

Figure 13.32   An older lesion of lupus profundus, demonstrating depression of the skin surface due to marked atrophy of the underlying fat.

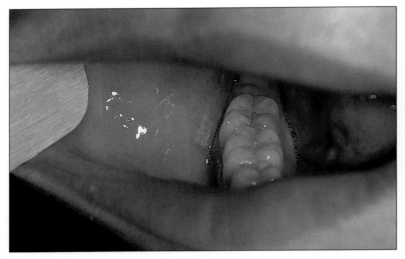

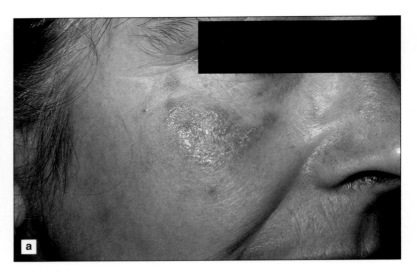

Figure 13.33 Lupus erythematosus of the buccal mucosa. This is difficult to distinguish clinically from lichen planus, and the diagnosis may depend on histologic features and the presence of skin lesions (see also Fig. 8.26).

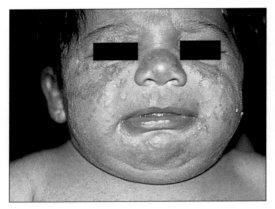

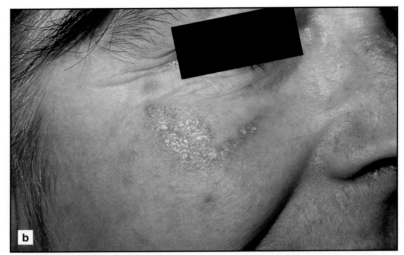

Figure 13.34 Neonatal lupus erythematosus typically affects the face, with SCLE- or DLE-type lesions. It tends to improve and usually clears by about 6 months, as the transplacentally acquired maternal antibody is gradually replaced by the infant's own antibody production. It may be associated with neonatal heart block, and the mother is usually Ro (SSA)-positive.

Figure 13.35 Topical tacrolimus has recently been used with success in discoid lupus erythematosus, as shown in this patient with a plaque that was resistant to strong topical corticosteroids.

sunbeds, and about half of the patients with LE in whom lesions can be artificially photoprovoked react in both the UVA and UVB ranges (see also Ch. 17).

The usual treatment for discoid lesions is a potent topical corticosteroid. Although these have potential risks of skin atrophy on the face, this is balanced against the potential for permanent scarring, particularly scarring alopecia in the beard area or scalp. Intralesional steroid injections may be useful for refractory discoid lesions, or isolated areas of LE profundus. Topical tacrolimus has recently been documented to be useful in DLE, and avoids the risk of corticosteroid atrophy (Fig. 13.35). SCLE or SLE may also require topical treatment along the same lines, but systemic therapy is also often required.

Antimalarials, usually hydroxychloroquine, are a useful adjunct to topical therapy in patients with troublesome DLE, in many patients with SLE (especially if photosensitivity is prominent), and especially in SCLE. They also appear to be useful in patients with thrombotic risk due to antiphospholipid syndrome (Fig. 13.36 and Ch. 14). Headache and nausea are the most common side effects, but most patients tolerate these drugs well. Hydroxychloroquine dosage should not be above 6.5 mg/kg lean body mass, as this increases the risk of ocular toxicity (chronic maculopathy). Mepacrine (Atabrine) does not have this ocular risk but causes yellowish or gray pigmentation (especially of palate and sclerae), and may cause a lichenoid drug eruption. In some patients, the two antimalarials used together appear to produce better results than either alone. Smoking markedly decreases the benefit from antimalarials: patients should be advised to stop.

In SLE, a variety of systemic agents may be used that are not usually necessary for the other types of LE. Systemic steroids should be started in acute severe LE on clinical suspicion, and adjusted on the basis of clinical response.

Azathioprine is commonly used as an immunosuppressive agent in SLE. It is generally well tolerated but causes dose-related hematologic toxicity (see Ch. 4 for details on use of azathioprine). Long-term azathioprine immunosuppression predisposes to skin cancers (see Chs 12 and 32), and hence is another reason for sun-avoidance measures in patients with LE.

Other immunosuppressive agents that may be used in LE include dapsone, methotrexate, gold, cyclophosphamide, retinoids, interferon, ciclosporin, pulsed methylprednisolone, intravenous gamma-globulin, thalidomide, and clofazimine. Dapsone produces a rapid response in patients with a rare bullous form of LE in which blisters arise on clinically normal skin, and is also useful in SCLE. Other agents, such as antihypertensives, are also commonly required for the systemic manifestations.

SCLERODERMAS

Scleroderma (tight skin) is a term used for a range of disorders in which tight, hard, sclerotic skin is the main feature, but it may also occur in other situations (Table 13.5). Some of these other disorders may be difficult to distinguish from autoimmune collagen vascular type scleroderma at times, especially conditions such as eosinophilic fasciitis. However, Table 13.5 gives some features that help to differentiated these, and they are all discussed elsewhere in the text. This section discusses the collagen vascular sclerodermas which can be classified as follows.

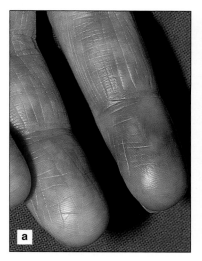
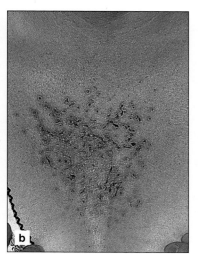

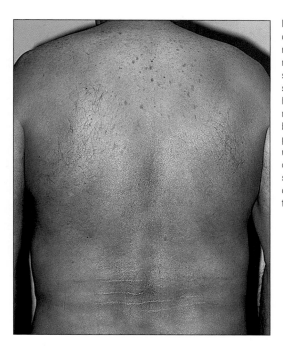

Figure 13.38 A more diffuse pattern of morphea, which might resemble the sclerodermatous skin of systemic sclerosis. However, diffuse morphea often has a brownish color, does not particularly affect the upper trunk (a common distribution for systemic sclerosis), and characteristically spares the periareolar region.

Figure 13.36 Antiphospholipid antibodies and LE. (**a**) Dusky fingers, with a livedo pattern, in a patient with a borderline antiphospholipid screen; she also had discoid lupus erythematosus lesions of scalp and V of neck (**b**) at presentation. Hydroxychloroquine is useful in this situation, not only for the photosensitivity, but also because it has an antithrombotic effect.

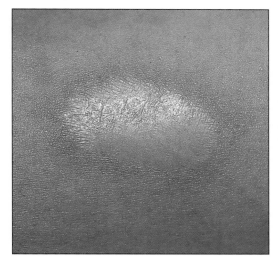

Figure 13.37 A typical lesion of early morphea. The center is ivory-colored and shiny, with loss of follicles, and there is a violaceous inflammatory border. This type of lesion may improve using strong topical steroids, although the white color usually persists.

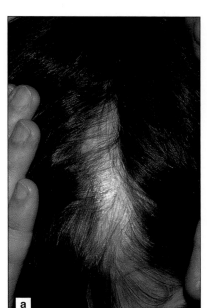

Figure 13.39 Morphea en coup de sabre (**a**). Involvement of the scalp, producing linear alopecia. This pattern generally extends on to the forehead and distorts the forehead crease lines when frowning. The scalp defect can sometimes be excised if necessary. (**b**) Less commonly, there are two (as shown here) or even three bands.

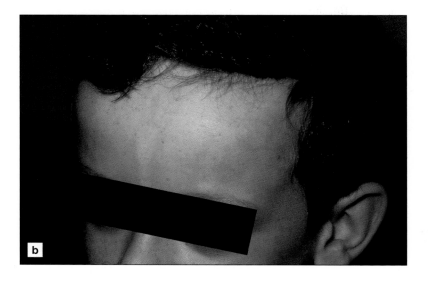

- Morphea (cutaneous scleroderma; Figs 13.37–13.42):
  - plaque,
  - linear,
  - guttate,
  - nodular,
  - profunda (deep morphea),
  - bullous, and
  - generalized (adult) and disabling pansclerotic morphea of childhood.
- Systemic scleroderma (Figs 13.43–13.54):
  - limited disease (acrosclerosis and CREST), and
  - diffuse disease (systemic sclerosis, SSc, or progressive systemic sclerosis, PSS).

Etiology and pathogenesis

The various forms of scleroderma listed here have different clinical courses, different human leukocyte antigen (HLA) and antibody associations, and probably different pathogenetic mechanisms. For example, ANA is often positive in linear morphea in children but not in other purely cutaneous sclerodermas. However, they all involve different degrees of microvascular obliteration, endothelial damage, and perivascular mononuclear inflammatory response, and increased deposition of collagen and matrix components in the skin.

Table 13.5   CAUSES OF SCLERODERMATOUS CHANGES IN THE SKIN

Disorder	Comments
Morphea (cutaneous scleroderma)	May be localized (plaque type), generalized, or specific variants (linear, en coup de sabre, nodular, guttate, profunda [deep], bullous).
Systemic scleroderma	Includes limited disease (acrosclerosis, CREST) and diffuse disease (systemic sclerosis or progressive systemic sclerosis). Distinction from generalized morphea is important: progressive systemic sclerosis usually affects the upper trunk predominantly.
Mixed connective tissue disease (MCTD) and other collagen vascular overlap syndromes	Many collagen vascular diseases may overlap with others; MCTD (see text) overlaps especially with CREST. Autoantibodies, other clinical features, and passage of time may all help to achieve a more precise diagnosis.
Postirradiation morphea	Usually affects the breast (Fig. 13.43); may resemble metastatic breast carcinoma, especially if it initially has an inflammatory stage.
Drug and toxin-induced pseudoscleroderma	Causes include bleomycin (usually acral pattern), L-tryptophan, 'toxic oil syndrome', polyvinyl chloride, silicosis. Localized scleroderma may be caused by vitamin K injections, silicone, or paraffin implants.
Atrophoderma of Pasini and Pierini	Usually affects low back, brownish color, firm but depressed below skin surface contour.
Graft-versus-host disease (GVHD)	Sclerodermatous change is characteristic of late-stage GVHD (Ch. 12), but the diagnosis is generally apparent from the history of marrow transplant.
Porphyria cutanea tarda (PCT)	Sclerodermatous change may occur (Fig. 13.44); the diagnosis is usually apparent from the other features of PCT (Ch. 17).
Dermatomyositis	Sclerodermatous change may occur; it is often patchy and mixed with more classic rash of dermatomyositis.
Eosinophilic fasciitis	Usually affects lower legs, with acute onset and often good response to prednisolone. A sufficiently deep biopsy (to include fascia) will usually show tissue eosinophilia. See Chapter 11.
Paraneoplastic fasciitis	May cause acral sclerotic change or tethering similar to that of eosinophilic fasciitis; changes are very resistant to treatment.
Carcinoid syndrome	Scleroderma-like areas may be apparent, and telangiectasia, but there is also flushing and weight loss.
Lipodermatosclerosis	Affects the foot and lower leg, especially above the medial malleolus in patients with chronic venous insufficiency (Ch. 15).
Diabetic stiff skin and cheirarthropathy	This generally has an acral predominance, without the telangiectasia of CREST; see Chapter 12.

CREST: calcinosis, Raynaud phenomenon, esophagus, sclerodactyly, telangiectasia.

Occasionally, there may be specific local factors that influence the development of morphea, such as the type that occurs as a late effect following radiotherapy (postirradiation morphea, see Fig. 13.42). This is typically related to treatment of breast cancer, and is unrelated to silicon breast implants, which have been (controversially) implicated as a cause of systemic sclerosis. Tick bites and *Borrelia burgdorferi* infection have also been linked with development of morphea, and treatment with penicillin has been advocated. Patients with porphyria cutanea tarda (PCT, see also Ch. 17) may also develop sclerotic plaques (Fig. 13.43) resembling morphea but usually have other features of PCT as well.

Clinical aspects, diagnosis, and investigations

Some identifiable subsets of the sclerodermatous disorders are discussed individually. Morphea is considered here, although it is not associated with Raynaud phenomenon, and does not have the same implications for general health as the other sclerodermatous disorders. For most variants in the scleroderma spectrum, the diagnosis is primarily clinical, with support from autoantibody tests and investigations to determine internal organ involvement, as appropriate. Skin biopsies can confirm skin thickening and sclerosis, but this is somewhat subjective and varies according to the body site; it can be useful to exclude deposition disorders such as scleredema (Ch. 11).

A clinically similar condition known as eosinophilic fasciitis is discussed in Chapter 11; it usually affects the lower legs. A malignancy-associated fasciitis syndrome has also been described.

Morphea

This is a disorder of localized scleroderma (Figs 13.37–13.42), which usually occurs as one or a few lesions, usually of several centimeters in diameter. The characteristic appearance is of a shiny ivory-white sclerotic area with surrounding purplish inflammatory erythema, which gradually fades with time (Fig. 13.37). The skin is palpably hard, a feature that may not be apparent with visual inspection alone. The lesions may soften or become more brown over a long period, and generally the only problems are itch in early lesions and the cosmetic aspects.

One or more localized plaques of morphea are by far the commonest pattern, but several variants occur, as listed earlier. Linear and en coup de sabre types are discussed in more detail below. *Guttate morphea* is a pattern in which there are multiple tiny spots; it may be difficult to diagnose with confidence. *Subcutaneous deep morphea (morphea profunda)* is uncommon but also poses particular diagnostic difficulties, as does *nodular morphea*, in which lesions resemble keloids. *Bullous morphea* is rare.

Generalized or *diffuse morphea* is rare and may be confused with systemic sclerosis; it involves a large proportion of the body surface area (often sparing around the nipples), and causes some skin tightness, but without

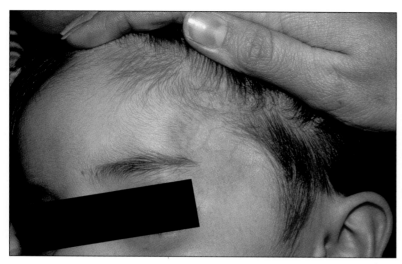

Figure 13.40 Parry–Romberg syndrome (progressive facial hemiatrophy) may occur in isolation or with lesions of morphea at other sites. Some authors view morphea en coup de sabre as an abortive form of this condition.

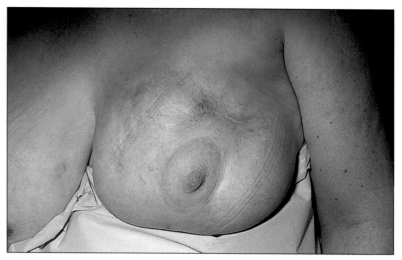

Figure 13.42 Postirradiation morphea is probably an underestimated condition. Its importance, apart from the cosmetic aspects, is the potential difficulty in excluding a sclerotic cancer recurrence on the breast, especially in early cases, when there may be inflammation resembling carcinoma erysipeloides.

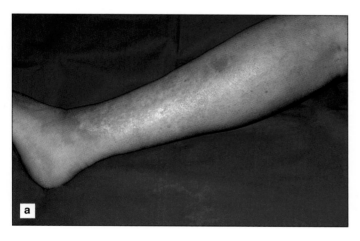

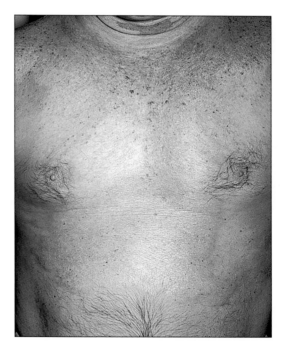

Figure 13.43 Sclerotic plaques due to porphyria cutanea tarda may resemble lesions of morphea, but affected patients may also have photosensitivity, blistering of exposed skin, and facial hypertrichosis. (Courtesy of Michael O. Murphy, M.D.)

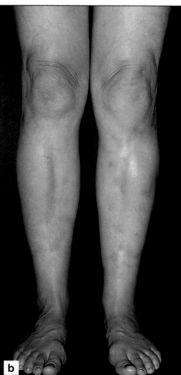

Figure 13.41 Rare types of morphea: linear and deep patterns. Linear morphea (**a**) is uncommon, and most frequently affects a single limb, although other body sites can be affected. On the leg, in particular, there is a risk of altered bone growth and flexion contractures. Some patients have a positive antinuclear antibody test. (**b**) Deep morphea extends into the fat but may have minor skin surface changes; it may present due to the hardness of the skin or the functional impairment. This patient responded to oral ciclosporin after periods using other topical and oral agents, but some cases may spontaneously resolve.

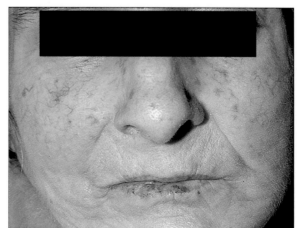

Figure 13.44 Scleroderma of the face, causing prominent mat telangiectases of the lips and cheeks. This pattern may be confused with hereditary hemorrhagic telangiectasia.

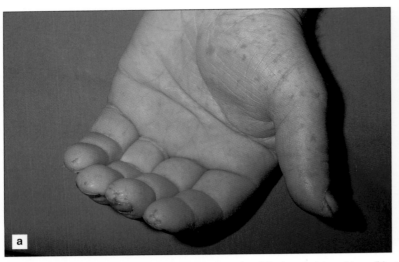

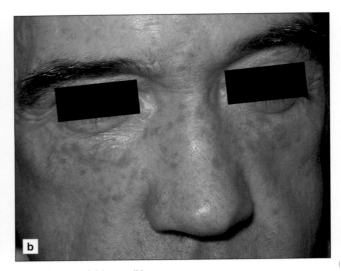

Figure 13.45 CREST syndrome with telangiectasia of the hands (**a**) and face (**b**), a common feature of this condition.

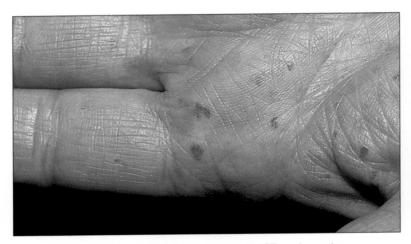

Figure 13.46 Mat telangiectasia of the hand in CREST syndrome. In some patients, this may precede other changes by several years.

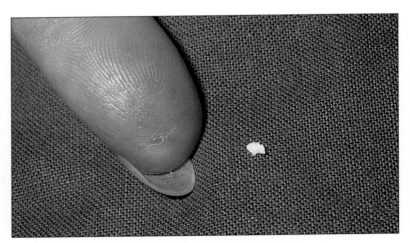

Figure 13.48 Calcinosis is one of the typical features of CREST syndrome. Occasionally, calcified material may be transepidermally eliminated from dystrophic fingertip skin, as shown in this case.

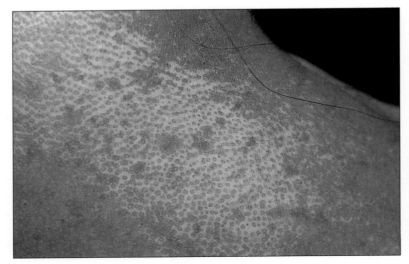

Figure 13.47 Scleroderma demonstrating a 'salt and pepper' pattern of brown spots on a white background. The brown areas may represent initial follicular sparing.

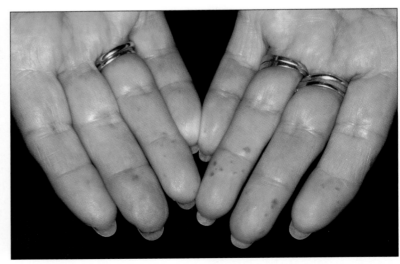

Figure 13.49 Scleroderma of the fingers, showing telangiectases and a dusky swollen finger (note that the changes of mixed connective tissue disease, Fig. 13.56a, may be identical).

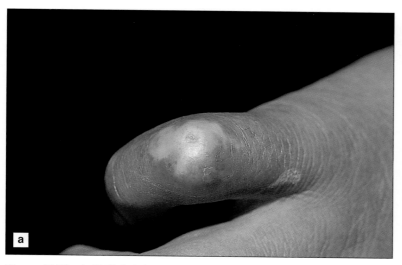

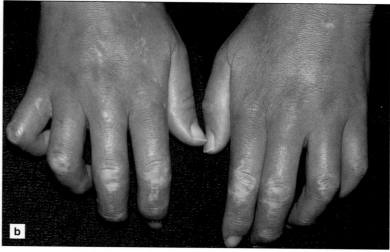

Figure 13.50 (**a,b**) Digital ulceration may occur in CREST or systemic sclerosis, may affect either the skin over joints or the finger pulps, and often leads to further tightness and pigment change if it heals (**a**). In this case, ulceration has occurred over the bony prominence of the proximal interphalangeal joint due to the flexion contracture and tight skin on the fingers in a patient with advanced and disabling contractures, causing a 'claw hand'.

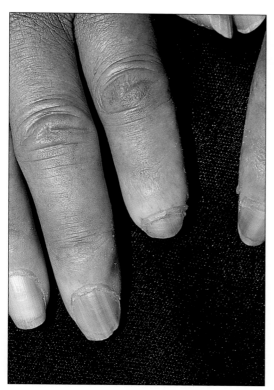

Figure 13.51 Pulp atrophy of digits, seen at an early stage in Figs 13.48 and 13.54, may progress with underlying bone resorption, leading to a shortened digit with a small fingernail, as shown here.

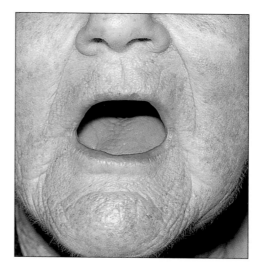

Figure 13.52 Perioral changes are common in CREST, and include telangiectasia (Fig. 13.44) and changes due to constriction of the lips (radial furrows and restricted mouth opening). Patients who wear dentures may find it difficult to insert these if mouth opening is impaired.

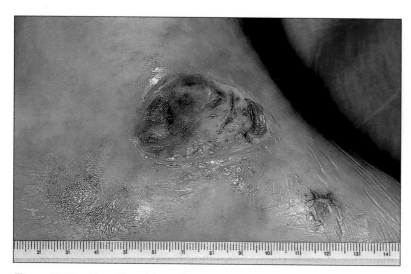

Figure 13.53 Ulceration of the ankle associated with tight, shiny skin in a teenaged patient with systemic sclerosis. Treatment with intravenous vasodilators may help in some such cases, but the response is often limited.

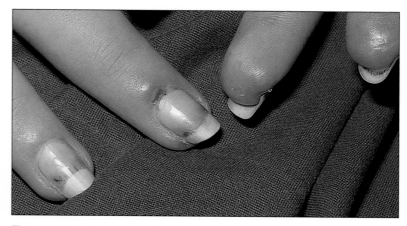

Figure 13.54 Periungual and finger pulp infarcts in a patient with acute onset of Raynaud phenomenon due to systemic sclerosis.

the internal involvement or relentless constriction of systemic sclerosis (Fig. 13.38). *Disabling pansclerotic morphea of childhood* is a similar process but has implications that do not apply in adults; sclerosis of the skin when growth is still occurring may lead to joint contractures and muscular atrophy.

Large studies suggest that about 5% of patients with morphea may develop systemic sclerosis, but some of these may actually have had localized skin lesions of systemic sclerosis from the outset, or may have had generalized morphea rather than systemic sclerosis. About 30% of patients with linear morphea have positive ANA, and morphea-like plaques occur in a similar proportion of patients with eosinophilic fasciitis. Antihistone antibodies are common in extensive morphea, but other antibodies (to topoisomerase I, centromere, SSA, SSB, or dsDNA) are not found.

Linear morphea

This uncommon variant of morphea is of importance due to involvement of underlying structures (Fig. 13.41). It usually affects a single limb, and may be associated with morphea plaques elsewhere. Deep fibrosis may affect fat and muscle, with melorrheostosis of the underlying bone, and joint contractures are common if the process extends across joints. Impaired bone growth may occur.

En coup de sabre morphea

This is a site-specific variant of linear morphea that affects the face, usually affecting the paracentral forehead and frontal scalp (Fig. 13.39). There is usually a single band, but may be more. It may be a variant of facial hemiatrophy (Parry–Romberg syndrome, Fig. 13.40).

Limited systemic sclerosis (CREST syndrome)

This variant of systemic sclerosis affects the hands, forearms, feet, face, and esophagus (Figs 13.44–13.46). The features that make up the acronym CREST are calcinosis, Raynaud phenomenon, esophageal involvement, sclerodactyly, and telangiectasia. Most patients have had Raynaud phenomenon for many years prior to any other symptomatic disease, although telangiectasia of the lips and fingers is prominent at an early stage in some individuals (and is morphologically similar to that of hereditary hemorrhagic telangiectasia). Nail fold telangiectasia (giant capillary loops) is usually prominent. Sclerosis around the mouth causes deep skin creases (radial furrows), and on the digits causes tight, shiny, bound-down skin with loss of hair, pigmentary variation, and is associated with loss of fingertip tissue and pulp infarcts. Esophageal involvement is usually manifest as reflux symptoms due to disordered motility causing abnormal peristalsis. Other gastrointestinal involvement, such as malabsorption due to small bowel involvement, is a late feature. Pulmonary hypertension is also a late feature.

The diagnosis is largely clinical. Serologic tests are useful, as most patients have a positive anticentromere antibody test; this test is less commonly positive in diffuse systemic sclerosis and uncommonly in primary Raynaud disease. Esophageal motility studies should be performed.

- Musculoskeletal—arthritis, myositis, and tendinitis.
- Pulmonary—basal fibrosis with restrictive defect, causing cough and exertional dyspnea.
- Gastrointestinal—esophageal symptoms as in CREST, reduced small intestinal motility (causing malabsorption), dilatation, and sacculation of the colon.
- Cardiac—pericarditis and myocardial fibrosis.
- Renal—severe hypertension and renal failure.

Investigations for internal disease are important and may need to be repeated at intervals, depending on symptoms. ANAs are positive in 95% of patients. Scl-70 (antibody to topoisomerase, producing a diffuse speckled nuclear fluorescence) is positive in 25–30%, and is associated with proximal sclerosis and lung disease; anticentromere antibody is positive in a smaller proportion and is associated with acral and less severe disease.

Mixed connective tissue disease and overlap syndromes

Mixed connective tissue disease does not neatly fit as any of the classic collagen vascular diseases, but has features that clearly belong within this overall category. Although some such patients may eventually fulfill criteria for systemic sclerosis or SLE, some patients have mixed features for prolonged periods. The most frequent features are Raynaud phenomenon, swollen hands with restricted movement of digits, sclerodactyly, arthralgia, and esophageal disease, but there may also be myositis, heliotrope rash, calcinosis, and other non-specific signs (Figs 13.55–13.57). A speckled pattern of ANA due to anti-U1RNP is typical but non-specific, and there should be negative tests to other more specific antibodies such as dsDNA, histones, Sm, Scl-70, SSA, and SSB. Pleurisy and pulmonary hypertension may occur, but severe renal or central nervous system disease is uncommon.

Overlap syndromes are those in which there appears to be a true association of different diseases, with sufficient features of each to have a firm diagnosis. Sjögren disease, in particular, may be associated with other disorders such as SLE, scleroderma, or rheumatoid arthritis. Some patients with childhood dermatomyositis may subsequently develop features of LE, and myositis may occur in LE.

Differential diagnosis

Plaque-type morphea is usually characteristic but, especially if not palpated, the inflammatory stage may be confused by the less experienced practitioner with tinea or other annular lesions (see Table 1.2). Older lesions may be referred non-specifically as 'pigmentary disturbance'. The guttate pattern of morphea may be difficult to distinguish from the similar-sized variant of lichen sclerosus. Morphea profunda clinically resembles deep variants of disorders such as sarcoidosis, granuloma annulare, and interstitial granulomatous dermatitis (see later in this chapter). The rare nodular variant resembles spontaneous keloids.

The puffiness and limited mobility of the hands in CREST should be differentiated from MCTD, from other causes and differential diagnoses of Raynaud phenomenon (Table 13.1), and from diabetic cheirarthropathy

---

PRACTICE POINT
- Palpation of the skin to assess firmness and texture is an integral part of the examination. Failure to do this will result in incorrect diagnosis and inappropriate treatment in patients with morphea.

Diffuse systemic sclerosis

Diffuse systemic sclerosis is manifest dermatologically by a more generalized sclerodermatous process, which particularly affects the upper trunk and distal limbs (Figs 13.47–13.54). There may be preceding Raynaud phenomenon, although in some patients the onset is abrupt and very rapidly progressive (the only subgroup in whom systemic steroids appear to be useful, probably because there is cutaneous inflammation and edema at this stage prior to fibrosis). In the initial stages of disease, for the first few years, there may be non-specific features of malaise and tiredness, with internal organ involvement in several systems.

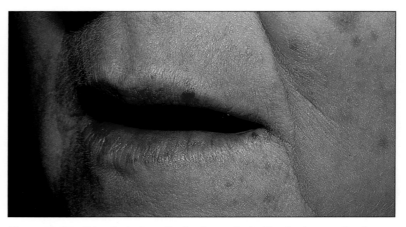

Figure 13.55 Telangiectasia on the lips in a patient with mixed connective tissue disease, a similar pattern to that seen in CREST.

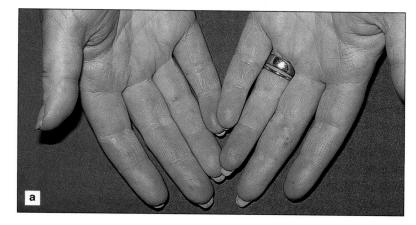

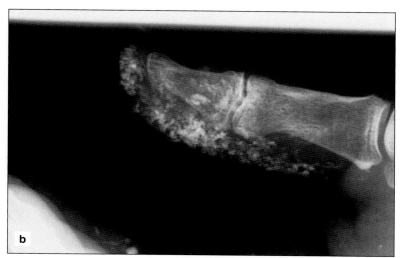

Figure 13.56　Mixed connective tissue disease, (**a**) presenting as a dusky blue discoloration of the hands, with cold skin and Raynaud phenomenon, and (**b**) showing marked radiologic evidence of calcification.

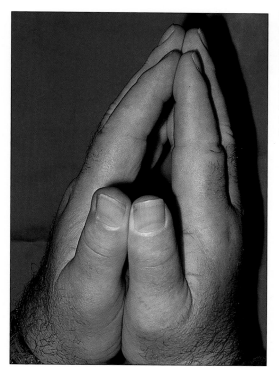

Figure 13.57　Mixed connective tissue disease, demonstrating the prayer sign (see also Fig. 12.17). The tight, puffy skin of the fingers prevents the hands from being pressed flat together when the wrists are extended to 90°.

(see Fig. 12.17). Telangiectasia in CREST may be difficult to distinguish from that of hereditary hemorrhagic telangiectasia, although the latter is usually manifest at a young age.

Generalized morphea and systemic sclerosis need to be distinguished because of the prognostic differences, and from the sclerotic disorders listed in Table 13.5 (which also provides some features that may help to make the diagnosis). Most disorders that may have scleroderma-like features usually have other features that readily distinguish them from scleroderma (such as blisters in PCT and flushing in carcinoid syndrome), but some may be similar to primary scleroderma processes (such as MCTD, eosinophilic fasciitis, and overlap syndromes). Other diffuse skin infiltrates, such as scleredema or scleromyxedema, may cause diagnostic problems, but both are rare, and biopsy will show mucin in these latter disorders.

Rare pediatric conditions such as stiff skin syndrome and congenital fascial dystrophy are unlikely to be confused with autoimmune sclerodermas.

Treatment

Many patients with localized lesions of morphea do not require any specific therapy other than explanation and reassurance; indeed, therapy is often not effective in established lesions. In the inflammatory stage, topical corticosteroids may have a role; these must be sufficiently potent to achieve penetration into the sclerotic skin. For more widespread cutaneous involvement, PUVA and UVA1 (a high-intensity long-wavelength UV treatment) can be effective, but the latter is not widely available.

Treatment of systemic sclerosis is complex, due to the multiple organs involved. Treatment of Raynaud phenomenon has already been discussed but, in addition, fingertip ulceration may require treatments such as mupirocin for secondary infection, and locally applied vasodilators such as glyceryl trinitrate.

Physiotherapy is important for skin and joint disease, with non-steroidal antiinflammatory drugs (NSAIDs). Immunosuppressive drugs (steroids if very acute, methotrexate, and cyclophosphamide) and antifibrotic drugs such as penicillamine have been recommended, with varying benefit. Colchicine, interferon, isotretinoin, and sulphasalazine have all been used with occasional apparent responses. Angiotensin-converting enzyme inhibitors are usually used for treatment of hypertension, in view of the associated renal arteriolar disease. Symptomatic treatment of reflux symptoms includes antacids, H_2 antagonists, and proton pump inhibitors. Malabsorption may, in part, be due to bacterial overgrowth and respond to appropriate antibiotics.

INTERSTITIAL GRANULOMATOUS DERMATITIS

Etiology and pathogenesis

This recently described rare entity is briefly discussed, as it has both striking clinical features and also a strong relationship with collagen vascular disease (especially with rheumatoid arthritis) or with the presence of autoantibodies (especially ANA, rheumatoid factor, and antithyroid antibodies).

Clinical

The main clinical and histologic features are apparent from the varied names that have been applied to this disorder: interstitial granulomatous dermatitis with plaques, interstitial granulomatous dermatitis with cutaneous cords and arthritis, and palisaded neutrophilic granulomatous dermatitis (of immune complex disease). The skin lesions are irregular plaques or linear bands, cutaneous and/or subcutaneous, often bizarre in appearance; they are typically symmetric, red-brown or violaceous, and situated on the flanks or in body folds.

Differential diagnosis

Clinically, the lesions may resemble morphea, lymphoma, or annular erythema; histologically, any granulomatous disorder may need to be considered (Ch. 11). Disorders that may be similar on both clinical and histologic grounds include sarcoidosis (Fig. 13.58), granuloma annulare, and granulomatous mycosis fungoides.

Treatment

Non-steroidal antiinflammatory drugs, oral corticosteroids, and immunosuppressive agents such as ciclosporin may be useful.

RHEUMATOID ARTHRITIS

Rheumatoid arthritis is not generally the province of the dermatologist, but there are several areas where skin manifestations may be involved (Fig. 13.59, Table 13.6).

DERMATOMYOSITIS

Etiology and pathogenesis

Dermatomyositis is an inflammatory eruption of the skin associated with myositis. It overlaps with polymyositis without skin involvement, but conversely may occur as an 'amyopathic' form with characteristic rash but no myositis. The skin changes most commonly precede or accompany the myositis.

About 25% of cases are paraneoplastic, mostly in patients aged over 40 years. A small proportion of cases are overtly autoimmune, being associated with other disorders such as LE, and many other 'idiopathic' cases will have some detectable autoantibodies (Table 13.7). Antibodies to various tRNA synthetases are infrequent but relatively specific, and correlate with clinical features such as fever, lung involvement, and polyarthropathy. A positive ANA is found in about 50% of patients.

Childhood dermatomyositis has several features that are uncommon in the adult variant, and may therefore have a different etiology; vasculitic lesions and cutaneous calcinosis are more common (and are now known to be associated with the presence of the tumor necrosis factor-α 308A allele), and gingival telangiectasia is often present.

Drug triggers of dermatomyositis or a dermatomyositis-like rash include hydroxyurea (skin features only), penicillin, sulfonamides, hydroxymethylglutaryl-CoA reductase inhibitors, and interferon-alpha.

Clinical features, diagnosis, and investigations

The rash of dermatomyositis is typically purplish and often has a streaky pattern, which may appear flagellate or zebra-striped. Notably affected body sites (Figs 13.60–13.68) are as follows:

- Around the eyes, with eyelid edema (heliotrope rash)—this may be an early (sometimes the only) feature.
- Dorsum of the hands, where it may produce streaks along the fingers (Gottron sign, also over knees and elbows) or may be accentuated over bony prominences (Gottron's papules).
- Upper trunk, where a V-of-neck photosensitivity distribution (V sign) or upper-back (shawl sign) may be apparent.
- Knees and elbows—underestimated sites that may cause diagnostic confusion (Fig. 13.67).

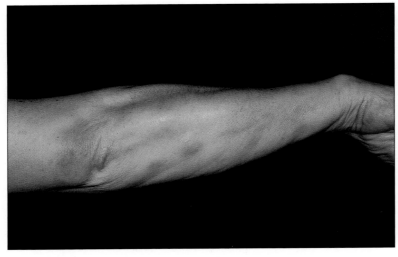

Figure 13.58 Nodules and a subcutaneous cord; the differential between interstitial granulomatous dermatitis versus subcutaneous sarcoidosis could not be made with certainty, but lesions resolved spontaneously. (Courtesy of Dr. L. Barco.)

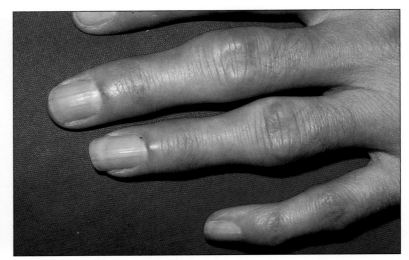

Figure 13.59 Rheumatoid arthritis (note the joint swelling) with small skin infarcts typical of rheumatoid vasculitis; this tends to parallel disease activity in the joints.

Table 13.6 SOME CUTANEOUS FEATURES ASSOCIATED WITH RHEUMATOID ARTHRITIS	
Feature	**Comments**
Rheumatoid ulcers	Due to rheumatoid vasculitis
Digital lesions, splinter hemorrhages, vasculitis	Due to rheumatoid vasculitis (Fig. 13.59)
Pyoderma gangrenosum	Relatively uncommonly associated with rheumatoid arthritis, but important therapeutically to distinguish them from vasculitic ulcers
Rheumatoid neutrophilic dermatitis	A relatively recently documented entity
Antiphospholipid syndrome	Rheumatoid arthritis is a cause
Rheumatoid nodules	Typical nodules on the elbow rarely cause a diagnostic problem, but small nodules (sometimes termed rheumatoid nodulettes) may present at unusual sites, and disorders such as multicentric reticulohistiocytosis may be in the differential of nodules plus arthritis
Amyloidosis	If secondary type, can sometimes be diagnosed in an aspirate of subcutaneous fat
Drug reactions	Includes urticarial and maculopapular, plus rarer conditions such as penicillamine-induced pemphigus

Table 13.7 AUTOANTIBODIES IN DERMATOMYOSITIS

Category	Antibodies	Comments
Myositis-specific antibodies (MSA)	Cytoplasmic: anti-aminoacyl tRNA synthetases (e.g. Jo1, PL7, PL12), anti-tRNA, anti-SRP Nuclear: Mi2	Antisynthetase and anti-tRNA antibodies are associated with the 'antisynthetase syndrome', which includes mechanic's hands, myositis, arthritis, Raynaud phenomenon, and interstitial lung disease. They can be positive in lupus erythematosus and in Sjögren syndrome. Anti-SRP is associated with polymyositis and poor response to treatment. Anti-Mi2 is associated with good prognosis dermatomyositis, and occurs in up to 20%. Anti-p155 and anti-Se have recently been linked with amyopathic disease.
Myositis-associated antibodies (MAA)	Anti-U1RNP, anti-Pm-Scl	Anti-U1RNP is usually positive in mixed connective tissue disease, and may be positive in several lupus erythematosus variants. Anti-Pm-Scl is positive in some sclerodermas.
Other autoantibodies that may be positive in patients with dermatomyositis	Tissue-specific autoantibodies: antimuscle antibodies, anti-endothelial cell antibodies. Antibodies associated with autoimmune diseases: antinuclear antibody (ANA), anti-SSA, anti-SSB, rheumatoid factor, antiphospholipid, antihistone	

tRNA, transfer RNA; SRP, signal recognition particle.

- Nail folds—telangiectasia of nail folds is a prominent feature, with 'giant' capillary loops being readily visible, and the cuticles are elongated and ragged.
- Scalp—itch and scaling are common, sometimes severe, and often not adequately considered.

Some patients have prominent poikilodermatous or scleroderma–like white areas within the rash, vasculitic lesions may occur (especially in children), and extensive subcutaneous calcification may be a feature of childhood dermatomyositis (Fig. 13.69). True photosensitivity may occur. Mechanic's hands, a pattern associated with antisynthetase antibodies, consist of fissuring, redness, and scaling, resembling a contact dermatitis (Fig. 13.68). Itch is a common, and sometimes dominant, feature of the rash. Occasionally, the facial rash may affect the nasolabial folds and resemble seborrheic dermatitis.

A small number of patients may have typical rash without ever having muscle symptoms, a situation known as 'dermatomyositis sine myositis' or 'amyopathic dermatomyositis'. This latter group may have a higher frequency of photosensitivity and associated autoimmune disease, and possibly have a lower risk of associated malignancy (discussed later), although this may be an artifact of analysis, as they constitute a minority of patients. It has been suggested that this diagnosis can be made with reasonable certainty only if the absence of muscle involvement continues for 2 years after diagnosis of the cutaneous rash, as some patients may have subtle or absent muscle disease for a period after presentation.

The muscle disease is symmetric and predominantly affects proximal muscle girdles. Difficulties in brushing hair, or in standing from a sitting position, are typical symptoms. The myositis is diagnosed on the basis of history, elevated muscle enzymes (creatine phosphokinase, aldolase, myoglobin, and urinary creatine:creatinine ratio), electromyography, and, if required, muscle biopsy. Less specific but often abnormal tests include the ESR. Autoantibody tests such as Jo-1 are also useful if positive.

Association with internal malignancy, and investigations

About 25% of patients with dermatomyositis have an underlying malignancy, with approximately equal proportions diagnosed before, after, and at the time of the skin eruption. Several studies have demonstrated that simple screening tests are adequate to identify the vast majority of malignancies, provided that any abnormal features in the history, examination, or simple tests are pursued. However, these conclusions predated ready availability of computed tomography (CT) or magnetic

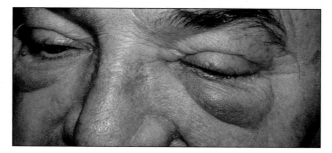

Figure 13.60 Eyelid edema may be an early and dramatic sign in dermatomyositis. It may mimic angioedema and contact allergies, but is less variable from day to day. Nail fold changes may be present even if the rash has not evolved at other cutaneous sites.

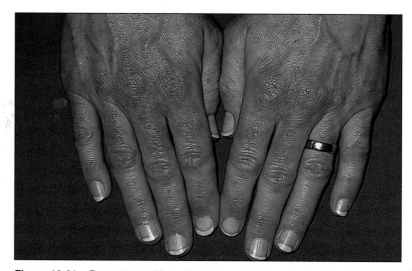

Figure 13.61 Dermatomyositis on the dorsum of the hands. A pattern of longitudinal purplish-colored stripes is common (Gottron sign).

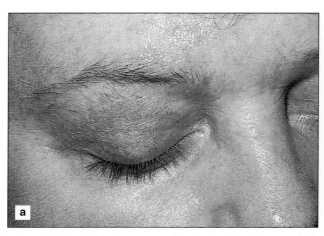

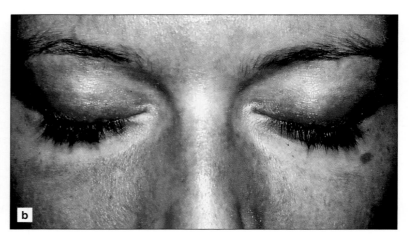

Figure 13.62 (**a**,**b**) Dermatomyositis showing the violaceous heliotrope rash, in these cases predominantly affecting the upper eyelid. Heliotropes are a type of plant with purplish-colored flowers. (Panel b courtesy of Dr. G. Dawn.)

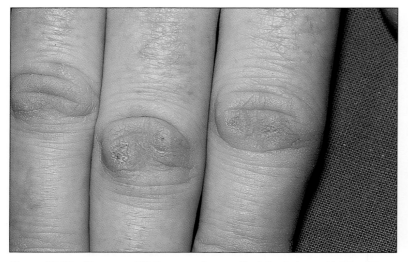

Figure 13.63 Close-up of Gottron papules over the interphalangeal joints of the fingers in a patient with dermatomyositis.

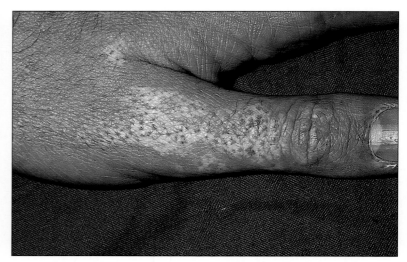

Figure 13.65 Poikilodermatous change on the thumb in a patient with dermatomyositis. The white sclerotic areas are reminiscent of scleroderma disorders.

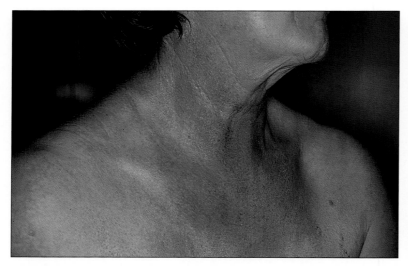

Figure 13.64 A photodistributed pattern of dermatomyositis in a patient without evidence of malignancy. Photoaggravation is relatively common, but rarely as limited to sun-exposed skin as in this case.

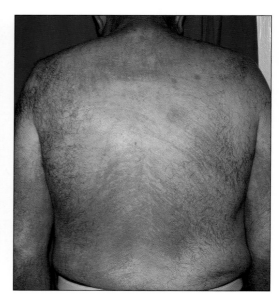

Figure 13.66 A streaky or 'flagellate' pattern of purplish or violaceous lesions on the trunk is strongly suggestive of dermatomyositis. In this case, there was an underlying non-Hodgkin lymphoma.

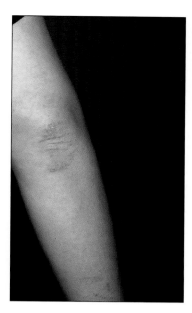

Figure 13.67   Rash on the elbow in a patient with dermatomyositis; the frequency of this is often underestimated, but it is important in differential diagnosis terms, as it often closely resembles the distribution (the knees are also affected) and the plaque morphology of psoriasis.

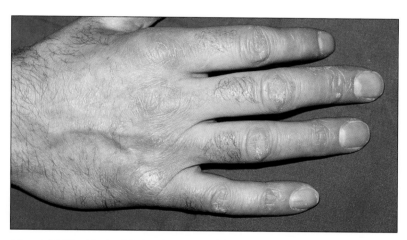

Figure 13.68   Mechanic's hands pattern of dermatomyositis, in a patient with associated interstitial lung disease. There is an appearance similar to chronic hand dermatitis, but with prominence of thickening over the finger joints.

resonance imaging (MRI) scanning, and it is uncertain to what extent these tests may be important in early detection of asymptomatic tumors: CT of chest, abdomen, and pelvis is increasingly performed in patients with dermatomyositis. Ovarian tumors, in particular, appear to be difficult to detect but are significantly linked with dermatomyositis. Bronchial (Fig. 13.70), colonic, and breast carcinomas are the most frequently associated tumors in patients with dermatomyositis, essentially reflecting their frequency in the general population; in South-East Asia, nasopharyngeal carcinoma is an important association.

A suggested approach to patients with probable dermatomyositis is shown in Table 13.8.

Differential diagnosis

This may include the following.

- Systemic lupus erythematosus—photosensitive pattern, nail fold changes, malaise, and arthralgia.
- Scleroderma and overlap diseases—rash of dermatomyositis may have sclerodermatous areas and nail fold changes.
- Psoriasis—especially if rash is prominent on hands, knees, or elbows.
- Photodermatoses—especially drug-related and photosensitivity dermatitis.
- Drug eruptions—especially hydroxyurea, which may produce a rash that mimics dermatomyositis.
- Dermatitis—mainly if prominent on the face (atopic; seborrheic; contact, especially reactions to eyedrops); also, contact dermatitis is in the differential of the mechanic's hands pattern.
- Graft-versus-host disease—may resemble dermatomyositis.
- Trichinosis—may present as myalgia with periorbital edema.
- Mycosis fungoides—poikilodermatous rash may resemble dermatomyositis.

Treatment

If there is an underlying malignancy, this should be treated, as usually the disease remits after curative surgery. Additionally, patients who respond poorly to treatment or relapse should be reinvestigated for this possibility.

Patients with amyopathic dermatomyositis may be treated with topical corticosteroids and oral antihistamine, and hydroxychloroquine can be useful in those with photosensitivity.

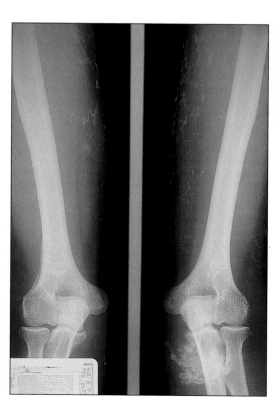

Figure 13.69
Radiograph showing subcutaneous calcification in dermatomyositis. This is a particular feature of the childhood variant of this disorder.

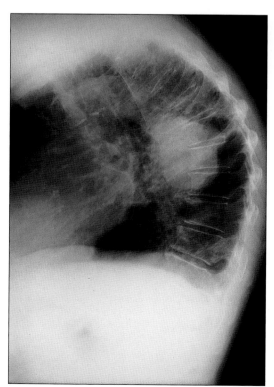

Figure 13.70
Malignant disease is present in about 25% of cases of adult dermatomyositis. The most frequent neoplasm in men is bronchial carcinoma.

Table 13.8   INVESTIGATIONS IN DERMATOMYOSITIS

Investigation	Reasons and comments
Thorough history and examination	Symptoms due to the disease; malignancy evaluation; possible drug triggers; include breast, rectal, and pelvic examination
Skin biopsy	To exclude cutaneous differential diagnoses, see bulleted list in Differential diagnosis section
Appropriate autoantibody screen	To evaluate likelihood of autoimmune collagen vascular disease etiology and overlap syndromes; specific antibodies, if respiratory symptoms
'Routine' blood tests	Malignancy evaluation; baseline for systemic therapy (complete blood count, chemistry, sedimentation rate, glucose)
Muscle enzymes; ideally muscle biopsy, electromyography	To detect or monitor muscle involvement
Malignancy evaluation	History and bloods as above, plus chest radiograph, stool for occult blood, abdominal and pelvic imaging (at least ultrasound, but increasingly computed tomography or magnetic resonance imaging)

Most commonly, myositis determines the need for systemic therapy, which is usually with systemic corticosteroids and immunosuppressive agents such as azathioprine, methotrexate (especially in adults), or cyclophosphamide (especially in children). Ciclosporin has also been used recently, and appears to be particularly useful in children. Intravenous gamma-globulin has been used, with good results in a few cases. Myositis in dermatomyosis may require urgent treatment, as it may affect respiratory muscles, leading to respiratory failure, or may cause dysphagia and a risk of aspiration pneumonia due to pharyngeal myositis. Note that respiratory symptoms due to muscle disease need to be distinguished from the interstitial lung disease that may also occur, or from symptoms due to an underlying bronchial carcinoma or metastases in some patients.

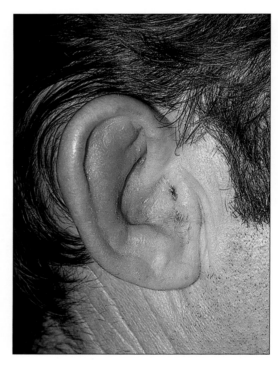

Figure 13.71
Relapsing polychondritis affecting the ear. Note the sparing of the lobe of the ear, in which there is no cartilage. Other cartilaginous tissue may be affected by this inflammatory process; in this case the patient also had chondritis of the nose, scleritis, and arthralgia.

PRACTICE POINTS
- Do not forget ovarian carcinoma as a cause of dermatomyositis; it may be difficult to detect.
- Beware of delayed development or deterioration of myositis.
- Lung disease in dermatomyositis may be directly or indirectly due to muscle disease, may be due to an underlying neoplasm, or may be due to interstitial lung disease.
- Repeat investigations for malignancy if symptoms alter.

RELAPSING POLYCHONDRITIS

General aspects, diagnosis, and investigations
This is probably an autoimmune disease involving antibodies against type II collagen in cartilage. It is associated in about 25% of cases with other disorders, such as vasculitis, rheumatoid arthritis, and Behçet syndrome.

Clinical features
The external ear is most commonly affected, presenting as sore, red, swollen ears, but with sparing of the non-cartilaginous earlobes (Fig. 13.71). Concurrent fever, arthritis, nasal soreness, and red eyes are all likely, although some patients have a very low-grade inflammatory process. Vasculitic lesions and erythema nodosum-like lesions may be a feature. Involvement of trachea and heart valves are less common but potentially fatal. The ears may become chronically swollen, and nasal bridge collapse similar to that of Wegener granulomatosis may occur. Non-specific markers of inflammation such as the ESR may be grossly elevated.

Differential diagnosis
The most likely feature to present to a dermatologist is the ear disease, for which the main differential diagnosis is infection (chondritis or perichondritis), trauma and related disorders such as auricular pseudocyst, and occasionally contact dermatitis; the specific sparing of the earlobe would be unlikely in the latter. Wegener granulomatosis is in the differential of the nasal features, but symptoms are usually intranasal and in the province of the otorhinolaryngologist. Disorders such as polymorphic light eruption, Jessner lymphocytic infiltrate, and sarcoidosis may all cause redness of the pinna but do not cause the tenderness of relapsing polychondritis.

Treatment
Significant lesions with fever and malaise are generally treated with systemic corticosteroids, and, if necessary, with other immunosuppressive agents such as azathioprine. Some cases with localized mild symptoms are controlled quite adequately with simple treatments such as NSAIDs.

SJÖGREN SYNDROME

This condition is not usually the province of the dermatologist but may cause skin lesions, and is discussed here, as it occurs secondary to LE and other collagen vascular diseases as well as occurring as an isolated entity. There may be differences between these primary and secondary forms; for example, a relatively new autoantibody, anti-α-fodrin, is much more commonly found in the primary than in the secondary form, and is especially associated with perniosis. More commonly tested autoantibodies that may be positive in Sjögren syndrome include anti-SSA (in about 50%), anti-SSB (25%), and less commonly some of the anti-tRNA synthetases.

Skin lesions in Sjögren syndrome occur in a minority, and seem to have a predilection for Japanese patients; the lesions are typically annular and on the face.

FURTHER READING

Beutner EH, Jablonska S, White DB, et al. Dermatologic criteria for classifying the major forms of cutaneous lupus erythematosus: methods for systemic discriminant analysis and questions on the interpretation of findings. Clin Dermatol 1993; 10: 443–56

Chlebus E, Wolska H, Blaszczyk M, et al. Subacute cutaneous lupus erythematosus versus systemic lupus erythematosus: diagnostic criteria and therapeutic implications. J Am Acad Dermatol 1998; 38: 405–12

Gilliam JN, Sontheimer RD. Distinctive cutaneous subsets in the spectrum of lupus erythematosus. J Am Acad Dermatol 1981; 4: 471–5

Kovacs SO, Kovacs SC. Dermatomyositis. J Am Acad Dermatol 1998; 39: 899–920

Provost TT, Ratrie H. Autoantibodies and autoantigens in lupus erythematosus and Sjögren's syndrome. Curr Probl Dermatol 1990; 2: 151–97

Santmyire-Rosenberger B, Dugan EM. Skin involvement in dermatomyositis. Curr Opin Rheumatol 2003; 15: 714–22

Sontheimer R. Management of autoimmune connective tissue disease. Dermatol Ther 2001; 14: 61–173

Sontheimer RD, Provost TT (eds) Cutaneous Manifestations of Rheumatic Diseases. Baltimore: Williams & Wilkins, 1996

Sontheimer RD, et al. Guidelines of care for cutaneous lupus erythematosus. J Am Acad Dermatol 1996; 34: 830–6

Tan EM, et al. The 1982 revised criteria for the classification of systemic lupus erythematosus. Arthritis Rheum 1982; 25: 1271–7

INTRODUCTION

This chapter discusses disorders in which there is either a breach of, or injury to, the blood vessel wall. In many instances, depending on severity, damage to the vessels will lead to extravasation of cellular blood contents.

Purpura is the extravasation of blood from vessels in the skin. It may have hematologic causes or hydrostatic causes, or may be related to vessel injury (Table 14.1). The latter may include physical damage (e.g. trauma), occlusion of vessels (e.g. prothrombotic or embolic disorders), or inflammation of the vessel walls (vasculitis). A useful concept in evaluating these possible causes in the skin is that inflammation (i.e. vasculitis) will produce local swelling as well as extravasation of erythrocytes, a combination termed palpable purpura and illustrated previously (Fig. 2.14).

Vasculitis occurs in several situations. It may be primary, the main topic of this chapter, or it may be associated with the collagen vascular or connective tissue diseases, such as lupus erythematosus, scleroderma, and dermatomyositis, discussed in Chapter 13. Dermatologists are most commonly faced with a pattern known as cutaneous small-vessel vasculitis (Fig. 14.1); an approach to this pattern will be outlined later.

Most primary vasculitides involve neutrophil polymorphs in at least some of their lesions. For this reason, neutrophilic dermatoses are also discussed here; they are often centered around vessels and may include a component of vessel wall inflammation, so there is a degree of pathologic overlap with vasculitis.

PURPURA

Classification

Tiny lesions of purpura are termed petechiae (lesions of up to a few millimeters), while large areas are termed ecchymosis (bruise). Causes overlap, but the pattern can be clinically useful; for example, abnormalities

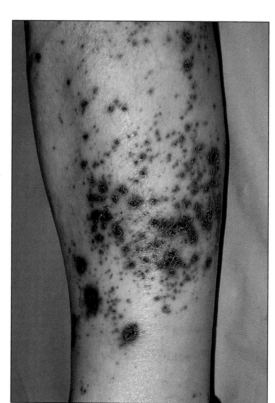

Figure 14.1
Cutaneous small-vessel vasculitis showing palpable purpuric lesions with necrosis and crusting. In this patient, very rarely, the trigger was extensive crusted scabies.

Table 14.1   CLASSIFICATION AND CAUSES OF PURPURA AND ECCHYMOSIS

Cause	Examples and comments
Platelet disorders	
Thrombocytopenia	Numerous causes
Abnormal platelet function	Especially due to drugs, uremia, myeloproliferative disease, inherited forms
Thrombocytosis	Mainly myeloproliferative disorders or isolated ('essential')
Coagulation disorders[a]	
Inherited	For example hemophilia
Drugs	For example anticoagulants
Localized	For example heparin injection sites, some insect bites
Metabolic	For example vitamin K deficiency, hepatic failure (decreased synthesis of clotting factors)
Thrombophilias	For example protein C deficiency, protein S deficiency
Disseminated intravascular coagulopathy and purpura fulminans	
Other intravascular causes of purpura	
Dysproteinemias	Hypergammaglobulinemic purpura (Waldenström), Sjögren syndrome
Cryoproteinemias	
Emboli	Crystal, fat, myxoma, infective
Non-thrombocytopenic vascular causes of purpura	
Raised intravascular pressure	Coughing, vomiting, stasis
Decreased support	Actinic ('senile') purpura, corticosteroid purpura, scurvy, amyloidosis, Ehlers–Danlos syndrome
Abnormal vasculature	For example purpura around vascular lesions
Non-thrombocytopenic toxin- and drug-induced purpura	
Purpura associated with infections	
Capillaritis (pigmented purpuric dermatoses)	
Vasculitis	
Associated with other dermatoses that are not usually purpuric	
Other causes of purpura or ecchymosis	
Physical and artefactual causes	
Multifactorial purpura associated with systemic diseases	
Easy bruising syndrome and purpura simplex	
Paroxysmal finger hematoma (Achenbach syndrome)	
Painful bruising (autoerythrocyte sensitization, Gardner–Diamond) syndrome	
Stigmata	

[a]Usually cause ecchymosis.

of clotting factors are most likely to cause bruising, whereas platelet defects often cause petechiae. A classification of purpura with examples of specific causes is provided in Table 14.1.

Capillary leakage
Bruises and purpura
This chapter is primarily a discussion of inflammatory disorders that affect blood vessels and that are likely to present to dermatologists or internists. However, extravasation of blood may occur in other settings (Table 14.1), including the following.
- Defects of coagulation: these usually produce overt bruising.
- Defects of platelet number or function: these usually cause non-palpable purpura.
- Abnormal vascular fragility: such as Ehlers–Danlos syndrome (Chs 19 and 22), scurvy (Ch. 12), solar purpura (Ch. 17), steroid purpura, amyloidosis (Ch. 11), and lichen sclerosus (Ch. 22).
- Unrecognized physical damage or stresses on vessels: such as talon noir (discussed in this section), bilateral hallux subungual hematomas, artefacts (such as suction purpura and pinch purpura), and cough purpura (Fig. 14.2).

Knowledge of colors in a bruise may be important, particularly in instances of suspected child abuse. Red color may be present at any age

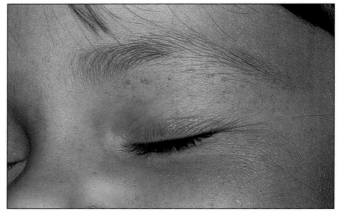

Figure 14.2 Purpura on the eyelids. This child had an upper respiratory illness 2 weeks previously, with severe coughing. This pattern of purpura is essentially the result of increased pressure due to the Valsalva maneuver, and mainly affects the poorly supported, thin skin of the eyelids. This process also occurs in systemic amyloidosis.

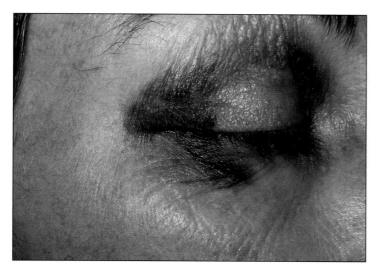

Figure 14.3 An ecchymosis (bruise), showing mixed colors about 24 h after the injury.

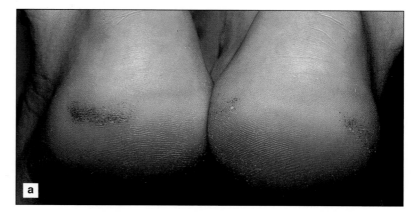

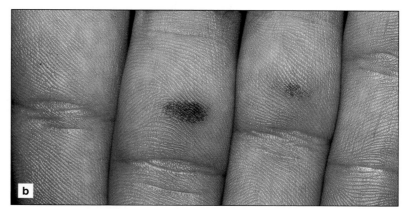

Figure 14.4 Talon noir. (**a**) Shear forces in this soccer player caused extravasation of blood at the lateral margins of the heel. (**b**) A similar change may occur on the hand.

of bruise, although it usually disappears by the end of the first week (Fig. 14.3). Yellow color takes at least 24 h to appear and green 48 h, these colors therefore indicating that the bruise is not fresh (delayed presentation is one feature of abuse).

Talon noir

This disorder is specifically discussed due to the diagnostic confusion it may cause. The lesions are multiple small, hemorrhagic, and thrombosed capillaries, which typically occur on the border of the heel in teenaged and young adult sportsmen due to shearing injury (Fig. 14.4). Similar lesions may occur on the sole of the foot over areas of irregularity in the soles of shoes, or on the hands if there is a frictional injury.

The lesions may be black and confused with melanoma, but close examination reveals the typical discrete, small spots of the damaged vessels. Some are diagnosed as warts. Less commonly, if they occur at sites on the foot other than the typical distribution on the heel, the differential diagnosis may include some forms of vascular occlusion, such as cholesterol emboli.

No treatment is required. The punctuate hemorrhages are gradually shed as the plantar epidermal turnover occurs.

Capillaritis (capillaropathy)

This term is applied to a group of disorders that share the common feature of erythrocyte extravasation and mild inflammatory changes around capillaries, sometimes with endothelial cell swelling but without frank vasculitis. In some cases, capillaritis occurs as a generalized self-limiting tendency following a viral infection or may be drug-triggered; some cases on the lower leg are clearly related to varicose veins.

Most types of capillaritis are idiopathic; the commonest variants occur mainly in children and young adults, and are often limited to the legs. A variety of eponymous names are applied, the commonest patterns being considered to be variants of disorders described by Majocchi or Schamberg. The main patterns are localized versions (with either prominent purpura or with predominantly golden-brown staining) and a generalized version (Figs 14.5–14.9).

Lichen aureus

This is probably the most common idiopathic capillaropathy, usually occurring in children. Lesions, which are generally solitary or few in number, are usually fairly well but not sharply circumscribed, and consist of multiple tiny red ('cayenne pepper') spots that gradually turn yellowish orange as iron pigment is deposited by breakdown of erythrocytes in the tissues (Fig. 14.5).

Schamberg disease

This also occurs in children, or in young adults. There are generally multiple lesions, mainly on the legs but sometimes extensive (Fig. 14.9). They have the purpuric component described for lichen aureus, but this

is generally less intense and the overall color of the lesions is brownish. There may be mild irritation of the skin and overlying fine scaling.

Purpura annularis telangiectatica (Majocchi disease)

This is a more florid disorder, in which the lesions are more overtly purpuric and usually arciform or annular, and hence may be confused with a vasculitis (Fig. 14.6). There is some overlap with the features of lichen aureus in older lesions.

Generalized capillaropathy

This can occur as a transient phenomenon, often lasting a few weeks then gradually fading (Figs 14.7 and 14.8). This sequence suggests that it may just be a type of viral exanthem, but no specific cause is usually identified, and systemic involvement is not clinically apparent.

Differential diagnosis

The lesions of Schamberg disease can be confused with eczema, particularly of discoid type, although the latter is much more pruritic. Vasculitis may need to be excluded. In younger children especially, the purpuric bruise-like appearance of some lesions may raise concerns about abuse.

Treatment

No treatment is very useful. Topical corticosteroids may be used if itch is a feature. Support stockings are felt to be useful if the lesions are particularly on the lower legs, and especially if there is any evidence of venous disease.

VASCULITIS

Classification

The classification of vasculitis is complex, for several reasons.

- The classification may be based on clinical patterns, on histologic features (such as the predominant size of vessels involved or the type of inflammatory infiltrate), on immunologic tests (for example, ANCA-positive vasculitides may be considered together), etc.

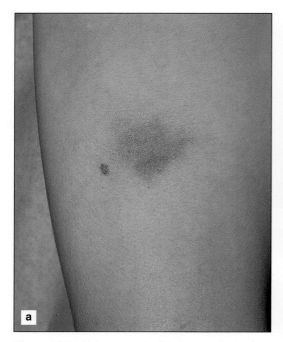

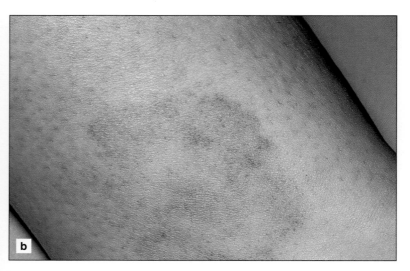

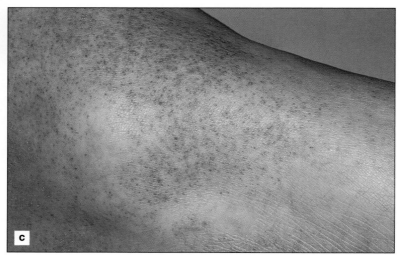

Figure 14.5 Lichen aureus, all lesions on the leg in different patients. This pattern of golden-brown lesion is most frequent in children, and is usually asymptomatic or mildly itchy when it first appears. (**a**) Typical morphology and site; (**b**) the golden-brown color of an older lesion; (**c**) a close-up view of early lichen aureus, demonstrating fresh pinpoint spots of capillary leakage, with a 'cayenne pepper' pattern.

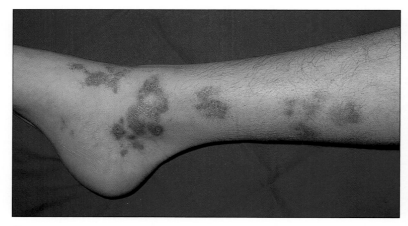

Figure 14.6 Purpura annularis telangiectoides (Majocchi disease) demonstrating annular and arciform lesions with a prominent purpuric component, on the leg of an otherwise well child.

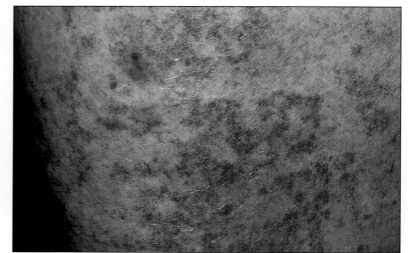

Figure 14.7 A more inflammatory and widespread capillaritis, in which there would be suspicion of true vasculitis features.

- There is overlap between many of the above (e.g. small-vessel neutrophilic cutaneous vasculitis is a feature of some large-vessel granulomatous vasculitides).
- Classifications based on systemic features of vasculitis correlate poorly with the type and extent of skin lesions.
- Some terminology is either of uncertain relevance or applied differently to the original descriptions (e.g. 'hypersensitivity vasculitis').
- Some disorders that may not be truly vasculitic overlap into the spectrum of vasculitis (such as the neutrophilic dermatoses).
- Some syndromes of vascular occlusion (such as cryoglobulinemia) are not initially inflammatory but cause secondary vasculitic inflammation.

- Some vasculitides overlap into other disease areas; for example, pityriasis lichenoides acuta, which has a lymphocytic vasculitis component, is in some cases associated with lymphoma (Ch. 33).

This chapter deals primarily with disorders that are generally accepted as 'mainstream' vasculitides, using headings that are designed to be clinically useful; it combines the predominant size of vessels involved with the clinical morphology of the skin lesions. A tentative classification is provided in Table 14.2.

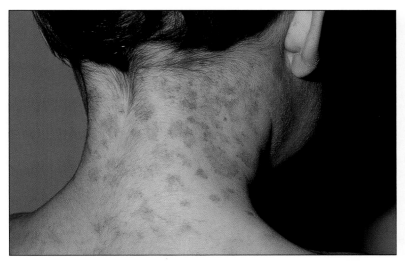

Figure 14.8 Capillaropathy on the neck of a child. He also had accentuation of lesions at sites of pressure from clothing and from a car seat belt. This presumably had a viral trigger, as the lesions faded over a few weeks.

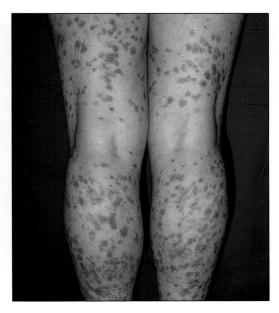

Figure 14.9 Older lesions of capillaropathy (Schamberg type) may look darker, probably because of some stimulation of overlying melanocytes, as occurs in venous stasis disease.

Table 14.2 CLASSIFICATION OF VASCULITIS	
Small-vessel vasculitis	**Larger-vessel vasculitis**
Cutaneous small-vessel vasculitis, not further classified Henoch–Schönlein purpura Essential mixed cryoglobulinemia Waldenström hypergammaglobulinemic purpura Associated with collagen vascular disease Urticarial vasculitis Erythema elevatum diutinum Eosinophilic vasculitis Rheumatoid nodules Reactive leprosy Septic vasculitis	Polyarteritis nodosa: microscopic polyarteritis, cutaneous form, systemic form Granulomatous vasculitis: Wegener granulomatosis, allergic granulomatosis of Churg and Strauss, lymphomatoid granulomatosis Giant cell arteritis: temporal arteritis, Takayasu arteritis Larger-vessel vasculitis with collagen vascular disease Nodular vasculitis

(From Barham KL, Jorizzo JL, Grattan B, et al. Vasculitis and neutrophilic vascular reactions. In: Burns DA, Breathnach SM, Cox NH, et al (eds) Rook's Textbook of Dermatology, 7th edn. Oxford: Blackwell Publishing, 2004.)

Antibodies

A number of tests involving antibodies are of importance in the investigation of vasculitis. Antinuclear antibody and other antibodies discussed in Chapter 13 are often tested, as many of the collagen vascular diseases have a vasculitic component. Direct immunofluorescence (discussed in Ch. 16 in the context of bullous dermatoses) is important to detect immune complex vasculitis, in which there are deposits of antibody in cutaneous blood vessels. The type of antibody may also be critical, for example IgA in Henoch–Schönlein purpura (HSP), discussed later.

Antiphospholipid and anticardiolipin antibodies are specifically discussed later in a section on the antiphospholipid syndrome.

Antineutrophil cytoplasmic antibodies (ANCAs) have become an important investigation in diagnosis of large-vessel vasculitides and are discussed in the relevant section of this chapter.

APPROACH TO VASCULITIS

The list of possible investigations in a patient with suspected vasculitis is potentially huge, given the large number of causes. Some suggestions for a logical approach are provided here and in Tables 14.3 and 14.4. This section is written from a dermatologic perspective, and the approach would be different in, for example, a patient suspected of having fever due to occult systemic vasculitis. Most vasculitis presenting due to cutaneous lesions is of small-vessel vasculitis type, in which about half will have no identifiable cause.

The main factors to consider in the approach to suspected vasculitis are as follows.

- Consideration of features that may indicate a serious vasculitis (either a serious cause or likely serious consequences).
- Which tests are required to reach a diagnosis.
- What treatment is necessary, and additional tests that may be necessary as a therapeutic baseline.
- Is it serious?

An important first step, as it dictates the urgency of referral or investigation, is to consider whether there are features of concern regarding significant systemic involvement, infective causes, or a need for systemic therapy. The most common clinically identifiable internal involvements in vasculitides are fever (which may indicate an infective cause or may be a consequence of internal vasculitis), arthralgia, and nephritis (hematuria and proteinuria). The questions listed in Table 14.3 may help.

Table 14.3   DOES THE PATIENT HAVE A SERIOUS VASCULITIS? QUESTIONS TO ASK

Is the patient otherwise well?	General malaise, fever, or organ-specific systemic symptoms should be considered; these may indicate either a systemic cause (such as infections) or may occur as a consequence of systemic vasculitis. Is the patient taking any new drugs for a medical condition?
Is there evidence of occult internal involvement?	In particular, it is important to perform urinalysis for evidence of hematuria or proteinuria; also, to consider cardiac murmurs that may be associated with subacute bacterial endocarditis.
Does the morphology of lesions suggest an occlusive or larger-vessel disease process?	For example, retiform non-inflammatory lesions, livedo, acral infarcts or cyanosis, larger nodules, broad areas of purpura or necrosis.
Does the pattern suggest an infective cause?	For example, predominance of pustular lesions. Also note the presence of fever, as discussed above.
Does the body site of lesions cause concern?	Is the pattern consistent with a cutaneous small-vessel vasculitis (CSVV)? This usually affects the lower half of the body primarily, especially the lower legs; more widespread lesions suggest a more severe process. Conjunctival or fundal involvement suggests the possibility of subacute bacterial endocarditis.
Does the skin damage of individual lesions warrant systemic therapy?	Small lesions of CSVV may not require aggressive therapy, whereas larger necrotic lesions may require active treatment.

Table 14.4   SOME INVESTIGATIONS TO DETERMINE THE CAUSE OF CUTANEOUS VASCULITIS

Investigation	Details
Basic bloods	Complete blood count; electrolytes, and renal and hepatic function; inflammatory markers (erythrocyte sedimentation rate, C-reactive protein)
Urinalysis	Plus 24-h urinary protein excretion if positive dipstick test
Skin biopsy	Of a *fresh* lesion, with direct immunofluorescence studies: confirms vasculitis and helps to distinguish vessel wall damage versus occlusive patterns
Autoantibodies	Antinuclear antibody (ANA), antineutrophil cytoplasmic antibody (ANCA), antiphospholipid, with or without others if connective tissue disorder suspected
Immunology tests	Complement levels (may be low in urticarial vasculitis or lupus erythematosus)
Infection screen	Depends on the situation; always required if there is fever or systemic malaise (may include blood cultures, throat swab, cerebrospinal fluid culture, viral serology, etc.)
Other blood tests	Cryoglobulins or electrophoresis, protein C, and protein S
Other investigations for systemic disease	Depends on history, clinical findings, and likely cause, for example chest X-ray, nasal or respiratory tract biopsy (Wegener granulomatosis), nerve conduction studies or biopsy and/or angiography (polyarteritis), etc.

PRACTICE POINTS
- Always consider infection as a cause of vasculitic lesions: treatment with immunosuppressive agents may be detrimental.
- Remember that fever, malaise, and other systemic symptoms may reflect either the cause or the effect of a systemic vasculitis.
- Always test for proteinuria and hematuria, even in the absence of any systemic symptoms.
- Drug-induced vasculitis accounts for a significant minority of cases of cutaneous small-vessel vasculitis.

Investigations to determine a cause

Investigations in any vasculitis with palpable purpura are directed toward both identifying a cause, and determining the presence and extent of internal organ involvement (see Table 14.3). Some suggested initial investigations to identify a cause of vasculitis are provided in Table 14.4.

As a general approach, it is reasonable to test full blood count, urinalysis, renal function, liver enzymes, and erythrocyte sedimentation rate (ESR) in all patients. Skin biopsy (discussed later) is also extremely helpful, especially if fresh lesions are present (Fig. 14.10). Tests for immunologic abnormalities (ANA, ANCA, rheumatoid factor, and other autoantibodies), complement levels, and cryoglobulins; tests for underlying infections or malignancy; and other organ-specific tests may be required, depending on the clinical severity and progression. For example, they are generally not necessary in a patient with a reasonably definite drug cause for cutaneous vasculitis and mild arthralgia, but some or all of these would be indicated for a patient with severe vasculitis or recurrent unexplained episodes.

Skin biopsy is a critical investigation in determining likely diagnostic territory and thus directing further investigations, and should always be performed in a patient who has ongoing new vasculitic lesions or who is unwell. It may not be necessary in, for example, an uncomplicated case of likely drug-induced vasculitis in an otherwise well patient in whom no fresh lesions are developing. When sending a skin biopsy, it is important to

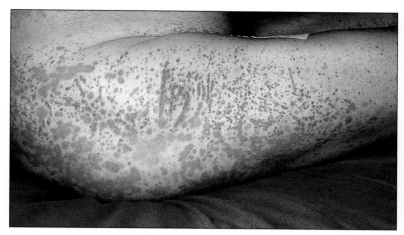

Figure 14.10 Vasculitis with mixed age of lesions; the red lesions are fresh and are more useful for histologic diagnosis than the older lesions represented by brown hemosiderin staining. Note the Koebner-like reaction of lesions along lines of scratch, in this instance probably just reflecting erythrocyte leakage from the trauma to small vessels. (From Lawrence CM, Cox NH. Physical Signs in Dermatology, 2nd edn. London: Mosby, 2002.)

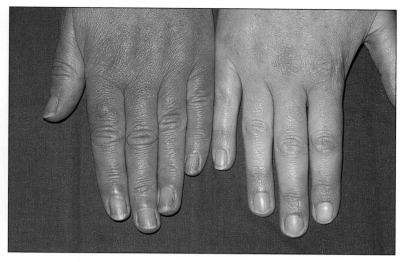

Figure 14.11 Acrocyanosis demonstrating diffuse dusky purplish color of the skin (left side of picture) compared with a control.

perform direct immunofluorescence, as a positive result confirms an immune-mediated process; positivity for IgA is specific for HSP. Note that immune deposits in the skin are destroyed within 12–24 h, so a fresh lesion must be biopsied for this evaluation to be meaningful. Potentially useful results from skin biopsy might include the following.

- Usually able to distinguish primary vessel wall damage from occlusion with secondary vasculitis.
- May be specific features, for example segmental changes in deeper skin arteries due to polyarteritis, eosinophilic infiltrate of Churg–Strauss syndrome, etc.
- Positive direct immunofluorescence confirms immunologic basis, for example IgA-positive in HSP.
- If occlusive, may be able to distinguish the type of occlusion, for example platelet ('white thrombi'), cryoglobulin, crystal (e.g. cholesterol emboli), and fungi (a particular risk if the lesions are necrotic and in an immunosuppressed patient).
- Consider sending additional biopsy samples, depending on the clinical situation, for example frozen tissue for histology (if cholesterol emboli are suspected) and tissue for culture (endocarditis, systemically unwell, or immunosuppressed patient).

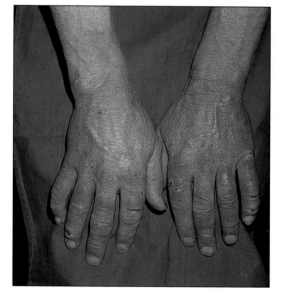

Figure 14.12 Acrocyanosis with chilblains (perniosis) over the proximal interphalangeal joints of the left hand.

> **PRACTICE POINTS**
> - Skin biopsy is crucial in investigation of cutaneous vasculitis.
> - Direct immunofluorescence should be included; it is crucial that this requires biopsy of fresh lesions.
> - Consider additional biopsy samples, depending on the clinical situation, for example frozen tissue for histology (suspected cholesterol emboli) and tissue for culture (necrotic lesions in immunosuppressed patient).
> - Make sure the biopsy includes deep dermis and some fat, so that larger vessels can be evaluated.

Investigations as a therapeutic baseline

Treatments for vasculitis are considered in more detail later. Some patients with mild small-vessel vasculitis may require only rest, without any active intervention. However, some patients will require significant immuno-suppressive or other drug therapy. It is therefore helpful to consider likely treatment, and to perform relevant baseline tests, as part of the initial work-up.

Many of the tests to determine a cause double as baselines for therapy with corticosteroids, dapsone, or immunosuppressive agents. Additionally, it may be appropriate to measure glucose and blood pressure (cortico-steroids), glucose-6-phosphate dehydrogenase level (dapsone), thiopurine methyltransferase level (azathioprine), etc.; see Chapter 4 for more details of individual agents.

LYMPHOCYTIC VASCULITIS

Primarily lymphocytic vasculitis is uncommon, although some disorders have a predominantly lymphocytic infiltrate in later stages (e.g. erythema nodosum, a panniculitis with perivascular inflammation in fat septae, Ch. 22). Pityriasis lichenoides et varioliformis acuta and lymphomatoid papulosis both have features of a lymphocytic vasculitis, and are discussed in Chapter 33. The capillaritis disorders discussed earlier are also lymphocytic, as are chilblains.

Chilblains (perniosis)
Etiology

These lesions are caused by cold, but not at subzero temperatures. They may occur in conjunction with acrocyanosis (Figs 14.11 and 14.12). Lesions may occur on the digits and other bony areas (at any age, Fig. 14.13) or over areas of fatty tissue (usually in older children and young adults, mainly women, Fig. 22.52).

Clinical

The lesions occur after cold exposure, but typically cause a hot throbbing quality of pain. They may last several weeks as red tender lumps, and occasionally develop small, necrotic, weeping areas.

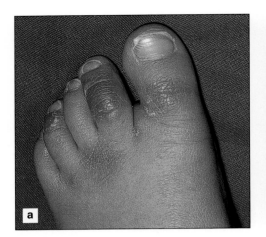

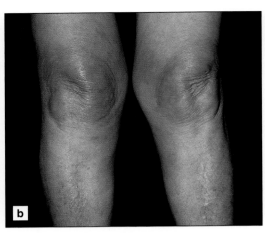

Figure 14.13 Chilblains (perniosis). (**a**) Chilblains on the toes of a young child. These lesions last for several weeks, and may be sore or itchy. (**b**) Perniosis on the knees of an adult. Symptoms are usually less marked at this site.

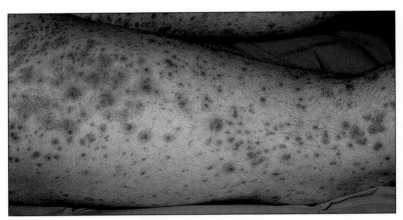

Figure 14.14 Henoch–Schönlein purpura: a typical pattern of palpable purpura at a typical site on the lower legs. This cannot be distinguished with certainty from other causes of small-vessel leukocytoclastic vasculitis on purely clinical grounds.

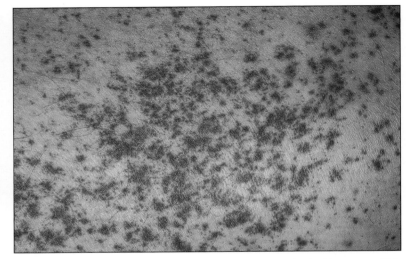

Figure 14.15 A more widespread semiconfluent pattern of palpable purpura. This urticated erythematous appearance is suggestive that Henoch–Schönlein purpura is the cause.

Differential diagnosis

The differential diagnosis of chilblains varies according to the sites affected.

Lesions affecting the digits may be associated with acrocyanosis, and may be confused with Raynaud phenomenon (in which the reperfusion phase may be tender, although the vasospastic whiteness of Raynaud phenomenon is not a feature of chilblains); alternatively, the tenderness and redness may suggest infection or paronychia.

On areas such as the thigh, overlying fatty tissue, the differential diagnosis includes neutrophilic vascular reactions such as erythema nodosum, nodular vasculitis, and other forms of panniculitis. An important diagnostic feature is that chilblains at such sites are markedly cold to touch.

Treatment

Explanation about warm gloves and clothing to prevent subsequent episodes is important. Non-steroidal antiinflammatory drugs (NSAIDs) may reduce symptoms, and nifedipine can abolish and prevent the digital type but is relatively unhelpful for lesions over fatty areas.

PRACTICE POINTS
- Chilblains of digits are probably underdiagnosed.
- Chilblains over fatty areas, despite their redness and throbbing pain, are notably cold to touch.

CUTANEOUS SMALL-VESSEL VASCULITIS (CSVV, LEUKOCYTOCLASTIC VASCULITIS)

General aspects

Many clinically diverse disorders include histologic features of small-vessel vasculitis (vessel-directed inflammation), including erythema multiforme (Ch. 11), erythema elevatum diutinum (this chapter), pityriasis lichenoides acuta (Ch. 33), drug-induced vasculitis, occlusive vasculitis, and HSP.

While many of these are morphologically distinct disorders, most CSVV presents with a clinical picture that does not in itself identify a specific cause. The features of palpable purpura, in some cases with associated urticarial lesions, pustules, or necrotic areas (Figs 14.14–14.20), are common to a wide range of disorders and etiologies. This section addresses the causes, relevant investigations, and main differential diagnoses of this constellation of features, in which the histologic correlate is a leukocytoclastic small-vessel vasculitis (leukocytoclasis implies the presence of fragmented nuclear remnants of neutrophil polymorphs in the perivascular and vessel wall infiltrate).

Etiology and pathogenesis

The main causes of CSVV are listed in Table 14.5.

Clinical

The skin lesions in most of these are similar. They occur primarily in dependent areas, mainly the lower legs. Individual lesions are usually a few millimeters to 1 cm in diameter, purpuric, often palpable, and may be necrotic. Blisters, usually hemorrhagic, may occur, and pustules (the latter especially in bacteremic causes of vasculitis). Larger necrotic areas may develop, especially around the ankles.

The presence of inflammation in early lesions helps to distinguish processes with primary vessel wall injury, compared with occlusive microvascular occlusion disorders. A primary vasculitis causes inflammation, with purpura as a secondary event, whereas inflammation occurs as the secondary event in microvascular occlusion disorders. Vasculitis lesions of any size are therefore palpable from the outset, whereas lesions

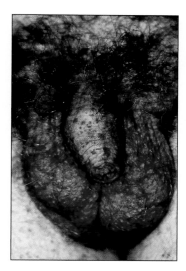

Figure 14.16 Henoch–Schönlein purpura affecting the genitalia. Lesions of buttocks and genitalia, along with lower leg lesions, are common in this disorder. (Courtesy of Dr. G. Dawn.)

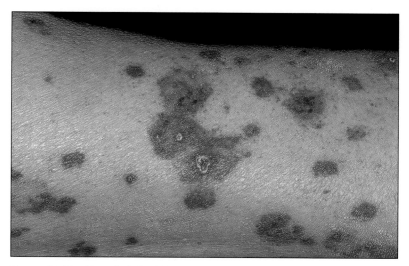

Figure 14.18 Henoch–Schönlein purpura demonstrating the retiform pattern of purpura. This occurs in other disorders, such as cryoglobulinemia, but the combination of retiform purpura with early inflammation is strongly suggestive of IgA-mediated vasculitis.

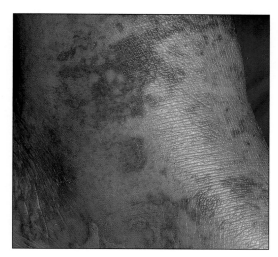

Figure 14.17 Close-up view of purpuric spots in a case of Henoch–Schönlein purpura. Note the reticulate pattern.

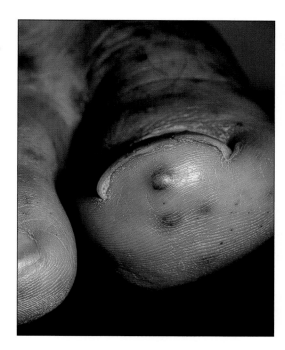

Figure 14.19 Henoch–Schönlein purpura on the feet, with a pustule.

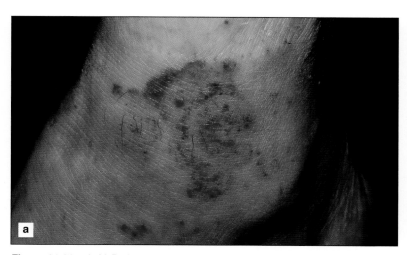

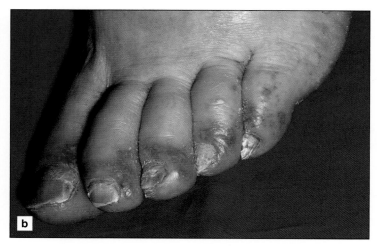

Figure 14.20 (**a**,**b**) Both annular lesions (**a**) and bullae may occur in several types of cutaneous small-vessel vasculitis, as shown here. (Panel b shows the same patient as in Fig. 14.1.)

Table 14.5   CAUSES OF CUTANEOUS SMALL-VESSEL VASCULITIS

Category	Examples and comments
Idiopathic	About 50% of cases
Henoch–Schönlein purpura	Defined by IgA deposition
Infections	Hepatitis B, hepatitis C, streptococcal, subacute bacterial endocarditis, bowel-associated dermatitis–arthritis syndrome, bronchiectasis, chronic meningococcemia or gonococcemia
Collagen vascular disease	Lupus erythematosus, rheumatoid disease (Figs 14.21 and 14.22)
Autoimmune diseases	Inflammatory bowel disease (especially ulcerative colitis)
Larger-vessel vasculitides	Cutaneous small-vessel vasculitis may occur in Wegener granulomatosis, Churg–Strauss syndrome, polyarteritis nodosa
Foods and drugs	Serum sickness, various drugs (see text)
Malignancy	Lymphoma, hematologic malignancy
Primarily occlusive microvascular disease	Vasculitis may occur as a secondary event
Other specific types of small-vessel vasculitis	Urticarial vasculitis, erythema elevatum diutinum, granuloma faciale

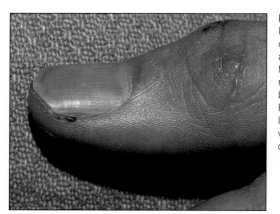

Figure 14.21 Bywater lesion of rheumatoid disease. This occurs around the nail fold or finger pulps as a deep nodule, which may become crusted. Histologically, there is a leukocytoclastic vasculitis with fibrinoid degeneration.

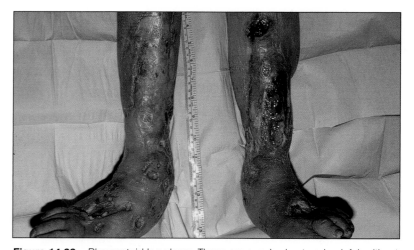

Figure 14.22   Rheumatoid leg ulcers. These are punched out and painful, without venous stasis changes, and therefore have the clinical appearance of arterial ulceration (see also Ch. 15).

Differential diagnosis

The main differential diagnosis issue is between the different causes of CSVV, and the distinction from disorders causing vascular occlusion.

Differentials of a small-vessel vasculitic process include the following.

- Large-vessel vasculitis with small-vessel skin lesions: for example Wegener granulomatosis.
- Disorders of microvascular occlusion: discussed later.
- Non-vasculitic causes of purpura: especially if the lower legs are affected or if the patient is unwell.
- Lesions with secondary hemorrhage: usually affecting the lower leg, for example bullous pemphigoid and cellulitis.
- Tiny angiomas that may not blanch on pressure: such as minute Campbell de Morgan spots, angiokeratomas, or angioma serpiginosum; these may mimic vasculitis, although such lesions are unchanging over days while vasculitic lesions will fade.
- Miscellaneous: excoriations and insect bite reactions.

Treatment of CSVV

The same principles apply to most causes of CSVV and to many of the specific patterns of vasculitis discussed later. Investigations should be performed to identify a treatable cause (see earlier text and Tables 14.3 and 14.4), the differential diagnosis should be addressed, and any identified cause such as medications should be specifically addressed. Rest, with elevation of the legs, may be sufficient therapy in many patients with mild vasculitis, and simple analgesics may be all that is required for arthralgia. Systemic corticosteroids are useful for arthralgia if sufficiently severe, and variably useful for renal or skin lesions; for cutaneous disease, this approach is usually reserved for more active necrotic or ulcerated lesions. Dapsone and colchicine are also useful as first-line or steroid-sparing therapy; azathioprine may be used for its steroid-sparing effect.

SPECIFIC TYPES OF SMALL-VESSEL VASCULITIS

'Allergic' or 'hypersensitivity' vasculitis

This is a somewhat historically confused term, as the original descriptions probably included individuals with a variety of disorders that would now be considered separately. It was separated from HSP, but as the latter was decreed to occur only in children, adult HSP was never diagnosed and would have been included as a hypersensitivity vasculitis. Some authors now use the term idiopathic vasculitis in place of hypersensitivity vasculitis, although ideally an idiopathic diagnosis should really be reached

due to microvascular occlusion initially consist of 'bland' non-inflamed lesions, often in a reticulate pattern, even though they may become edematous or inflamed later. Evaluation of early lesions is therefore important in directing the most profitable avenues of investigation. The combination of early inflammation and a reticulate or retiform patterning (Figs 14.17 and 14.18) is suggestive of IgA-mediated vasculitis (HSP).

by exclusion of specific causes. Generally, no cause is identifiable in about 50% of patients with CSVV.

Drug-induced purpura and vasculitis

Most cases of drug-induced vasculitis are not clinically distinguishable from other causes of a small-vessel vasculitis, but are discussed separately, as drugs should always be considered in the differential diagnosis of a vasculitic rash. In most cases, the pattern is of a predominantly lower leg, small-vessel disease. Potential causative agents include the following.

- Antibiotics: co-trimoxazole, penicillins, and isoniazid.
- Rheumatology: aspirin, NSAIDs, allopurinol, and gold.
- Cardiology: thiazides, furosemide, streptokinase, and diltiazem.
- Psychiatry: chlorpromazine.
- Neurology: hydantoins and barbiturates.
- Endocrine: carbimazole, thiouracils, and sulfonylureas.

Henoch–Schönlein purpura

Henoch–Schönlein purpura is the characteristic type of small-vessel leukocytoclastic vasculitis. Lesions are as described earlier. Early lesions often have an urticated component or an inflammatory retiform pattern (Figs 14.17 and 14.18).

Different criteria for the diagnosis make literature assessment difficult (e.g. some authors still restrict the diagnosis to childhood). However, the most logical approach appears to be for the term HSP to apply to IgA vasculitis.

There are several studies documenting preceding sore throat and upper respiratory tract infection (especially in children, most commonly streptococcal infections) and familial clustering. In adults, drug treatments are also implicated, commonly antibiotics such as penicillins.

The classic clinical associations are with arthralgia, gastrointestinal involvement (which may present as pain, bleeding, or intussusception, especially in children), and nephritis (IgA nephropathy). A common feature of HSP is recurrent episodes after initial improvement, which may occur on several occasions. In most cases, the overall tendency is toward improvement, but follow-up with monitoring of blood pressure and urinalysis is required.

Urticarial vasculitis

Urticarial vasculitis (Fig. 14.23, see also Ch. 9) is characterized by urticarial lesions that persist for more than 24 h, by comparison with ordinary urticaria, in which the lesions are more transient. The lesions are often more angular or stellate in shape compared with the circles and arcs of ordinary urticaria, and there may be associated purpura or bruising, although this can also occur in ordinary urticaria (especially if scratched due to itch). Pain may be present rather than the itch of more typical urticaria. There may be associated livedo reticularis, vasculitis, episcleritis, arthritis, nephritis, and other internal organ involvement.

Urticarial vasculitis may occur in association with various immune abnormalities, such as systemic lupus erythematosus (SLE), Sjögren

syndrome, mixed cryoglobulinemia, IgA myeloma, and monoclonal IgM gammopathy (Schnitzler syndrome). Viral infections, such as infectious mononucleosis and hepatitis C, may cause urticarial vasculitis without associated cryoglobulinemia. The most important association is with low complement levels, as this group has a high frequency of SLE (about 50%) and multisystem disease. This is known as the hypocomplementemic urticarial vasculitis syndrome (HUVS). Most such patients are women, and nearly all have immunoreactants at the basement membrane zone on direct immunofluorescence (positive lupus band). By contrast, normocomplementemic urticarial vasculitis patients have a less prominent female predominance, only a few percent have SLE, and the prognosis is generally better.

The most important differential diagnosis is from 'ordinary' urticaria (Ch. 9), and making the distinction between normocomplementemic urticarial vasculitis and HUVS.

Treatments include antihistamines (usually relatively unhelpful, by contrast to in ordinary urticaria), corticosteroids, dapsone, colchicine, and hydroxychloroquine.

PRACTICE POINT

Features that suggest urticarial rather than ordinary vasculitis include:

- associated purpura,
- pain rather than itch,
- individual lesion duration longer than 24 h, and
- associated systemic symptoms such as joint pain.

Waldenström hypergammaglobulinemic purpura

This disorder (Fig. 14.24) is probably underdiagnosed. It is typically a transient eruption that affects the lower legs in young women, often provoked by exercise, heat, and prolonged sitting or standing. It may occur over many years.

The lesions are petechial, occasionally palpable, and last for a few days, with some residual staining as they resolve. They are often asymptomatic but sometimes itch or burn when the eruption appears. Many patients are otherwise well, but some have arthritis, Sjögren syndrome, sarcoidosis, or other systemic diseases, and mild anemia is common.

Platelet counts and tests of clotting are normal, but ESR is often elevated, and there is a polyclonal increase in gamma-globulins (usually IgG) and sometimes positive antinuclear antibody or rheumatoid factor tests. Deposition of IgM, IgG, or complement C3 may be demonstrated in skin biopsies.

The differential diagnosis may include many causes of CSVV, or of simple purpura or capillaritis.

Treatment is often not required other than avoiding likely triggers, and the risks and costs of plasmapheresis or immunosuppressive therapy often outweigh the advantages. Aspirin and other antiplatelet agents are helpful in some cases.

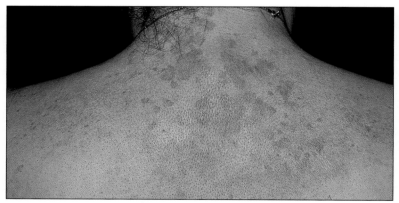

Figure 14.23 Urticarial vasculitis lesions on the nape of the neck and upper back. These may be more irregularly shaped than ordinary urticarial lesions, are more likely to have a purpuric component, and each lesion may often last a few days.

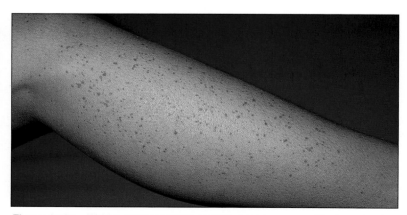

Figure 14.24 Waldenström hypergammaglobulinemic purpura. The lower leg in young women is a typical site of involvement. Lesions may be provoked by exercise.

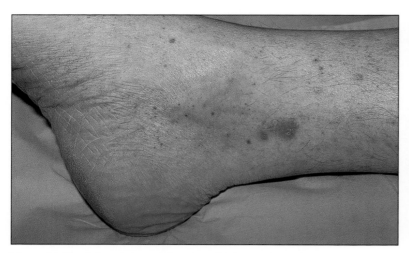

Figure 14.25 Subacute bacterial endocarditis in a patient with a prosthetic heart valve. Small vasculitic lesions of this type are common with this type of immune complex disease, and may be quite subtle. Histologically, the features are of a non-specific, small-vessel leukocytoclastic vasculitis.

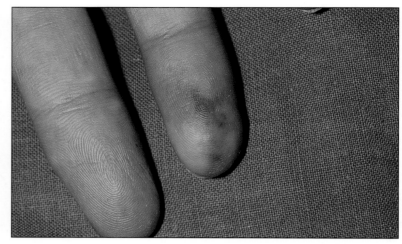

Figure 14.27 Subacute bacterial endocarditis demonstrating an Osler node of the finger pulp. These lesions may be embolic, as they have recently been demonstrated to contain bacteria.

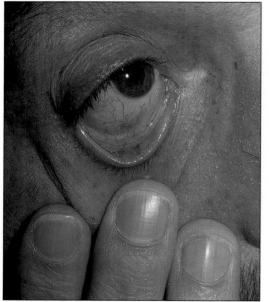

Figure 14.26
Subacute bacterial endocarditis (SBE) in the same patient as shown in Figure 14.25. Conjunctival lesions, as shown here, and retinal vasculitis are uncommon in Henoch–Schönlein purpura or drug-related small-vessel vasculitis, and support a presumed diagnosis of SBE. Examination of fundi is diagnostically important in this disorder.

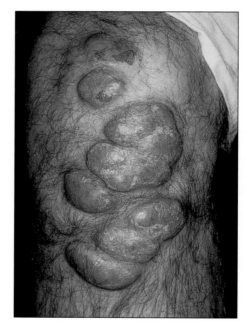

Figure 14.28 Erythema elevatum diutinum. Old lesions may be quite large and fibrotic, as shown here. The knees and other bony prominences are a common site. (Courtesy of Gary W. Cole, M.D.)

Bacterial endocarditis

The clinical picture in subacute bacterial endocarditis (SBE) is primarily due to immune complex disease causing a small-vessel leukocytoclastic vasculitis (Figs 14.25 and 14.26). This is accompanied by splinter hemorrhages, retinal or conjunctival hemorrhages or edema, and lesions on the hands and fingers (Osler nodes, Fig. 14.27, and Janeway lesions). The presence of bacteria has been documented in the latter lesions, suggesting that at least some of the features of SBE are due to infective emboli.

Erythema elevatum diutinum

This disorder is rare in the UK but may be more common in the USA. Some cases are associated with paraproteinemias, usually of IgA type. Histologically, there is a leukocytoclastic vasculitis with mixed inflammatory infiltrate that may contain neutrophils, eosinophils, and plasma cells.

Lesions are purplish and sometimes purpuric, often with discoid or annular morphology and a yellowish margin. They tend to occur over bony prominences of the hands, knees (Fig. 14.28), and face. Older lesions are more brown. Variation in intensity in relation to temperature change and premenstrual exacerbations may occur.

Treatment is usually with topical corticosteroids or systemic dapsone.

Granuloma faciale

This disorder occurs typically on the face, but is actually vasculitic rather than granulomatous. Lesions are (usually solitary) brownish plaques

(Fig. 14.29), which have a benign behavior. Dapsone is usually recommended to treat this process, but some cases respond fully to strong topical steroids or intralesional steroid.

INTRAVASCULAR OCCLUSIVE CAUSES OF VASCULITIS-LIKE LESIONS

Several varied disorders may cause intravascular occlusion, which mimics vasculitis. Indeed, many of these disorders cause inflammation and a secondary vasculitis. The features include varying degrees of livedo (Fig. 14.30); dusky, necrotic, or ulcerated extremities (Fig. 14.31); large acute necrotic lesions; and internal organ involvement. The relevant disorders include the following.

- Cold-precipitating proteins.
- Other hyperviscosity disorders, such as paraproteinemias.
- Platelet plugging: thrombocytosis and myeloproliferative disease.
- Thrombophilic disorders due to abnormalities of the clotting cascade (e.g. protein C deficiency, purpura fulminans, disseminated intravascular coagulopathy, and coumarin necrosis; see also Chs 12 and 18).
- Antiphospholipid syndrome.
- Vascular coagulopathies: for example Sneddon syndrome.
- Embolic vasculitis.

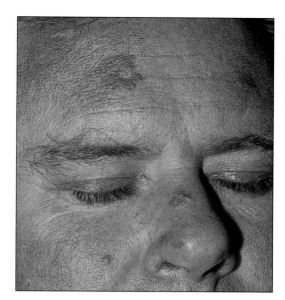

Figure 14.29
Granuloma faciale, which has a typical brown and rather granulomatous appearance. Histologically, this has mild vasculitic features.

Livedo

Livedo reticularis and livedo racemosa are descriptive terms applied to a net-like or 'chicken wire' reticulate patterning of vascular lesions (Figs 14.30 and 14.32). The terms overlap in common usage; some view them as identical, others use livedo racemosa when the network pattern is broader and more clearly defined. These terms have been applied to a confluent physiologic pattern (seen best in babies and young women, and capable of blanching with pressure), a rare congenital abnormality (cutis marmorata telangiectatica, Fig. 19.17), and a more patchy 'broken livedo' pattern that occurs in some vasculitides and vasoocclusive disorders (when it may be associated with necrosis and ulceration). This last patchy and potentially necrosing pattern is indicative of several potential underlying vascular disease processes, including the following.

- Polyarteritis nodosa (see later) and other large-vessel vasculitis.
- Vasculitis in connective tissue diseases: lupus erythematosus, rheumatoid, and mixed connective tissue disease.
- The causes of intravascular occlusion listed earlier (some are specifically discussed in this chapter also).
- Vasospasm (e.g. due to long-term amantadine).

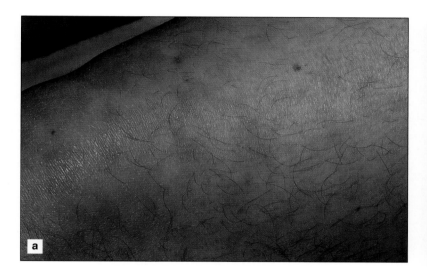

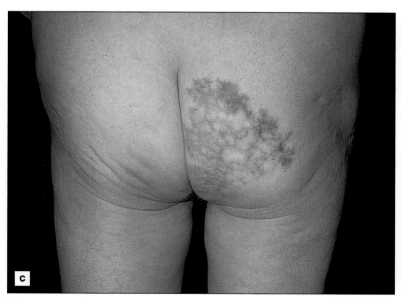

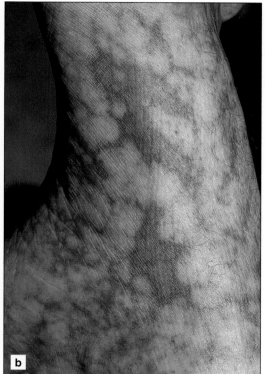

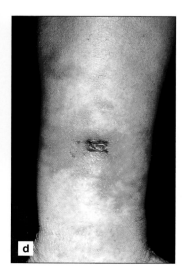

Figure 14.30   Examples of livedo. (**a**) Patchy faint livedo in a patient with positive antinuclear antibody but no clear clinical diagnosis. (**b**) Vasculitis with a prominent livedo patterning on the leg. (**c**) Typical chicken wire appearance of livedo. This was a fixed lesion that occurred in a patient who had a renal transplant operation, with no subsequent livedo elsewhere, and was felt to represent a gluteal artery occlusion. (**d**) Vasculitic ulcer with adjacent livedo. See also Fig. 18.53. (Panel d courtesy of Dr. G. Dawn.)

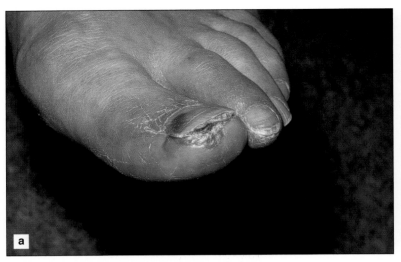

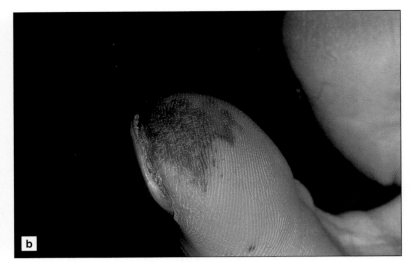

Figure 14.31 Acral changes of hyperviscosity syndrome. (**a**) A dusky blue toe. This is a common feature in occlusive types of vasculitis. (**b**) A purpuric fingertip lesion due to occlusive vasculitis. This patient had lesions of several fingers and toes of both hands and feet, with no cause demonstrated despite extensive investigation. Treatment with aspirin prevented further fresh lesions.

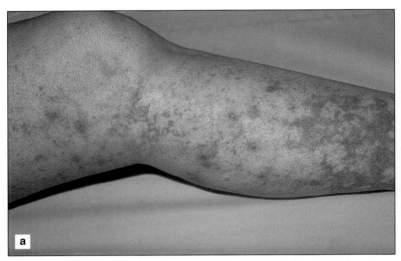

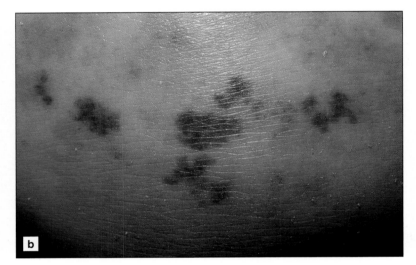

Figure 14.32 (**a**) Cryoglobulinemia presenting as a livedo pattern on the leg with exacerbations over many years. Hepatitis screen was negative, and lesions occurred over many years despite a series of immunosuppressive therapies. (**b**) Cryoglobulinemia presenting with rather retiform purpuric lesions on the knees. By contrast to the retiform purpura that occurs in Henoch–Schönlein purpura, these cryoglobulin lesions have no urticated or inflammatory component.

- Primary idiopathic livedoid vasculopathy.
- Metabolic: calciphylaxis (Ch. 12), hyperoxaluria, and homocystinuria.

Cryoglobulinemia and other cold-precipitating proteins
Cryoglobulinemia
Cryoglobulins are cold-precipitating proteins in the circulation, which fall into three classes.
- Type I: monoclonal IgM or IgG cryoglobulin.
- Type II: mixed cryoglobulin (monoclonal rheumatoid factor against polyclonal IgG).
- Type III: mixed polyclonal cryoglobulin.

The most common disorder is that due to type II or type III mixed cryoglobulinemia, which is now recognized to occur secondary to hepatitis C infection in about 50% of cases (conversely, about 2% of patients with hepatitis C infection will develop cryoglobulins). Other cases occur secondary to connective tissue disorders, hematologic malignancies, and other infections or causes of chronic antigenemia.

The clinical features of this disorder are purpuric vasculitis due to intravascular occlusion, arthralgia, and systemic vasculitis causing nephritis, neuropathy, hepatitis, and pneumonitis. The cutaneous lesions (Fig. 14.32) typically affect acral sites and may cause livedo, purpuric lesions, ulceration, duskiness of digits ('purple toe' or 'blue toe' syndrome), or gangrene.

Treatment includes preventive measures such as avoiding peripheral cooling, non-specific therapies such as high-dose systemic steroids, and a variety of immunosuppressive and cytotoxic therapies (such as azathioprine, cyclophosphamide, chlorambucil, fludarabine, and 2-chlorodeoxyadenosine). Plasmapheresis may be used to reduce circulating levels of cryoglobulin. Interferon and ribavirin is probably the treatment of choice for patients with underlying hepatitis C infection. Immunosuppressive agents and chemotherapy may be required for underlying connective tissue disease or lymphoma.

Cryofibrinogenemia
This is a rare disorder that may be secondary to hematologic and other malignancies or may occur in isolation (Fig. 14.33). The cutaneous features are the same as in cryoglobulinemia.

Treatments are similar to those for cryoglobulinemia, but fibrinolytic therapy with stanozolol can also be extremely effective.

Embolic occlusion
Etiology and pathogenesis
Embolic vasculitis may have several causes, including the following.
- Bacterial endocarditis (see earlier) and infective emboli (Fig. 14.34).
- Cholesterol emboli.

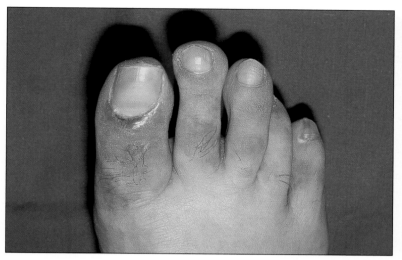

Figure 14.33 Idiopathic cryofibrinogenemia, demonstrating a dusky blue color with some infarction of the periungual skin. This responded to stanozolol and low-dose prednisolone.

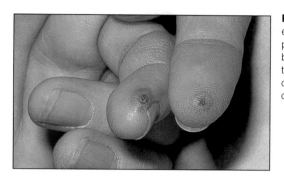

Figure 14.34 Infective emboli causing fingertip pustules. These should be cleaned and pierced to obtain bacteriology cultures of the pus content.

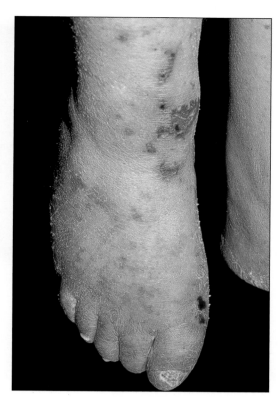

Figure 14.35 Cholesterol emboli. Embolic fragments of larger vessels lodge in the extremities, causing decreased blood flow, pain, a livedo pattern, and necrosis. Angiography or other manipulation of the vessels may precipitate this condition, as may antithrombotic and anticoagulant drugs of various types.

- Cardiac myxoma, which may be associated with cutaneous myxomas, blue nevi, spotty pigmentation, or endocrine disease (Carney complex or LAMB [lentigines, atrial myxomas, mucocutaneous myxomas, blue nevi] syndrome).
- Fat emboli.

Clinical

The features vary to some extent, depending on the cause, but include livedo, infarcts, purpuric lesions, ulcers, and blisters. Endocarditis (see earlier) and cholesterol emboli (below) are the commonest causes. Cardiac myxoma may cause fever, malaise, and cardiac murmurs. Fat emboli occur in the context of a recent fracture, and may also affect other organs, such as lungs.

Cholesterol emboli

Cholesterol emboli most typically arise from the lower aorta or femoral vessels, and hence affect one or both legs. They may be dislodged during arteriography or arterial surgery, or after cardiopulmonary resuscitation, and should be strongly suspected in cases of apparently unilateral foot vasculitis. However, this condition causes most diagnostic difficulty when there are spontaneous recurrent episodes of embolization or episodes affecting both lower legs. The process may occur after use of anticoagulants or thrombolytic therapy.

The cutaneous signs include livedo reticularis, purpuric rash, decreased perfusion manifest as a dusky extremity or extremities or as gangrene, and ulcers or infarction (Fig. 14.35). Myalgia and renal involvement (hypertension; hematuria or proteinuria, or renal failure) may occur, as may involvement of the brain (stroke), eyes (acute loss of vision), or gastrointestinal tract (abdominal pain, diarrhea, and gastrointestinal blood loss). The majority of patients have palpable distal pulses.

The characteristic pathologic lesion is the presence of cholesterol clefts, seen as needle-shaped defects in arteriolar walls in the histologic specimen (the cholesterol dissolves out during standard tissue processing). In acute lesions, the clefts are surrounded by inflammation, and there may

be associated eosinophilia, hypocomplementemia, elevated ESR, and occasionally a positive ANCA; all these may suggest immunologic vasculitides such as polyarteritis nodosa.

If minor, supportive treatment may be all that is needed. Otherwise, surgery may be needed.

Antiphospholipid syndrome
Etiology and pathogenesis

The antiphospholipid syndrome (APS) is a constellation of features that occur due to anticardiolipin antibodies or the lupus anticoagulant, together known as antiphospholipid antibodies (aPL). These are a heterogeneous group of antibodies, which may explain the wide range of clinical manifestations; indeed, some individuals with positive antibody tests never develop any clinical disease. The two antibody systems are distinct but often coexist.

The APS may occur as a primary disorder or associated with a huge range of conditions (Table 14.6), of which the main one is lupus erythematosus.

Clinical

Clinical manifestations are due to arterial and venous thromboses in various organs, and probably direct effects on phospholipids in other tissues, such as placenta and brain. Features include the following.

- Neurologic: stroke, multiinfarct dementia, Sneddon syndrome, and retinal infarction.
- Cardiovascular: deep venous thrombosis, thrombophlebitis, myocardial infarction, and valve defects.
- Renal: microangiopathy and renal arterial thrombosis.
- Other viscera: hepatic infarction, adrenal infarction, and mesenteric ischemia.
- Skin (Fig. 14.36): livedo reticularis, vasculitis, digital necrosis, ulcers, and Degos disease.
- Obstetric: recurrent abortions.
- Hematologic: thrombocytopenia and abnormal clotting tests.

Full laboratory evaluation is relatively specialized, but prolongation of the kaolin partial thromboplastin time (KPTT) or dilute Russell viper venom time (dRVVT) are readily available screening tests. Different types of aPL can be measured (anticardiolipin antibody and lupus anticoagulant), and other antibodies may also be markers for this condition (such as the type M5 antimitochondrial antibody).

Table 14.6 DISORDERS ASSOCIATED WITH ANTIPHOSPHOLIPID ANTIBODIES

Type of disorder	Examples
Collagen vascular	Systemic lupus erythematosus, drug-induced lupus erythematosus, rheumatoid arthritis, systemic sclerosis, dermatomyositis, Sjögren syndrome
Vasculitides	Behçet syndrome, giant cell arteritis
Hematologic	Autoimmune hemolytic anemia, thrombocytopenic purpura, myelodysplasia, monoclonal gammopathies, macroglobulinemia, lymphomas, thymoma
Infections	Tuberculosis, syphilis, endocarditis, AIDS

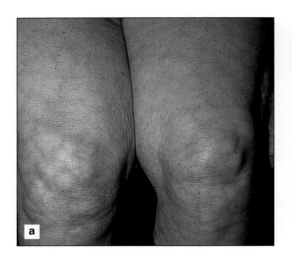

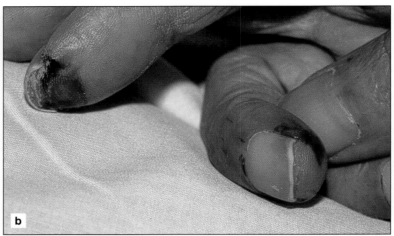

Figure 14.36 Antiphospholipid syndrome. The clinical presentations of this disorder are protean and include those shown here. (**a**) Broad bands of livedo around the knees in a patient with anticardiolipin antibodies; physiologic livedo has a finer patterning and less obvious lesions. (**b**) Digital infarcts, a non-specific feature of several vascular occlusion disorders.

Differential diagnosis

This includes other causes of livedo, vascular occlusion, and vasculitis.

Treatment

Treatment of APS remains a contentious issue, as even high-titer antibodies do not necessarily lead to clinical disease; in such cases, the dangers of aggressive anticoagulation may outweigh the potential benefits. In patients anticoagulated with heparin, the doses required to achieve benefit may be higher than usual. Even on treatment, catastrophic APS (which may be provoked by infection) can still occur, and stopping anticoagulants may lead to thrombotic episodes. Aspirin is commonly used, warfarin or long-term subcutaneous heparin is appropriate for treatment of thrombosis but more debatable for long-term prophylaxis, and oral steroids are probably beneficial in pregnancy but less appropriate in the long term. Plasmapheresis and immunosuppressive agents may be useful in some cases, and hydroxychloroquine has been shown to reduce the risk of thromboses in patients with SLE and anticardiolipin antibodies.

Vascular coagulopathies

Sneddon syndrome, Degos disease, and idiopathic livedoid vasculopathy, all disorders that may cause livedo reticularis, are difficult to classify on an etiologic basis. Antiphospholipid antibodies are demonstrable in some cases, but not all. They are best considered to involve abnormal thrombotic mechanisms at the microvascular level.

Sneddon syndrome

This eponymous name was applied to patients with generalized reticular livedo associated with cerebrovascular accidents. It appears to have a variety of pathogenetic mechanisms. About 20% of patients will be found to have aPL (discussed earlier). A further 30% have antiendothelial cell antibodies, alone or with aPL.

Patients are typically young women. Widespread livedo (Fig. 14.37) is the characteristic cutaneous feature, which may be accompanied by

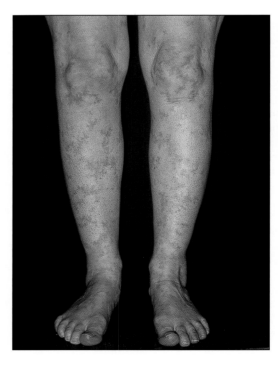

Figure 14.37 Sneddon syndrome. Livedo on the legs in a patient with previous mononeuritis multiplex. The lesions respond poorly to treatment, because there is no significant inflammatory component that can be potentially modified.

digital ischemia or infarction. Neurologic features include cerebrovascular accidents, but also peripheral nerve problems such as mononeuritis multiplex. Hypertension may also occur.

This condition is relatively refractory to therapy, and tends not to respond to steroids or immunosuppressive agents, as there is no inflammatory vasculitis. Anticoagulants, antifibrinolytic agents, and antiplatelet agents are all used (see section on idiopathic livedoid vasculopathy, later in this chapter), as well as vasodilators (see Raynaud phenomenon, Ch. 13).

Figure 14.38 Degos disease (malignant atrophic papulosis) showing a typical porcelain-white atrophic area due to an endarteritis. This is not a neoplastic disorder, but gastrointestinal involvement may be lethal, hence the use of the term malignant.

Malignant atrophic papulosis (Degos disease)

This is a rare disorder in which non-inflammatory thrombosis of dermal vessels causes characteristic small papules that progress to form ivory-white atrophic scars (Fig. 14.38). Classically, the lesions are associated with internal involvement of gastrointestinal tract or nervous system, causing gastrointestinal infarction and bleeding, or cerebrovascular accidents. However, it is likely that 'less exciting' cases limited to the skin are relatively underreported.

Treatment with fibrinolytic agents may be helpful, but generally the response is poor. Morphologically similar lesions may occur in other disorders, such as dermatomyositis.

Idiopathic livedoid vasculopathy

The etiology of this disorder is unknown, but it is probably due to intravascular thrombotic occlusion (of several etiologies) with secondary vasculitic features, rather than to a primary vessel wall inflammation. Some patients clearly have venous stasis disease, in which case the livedo change with white scarring is often termed atrophie blanche (although this term is purely a description, and applies equally to any cause of livedoid vasculopathy; Fig 14.39a).

The typical features are livedo racemosa, ulceration, and necrosis (Fig. 14.39b). Pain is a prominent feature, and may be seasonal (livedo reticularis with summer or winter ulcerations). White, stellate scars occur at sites of previous ulceration.

Treatment is difficult. Antiinflammatory and immunosuppressive agents are relatively unhelpful. Various combinations of fibrinolytic, anticoagulant, and antiplatelet agents are used, including aspirin, dipyridamole, oxpentifylline, and heparin. Danazol appears to be a particularly useful fibrinolytic agent in this disorder, but does have androgenic side effects, such as amenorrhea in women.

Disseminated intravascular coagulation (DIC)

This disorder typically occurs in a patient who is profoundly ill. The normal inhibition of clotting mechanisms leads to intravascular coagulation associated with consumption of platelets and clotting factors. Associated or underlying diseases include gram-negative sepsis and shock. Patients with defects in protein C or S are predisposed.

Widespread areas of necrosis are seen. The distal extremities are usually affected first, but the condition, if unchecked, will spread centrally (Figs 14.40 and 14.41).

Treatment usually needs to occur in an intensive care unit setting. Pressors, fluid support, administration of fresh frozen plasma, fibrinogen, and platelets, as well as treatment of any underlying condition, are needed. Activated protein C (APC), a natural anticoagulant, is showing benefit in treating patients with DIC, but mortality remains high.

PRACTICE POINTS

- Livedo in combination with acral duskiness or ulceration strongly suggests the possibility of a disorder of microvascular occlusion.
- Livedo with thrombosis and a history of fetal loss strongly suggests the possibility of antiphospholipid syndrome.
- To exclude a disorder of cold-precipitating proteins, blood samples must be kept at body temperature until they are processed in the laboratory.
- Acral duskiness and/or ulceration following cardiovascular interventions, including thrombolysis or commencing anticoagulation, should raise the possibility of cholesterol embolization, a syndrome with very diverse systemic manifestations in which acute renal failure, stroke, and loss of vision may all result.

MEDIUM- AND LARGE-VESSEL VASCULITIS

General aspects, diagnosis, and investigations

The typical medium- and large-vessel vasculitides of dermatologic importance are polyarteritis nodosa, Wegener granulomatosis, and Churg–Strauss disease. In each of these, there may also be small-vessel disease. Lymphomatoid granulomatosis is a rare disorder in which there is

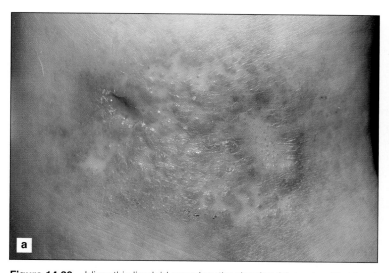

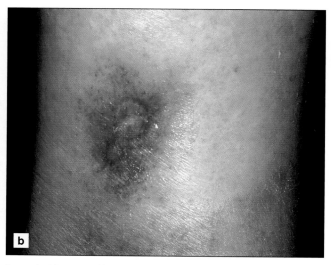

Figure 14.39 Idiopathic livedoid vasculopathy showing (**a**) an atrophie blanche pattern of white scar with punctuate vessels, and (**b**) a more livedoid pattern with ulceration.

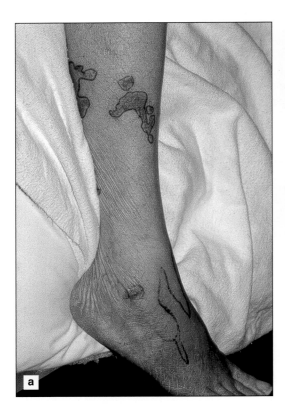

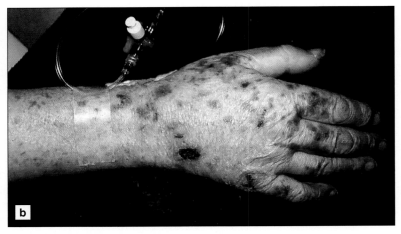

Figure 14.40 (**a**,**b**) Disseminated intravascular coagulation causing a livedo patterning of necrotic areas. (Panel b courtesy of Dr. G. Dawn.)

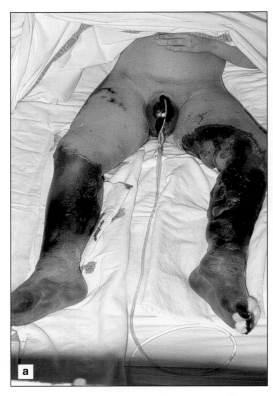

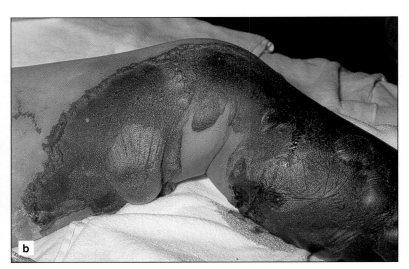

Figure 14.41 (**a**,**b**) Disseminated intravascular coagulation: a more severe case with confluence of lesions, widespread vascular occlusion, and necrotic areas of skin. Death is common in severe cases; amputation or permanent deformity of limbs may occur in survivors if the pattern is mainly acral, as shown here. (Courtesy of O. Dale Collins III.)

necrotizing vasculitis of large vessels, but this has a poor prognosis, as it may progress to frank lymphoma; it is discussed in Chapter 33. Other large-vessel vasculitis rarely presents to dermatologists, but occasionally forehead or scalp ulceration due to temporal arteritis may be seen initially in dermatology departments.

Nodular lesions occur in medium- and large-vessel vasculitis of numerous types (Fig. 14.42) due to the presence of necrotizing lesions; for example, they are a feature of cutaneous polyarteritis nodosa and of the granulomatous lesions of Wegener granulomatosis. In such cases, they usually occur with other vasculitis features, such as livedo or small-vessel palpable purpura. They also occur in panniculitis (Ch. 22) and erythema induratum (Ch. 11). However, the term nodular vasculitis is generally unhelpful, as it is descriptive rather than identifying a cause.

Antineutrophil cytoplasm antibodies

Antineutrophil cytoplasm antibodies are primarily of relevance in large-vessel vasculitis, although they also occur in other disorders. The main patterns are as follows.

- c-ANCA (cytoplasmic): this is mainly due to antibodies against proteinase-3, a serine protease present in neutrophil cytoplasmic granules. It has high specificity for Wegener granulomatosis, including those who present initially with necrotizing crescentic glomerulonephritis, and is related to disease activity. The majority of patients with a vasculitic component in Wegener granulomatosis will give a positive c-ANCA result, but this drops to a third of patients in clinical remission. It is often also positive in microscopic polyarteritis and in Churg–Strauss syndrome, as well as in some forms of glomerulonephritis (Fig. 14.43).

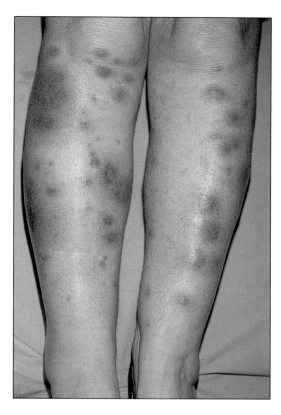

Figure 14.42 Nodular vasculitis. These lesions had a distribution suggestive of erythema nodosum, and close-up morphology suggestive of Sweet disease. Nodular vasculitis is best approached as a descriptive term rather than a diagnosis.

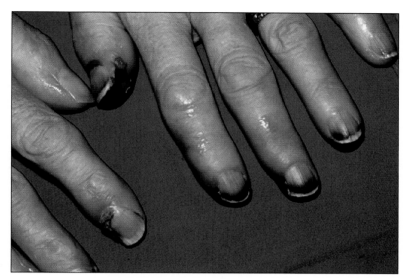

Figure 14.43 Fingertip necrosis in a patient with glomerulonephritis and positive proteinase-3 c-ANCA serology.

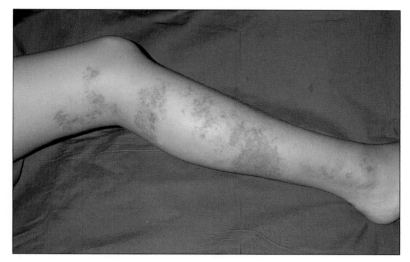

Figure 14.44 Polyarteritis nodosa, showing a pattern of patchy 'broken' livedo on the lower leg.

- p–ANCA (perinuclear) is less specific; in most cases, it is due to antibodies against myeloperoxidase (MPO), but it may also be due to antibodies against enzymes such as elastase, cathepsin, and lysozyme. These granules are actually cytoplasmic, but ethanol fixation of neutrophils allows permeation into the nucleus, hence the perinuclear pattern. Positive results may occur in a variety of autoimmune conditions, but anti-MPO is associated with microscopic polyarteritis, Churg–Strauss syndrome, drug-induced systemic vasculitis (such as that due to thiouracils), and small-vessel vasculitides of lung and kidney.

- Atypical ANCA (x-ANCA, atypical p-ANCA) also produces perinuclear positivity, which looks similar to p-ANCA on ethanol-fixed neutrophils but differs by having no associated granular cytoplasmic positivity on formalin-fixed neutrophils. It is associated with inflammatory bowel disease (IBD) and liver disease.

Polyarteritis nodosa

Polyarteritis nodosa (PAN) is a spectrum of disease affecting small- to medium-sized vessels, causing a leukocytoclastic vasculitis with segmental infarction of the vessel walls (Figs 14.44 and 14.45). Neutrophilia, positive rheumatoid factor, elevated ESR, hypergammaglobulinemia, and positive hepatitis B serology are all common features. Three patterns are now felt to occur, but clinical overlap between the patterns can cause diagnostic problems.

Microscopic PAN

This disorder typically presents as glomerulonephritis; one-third of patients have pulmonary involvement, which may present with alveolar hemorrhage. The skin is involved in one-third of patients, usually with palpable purpura or ulceration of the legs. Peripheral neuropathy, pericarditis, and ocular involvement may occur. ANCA is positive in 90% of patients, approximately equally divided between p-ANCA and c-ANCA.

Cutaneous PAN

This affects predominantly small arterioles, and causes tender nodules, livedo, and ulceration. Fever, myalgia or arthralgia, and neuropathy all occur fairly frequently, but severe systemic disease is not a feature. Digital gangrene can occur.

Classic PAN

This disease occurs predominantly in men. Some cases appear to be triggered by infections such as hepatitis B or streptococcal disease; it may occur due to drugs such as amphetamines, and some cases are associated with hairy cell leukemia. It affects small- and medium-sized arteries, and small-vessel vasculitis is not a feature. Skin involvement is therefore uncommon in classic PAN, and is usually either palpable aneurysms or acral ulceration and necrosis. Oral lesions include papules, nodules, and ulcers. More typical features are fever, myalgia, arthralgia, hypertension, and neuritis, which may be of mononeuritis multiplex type. Renal or hepatic arterial aneurysms are demonstrated in two-thirds of patients, and mesenteric arterial aneurysms in one-third. However, visceral microaneurysms can occur in other vasculitides (such as Behçet syndrome) and in bacterial endocarditis, hereditary hemorrhagic telangiectasia, and emboli from atrial myxoma. ANCA is positive in only about 30% of patients with classic PAN, p-ANCA more commonly than c-ANCA.

Differential diagnosis

This is wide when all presenting features are considered. In the skin, the differential is from other causes of livedo, vascular occlusion, and vasculitis, as already discussed.

Treatment of PAN

Classic systemic PAN has a poor prognosis due to renal disease, hypertension, and bowel infarction. Renal and lung involvement may be severe in microscopic PAN. In both of these, treatment is with systemic steroids,

283

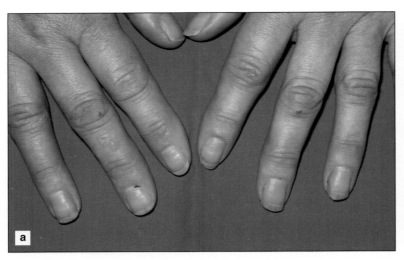
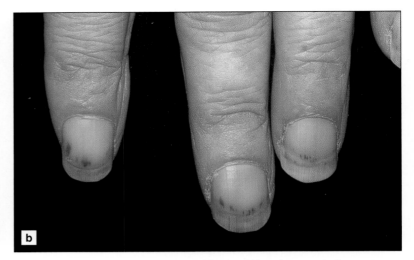

Figure 14.45 Polyarteritis nodosa, lesions on the hands: (**a**) scattered necrotic papules, and (**b**) splinter hemorrhages in several fingers. Although trauma is the most common cause of splinter hemorrhages, lesions affecting several digits in individuals who are not performing manual tasks are very suggestive of a systemic cause.

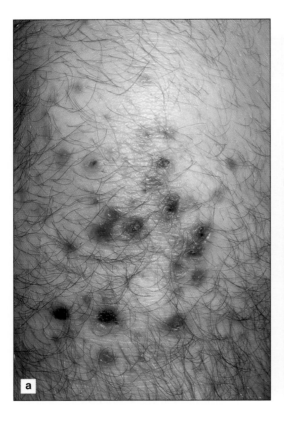
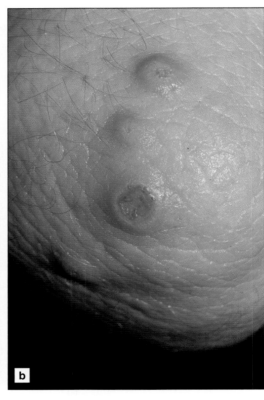

Figure 14.46 Vasculitis due to Wegener granulomatosis. (**a**) Necrotic lesions due to small-vessel vasculitis of skin; (**b**) more nodular lesions, suggesting a medium or large vessel vasculitis process.

cyclophosphamide, or azathioprine, along with treatment of effects such as hypertension, and treatment of underlying diseases (such as interferon for hepatitis). Cutaneous PAN is often chronic, and symptoms occur due to tender nodules, myalgia or arthralgia, and neuropathy. Steroids and NSAIDs are useful in some patients.

Wegener granulomatosis
Etiology and pathogenesis
Wegener granulomatosis is a triad of respiratory tract granulomas, renal granulomas, and vasculitis of small to medium arteries and veins, which may affect various organs. The etiology is unknown, although infectious foci may be important in the lung. It follows a variable course, the prognosis being determined mainly by renal involvement, although some patients have no demonstrable renal disease.

Clinical features
The initial presentation is often with nasal symptoms of discomfort and bleeding, which may cause cartilage destruction and collapse of the nasal bridge. In the skin, the initial lesions may be a small-vessel leukocytoclastic

vasculitis, which is purpuric but without any granulomatous component, or may resemble PAN; the features therefore range from a small-vessel vasculitis to nodules and ulcers (Figs 14.46 and 14.47). Other features include pyrexia, malaise, otitis media, neuropathies, and vasculitis of other organs. ANCA, usually c-ANCA, is positive in over 90% with active systemic Wegener granulomatosis, and the positivity usually decreases with clinical improvement. Biopsies of skin, kidney, and other organs may be required to confirm the type of vasculitis, although renal biopsy usually demonstrates glomerulonephritis rather than granulomatous vasculitis, and investigations of organ damage are as for other vasculitides. Neutrophilia, anemia, positive ANA and rheumatoid factor, and elevated C-reactive protein and ESR are all common.

Differential diagnosis
Wegener granulomatosis often presents with nasal rather than cutaneous symptoms. However, it may cause a small-vessel vasculitis of skin (and is therefore part of the differential of CSVV), or may cause non-specific cutaneous ulceration that may suggest a primary skin infection, or pyoderma gangrenosum (see later).

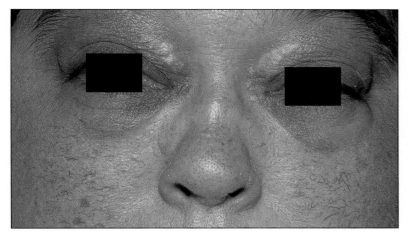

Figure 14.47 Wegener granulomatosis. There is a marked depression of the nasal bridge due to preceding inflammation.

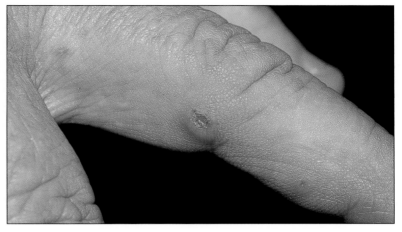

Figure 14.48 Churg–Strauss syndrome, with ulceration on the side of a finger.

Treatment

The disorder is usually treated with systemic corticosteroids and immunosuppressive agents, typically cyclophosphamide. Nasal spray steroids may be useful, and intralesional steroids for skin nodules. Long-term co-trimoxazole reduces morbidity and mortality, even in the absence of overt chest infections.

Churg–Strauss syndrome
Etiology and pathogenesis

This disorder, also termed allergic granulomatosis, is a multisystem vasculitis of small- to medium-sized vessels, with asthma and eosinophilia of uncertain etiology.

Clinical

Skin lesions occur in about 50% of patients (Figs 14.48 and 14.49), and may be the presenting feature in about 10% of these (usually a purpuric vasculitis). The skin lesions that occur include a leukocytoclastic vasculitis (which may be ulcerated, necrotic, bullous, or resemble erythema multiforme), necrotizing granulomas, livedo reticularis, and nodules due to panniculitis. Systemic features include asthma, allergic rhinitis, peripheral neuropathy (may be mononeuritis multiplex), arthralgia or myalgia, cardiac failure, hypertension, pericarditis, and abdominal pain. There is marked eosinophilia, often elevated IgE, and often positive ANCA (usually p-ANCA).

Differential diagnosis

The skin lesions may mimic any cause of vasculitis or livedo, although they are often relatively subtle or non-specific. Lesions around the elbows are rather suggestive of Churg–Strauss syndrome. The most important differential diagnosis is that of the asthma component, or of associated systemic vasculitis (such as mononeuritis multiplex). An important issue in differential diagnosis is the apparent provocation of Churg–Strauss syndrome with use of leukotriene antagonists. Whether this is correct is uncertain; it is more likely that such cases were actually those that presented with milder asthma symptoms and were not initially recognized.

Treatment

There is typically a good response to oral steroids, but other immunosuppressive agents may be required (azathioprine, chlorambucil, and cyclophosphamide).

NEUTROPHILIC DERMATOSES

This comprises a group of disorders, with some overlapping clinical and histologic features, which are characterized by a predominantly perivascular neutrophilic infiltrate that may exhibit leukocytoclasis (fragmented nuclear remnants in the tissues) and some endothelial swelling, but most do not have a true vasculitis.

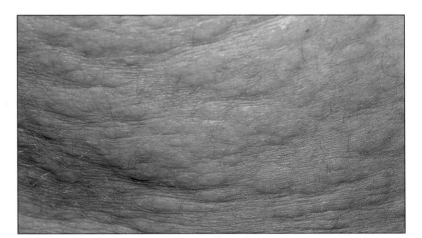

Figure 14.49 Churg–Strauss syndrome. This patient, with asthma and peripheral eosinophilia, developed infiltrated papules and plaques on the trunk.

These disorders are important for several reasons. They often have rather dramatic clinical features, are often accompanied by systemic malaise and neutrophilia, and many of them may be associated with significant internal disease. In some instances, such as rheumatoid neutrophilic dermatosis (which is not discussed further here), the internal association is with a specific disease entity. More commonly, the reaction does not identify a specific cause but raises the suspicion of one of several internal disorders. In particular, many of this group of neutrophilic dermatoses are associated with leukemia and other hematologic malignancies; in this context, they can even occur during periods of therapeutic granulocytopenia.

Acute febrile neutrophilic dermatosis (Sweet syndrome)
Etiology and pathogenesis

This disorder was described in 1964. It is characterized histologically by a predominantly neutrophilic infiltrate, classically without vasculitis, although this has been demonstrated in some cases. Associated disorders include the following.

- Malignancies of various types: especially myeloid disorders (leukemias, myeloproliferative disorders, and polycythemia rubra vera), other hematologic disorders (myeloma and gammopathies), less commonly solid tumors (especially breast cancers).
- Endocrine disorders: such as thyrotoxicosis and in pregnancy.
- Autoimmune disorders: lupus erythematosus, Sjögren syndrome, inflammatory bowel disease, and chronic active hepatitis.
- Infections: especially upper respiratory tract infections (the most common association in early case series).

• Drugs: for example lithium, all-*trans* retinoic acid, and granulocyte colony-stimulating factor.

Clinical features

The eruption is of acute onset, often with associated fever and neutrophilia (as suggested by the name), although these are not invariably present; the neutrophilia may be limited to the tissue infiltrate. Women are most commonly affected. The lesions are well-demarcated, elevated, inflammatory plaques, usually multiple, which may be studded with pustules or yellowish papules termed pseudopustules (Figs 14.50–14.56). The neck, trunk, and upper limbs are the most frequent sites. There may be associated conjunctivitis. Non-specific features such as malaise, elevated ESR, and elevated C-reactive protein are common but constitute only minor diagnostic criteria. Biopsy confirmation is often appropriate, and underlying disorders should be sought with appropriate investigations. This is particularly important in the small minority who get chronic lesions or recurrences. In any patient with neutrophilia, it is useful to check a convalescent blood count to ensure that this has resolved and does not represent a leukemic process. Occasionally in leukemia-associated Sweet disease, there may be atypical granulocytes in the skin biopsy.

In some instances, lesions may essentially be confined to the backs of the hands. Such lesions may ulcerate, may resemble a vasculitis or pyoderma gangrenosum, and may leave scarring when they resolve. This disorder has a neutrophilic infiltrate and may show more necrotic vascular changes than are typical of Sweet syndrome; it has been termed *pustular*

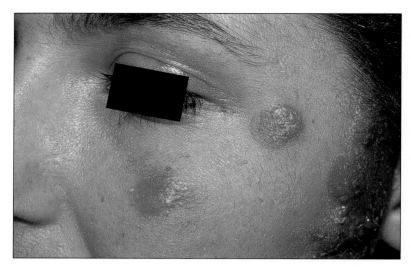

Figure 14.52 A minority of patients with Sweet syndrome have recurrent episodes or chronic lesions, as in this patient. Treatment with dapsone was administered.

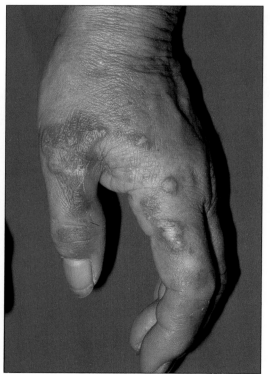

Figure 14.53 Frank pustular lesions may occur in Sweet syndrome, although some authors would view this acral pattern as a specific variant of pustular vasculitis. These lesions may leave a rather rippled pattern of scarring.

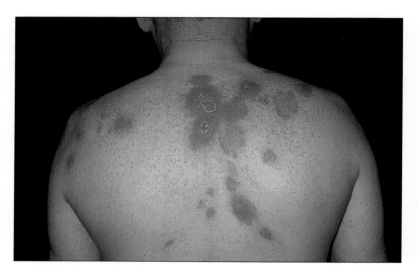

Figure 14.50 Sweet syndrome. Discrete, very inflammatory plaques on the upper back.

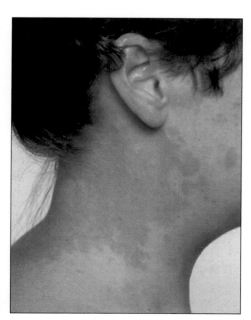

Figure 14.51 Sweet syndrome: a case with rather more confluent lesions, which may be confused with erythema multiforme. This patient had thyroid disease, which is associated with Sweet syndrome.

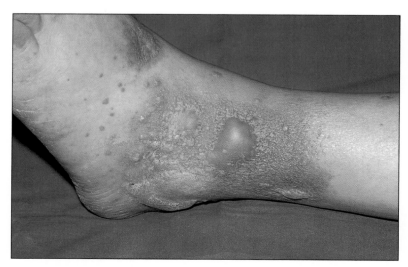

Figure 14.54 Sweet disease in a patient with myelodysplasia; sometimes in hematologic disease, there may be bullous lesions and an overlap with the appearances of pyoderma gangrenosum.

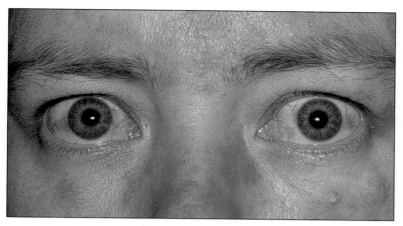

Figure 14.55 Ocular inflammatory changes may occur as part of the spectrum of Sweet syndrome, in this case in a patient with exophthalmos due to thyrotoxicosis.

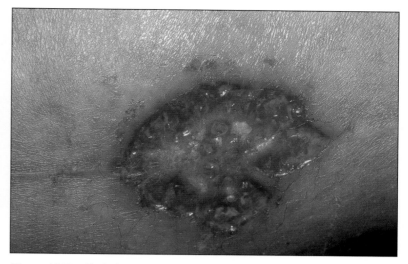

Figure 14.57 Typical ragged inflammatory ulceration of pyoderma gangrenosum.

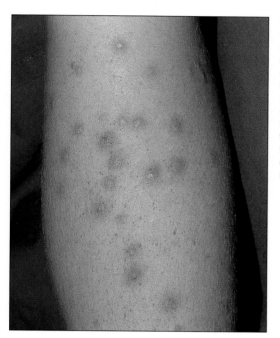

Figure 14.56 Pseudopustular lesions representing part of the spectrum of neutrophilic dermatoses, in a patient with exacerbation of inflammatory bowel disease. The lesions resembled pustules but were solid and sterile; the yellowish color was due to the intense neutrophilic infiltrate.

vasculitis of the dorsal hands but is probably a variant of Sweet disease and should be managed accordingly (usually with prednisolone or dapsone).

Differential diagnosis

This includes the following.

- Erythema multiforme: probably the most commonly suggested diagnosis.
- Lupus erythematosus (especially the tumid form) and Jessner lymphocytic infiltrate (Ch. 11): both differentials apply mainly to facial lesions.
- Erythema nodosum: especially if lesions are smooth-surfaced and mainly on distal limbs.
- Primary skin infections: such as staphylococcal infection.
- Other common inflammatory dermatoses: for example tinea and acute-onset psoriasis.

Treatment

Underlying conditions should be treated as required. The lesions may respond to strong topical corticosteroids, although a short course of oral corticosteroids is often helpful to treat the associated fever and malaise (usually at moderate 10–20 mg doses). Dapsone may be required in more persistent cases. Doxycycline, ciclosporin, colchicine, and potassium iodide have all been used.

Pyoderma gangrenosum
Etiology and pathogenesis

Pyoderma gangrenosum (PG) is important as, although it can occur in isolation, it is strongly associated with underlying medical disorders. The three main groups are:

- IBD;
- hematologic disorders, especially myeloproliferative malignancies; and
- inflammatory joint disease.

Pyoderma gangrenosum occurs in 1–2% of patients with ulcerative colitis (UC), and is five times as common in UC compared with in Crohn disease; IBD accounts for about 50% of cases of PG. The other important causes are hematologic malignancies (leukemias and myeloproliferative disorders, myelofibrosis, and paraproteinemias), but a few cases occur in patients with inflammatory joint disease such as rheumatoid arthritis. Other rare gastrointestinal associations include chronic active hepatitis and carcinoid tumor. Although it may parallel the course and severity of the gastrointestinal disease, PG may occur in patients without contemporary gastrointestinal symptoms. The fact that it has been reported up to 10 years after panproctocolectomy is clear evidence that a diseased bowel does not need to be present for PG to occur, and suggests that this disorder is related to the colitis phenotype itself.

Clinical features

The characteristic lesion of PG is a rapidly evolving, tender, inflammatory skin ulcer (Figs 14.57–14.63). This may initially appear as a pustule or small nodule, but rapidly breaks down to form a necrotic ulcer that typically has a bluish, undermined ulcer edge and surrounding inflammation. Lesions may occur at any site, but the commonest is the lower leg. Lesions at less common sites may cause diagnostic uncertainty; PG of the face or scalp is particularly difficult to diagnose with confidence.

Pyoderma gangrenosum should always be considered in cases of peristomal ulceration, even if the stoma was not as a consequence of IBD, although this is much the most frequent association.

Ulcers of PG are usually solitary but may be multiple. They often occur at sites of minor injury (a process known as pathergy). Less commonly, verrucous, pustular, or punched-out necrotic areas may be the dominant lesion.

Differential diagnosis

The main differentials are as follows:

- Vascular causes of ulceration.
- Infective causes of ulceration: especially deep fungal infections.
- Vasculitis.
- Tumors: especially if pyoderma occurs on the face or scalp.
- Artifact: especially facial or breast lesions.

Treatment

Gentle debridement of the ulcer may be helpful, but attempts at excisional surgery should be avoided in any form or site of PG, as it typically exhibits a pathergic response and recurs.

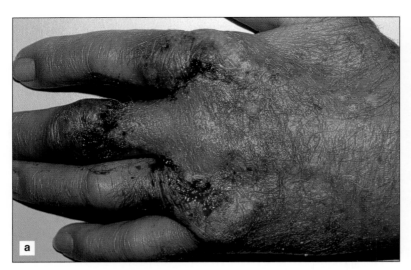

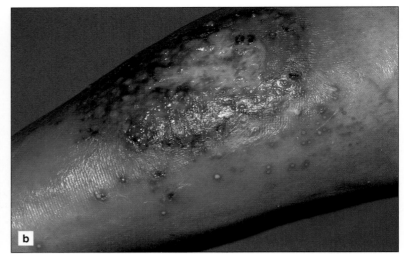

Figure 14.58 Pustular macerated lesions are typical of rapidly progressing lesions of pyoderma gangrenosum, shown here (**a**) on the hand and (**b**) on the leg.

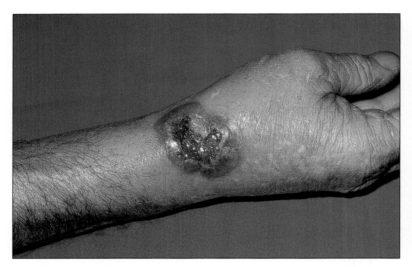

Figure 14.59 A bolstered blue border around a painful and progressive ulcer is very suggestive of pyoderma gangrenosum.

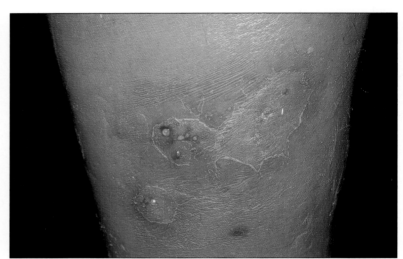

Figure 14.61 A chronically inflamed area of pyoderma gangrenosum with discharging areas. Clinically, this could be an area of panniculitis, as the discharge has the oily appearance that occurs with liquefied fat.

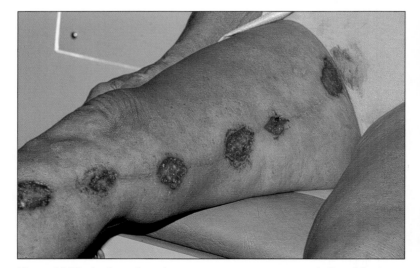

Figure 14.60 Lesions of pyoderma gangrenosum may occur at sites of tissue injury (pathergic response), in this case at sites of stripping of varicose veins.

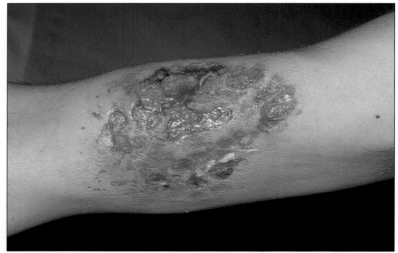

Figure 14.62 Cribriform scarring is typical of pyoderma gangrenosum. The scar has small perforations or pits, resembling a colander.

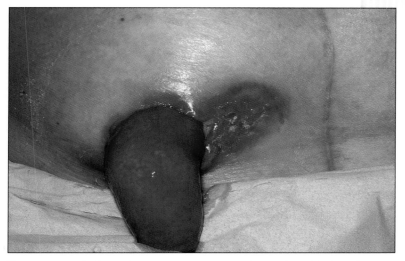

Figure 14.63 Peristomal pyoderma gangrenosum in a patient with ulcerative colitis; this is a difficult management problem, and may initially be misdiagnosed as a dehisced or infected wound.

Some lesions respond to strong topical or intralesional steroid injection, or to topical tacrolimus, but systemic therapy is often required. The choice of systemic therapy may depend on the treatment required for any underlying disorder, as this may lead to resolution of PG; for example, if the patient has severe active IBD that requires infliximab infusions, then this is likely to heal the PG. In some cases, combining systemic and topical therapy, or combining systemic agents with a different spectrum of side effects (Ch. 4), can be useful to limit doses. Systemic treatment options include the following.

- Corticosteroids: usually prednisolone at doses of 40 mg daily or greater.
- Immunosuppressive agents: the greatest experience is with ciclosporin, but azathioprine, dapsone, cyclophosphamide, or mycophenolate mofetil can all be effective.
- Other antiinflammatory regimens: such as minocycline or oxytetracycline.
- Plasmapheresis.
- Cytotoxic agents: such as chlorambucil.
- Infliximab infusions: these have been used more recently with success.

Peristomal PG causes particular management problems, as many topical agents are difficult to apply while still achieving adhesion of the stoma appliance. The topical and systemic options are as for PG at other sites, but topical agents may need to be formulated in more adhesive vehicles.

PRACTICE POINTS

- Neutrophilic dermatoses are often associated with internal disease; hematologic malignancy, in particular, may be occult.
- Always consider the possibility of unusual infections when making a diagnosis of pyoderma gangrenosum, especially in areas where deep fungal infections are at all frequent.
- Pyoderma gangrenosum may occur in patients with a history of ulcerative colitis, even if the colon has been removed.
- Always consider a diagnosis of pyoderma gangrenosum in patients with peristomal ulceration, and avoid surgical intervention other than a small biopsy if the diagnosis requires confirmation (e.g. to exclude a neoplasm).

Behçet disease
Etiology and pathogenesis

Behçet disease is an uncommon multisystem disorder of uncertain etiology, which is most common in Japan and eastern Mediterranean countries. It is strongly associated with human leukocyte antigen (HLA)-B51, especially in areas of high prevalence or with high frequency of ocular disease in affected individuals (such as Japan and Turkey). Early skin lesions have a perivascular neutrophilic tissue reaction or small-vessel vasculitis; later lesions may be lymphocytic. It may be best viewed as a disorder that lies between neutrophilic dermatoses and vasculitides.

Clinical features

The diagnosis of Behçet disease is clinical, as there are no specific laboratory tests. Diagnostic criteria are listed in Table 14.7. The development of lesions at the sites of needle prick injury (known as a positive pathergy test) is common in Turkish people but less so in the UK or USA. In some populations, the increased frequency of HLA-B51 is useful diagnostic support.

In most patients, the earliest feature is oral ulceration. Other features may take many years to become apparent. It is likely that milder cases also occur; for example, it is not uncommon to see individuals who have occasional aphthous ulcers, or a severe solitary episode of genital ulceration (even multiple episodes), but with no other features (see Ch. 20). Such patients do not meet the diagnostic criteria in Table 14.7, but perhaps these criteria suffer from the limitation that patients without oral lesions are excluded. Skin lesions include the ulcers discussed earlier, papulopustules and acneiform lesions, pseudofolliculitis, vasculitis (see Fig. 20.5), and erythema nodosum.

Ocular features, typically iritis, occur in about 50% of patients and are most frequent in males; retinitis is the potentially most severe ocular feature, which may lead to blindness.

Arthritis is usually episodic and mono- or oligoarticular, usually affecting the knees.

Differential diagnosis

The differential includes various causes of oral and/or genital ulceration, including severe idiopathic ('major') aphthous ulceration, herpangina, herpetic gingivostomatitis, Crohn disease, various sexually transmitted diseases, and artefactual ulceration.

Treatment

This varies according to disease severity. Topical agents that may be helpful for oral aphthae include various types of corticosteroid application (lozenges, pastes, and mouthwash) or sucralfate rinse. Topical steroids or local application of sucralfate can help genital lesions. Intralesional steroid injection can be very effective for localized oral or genital ulceration. In patients with vasculitis, immunosuppressive therapy is used and may include corticosteroids, azathioprine, ciclosporin, colchicine, dapsone, and others. Thalidomide is particularly useful for orogenital ulceration, but has the potentially irreversible side effect of peripheral neuropathy and is strictly contraindicated in pregnancy; it therefore requires monitoring by repeated nerve conduction studies and would not generally be considered a first-line treatment.

Other neutrophilic dermatoses
Bowel-associated dermatosis–arthritis syndrome

Although originally described as the bowel bypass syndrome, this entity is due to antigenic stimulus from bowel bacteria leading to immune

---

Table 14.7   INTERNATIONAL STUDY GROUP CRITERIA FOR BEHÇET DISEASE

Major symptoms	Recurrent oral aphthae (> 3 times a year)
And at least two minor criteria from:	Genital ulcers Ophthalmic involvement: uveitis, iritis, retinitis Skin lesions: erythema nodosum, folliculitis, sterile pustules, aphthous ulcerations Positive pathergy test

(From International Study Group for Behçet's disease. Criteria for diagnosis of Behçet's disease. Lancet 1990; 335: 1078–80.)

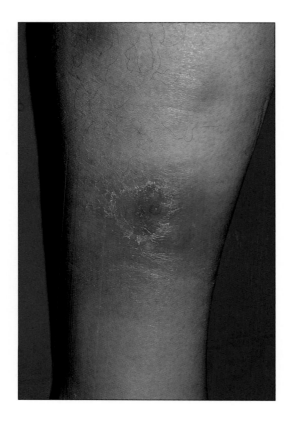

Figure 14.64 Bowel-associated dermatitis–arthritis syndrome. Some lesions resemble erythema nodosum; the most inflammatory lesion has ulceration reminiscent of pyoderma gangrenosum.

complex formation, and occurs in other situations where there is bacterial overgrowth.

The clinical features are a purpuric and pustular skin eruption, with crops of lesions associated with arthralgia, arthritis, myalgia, fever, and malaise. Lesions resembling erythema nodosum (Fig. 14.64), and ulceration (PG) may also be prominent. Raynaud phenomenon and nephritis may occur. Treatment is with appropriate antibiotics and resolution of the underlying bowel defect if possible; corticosteroids and immunosuppressive therapy may also be required (as for PG).

Subcorneal pustular dermatosis (Sneddon–Wilkinson disease)
This is a neutrophilic dermatosis but is not centered around vessels; it is clinically manifest as blistering and is thus discussed in Chapter 16.

FURTHER READING

Asherson RA, Cervera R. Antiphospholipid syndrome. J Invest Dermatol 1993; 100:21S–27S.

Barham KL, Jorizzo JL, Grattan B, et al. Vasculitis and neutrophilic vascular reactions. In: Burns DA, Breathnach SM, Cox NH, et al, eds. Rook's textbook of dermatology, 7th edn. Oxford: Blackwell Publishing; 2004: 49.1.

Callen JP. Cutaneous vasculitis: relationship to systemic disease and therapy. Curr Probl Dermatol 1993; 5:45–80.

Cox NH, Piette WW. Purpura and microvascular occlusion. In: Burns DA, Breathnach SM, Cox NH, et al, eds. Rook's textbook of dermatology, 7th edn. Oxford: Blackwell Publishing; 2004: 48.1.

Fiorentino DF. Cutaneous vasculitis. J Am Acad Dermatol 2003; 48:311–340.

Ghate JV, Jorizzo JL. Behçet's disease and complex aphthosis. J Am Acad Dermatol 1999; 40:1–18.

Gibson GE, Su WP, Pittelkow MR. Antiphospholipid syndrome and the skin. J Am Acad Dermatol 1997; 36:970–982.

Goeken JA. Antineutrophil cytoplasmic and anti-endothelial cell antibodies: new mechanisms for vasculitis. Curr Opin Dermatol 1995; 2:75–81.

Huang W, McNeely MC. Neutrophilic tissue reactions. Adv Dermatol 1997; 13:33–63.

Lotti T, Ghersetich I, Comacci C, et al. Cutaneous small-vessel vasculitis. J Am Acad Dermatol 1998; 39:667–687.

Nahass GT. Antiphospholipid antibodies and the antiphospholipid antibody syndrome. J Am Acad Dermatol 1997; 36:149–168.

Piette WW. Primary systemic vasculitis. In: Sontheimer RD, Provost TT, eds. Cutaneous manifestations of rheumatic diseases. Baltimore: Williams & Wilkins; 1996: 177–232.

Powell FC, Su WPD, Perry HO. Pyoderma gangrenosum: classification and management. J Am Acad Dermatol 1996; 34:395–409.

Von den Driesch P. Sweet's syndrome (acute febrile neutrophilic dermatosis). J Am Acad Dermatol 1994; 31:535–556.

15 Vascular Disorders

INTRODUCTION

The vascular system provides a constant supply of nutrients and oxygen to keep the skin healthy and functioning. It also provides heat and removes carbon dioxide and other unwanted metabolic products. Arterial occlusion causes rapid necrosis. Impaired arterial supply results in cool, dry, lifeless skin. Impaired venous return causes swelling and irritation of the tissue. Both these processes can result in ulceration of the skin. Vascular malformations may be present congenitally; acquired vascular growths are common. Flushing is covered in Chapter 12. Diascopy (Fig. 15.1) is a quick way of verifying that a lesion is primarily vascular; most vascular lesions are compressible.

Discussion of vascular disorders includes both primarily anatomic abnormalities (malformations), various tumors (benign, reactive, and malignant), predominantly functional problems (such as abnormal reactions to cold), and mixed or degenerative conditions such as arterial disease or venous disease. Malignant vascular tumors are discussed in Chapter 33.

CLASSIFICATION OF VASCULAR ANOMALIES AND TUMORS

This is a complex area, and a detailed discussion is beyond the scope of this book. Some relevant modern references are provided.

There is a fundamental division into:
- non-proliferative lesions (malformations), and
- proliferative lesions (angiomas and other tumors), which may be further subdivided into congenital and acquired, and also into benign, reactive, and malignant types.

Distinction between these has led to historical confusion. For example, the term cavernous hemangioma has been applied to both venous malformations and to true angiomas, but is important in predicting outcome and both the need for and the choice of therapy. This is most relevant in the neonate and childhood in differentiating between a venous malformation and a deeply situated angioma, and is discussed further later in this chapter. Various radiologic tests, immunohistochemistry, and genetic analyses may be necessary to correctly label or to determine the extent of internal organ involvement by such lesions.

Occasionally, malformations and proliferations may coexist even within the same lesion. Examples include nodules within a capillary malformation (port wine stain), most of which develop gradually over time, but pyogenic granulomas may appear suddenly; similarly, spindle cell hemangioendotheliomas may occur on a background of Maffucci syndrome (a rare venous malformation).

Table 15.1 gives a simplified classification.

VASCULAR MALFORMATIONS

Capillary malformations
These include the following.
- Port wine stain and associated syndromes.
  - Sturge–Weber syndrome
  - Klippel–Trenaunay syndrome
  - Proteus syndrome (Ch. 19)
- Cutis marmorata telangiectatica congenita

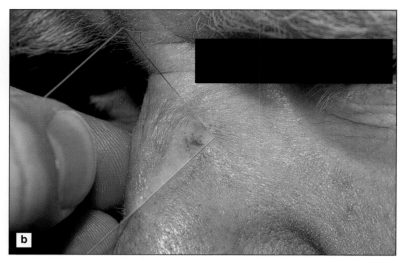

Figure 15.1 (**a,b**) Diascopy. One quick way of confirming that a lesion is vascular is through diascopy. A clear glass slide is applied to the lesion. With vascular lesions, the red color of contained blood may be completely removed (or nearly so). In addition, the lesion often compresses to a much smaller size.

Table 15.1 CLASSIFICATION OF VASCULAR ANOMALIES

Type of lesion	Subdivision	Example(s)	Comments
Malformations and ectasias (non-proliferative)	Capillary (red)	Port wine stain	Also various syndromes that include port wine stain; see text, this chapter
		Spider angioma	See text, this chapter
		Telangiectasias	See text, this chapter
		Others	Cutis marmorata telangiectatica congenita, phacomatoses (pigmented lesions with vascular anomalies)
	Venous (blue)	Blue rubber bleb nevus syndrome	Note internal organ involvement
		Glomuvenous malformation	Also termed multiple glomangiomas, multiple glomus tumors
		Venous lake	May be solitary (usually on the lip) or multiple (usually solar-damaged face and neck skin)
	Arterial and mixed malformations	Arterial	Includes arterial malformation and arteriovenous fistula
		Mixed	Various combinations of arterial, venous, capillary, and lymphatic malformations, subdivided into fast-flow and slow-flow types
	Lymphatic	Small cyst–type lymphangiomas	Lymphangioma circumscriptum
		Large cyst–type lymphangiomas	Cystic hygroma
Angiomas and tumors (proliferative)	Benign, congenital	Hemangioma, kaposiform hemangioendothelioma, tufted angioma (some)	See text, this chapter
	Benign, acquired	Cherry angioma, pyogenic granuloma, tufted angioma (some), targetoid hemosiderotic hemangioma, spindle cell hemangioendothelioma, angiolymphoid hyperplasia with eosinophilia, unilateral nevoid telangiectasia	See text, this chapter
	Reactive	Kaposi sarcoma	See also Chapters 12 and 33
	Malignant	Angiosarcoma, epithelioid hemangioendothelioma	Chapter 33

- Telangiectasias and spider angioma (discussed as a separate section of this chapter)

Lesions that constitute vascular ectasias rather than malformations, such as erythema nuchae, are described in Chapter 19.

Port wine stain

A flat, red or pink patch is characteristic of a port wine stain (PWS), a congenital vascular patch comprising superficially located dermal vessels. At birth, a PWS cannot always be distinguished from a hemangioma, which will proliferate into a vascular plaque in the ensuing weeks. It often follows a dermatomal distribution and, when located about the eyes, it may signify internal abnormalities (Figs 15.2 and 15.3).

Facial PWS involving the V1 dermatome (forehead, upper and lower eyelid, and side of the nose) may be associated with ocular abnormalities (e.g. glaucoma and choroidal angioma) with or without Sturge–Weber syndrome (Fig. 15.4, see also text below and Fig. 5.6); for PWS in this distribution, ophthalmologic examination initially and every 6 months is recommended.

Laser (usually tunable dye) therapy, even in infancy, is recommended for cosmesis. Treatment in infancy is recommended because of a smaller surface area and greater lightening of lesions. In one study, lesions greater than 20 cm² and lesions in patients older than 1 year of age were less likely to clear. Complete clearing is often not achieved, but the PWS is converted to mild erythema. PWSs of V2 respond slightly less well to the tunable dye laser than elsewhere on the face. If untreated, the PWS may become raised, irregularly surfaced, and deeply colored later in life. Vascular nodules are commonly seen in middle age in untreated lesions (Fig. 15.5).

Port wine stains that tend to respond less well are red-purple, dark or nodular, non-facial, and especially acral. Those on the lower leg or foot are the most difficult to clear. The larger the lesion (e.g. > 20 cm²), the less likely it is to clear.

Sturge–Weber syndrome

The Sturge–Weber syndrome (SWS) is a non-inherited disorder that combines a facial PWS involving the V1 dermatome (forehead, upper and lower eyelid, and side of the nose; Fig. 15.6), seizures (usually within the first year of life), and ipsilateral leptomeningeal angiomatosis. Other associations include mental retardation and glaucoma. If the PWS is in the V2 (upper lip and cheek) or V3 (lower lip, chin, jawline, ear, and preauricular) dermatome without involvement of V1, there is no need to consider SWS. (Note: there is some difference in the location of V1 and V2 regarding the lower eyelid, making for some disagreement in recent studies.) If V1 (eyelid or the side of the nose) is involved, one does need to rule out the SWS (V1 alone approximate risk 10%; V1, V2, and V3 together, approximate risk 30%). Full V1 involvement or bilaterality represents a higher risk. An ophthalmologic examination should be obtained to exclude glaucoma, which is more likely when there is involvement of both the upper and lower eyelids by PWS.

Treatment requires a multidisciplinary approach. Magnetic resonance imaging (MRI) may be used to diagnose SWS and delineate central

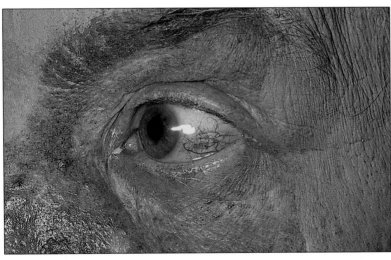

Figure 15.2 Ocular changes with port wine stain.

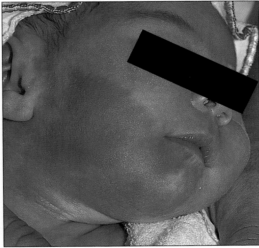

Figure 15.4 Facial port wine stains (PWSs) involving V1 may be associated with ocular abnormalities (e.g. glaucoma and choroidal angioma) with or without Sturge–Weber syndrome. The child shown here with a PWS of V3 is at risk for neither. Cosmesis is the main concern.

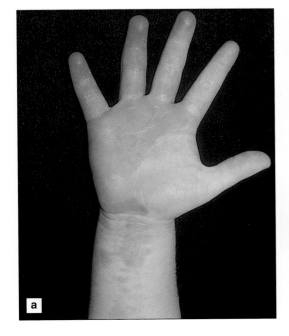

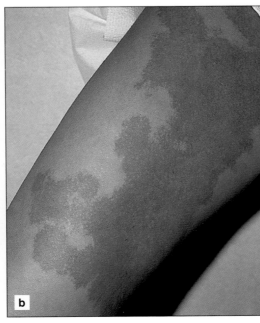

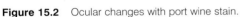

Figure 15.3 Port wine stain: (**a**) on the arm, palm, and several fingers, and (**b**) on the leg.

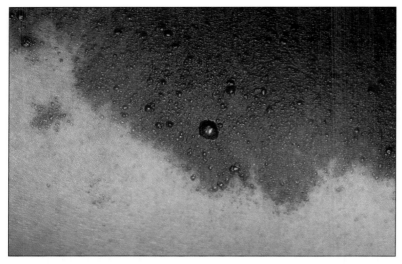

Figure 15.5 If untreated, PWS may become darker red, thickened, and irregular-surfaced, with nodularity.

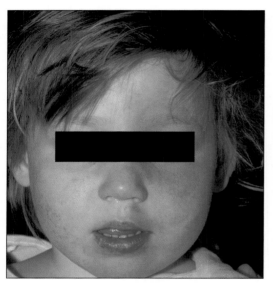

Figure 15.6 Sturge–Weber syndrome (SWS). If the port wine stain is in the V2 (upper lip and cheek) or V3 (lower lip, chin, jawline, ear, and preauricular) dermatome without involvement of V1, there is no need to rule out SWS. Involvement of V1, V2, and V3, as shown here, significantly increases the risk of SWS.

nervous system involvement. An ophthalmologic examination should be obtained initially and every 6 months. Laser treatment of the cutaneous component is discussed in the preceding section on PWS.

Klippel–Trenaunay syndrome

Klippel–Trenaunay syndrome combines a nevus flammeus and ipsilateral hypertrophy of the underlying soft tissue and bone. Onset is at birth or soon after, and more boys than girls are affected. Other reported associations including lymphatic obstruction, spina bifida, polydactyly, and syndactyly. Blood in the urine or stool may develop from bladder, colonic, or rectal lesions. Venous thromboembolism (e.g. pulmonary embolism) is not uncommon, and superficial thrombophlebitis may occur. Varicose veins present in the majority and symptomatically cause pain and swelling (Fig. 15.7). The lower limb is involved in the majority of cases.

In one study, the presence of a geographic (versus blotchy) stain was highly correlated with an underlying lymphatic abnormality. In addition, the complication rate was higher in patients with a geographic stain. The definitions were as follows. A geographic stain was extremely sharply demarcated, the shape was irregular (resembling a country or continent), and the color was dark red or purple in most cases. A blotchy or segmental stain had an indistinct border from normal skin in some areas, was often large with a segmental distribution, and was light pink or red-pink in color. Inheritance appears to be multifactorial, with a range of vascular malformations found in family members. If an arteriovenous fistula is associated, the term Klippel–Trenaunay–Weber syndrome is used.

Magnetic resonance imaging of the leg to detect arteriovenous malformation (AVM), and arteriogram if the MRI is positive or suggestive, has been advocated, although its necessity is debated. In one study of 22 patients, none had an AVM. The limb length abnormality should be evaluated by radiography. Leg discrepancy may be hidden by compensatory scoliosis. In one study, limb length discrepancy rarely increased after 12 years of age.

A multidisciplinary approach to therapy is needed, involving an orthopedic surgeon, a vascular surgeon, and a dermatologist, especially one able to perform laser surgery. Compressive stockings are probably the best approach for symptomatic relief of pain and swelling. Vein stripping often fails to relieve symptoms and may make matters worse. A lymphedema pump may be used for severe edema. If surgical intervention is necessary, it should be done only by a specialist. For leg length abnormalities, shoe elevators and epiphyseal surgery to slow growth of the longer limb can be

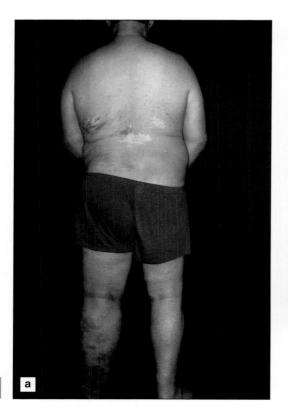

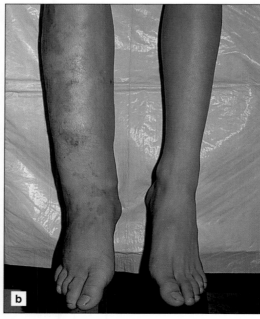

Figure 15.7 Klippel–Trenaunay syndrome. (**a**) This patient had unequal leg lengths, causing compensatory scoliosis. He suffered from recurrent cellulitis, presumably secondary to lower leg swelling and tinea pedis. Chronic low-dose penicillin prevented further bouts of cellulitis. (**b**) A congenital nevus flammeus (also known as port wine stain) along with ipsilateral hypertrophy of the bones and soft tissue occur together in this syndrome. An extremity is usually affected. Varicose veins develop later in the majority and can cause pain and swelling. (Panel b courtesy of Michael O. Murphy, M.D.)

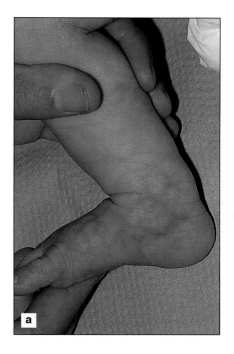

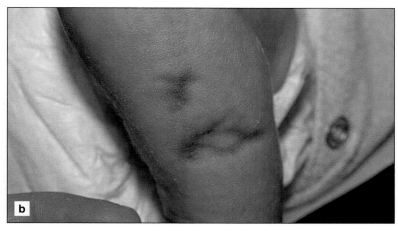

Figure 15.8 Cutis marmorata telangiectatica congenita. (**a**) A mild case with only reticulate erythema and slight atrophy. (**b**) More atrophy is apparent here. Note the reticulate pattern.

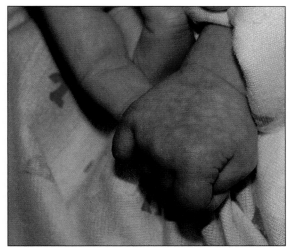

Figure 15.9 Cutis marmorata on the hand of a newborn. This change is entirely benign.

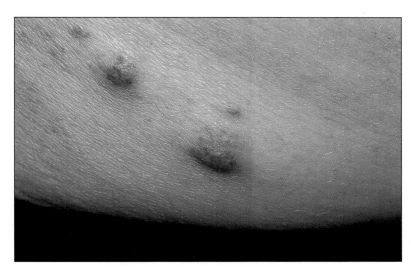

Figure 15.10 Blue rubber bleb nevus syndrome. Patients with this condition develop multiple bluish or purple papules and nodules on all areas of the body. Lesions may range in size from several millimeters to several centimeters in diameter.

done. Some have recommended that patients with Klippel–Trenaunay syndrome avoid taking estrogens (e.g. oral contraceptives) because of the increased risk of thromboembolism and antithrombotic prophylaxis after any surgery. Venous malformations have been treated successfully by sclerotherapy, but this approach requires a specialist trained in using this modality for larger vessels. Color echo-Doppler ultrasonography-guided sclerotherapy with polidocanol microfoam has been very effective in treating the venous malformations of patients.

Port wine stain of the leg usually does not respond well to pulsed dye laser, but occasionally it does, and one report suggested waiting 4–5 months between treatments.

Cutis marmorata telangiectatica congenita

Congenital persistent cutis marmorata, skin atrophy, ulceration, telangiectasia, and phlebectasia may all be seen in cutis marmorata telangiectatica congenita (CMTC) (Fig. 15.8). Many patients have no associated abnormalities, but body asymmetry, PWS, glaucoma, aplasia cutis congenita, and cleft palate may all occur. When macrocephaly is associated, the term macrocephaly cutis marmorata telangiectatica congenita is used. When the changes overlie an eye, glaucoma may be found. The cutaneous lesions may persist, improve, or resolve over time.

The differential diagnosis includes the entirely benign entity cutis marmorata (Fig. 15.9). This condition is a reticular red pattern of the extremities that represents physiologic variations in blood content of the skin; it is accentuated by cold temperature. Rarely, neonatal lupus may mimic CMTC.

VENOUS MALFORMATIONS

Venous malformations, cutaneomucosal venous malformations, and blue rubber bleb nevus syndrome
Etiology and pathogenesis

Venous malformations are generally apparent at birth, a minority being familial. They are usefully divided into two main groups.

- Venous malformations—these may have deep local extension but do not have an association with separate internal lesions.
- Cutaneomucosal venous malformations (CMVM)—in which similar lesions affect mucosae such as the gastrointestinal tract, and other organs such as the liver, pancreas, and spleen. On the basis of familial cases, mutation in the gene *VMCM1* on chromosome 9p.21, coding for the protein TIE2/TEK, has been identified as the cause in most familial cases but not in all.

It has recently been suggested that the blue rubber bleb nevus syndrome (Bean syndrome) may be a variant of CMVM.

There is also some overlap with Maffucci syndrome.

Clinical

Multiple, protuberant, blue, compressible, cutaneous nodules are characteristic (Fig. 15.10). Most patients are white and the onset is usually at birth or in childhood. The lesions may be noted on ultrasound in the prenatal period.

Extracutaneous venous malformations may occur virtually anywhere but characteristically affect the gastrointestinal tract and skeletal system. The gastrointestinal tract involvement may cause chronic asymptomatic blood loss or life-threatening hemorrhage. Subcutaneous masses may be noted. MRI or other imaging studies may be needed. Limb lesions may cause hypertrophy, and osseous lesions may cause joint pain or bony erosion.

Differential diagnosis
The main differentials are as follows.
- Other types of vascular malformation, especially glomuvenous malformation (discussed later). Mixed types of malformation cause particular difficulty, as they may have red (superficial and capillary) as well as blue (deeper and venous) colors.
- Deeply situated (therefore blue-colored) infantile hemangiomas (IHs)—features that may help in distinguishing venous malformations from IHs include the following.
  - Sex incidence—equal in venous malformations, female excess in IHs.
  - Color—either may be blue, but a red patch at birth suggests IH.
  - Course—significant proliferation then involution occurs in IHs; venous malformations are usually obvious at birth and are more stable over time.
  - Pathology—IHs have small dense vessels that stain positive with proliferation markers and Glut-1.
  - Radiology—several differences may be apparent.
  - Genotyping—an advancing field; see etiology section earlier in this section.
- Other vascular lesions—for example Kaposi sarcoma.

Treatment
No treatment is needed. If treated early in the macular stage, the pulsed dye laser can remove each lesion. Otherwise, surgery is the only remedy.

Glomuvenous malformation (multiple glomangiomas, multiple glomus tumors)
Glomuvenous malformations (GVMs; Fig. 15.11) are inherited in about two-thirds of cases, and are due to mutations in the *VMGLOM* gene on chromosome 1p21–22, a gene that appears to alter differentiation of vascular smooth muscle cells via its protein product, glomulin. The lesions may develop in childhood, adolescence, or adulthood. Many are similar to venous malformations but have sometimes abundant, glomus cells histologically. The term multiple glomus tumors is technically incorrect and would be best dropped.

A recent study used clinical criteria, histology, and mutations in the *TIE2* or glomulin gene to separate these entities, with the following results.
- Glomuvenous malformations are often inherited (64%), whereas this applies to only just over 1% of venous malformations.
- Glomuvenous malformations are mainly acral and in the skin and subcutis, whereas venous malformations are around joints or involve deeper tissues such as muscle.
- Glomuvenous malformations are often multilobular, cobblestoned or plaque-like, and are not easily compressed, whereas venous malformations are softer, blue, and compressible.
- Compression may aggravate the associated pain of GVMs if this is present, while venous malformations are more likely to be painful on waking or after physical activity.

No treatment is needed. Excision may be done for painful lesions if not extensive. Infrared coagulation has been used.

Venous lake
Dark-blue, soft, compressible, benign, vascular papules in the sun-exposed skin of an elderly person are characteristic of venous lakes (Fig. 15.12). The ears, lips, and face are favored sites. They are often solitary and up to about 5 mm in diameter when they occur on the lip, but are often smaller and multiple at other facial sites. Treatment with cryotherapy or electrocautery (with risk of a scar) may be tried. Pulsed, tunable dye and argon lasers have been used, as has infrared coagulation. Sclerotherapy with polidocanol was effective in the treatment of lip venous lakes.

Arterial and mixed malformations
Arteriovenous malformations account for about 5% of vascular anomalies. Arteriovenous fistulae are usually traumatic or created surgically (e.g. for hemodialysis access).

PRACTICE POINTS
- Most vascular malformations can be compressed: this is particularly helpful in diagnosis of darker lesions, such as venous lakes, which may otherwise be diagnosed as melanocytic.
- In distinguishing between glomuvenous malformations (without internal involvement) versus blue rubber bleb nevus syndrome (with likely gastrointestinal involvement and risk of internal bleeding), firm or tender lesions suggest the former, while oral mucosal lesions indicate the latter.

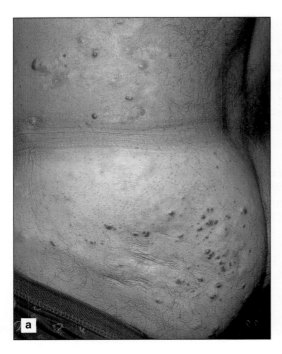
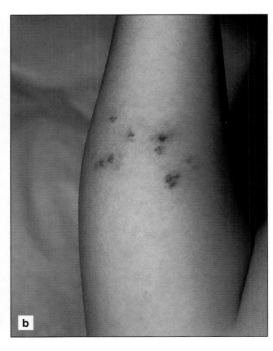

Figure 15.11 Glomuvenous malformation (GVMs). (**a**) GVMs on the buttocks and trunk. (**b**) GVM on the arm of a child.

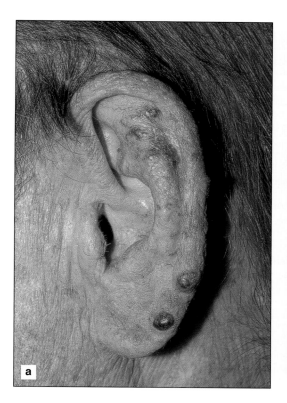

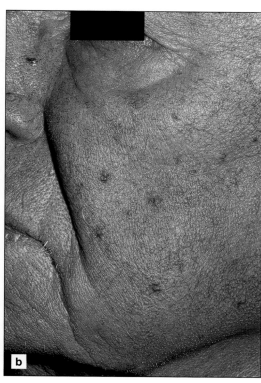

Figure 15.12 Venous lakes. These soft, compressible blebs are common in the elderly. The lips, ears (**a**), and face (**b**) are common sites.

ANGIOMAS AND TUMORS

The types of angioma are outlined in Table 15.1, and the differential diagnosis of commoner vascular or angiomatous papules and nodules applicable to this section is presented in Table 15.2.

Congenital and infantile hemangioma
Etiology and pathogenesis
Most IHs appear after birth, grow rapidly, and regress slowly. They are found in 6–10% of white infants, and are more common in preterm infants and in girls (ratio 3:1). They are also found at increased frequency in children whose mothers had undergone chorionic villus sampling. There are rare kindreds in which hemangiomas are common, following an autosomal dominant inheritance pattern. Some of these kindreds have vascular malformations as well. It is presumed that there are genetic mutations in these families.

Some hemangiomas have a higher risk of internal associations and complications. Variants that should alert the clinician include the following.

- Large facial hemangiomas—these may be part of the PHACE(S) syndrome, a neurocutaneous syndrome including posterior fossae brain abnormalities, hemangiomas, arterial anomalies, coarctation of the aorta and/or other cardiac anomalies, eye abnormalities, and sternal defects in some cases.
- Segmental hemangiomas—the most common sites of internal abnormalities associated with segmental hemangiomas in one study were the liver, gastrointestinal tract, brain, mediastinum, and lung.
- A plaque-like hemangioma that spans the lumbar midline—this may be associated with a tethered spinal cord (also with genitourinary abnormalities). Like other hemangiomas, the lumbar hemangioma will regress over time, so this entity must be recognized in infancy before serious neurologic damage occurs. MRI is useful in imaging an infant with a significant midline lesion.
- Multiple small scattered angiomas—also termed neonatal hemangiomatosis, which is commonly associated with hepatic angiomatosis and is classically manifest as a triad of hepatomegaly, heart failure, and anemia (sometimes with low-grade thrombocytopenia but usually with normal liver enzyme tests). MRI is useful for diagnosis and monitoring, but there is a high mortality rate. In those who survive, the internal lesions regress.

Congenital hemangiomas, as the name implies, are present at birth. They have typically reached their maximum size at birth and do not have an accelerated postnatal growth phase. Under this category, two subsets have been described.

- Rapidly involuting congenital hemangiomas (RICH), which typically involute by 12–24 months (sometimes regression even starts in utero).
- Non-involuting congenital hemangiomas (NICH), which stay stable in size.

Both subtypes affect boys and girls equally.

Potential complications of larger hemangiomas include ulceration, bleeding, infection, and high-output cardiac failure. Hemangiomas overlying the anterior neck may be associated with airway involvement and obstruction. Ultrasound with color flow imaging and MRI are useful non-invasive imaging procedures. Arteriography is only rarely needed. Hemangiomas are quite common, but only those on the midline of the neck or back routinely require imaging.

The Kasabach–Merritt phenomenon has classically been linked to hemangiomas but is actually now felt to occur in kaposiform hemangio-endothelioma or tufted angioma (indeed, the precursor skin lesion is clinically very minor in most cases); the condition consists of a consumptive coagulopathy with thrombocytopenia, and has a high mortality rate. A lymphatic component in such lesions has been implicated.

Clinical
At birth, a barely visible, white, anemic stain; a faint, telangiectatic lesion; a blue spot mimicking a bruise; or, rarely, a full-grown hemangioma may be present (Figs 15.13 and 15.14). Hemangiomas usually present within the first month of life. Generally, they may be separated into a superficial (bright red, arising from the dermis), a deep (blue, arising from subcutaneous tissue), and a mixed type. If untreated, resolution to normal skin, slight redness, telangiectases, wrinkling, or sagging occurs in 50% by 5 years and 70% by 7 years.

Some hemangiomas develop in utero and present as congenital hemangiomas. Rarely, these tumors may be picked up on ultrasonography. Growth after delivery is usually not seen. Rapid involution may occur, although some have necessitated treatment with prednisone or excision.

Differential diagnosis
This falls into several main categories.
- Early, flat, pale-pink lesions may resemble nevus flammeus or PWS.

Table 15.2 DIFFERENTIAL DIAGNOSIS OF VASCULAR PAPULONODULES (EXCLUDING NEONATAL ANGIOMATOSES)

Lesion	Main features	Comments
Capillary hemangioma	Bright red, unless patient is cyanosed; usually multiple; may be associated 'minute' lesions	Rarely a diagnostic problem; tiny lesions may be confused with purpura or vasculitis, or with angiokeratomas
Congenital and infantile hemangiomas	Present at or soon after birth	Some are difficult to distinguish from malformations
Nodules within a capillary malformation (port wine stain)	May develop gradually over time, but pyogenic granulomas may appear suddenly	Usually multiple, cobblestoned; may need biopsy to confirm benign nature
Pyogenic granuloma	Usually acral or facial, often crusted and bleed easily, solitary (occasionally grouped 'satellite' lesions), commonly in children or during pregnancy	May be confused with several malignant tumors; amelanotic melanoma is the most important
Glomus tumor (solitary or multiple forms)	Typically red and painful if solitary (especially subungual); multiple lesions are more blue, and tenderness is variable	Various tender skin lesions are in the differential (Table 15.2); the multiple form (glomangiomas) is very similar to blue rubber bleb nevus syndrome
Blue rubber bleb nevus syndrome	Multiple blue lesions	Closely resembles glomangiomas
Targetoid hemosiderotic hemangioma	Solitary, may have elevated central nodule and bruising around it	Solitary angiokeratoma, bleeding in or around other angiomas (or lymphangiomas, aneurysmal fibrous histiocytoma), large spider nevi
Venous lake	Blue, compressible; solitary (especially on the lip) or multiple; mainly head and neck	May be confused with angiokeratomas, occasionally with melanocytic lesions
Angiokeratomas (solitary or multiple forms)	Typically dark blue–purple color; often lower leg, but specific variants at other sites (Fordyce type, Fabry disease; see text)	May be confused with melanocytic lesions, occasionally with vasculitis
Angioma serpiginosum	Clustered small lesions, may have midline cut-off	Main differentials are multiple minute capillary hemangiomas, Fabry disease, capillaritis, and purpura
Angina bullosa hemorrhagica	Intraoral, see Chapter 20; solitary; may be recurrent; dome-shaped and sharply defined	Could be confused with intraoral Kaposi sarcoma, but the latter produces vague expanding macules or plaques
'Blood blister'	Usually obvious preceding trauma, but not always	May resemble angioma (early lesions) or melanoma (older lesions)
Angiolymphoid hyperplasia with eosinophilia	Often head and neck, may have cobblestoned surface	May resemble various angiomas or basal cell carcinoma; in east Asian people, Kimura disease has some similarity but is more aggressive
Kaposi sarcoma	Mostly HIV-associated and multiple; see text, this chapter, and Chapters 12 and 33	Look in the mouth for palatal lesions, or for candidiasis
Angiosarcoma	Usually starts as a flat patch or just raised plaque, may develop nodules; usually head and neck, in older subjects	Main differential is sporadic type of Kaposi sarcoma or other neoplasms
Various neoplasms	A red vascular appearance is particularly likely in amelanotic melanoma, Merkel cell tumor, poorly differentiated squamous cell carcinoma, atypical fibroxanthoma, and metastatic renal cell carcinoma; local skin involvement or metastases from breast carcinoma may appear telangiectatic	Biopsy any pyogenic granuloma–like lesion if in doubt or if the site or age group is unusual
Vasculitis	May cause large blood and necrotic tissue–filled lesions	Usually acute onset and associated with overtly vasculitic lesions

- Deep or large hemangiomas may be difficult to distinguish from vascular malformations, although this is clear in most cases by the fact that the lesion is proliferative, typically during the first 3–9 months and rarely beyond 18 months (Fig. 15.14).
- Other rarer congenital vascular lesions may resemble hemangiomas, for example kaposiform hemangioendothelioma, congenital-type tufted angioma, and infantile myofibroma.
- Other nodules and tumors, for example nasal glioma (Ch. 19) and rhabdomyosarcoma. The latter might be suspected in any hemangioma that seems excessively firm, and deserves careful evaluation and biopsy if necessary.
- Non-vascular eruptions—multiple small hemangiomas could be confused with rarities such as blueberry muffin baby (Ch. 19), but the hemangiomas in such cases are usually quite red in color compared with the dusky blue color in blueberry muffin baby.

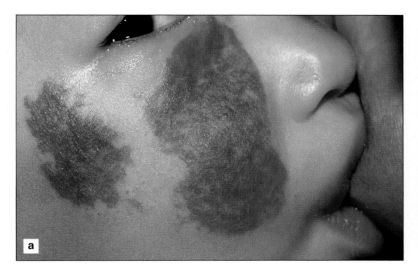

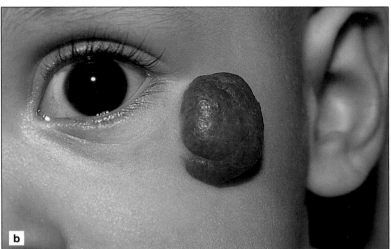

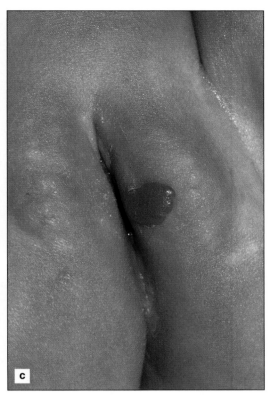

Figure 15.13 Congenital and infantile hemangiomas (IHs). (**a**) A superficial variant of an IH. Note the slightly raised and irregular surface in contrast to a port wine stain. (**b**) If this periocular hemangioma were to grow to the point that it obstructed vision, treatment would be mandatory. Otherwise, permanent visual impairment could result. (**c**) Hemangioma in a premature infant girl.

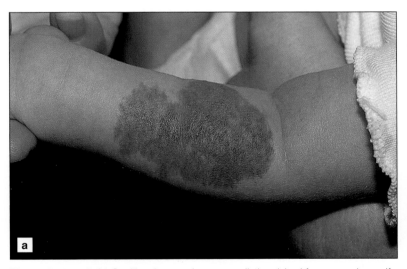

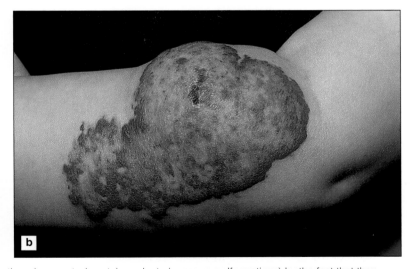

Figure 15.14 (**a,b**) Capillary hemangiomas are distinguished from vascular malformations (e.g. port wine stain and arteriovenous malformations) by the fact that they proliferate, typically during the first 3–9 months of life. The first picture (**a**) shows a lesion at birth that could be either a port wine stain or a hemangioma. (**b**) The appearance of the same lesion several weeks later gives the answer.

Treatment

There is great pressure to act, but the majority of hemangiomas should be left alone. (Some have advocated intralesional corticosteroids regardless of the size or age of the patient.) To protect the area and promote healing when a lesion is located on an extremity, a self-adherent stretch bandage may be applied at home over a snug but not tight non-adherent dressing.

Ulceration may occur in approximately 5% of lesions, especially those of the lips and anogenital area. For these, routine cleansing, topical antibiotics, and possibly a dressing or oral antibiotics are indicated. Healing should occur within 2–3 weeks. Use of the pulsed dye laser for ulcerative hemangiomas has been recommended, but not proved in controlled studies. For ulcerated hemangiomas on the extremities, saline or Burow solution, followed by an antibiotic ointment, adherent pad, and a compressive wrap, has been recommended as being able to heal most ulcers within 2 weeks.

The so-called alarming hemangiomas require aggressive therapy. Hemangiomas are alarming if they are compromising, or threatening to compromise, vision, breathing, or eating, or are causing gastrointestinal bleeding, congestive heart failure, or extensive skin ulceration. For such

299

lesions, a corticosteroid given either intralesionally or systemically (e.g. prednisone 2–4 mg/kg per day for 3 weeks, then tapered over 2 weeks) is the first-line treatment. One should monitor for growth retardation, blood pressure elevation, and immunosuppression. The administration of live vaccines (e.g. polio vaccine) during treatment should be avoided. Ensure that the patient has not recently been exposed to varicella. Some combine prednisone and the pulsed tunable dye laser (PTDL). In one study, prednisone (5 mg/kg per day divided four times daily and given for 2 weeks, then tapered) was excellent, and better than 3 mg/kg per day. Side effects included moon facies and delayed growth in a few. Catch-up growth occurred in all those so affected.

The pulsed dye laser has definite limitations but can be helpful for small, superficial lesions and for some large, plaque-like lesions if treatment is started early enough. This laser can, at times, induce ulceration and, rarely, shallow scarring.

Interferon-alpha is effective in the treatment of hemangiomas but has been found to cause spastic diplegia in a small percentage of patients treated. The risk is highest in patients below 1 year of age, and thus it should be reserved for life-threatening conditions unresponsive to other therapies.

PRACTICE POINTS
- Reassurance is the best treatment for most infantile hemangiomas.
- Consider the possibility of associated internal lesions or other malformations in those with large facial hemangiomas, scattered small lesions, and segmental or midline trunk lesions.
- The diagnosis of hemangioma should be reconsidered in cases where the lesion is abnormally firm. Rhabdomyosarcomas may masquerade as 'firm hemangiomas'.

Capillary hemangiomas (cherry angiomas, Campbell de Morgan spots)

Etiology and pathogenesis

Capillary hemangiomas, also known as Campbell de Morgan spots, are vascular growths that affect almost every adult over 40. In one study of adults aged 30–39 years, 90% of the men and 65% of the women had at least one cherry angioma.

Clinical

Most adults over 40 have one or more red vascular papules on the trunk (Fig. 15.15). Sometimes, they appear almost 'petechial' as 1–2-mm red macules. These are also called minute Campbell de Morgan spots. Some angiomas, particularly those on the face, may have a significant arterial feeder vessel that gives them a surrounding flare (Fig. 15.16), much like spider angiomas.

Differential diagnosis

Darker lesions, or those that transiently turn black due to intralesional bleeding from inadvertent trauma, have been confused with melanoma (if bruising is frequent, consider targetoid hemosiderotic hemangioma, which is discussed later).

The multiple minute form may resemble angioma serpiginosum (discussed later) if extensive, and occasionally give rise to concern about vasculitis, meningococcemia, etc., as they are too small to blanch with diascopy.

Less likely differentials for a larger solitary lesion include pyogenic granuloma, glomus tumor, and other vascular neoplasms, and for multiple lesions include Kaposi sarcoma or bacillary angiomatosis.

Treatment

No treatment is usually needed, although electrodesiccation is effective. Cryotherapy, especially with a probe to press blood from the lesion, may be tried.

Pyogenic granuloma

Etiology and pathogenesis

A pyogenic granuloma is a rapidly growing benign vascular tumor that histologically resembles vascular proliferation in healing tissue. They are more common in pregnancy. The vast majority occur in the skin, but they

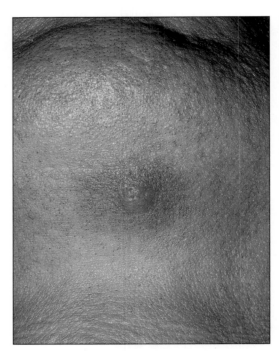

Figure 15.16 Angioma with flare of surrounding dilated vessels, in the beard area under the chin. Some angiomas of the face have a significant flare about them. An arterial vessel often feeds these lesions, similar to a spider angioma.

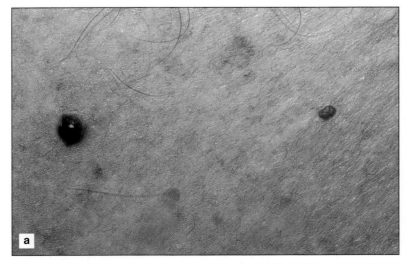

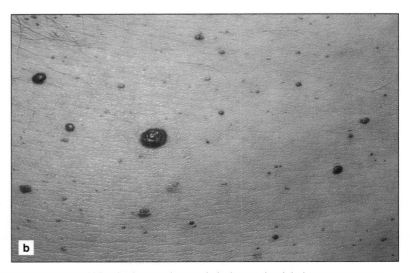

Figure 15.15 Capillary hemangiomas. (**a**) The red lesion on the left contains relatively more oxygenated blood, whereas the purple lesion on the right has more venous blood. (**b**) Multiple lesions, from papules to pinpoint petechia-like lesions, are present.

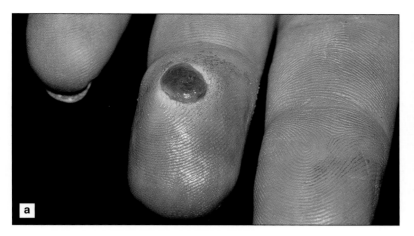
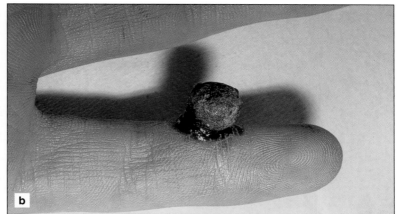
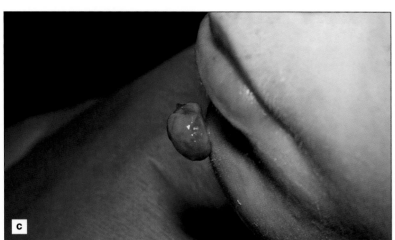
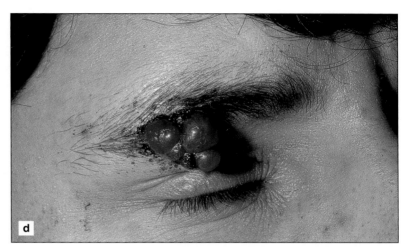

Figure 15.17 Pyogenic granuloma. (**a**) This is the classic appearance of a red, friable nodule growing rapidly on the finger. There is often a portion that extends under the skin laterally. (**b**) Pyogenic granuloma on the finger. This lesion is more dry and crusted. (**c**) Pyogenic granuloma on the chin of an adult. The fingers, lip, palms, soles, and face are typical sites. (**d**) Pyogenic granuloma of the eyebrow.

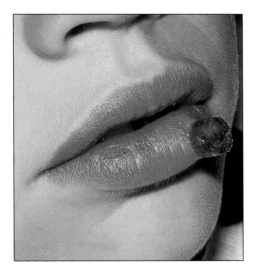

Figure 15.18 Pyogenic granuloma on the lip of a child.

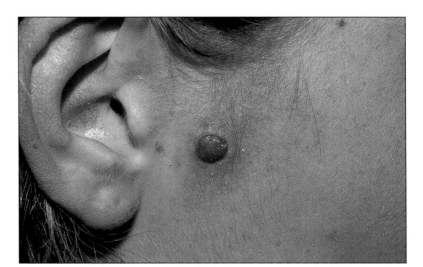

Figure 15.19 Pyogenic granuloma. These may develop in a port wine stain as shown here.

may occur in the oral mucosa (especially during pregnancy) and rarely in the gastrointestinal tract, a rare cause of gastrointestinal bleeding.

Clinical
The sudden appearance of a vascular, friable papule that bleeds easily, on the finger, palm, sole, head, or neck, is characteristic of a pyogenic granuloma (Figs 15.17–15.19). An epidermal collarette may be prominent. The parents may apply layer on layer of bandages to control the bleeding, giving rise to the 'bandage sign'.

Differential diagnosis
On rare occasions, a nodular melanoma may be mistaken for a pyogenic granuloma (Figs 15.20 and 15.21). Thus all specimens should be sent for

histologic examination. Older lesions may be difficult to distinguish from other types of angioma or vascular neoplasms.

Treatment
Local anesthesia followed by shave biopsy, curettage, and electrocautery is usually curative. If the lesion is not fully curetted, control of bleeding may be difficult and recurrence common; if at a technically easy site, a formal elliptic excision may be preferred in the first instance for this reason. This procedure runs smoothly for the teenager or adult, but young children rarely cooperate. Use of the papoose (flat board with cloth wraps to hold the child still) is often needed. Lesions on the finger may benefit from a tourniquet to prevent bleeding. Wound care should consist of leaving the

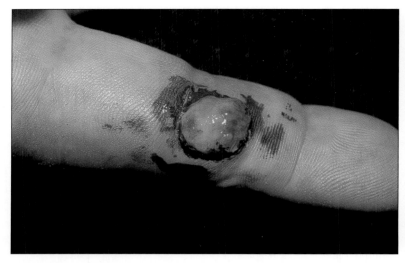

Figure 15.20 Pyogenic granuloma mimicking melanoma. The finger is a characteristic site of the pyogenic granuloma. Silver nitrate has been applied in a failed attempt to eradicate the lesion.

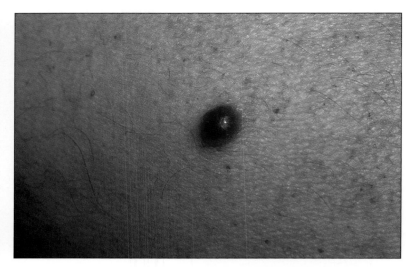

Figure 15.22 Solitary glomus tumor. This vascular lesion may be single or multiple. Lesions are often painful, and the subungual area is a common site.

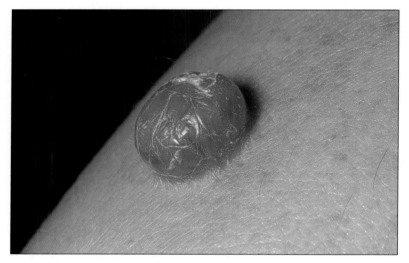

Figure 15.21 Pyogenic granuloma. This pyogenic granuloma is less common, as it is large and does not have a friable, bleeding surface. A biopsy is mandatory to exclude an amelanotic melanoma (compare with Fig. 15.20).

Table 15.3	DIFFERENTIAL DIAGNOSIS OF PAINFUL SKIN TUMORS
Glomus tumor	
Angiolipoma	
Neurilemmoma (schwannoma)	
Eccrine spiradenoma	
Leiomyoma	
Angioleiomyoma	

area open to dry. Keeping it moist may increase the likelihood of recurrence.

Patients or parents should always be told of the small risk of recurrence. If recurrence does occur, the same procedure may be tried again, or elliptic excision, including a small amount of dermis, may be done. Cryotherapy can be useful for some lesions or for recurrences but requires long freeze times and matching discomfort. Alternatively, one, two, or three treatments with the flash lamp-pumped pulsed dye laser were successful in 91% of children in one series. The site and age group need to be typical, and the diagnosis certain, if destructive therapies are to be used.

The eruption of multiple lesions after treatment of a single one (satellitosis) occurs rarely. In the case of a giant pyogenic granuloma with satellitosis, an oral steroid was successfully employed.

PRACTICE POINTS

- Remember that neoplasms, for example amelanotic melanoma, Merkel cell tumor, or cutaneous metastases, may appear vascular and in particular may mimic pyogenic granuloma. Always query the diagnosis of pyogenic granuloma if the site is unusual, and always get histologic confirmation.
- A painful, red, subungual tumor is probably a glomus tumor.
- A rapidly developing moist or crusted red tumor affecting the periungual skin or distal part of a finger is probably a pyogenic granuloma.

Glomus tumor (solitary)
Etiology and pathogenesis
Glomus tumors are benign vascular lesions that arise from the neuro-myoarterial apparatus. The glomus body from which they originate contains an afferent arteriole, a connecting vessel (Sucquet–Hoyer canal), a primary collecting vein, smooth muscle cells, and epithelial-type cells (glomus cells), surrounded by a fibrous capsule.

Clinical
A solitary blue-red vascular papulonodule is typical (Fig. 15.22). It often occurs under the nail, where a bluish red discoloration overlying a subungual papule is characteristic. Pain may occur spontaneously, after contact, or after change to cooler temperature. Exact localization of the tumor may be difficult. Radiography may show bony erosion of the distal phalanx. Ultrasound and high-resolution MRI have been used.

Multiple glomus 'tumors' (more correctly, GVMs) are rather different, as discussed previously.

Differential diagnosis
Other angiomas may be in the differential, and subungual melanoma may be considered but does not have the characteristic pain of a glomus tumor at this site. There are several causes of a painful tumor that should be considered in the differential of glomus tumor at other skin sites (Table 15.3).

Treatment
Excision is curative but usually involves removal of the nail for subungual lesions, which may be technically difficult to remove.

Targetoid hemosiderotic hemangioma
The targetoid hemosiderotic hemangioma (THH) is a solitary vascular tumor that clinically has a 'targetoid' appearance (Fig. 15.23). Specifically,

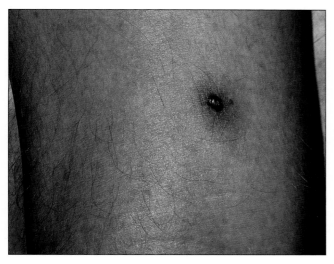

Figure 15.23 Targetoid hemosiderotic hemangioma. Note the central vascular papule with the surrounding ecchymosis. (Courtesy of Fred Fehl, M.D.)

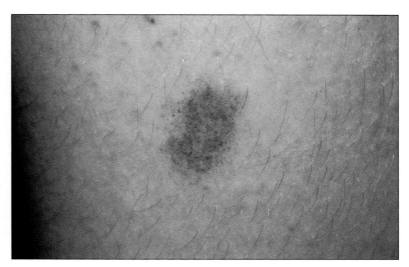

Figure 15.25 Angioma serpiginosum. It is said that this childhood vascular lesion is more common in females and is most often found on the extremities. Note the presence of pinpoint red papules and the absence of a serpiginous component.

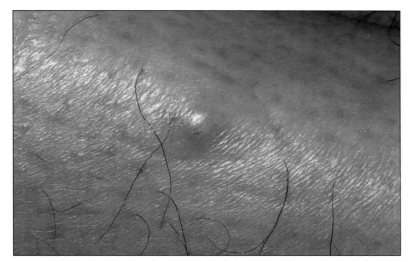

Figure 15.24 Spindle cell hemangioendothelioma.

there is a central violaceous papule with a surrounding ecchymotic or brown ring that can enlarge or disappear. The central papule may have a cobblestoned morphology that resembles a raspberry. It is postulated that both solitary angiokeratomas and THH are variants of the same process in which trauma induces a dilatation of vascular elements. THH, in general, is larger than solitary angiokeratoma. The differential diagnosis includes the following.

- Solitary angiokeratoma.
- Bleeding in and around other angiomas or small lymphangiomas, or occasionally around rarer lesions such as aneurysmal fibrous histiocytoma.
- Large spider nevi may have a raised central nodule with a telangiectatic halo.

If there is any question of the possibility of an atypical pigmented lesion, a biopsy should be performed. Otherwise, no treatment is needed. Shave biopsy with cautery of the base or simple excision may be performed.

Spindle cell hemangioendothelioma
See Fig. 15.24.

Angioma serpiginosum
This benign vascular lesion (Fig. 15.25) usually has its onset in childhood. It usually progresses over several years and then remains stable. Most patients are female, and the lower extremity is preferred. From a distance, the lesion may appear as diffuse redness, but on close inspection, multiple pinpoint, angiomatous, red papules are seen. They do not blanch on pressure. Despite its name, there is no serpiginous component. The appear-

ance of angioma serpiginosum may at times be similar to capillaritis, but the former is stable over time or slowly progressive, whereas capillaritis will either resolve or wax and wane over time. Unilateral nevoid telangiectasias may have a similar age of onset and be vascular and asymmetric in clinical presentation, but close inspection will show the individual lesions to be telangiectasias. No treatment is needed, but laser can reduce the appearance of the lesions.

Kaposi sarcoma
Etiology and pathogenesis
Kaposi sarcoma is one of two cutaneous vascular proliferations derived from lymphatic endothelial cells (the other being angiosarcoma). Kaposi sarcoma is divided for clinical purposes into HIV-associated and classic, but both are associated with infection by the human herpesvirus 8.

Clinical
A reddish blue to purple papulonodule or plaque beginning on the toe or sole of a man of southern or eastern European descent is characteristic (Fig. 15.26). Slow progression may occur, with lesions ascending the leg to all parts of the body. Internal involvement is most common in the gastrointestinal tract. Many other organs may be involved (e.g. bone) but, because of the slow progression of the disease, most patients die of unrelated causes.

Differential diagnosis
If the lesion is solitary, the differential is more broad (see Table 15.3). For multiple lesions, particularly on the lower extremities, the differential is more limited. One might consider an angiosarcoma (Fig. 15.27) or possibly metastatic disease, as it can mimic a vascular lesion.

Treatment
HIV infection should be excluded. Cryotherapy, curettage and dilatation, or excision may be performed for small lesions. Radiation therapy is also effective. Intralesional interferon alpha-2a has been used. If classic Kaposi sarcoma develops on the legs of an elderly patient with some circulatory insufficiency and radiation therapy is used (at times repeatedly for recurrent disease with the potential for overlapping fields), stasis dermatitis or radiation dermatitis, with the potential for ulceration, may result.

Intralesional vinblastine may be used (vinblastine 0.2 mg/mL, 0.1–0.3 mL/lesion monthly, as needed).

Angiolymphoid hyperplasia with eosinophilia
Etiology and pathogenesis
Angiolymphoid hyperplasia with eosinophilia (ALHE) is an unusual vascular proliferation that tends to occur in the head and neck, particularly about the ears, of adults. Although human herpesvirus 8 DNA has been

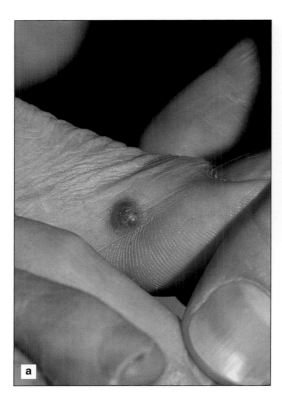

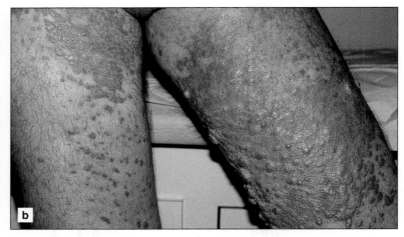

Figure 15.26 Kaposi sarcoma, classic type. (**a**) A vascular lesion on the leg or foot of an older patient should raise the suspicion of classic Kaposi sarcoma. (**b**) Extensive lesions. (Courtesy of Michael O. Murphy, M.D.)

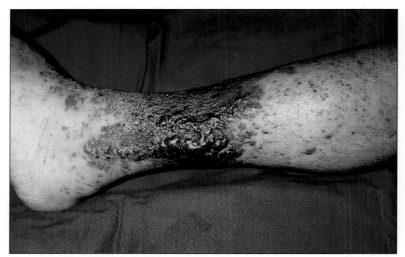

Figure 15.27 Angiosarcoma.

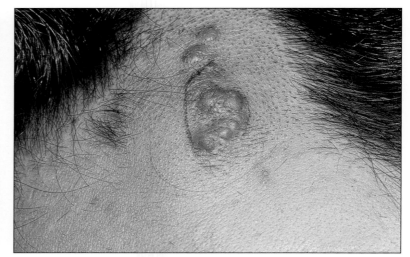

Figure 15.28 Angiolymphoid hyperplasia with eosinophilia. This unusual benign, vascular proliferation is found most commonly on the ear and scalp. Dilated vessels and eosinophils are seen histologically. (See also Fig. 11.3.) (Courtesy of Duane Whitaker, M.D.)

reported in at least one case of ALHE, a larger series failed to show any connection.

Clinical

The ear and preauricular areas are most commonly affected by the red (less often, grayish or skin-colored) papulonodules of ALHE (Fig. 15.28). The head and neck may also be affected. Widespread papules mimicking prurigo nodularis have been reported. Peripheral eosinophilia is often seen. Ulceration and bleeding may occur. Work-up should include a complete blood count, a skin biopsy, and a lymph node examination.

Differential diagnosis

Kaposi sarcoma as well as angiosarcoma of the head and neck should be considered. Some lesions resemble basal cell carcinoma. Kimura disease must be considered, as it has a similar histologic picture. However, its lesions are typically larger, deeper nodules with normal overlying skin and often with lymphadenopathy. A biopsy is always necessary to establish the diagnosis.

Treatment

Excision, intralesional steroids, cryotherapy, electrodesiccation, or laser have been used. Mohs surgery is reported to be very effective, with the

characteristic cells readily identified in frozen sections. Two cases related to elevated female hormones (birth control pill and pregnancy) resolved or improved after the exposure stopped (stopping 'the pill' and after delivery, respectively). Multiple treatments with the pulsed dye laser have been helpful for superficial lesions. Radiation therapy was successful in one case without any side effects after 9 years of follow-up.

TELANGIECTASES

Spider telangiectases

Spider angiomas (spider telangiectases) are very common in children, in pregnancy, and in patients with liver disease (Figs 15.29 and 15.30). They are usually facial and solitary or few in number in the childhood type, but may be extensive in liver disease, in which they are particularly common on the upper trunk. Any adult who develops significant spider telangiectasias should have liver transaminases measured.

An arcade of vessels radiating out from a central arteriole is the characteristic appearance. Compressing the central point blanches the arcade.

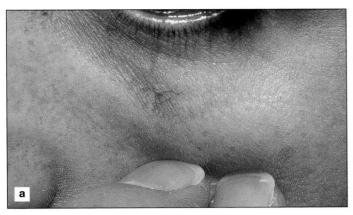

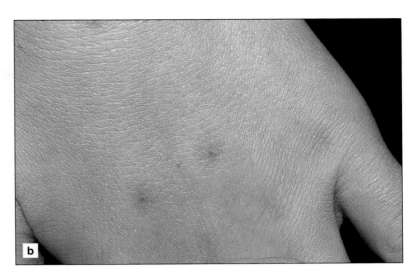

Figure 15.29 Spider telangiectases in children. (**a**) This spider web of vessels emanating from a central arteriolar source occurs classically on the upper cheek in children. (**b**) Multiple spider angiomas in a child. The dorsa of the hands are common places for spider angiomas in a child.

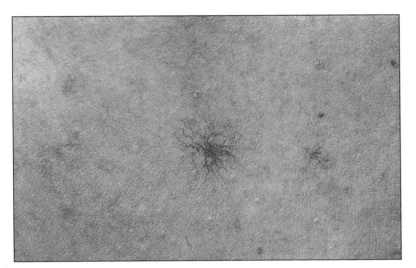

Figure 15.30 Spider telangiectases in an adult. The finding of multiple spider angiomas on the chest of an adult should prompt a search for liver disease.

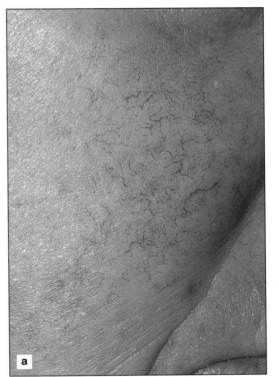

This radiating pattern is not seen in the other telangiectatic disorders discussed in this section. The area just below the eye on the upper cheek is a very characteristic site for spider telangiectases in children. The rest of the face, chest, and hands may be affected as well.

No treatment is needed, and most of these lesions will fade over time. Light electrocautery with an epilating needle is quite effective. The tunable dye laser has also been used.

Benign (facial) telangiectases

Multiple telangiectasias are common on the face of fair-skinned adults. Presence on the area about the nose and cheeks is common. This is often an isolated finding, unrelated to rosacea (Fig. 15.31). Solar damage is probably important.

Costal fringe

An arcade of telangiectases (Fig. 15.32) on the trunk, often near the costal margin but also elsewhere on the trunk, is characteristic of this benign skin change of the elderly. The telangiectases tend to be blue rather than bright red as occurs in many other telangiectatic disorders. No treatment is needed.

Unilateral nevoid telangiectasia

Telangiectasias in this condition develop in a segmental or 'nevoid' distribution. The onset of this condition is often associated with an elevation in hormones, for example at puberty or during pregnancy (in the latter cases, some will disappear or fade after delivery, so treatment should be avoided).

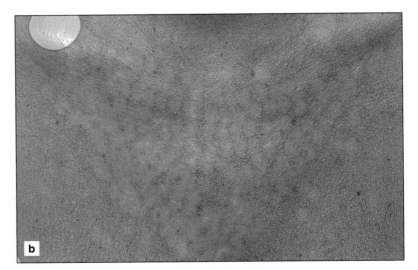

Figure 15.31 Benign telangiectasia. (**a**) Facial telangiectases. (**b**) Partial pulsed dye laser treatment of telangiectases of the chest. Note the multiple, relatively avascular areas on this woman's chest, each of which represented one pulse from a dye laser. Obviously, more treatments were needed.

Often, no treatment is necessary other than reassurance that this is a type of birthmark made apparent by the effects of estrogen. The pulsed dye laser was surprisingly ineffective in one study, with new lesions recurring soon after treatment.

Hereditary hemorrhagic telangiectasia
Etiology and pathogenesis
Patients with hereditary hemorrhagic telangiectasia (HHT), also known as Osler–Weber–Rendu disease, develop multiple cutaneous telangiectasias as well as AVMs internally. The inheritance is autosomal dominant with incomplete penetrance. Mutations in one of two chromosomal sites can cause HHT. In HHT-1, mutations at chromosome 9 alter the protein endoglin. In HHT-2, mutations at chromosome 12 alter the protein activin receptor-like kinase-1 (ALK-1). Both ALK-1 and endoglin are receptors for transforming growth factor-β (TGF-β) and are expressed primarily in arterial endothelial cells. Endoglin and ALK-1, as well as other TGF-β signaling components, are essential during angiogenesis.

Vascular abnormalities may affect the liver (portal hypertension), spleen, lung (pulmonary AVM and hemoptysis; Fig. 15.33), gastrointestinal tract (gastrointestinal bleeding and anemia), and urinary tract (hematuria). Central nervous system abscess may occur, presumably from pulmonary AVMs that do not filter venous septic foci.

Clinical
The classic patient experiences recurrent epistaxis at a young age. Later, telangiectatic mats develop on the tongue, lips, fingertips, and elsewhere (Fig. 15.34).

Differential diagnosis
There is very little doubt of the diagnosis for the patient who develops epistaxis in childhood, followed by the classic cutaneous telangiectasias. The main difficulty is that some children have multiple telangiectases clinically resembling HHT, usually on the dorsal forearms and hands, without epistaxis or other bleeding; it is difficult to know whether this represents a milder variation of HHT (possibly due to an as yet undescribed mutation). Adults with CREST syndrome (calcinosis, Raynaud phenomenon, esophageal dysfunction, sclerodactyly, and telangiectasia; Ch. 13) can appear nearly identical to patients with HHT as they can have telangiectasias on the face and fingers.

Treatment
Many complications involving the brain, liver, and lung can develop. Thus a multidisciplinary approach to therapy is needed, with the primary risks being outside the dermatologist's arena. The cutaneous telangiectases may be treated with laser. DNA testing is now available, and so relatives may be screened, thus saving on radiologic imaging. Only those relatives with a positive genetic analysis need further evaluation of internal organs.

Telangiectasia macularis eruptiva perstans
This variant of mastocytosis presents with telangiectatic macules, often on the trunk, of a woman (Fig. 15.35). Special stains may be needed to help identify the mast cells histologically. Clinically, one sees 5–10-mm pink-brown telangiectatic macules, predominantly on the trunk. Itching may vary from mild to intense. Gentle scratching may elicit Darier sign. The

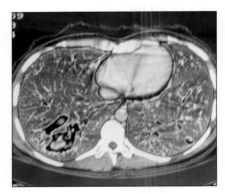

Figure 15.33 Pulmonary arteriovenous malformations are relatively common in patients with hereditary hemorrhagic telangiectases.

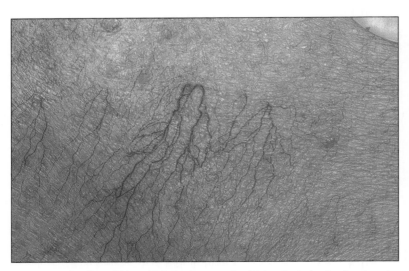

Figure 15.32 Costal fringe. This benign arcade of telangiectasias is often found incidentally while treating other problems.

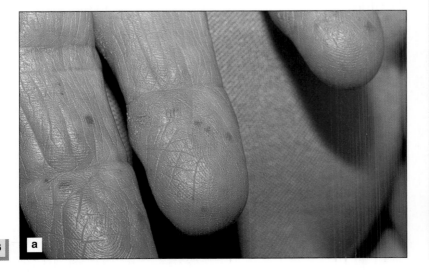

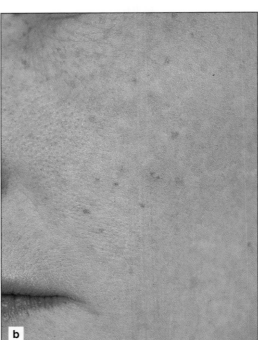

Figure 15.34 Hereditary hemorrhagic telangiectasia. (**a**) The patient is born with a tendency to develop multiple telangiectases, usually on the face and hands. Epistaxis (nose bleeds) are extremely common in early childhood. (**b**) Multiple lesions on the face.

a

b

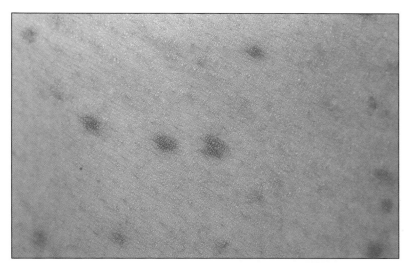

Figure 15.35 Telangiectasia macularis eruptiva perstans. Fine telangiectasias coalesce to form small mats on the skin. An aggregate of mast cells in the skin is the cause.

forms of mastocytosis and its investigation, differential diagnosis, and therapy are discussed in Chapter 11.

For treatment, a potent topical steroid may be very effective. For example, clobetasol (0.05% cream applied to one section of the body every day for 1 month) can nearly clear lesions. Then another section of the body should be treated, while applying maintenance to the initial area (e.g. initially once a week down to once a month). It is important not to coat the body daily with a potent topical steroid, so as not to suppress the hypothalamic–pituitary axis. In addition, it is important to avoid prolonged daily use of such a potent topical steroid, as it may induce atrophy and telangiectasias.

The 585-nm flash lamp-pumped dye laser cleared all treated lesions without scarring after one treatment in one study. Doxepin given pre- and postoperatively provided the best mast cell-mediator blockade. Its effects seem to be secondary to reducing the vasculature and not via an effect on the mast cells. Any itching should be treated with a non-sedating antihistamine. PUVA may be tried. Total skin electron beam completely cleared one patient's condition.

Generalized essential telangiectasia

Telangiectases develop in the skin of patients with this benign condition. Only small areas or the entire body, including the eyes, may be involved (Fig. 15.36). Inheritance patterns and clinical variants have yet to be fully defined. No systemic bleeding is usually associated, although cases have been described with similar lesions in the stomach, and one patient did develop gastrointestinal bleeding associated with a watermelon stomach.

Hereditary hemorrhagic telangiectasia should be excluded, and a screen for liver abnormalities should be done. Individual lesions may respond to laser therapy, but treating the entire patient is usually impractical.

Other telangiectasias

- Rosacea (Ch. 10) and solar damage are common causes of facial telangiectases.
- Venous hypertension is discussed later in this chapter. A 'venous flare' of blue telangiectatic vessels may occur on the feet or ankle region, sometimes with a radiating pattern.
- Extensive telangiectasia may occur in Cushing syndrome; similarly, potent topical corticosteroids may induce local atrophy and telangiectasias if overused.
- Some rare genodermatoses feature telangiectasia, notably ataxia telangiectasia.

ANGIOKERATOMAS

Angiokeratoma of Fordyce

Small, 1–6-mm, vascular, red papules on the scrotum of an older man or the labia majora of an older woman are characteristic (Fig. 15.37). No treatment is needed.

Solitary angiokeratoma

Localized angiokeratomas are usually solitary and develop in young adults, most commonly on the legs. Occasionally, multiple lesions (often in a localized zone of the skin on legs or feet) may occur. Lesions range in size from 3 to 10 mm. Early on, they are usually red, but in later years may become blue-purple and occasionally may clot, resulting in a dark blue or black lesion than can be mistaken for melanoma (Figs 15.38 and 15.39). If necessary, a biopsy should be performed. Otherwise, no treatment is needed.

Angiokeratoma corporis diffusum (Fabry disease)
Etiology and pathogenesis

Angiokeratoma corporis diffusum, also known as Fabry (or Anderson–Fabry) disease, is caused by a deficiency of the lysosomal hydrolase α-galactosidase, leading to progressive accumulation of uncleaved glycosphingolipids, predominantly trihexosylceramide. Inheritance is X-linked, and the condition is most severe in men. Most patients are diagnosed in childhood or early adult life.

The patient develops widespread cutaneous angiomas (Fig. 15.40) as well as systemic abnormalities (e.g. myocardial infarctions, chest pain,

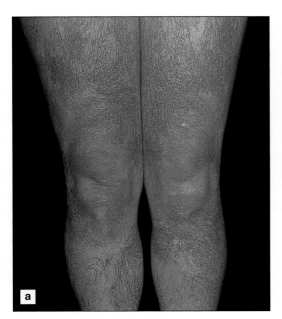

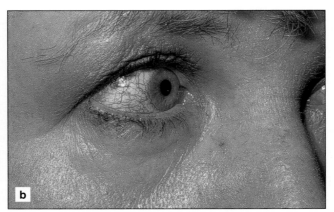

Figure 15.36 Generalized essential telangiectasia. (**a**) Innumerable telangiectases cover the legs. (**b**) The same patient as in (a) displaying generalized essential telangiectasia involving the eyes.

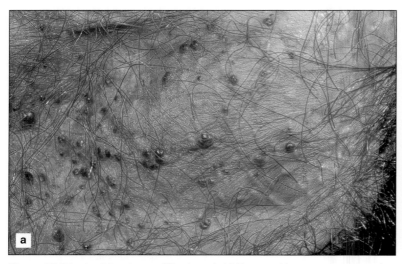

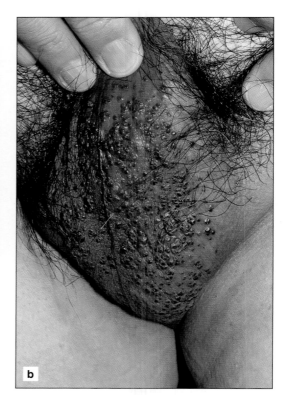

Figure 15.37 Angiokeratoma of Fordyce. (**a,b**) These red bumps are commonly seen on the scrotum of men. These vascular papules occur on the labia majora as well.

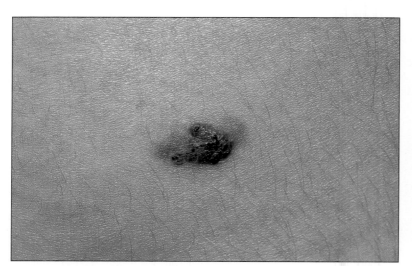

Figure 15.38 Solitary angiokeratoma.

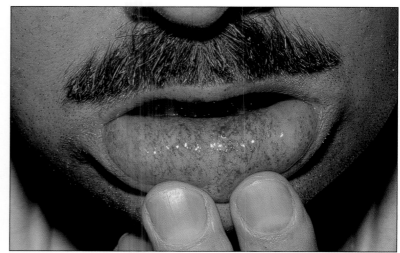

Figure 15.40 Fabry disease. The presence of multiple, small, dark-red to black, sometimes verrucous papules is characteristic of angiokeratoma corporis diffusum. It may occur idiopathically or be associated with various syndromes, most of them hereditary lysosomal storage diseases.

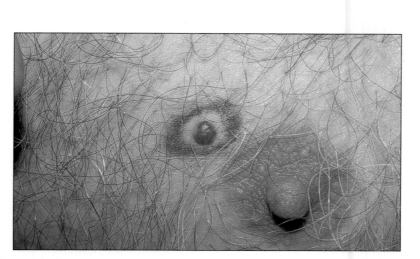

Figure 15.39 Thrombosed angiokeratoma. These lesions may thrombose, mimicking melanomas. Sometimes, unusual halos of blood surround the lesion.

dysrhythmias, renal failure, cerebrovascular accident, seizures, and cerebral hemorrhage). Patients may experience episodic bouts of painful, burning palms and soles, often described as 'burning, sharp, pins and needles-like'. There is often an intolerance to heat or cold and the inability to sweat, as well as high-frequency neurosensory hearing loss. Slit-lamp examination shows posterior capsular spokes, termed cornea verticillata.

The diagnosis may be confirmed by measuring the enzymatic levels of α-galactosidase (e.g. from skin fibroblast homogenates). Prenatal diagnosis is possible.

The primary cause of death is renal, and without renal transplantation or dialysis the mean age of death is about 40 years. Cardiac events are another source of mortality.

Clinical

The patient experiences the onset in childhood of innumerable tiny red papules (angiokeratomas) in bathing trunk distribution. Lesions may be grouped and, in mild cases, only a limited number of lesions develop in the scrotum, thighs, and about the umbilicus. The other features have already been described.

Differential diagnosis

Deficiency of other enzymes, such as β-galactosidase, α-fucosidase, and α-sialidase, may produce identical cutaneous angiokeratomas; these should be measured in patients with normal α-galactosidase levels.

The main other differentials are multiple minute capillary hemangiomas, angioma serpiginosum, capillaritis, and other purpuric disorders. The scrotal lesions are indistinguishable from angiokeratomas of Fordyce, but the family history, lesions at other sites, and the age group at which most patients present should readily distinguish the two.

Treatment

Enzyme replacement therapies for the human enzyme α-galactosidase A are now available. They can decrease pain, increase the ability to sweat, improve the tolerance to temperature change, improve cardiac function, etc. (although the effect on the visible skin angiokeratomas is often less apparent). Enzyme replacement therapy should begin as soon as possible.

HEAT- AND COLD-INDUCED LESIONS

Erythema ab igne
Etiology and pathogenesis

Erythema ab igne (EAI) is a reticulated pattern of thermal damage to the skin. The damage occurs preferentially in the border areas between the blood-dispersing arterial zones, because the heat dispersion in these areas is low.

Clinical

A reticulated pattern of erythema and later hyperpigmentation (Fig. 15.41a) at the site of chronic thermal exposure (e.g. from a heater, heating pad, laptop computer, or fire) is characteristic. Rarely, bullous lesions may occur. Typical forms of EAI include that of the shins in a patient who huddles near a fire (much the commonest pattern), facial EAI in cooks, or low back EAI in patients with low back pain who frequently use hot water bottles. A special recliner with a built-in heating element has caused EAI in two patients. EAI should always prompt an inquiry as to the source of the heat, and if it is to relieve pain, what the source of the pain is. Underlying pancreatitis, splenomegaly, or cancer (Fig. 15.41b), all

resulting in pain, have been found in this manner. There is an increased risk of squamous cell carcinoma and, rarely, Merkel cell carcinoma.

Treatment

If the heat is avoided, the pattern may resolve over time. 5-Fluorouracil has been recommended to eliminate keratinocyte atypia and may make malignant change less likely.

Raynaud phenomenon

Sharply demarcated blanching occurs initially, followed by cyanosis and subsequently hyperemia in Raynaud phenomenon (see Ch. 13).

Perniosis

Acral, pruritic, often painful, purplish papules, patches, and plaques in a patient exposed to a cold, damp environment are characteristic (Fig. 15.42). There may be background acrocyanosis if the extremities are affected. The perniosis lesions themselves spontaneously resolve over a few weeks. Home heating and warm clothes prevent recurrences. Nifedipine may be used in severe cases.

Neutrophilic eccrine hidradenitis is a possible differential diagnosis of perniosis on the feet in children but typically affects the sole rather than the digits. The chilblain pattern of lupus erythematosus (Ch. 13) may be considered but usually has more surface change and affects most or all digits, whereas just one or two tend to be involved in perniosis.

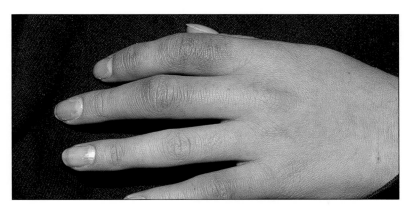

Figure 15.42 Perniosis. These painful erythematous plaques occurred on the fingers and toes of a young girl exposed to the cold for several days.

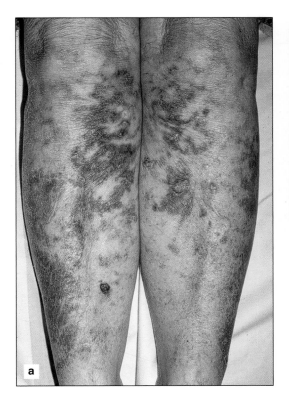

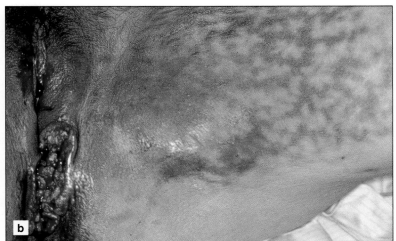

Figure 15.41 Erythema ab igne (EAI). (**a**) Lesions on the shins. A reticulated pattern of erythema and hyperpigmentation develops in areas chronically exposed to heat. Thermal damage develops in border areas between blood-dispersing arterial zones. (**b**) EAI of the thigh. This 41-year-old woman also had a squamous cell carcinoma arising from the anus. (Courtesy of Paul Koonings.)

ARTERIAL DISEASE

Acute arterial insufficiency
Large-vessel obstruction
If a large embolus occludes a large vessel, the distal leg turns acutely white, as shown in Fig. 15.43. This is a medical emergency, and the vascular surgeon should be consulted.

Diabetic foot
Diabetes mellitus can cause both a microangiopathy as well as atheroma of large vessels. Impaired arterial blood supply and even gangrene may result (Fig. 15.44 and see Fig. 12.9).

Arterial ulcers
Progressive impairment of arterial blood supply severely compromises the function of the skin. The skin of the lower extremities often exhibits pallor, cyanosis, loss of hair, and brittle or deformed nails. As the condition progresses, ulcers may develop.

The classic arterial ulcer does not occur on the medial ankle (where the venous ulcer is typical), but instead occurs on the toes, shins, or dorsa of the foot (Fig. 15.45). Ischemic ulcers are often dry and punched out. Features of venous disease (brown pigmentation, stasis dermatitis, or lipodermatosclerosis) are absent. Elevation or compression bandaging will worsen symptoms of arterial disease. The differential diagnosis of leg ulcers is listed in Table 15.4.

Unfortunately, a component of both arterial and venous disease may coexist in many patients, so the physical signs may be mixed.

Treatment of arterial ulcers may be difficult. Investigations by a vascular surgeon are typically required. Pressure should be avoided, and the nutritional and health status of the patient should be optimized. Any secondary infection should be addressed, and local wound care to promote healing should be provided. A specialist vascular nurse is often an asset in treating patients. Despite all these measures, healing often does not occur unless the arterial blood supply is improved with surgery. Excision and grafting may be necessary.

PRACTICE POINTS
- Chronic leg ulcers are often best treated by a team of specialists, including the surgeon, wound care nurse, and dermatologists.
- Compression is the most important aspect of treating venous ulcers but will worsen arterial ulcers.

Thrombophlebitis
Superficial thrombophlebitis may present to vascular surgeons, dermatologists, or generalists. Most cases are related to varicose veins, less commonly associated with deep venous thrombosis. Cases may be misdiagnosed as localized cellulitis or as solitary lesions of erythema nodosum due to the tenderness and erythema. However, lesions are often localized over areas

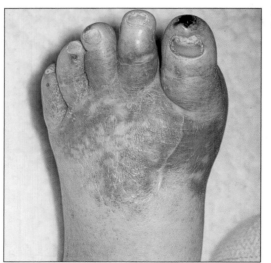

Figure 15.43 Acute arterial insufficiency.

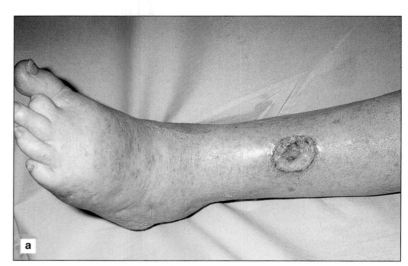

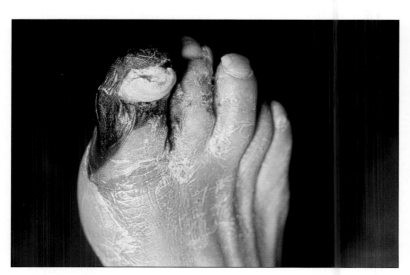

Figure 15.44 Diabetic foot with gangrene.

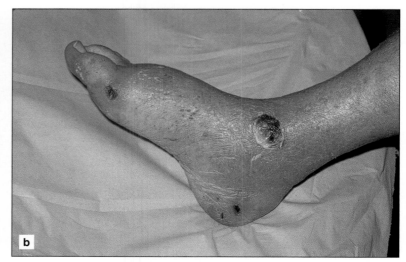

Figure 15.45 Arterial ulcer. (**a**) A pretibial ulcer without associated pigmentation, stasis changes, or lipodermatosclerosis is typical. (**b**) Arterial ulcer after occlusion of the popliteal end of a femoral–popliteal graft.

Table 15.4 CAUSES OF LEG ULCERATION

Type of mechanism	Examples: common to moderately common	Examples: less common or rare
Venous disease	Varicose veins, deep vein thrombosis, other venous obstruction, ulcerated superficial thrombophlebitis	Congenital vascular malformations, Klippel–Trenaunay syndrome, ruptured varices
Arterial disease	Atherosclerosis, diabetes	Cholesterol emboli, obstruction (e.g. fat emboli), hypertensive ulcer, arteriovenous fistula
Vasculitis and neutrophilic dermatoses	Pyoderma gangrenosum, rheumatoid ulcers, small-vessel leukocytoclastic vasculitis (including Henoch–Schönlein purpura)	Other connective tissue disease (systemic lupus erythematosus, systemic sclerosis) and vasculitides, livedoid vasculopathies
Other dermatoses and metabolic causes	Necrobiosis lipoidica, immunobullous diseases (e.g. pemphigoid)	Scleroderma, calciphylaxis
Genetic predisposition	(See hematologic causes, below)	Klinefelter syndrome, prolidase deficiency
Hematologic disorders and hyperviscosity	Sickle cell disease, thalassemia (common causes in some parts of the world)	Thrombophilias (Ch. 14), cryoglobulinemia, hypergammaglobulinemias, spherocytosis, myeloproliferative disorders
Infections	Streptococcal cellulitis, leprosy, tropical ulcer, Buruli ulcer	Osteomyelitis, fungal infections, mycobacterial infections, leishmaniasis, necrotizing fasciitis
Peripheral neuropathy	Leprosy (common in some parts of the world), diabetes	Spina bifida, spinal injury, other spinal disorders
Trauma and extrinsic	Direct injury, pressure, burns, chemical injury (e.g. sclerotherapy, caustics such as cement), bites and stings (insects, snakes, stingray, etc.)	Intravenous drug use, dermatitis artefacta
Neoplasia	Basal cell carcinoma, squamous cell carcinoma	Merkel cell carcinoma, Kaposi sarcoma, melanoma, malignant fibrous histiocytoma
Iatrogenic	After therapeutic radiation	Hydroxyurea

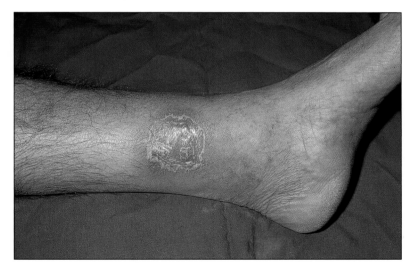

Figure 15.46 Thrombophlebitis. A linear ridge was palpable under this discoid area, demonstrating the importance of palpation. Presumably, a superficial thrombophlebitis extended into the perforator vessel at this site.

of perforating veins at the ankle (Fig. 15.46), or linear induration may be palpable following the course of a vein. Migratory thrombophlebitis is associated with internal neoplasia (especially of the pancreas; see Ch. 12) but also occurs due to oral contraceptives, anticardiolipin antibodies, and thrombophilia (e.g. protein C or S deficiency), and in Behçet disease (see Ch. 14).

Treatment is usually symptomatic (elevation, support stockings, and non-steroidal antiinflammatory agents), but anticoagulant drugs and fibrinolytic agents may be required.

Cholesterol crystal embolization

This is an arterial wall disease etiologically, but usually presents in the skin as a livedo, or vasculitic or embolic disorder, and is discussed in Chapter 14.

VENOUS DISEASE

Varicose veins

The venous system is lined with one-way valves that direct blood back to the heart. With age, or as a result of inherited poor or absent valves, these valves may become progressively incompetent. Dilated or varicose veins result.

Large varicose veins (Fig. 15.47) and smaller telangiectases (spider veins) occur on the legs. One of the first signs of venous insufficiency is the ankle flare (Fig. 15.48), which appears as a crown of dilated venules about the medial ankle. Occasionally, a superficial varicosity may ulcerate through the skin, with significant bleeding.

Investigation to define the origin and extent of the varicose veins and the competence of the deeper venous system can involve physical examination, blood pressure measurement, Doppler ultrasound, and phlebography. Sclerotherapy may be helpful for smaller vessels, surgery for larger lesions. An intense pulsed light source is effective for leg veins of 0.1–3 mm in diameter, with most cases showing better than 50% clearance.

Acroangiodermatitis

This disease is a vascular lesion of the extremities, clinically resembling Kaposi sarcoma. It may occur in the setting of venous insufficiency or it may arise over either a congenital vascular malformation or an acquired arteriovenous fistula (Fig. 15.49).

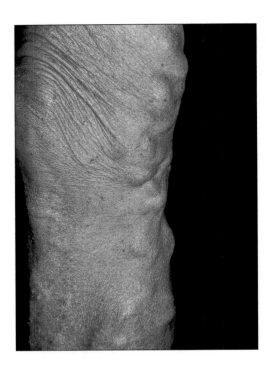

Figure 15.47 Varicose veins.

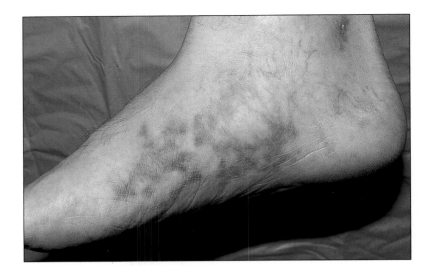

Figure 15.49 Acroangiodermatitis in the setting of venous insufficiency.

In severe cases, ulceration may develop. A venous ulcer is most common just above the medial malleolus. This is where venous hypertension is the highest. The ulcer is usually moist. The edges may be raised up or relatively level with the base of the ulcer. The surrounding skin may be eczematous. An odor may result from infection or simple colonization (Fig. 15.52).

Differential diagnosis

The differential diagnosis of leg ulceration is given in Table 15.4.

Venous eczema is usually apparent by its distribution, but asteatotic eczema, eczema due to sudden development of leg edema, and contact dermatitis (either primary or as a complication of treating venous eczema or ulcers) need to be excluded.

Bacterial colonization of ulcers may need to be distinguished from local cellulitis.

Treatment

Leg edema *must* be controlled or prevented. Prolonged standing should be avoided. Walking is allowed. Elevate the legs, ankle above the heart, for 20 min every 2–3 h. Elevate the foot of the bed 2–3 inches. Compression stockings or bandages from the mid-foot (including the heel) to just below the knee are essential. A three- or four-layer compression bandage (multilayer elastic compression) is very helpful in treating both stasis dermatitis and stasis ulcer. However, an ankle:brachial systolic pressure ratio should be calculated. If significantly lower than 0.8, then arterial compromise is present and compression therapy should not be used; compression should be used with caution if the ratio is between 0.8 and 1.0.

Salt restriction may be needed to control swelling. Diuretics may be appropriate for some patients with cardiac disease causing edema. Medium-potency topical steroid ointments twice daily are useful for eczematous changes. Soaks twice a day are helpful if the skin is exudative. Scratching should not be allowed.

If ulceration has developed, wound care must be carried out, including daily wound cleansing followed by application of an occlusive dressing. Stop all topical salves except those absolutely necessary, as allergic contact dermatitis is common. Once the ulcer is clean, a four-layer bandage can be applied for a week at a time.

Both superficial and deep venous incompetence occur, and sclerotherapy or surgery may speed healing and/or reduce recurrences. The lesion should be monitored for secondary infection by both bacteria and *Candida*. Any putrid smell may be combated with metronidazole gel. If the ulcer is uninfected, a plaster boot (e.g. Unna boot) may be applied and changed every 1–2 weeks.

Pentoxifylline 400–800 mg t.i.d. when combined with compression does seem to improve healing rates.

Atrophie blanche

A stellate white scar is seen on the ankle. Many consider atrophie blanche to be the scarred end point of various diseases (Fig. 15.53).

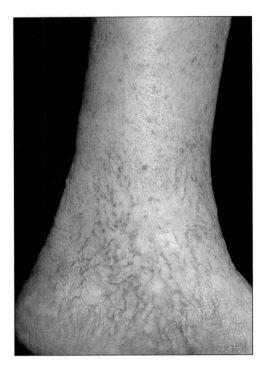

Figure 15.48 Ankle flare. A crown of dilated venules about the medial ankle is a sure sign of underlying chronic venous insufficiency. No treatment is needed, but appropriate work-up and therapy for chronic venous insufficiency may be needed at some point. (Sclerotherapy may be used in appropriate cases.)

Stasis dermatitis and venous ulceration
Etiology and pathogenesis

Stasis dermatitis is an eczematous condition of the leg that results from edema. If the stasis is severe, ulceration may result. The calf pump mechanism ensures adequate blood flow through the lower leg. When the calf muscle contracts, the blood is forced out and back to the heart. When the muscle relaxes, reflux of blood is prevented by venous valves. If either the superficial or deep venous valves are incompetent, venous hypertension occurs. If the muscle does not contract adequately in the first place, musculoskeletal calf pump dysfunction may occur. Osteoarthritis, stroke, rheumatoid arthritis, or obesity are common causative factors.

Clinical

The patient will present with swollen legs and a red, scaly rash over the medial part of the ankle (Figs 15.50 and 15.51). The entire lower leg may be involved. In later stages, the skin may develop a red-brown hue secondary to hemosiderin deposition. Allergic contact dermatitis to topical medication may complicate the clinical picture. Lipodermatosclerosis may also be present.

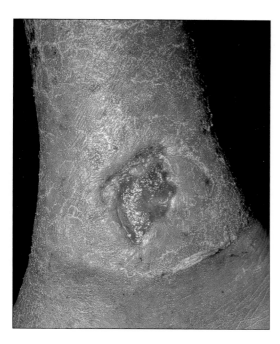

Figure 15.50 Stasis ulcer. Any ulcer in this location with surrounding edema, redness, and scale is typical of a stasis ulcer.

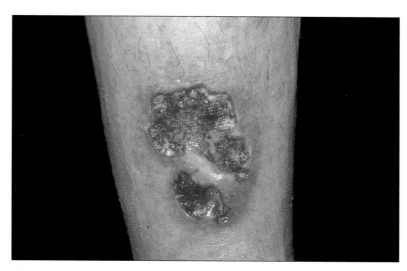

Figure 15.52 Basal cell carcinoma. This chronic ulcer of the shin was treated for 2 years as a venous ulcer. A biopsy should be performed on any non-healing leg ulcer.

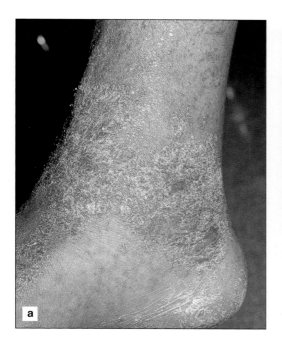

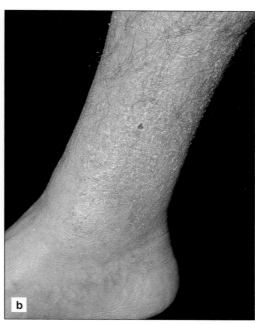

Figure 15.51 Stasis dermatitis. (**a**) Red, scaly changes over the medial ankle have developed in this older man with impaired venous circulation. (**b**) A leg that served as the donor site of a vein graft is at increased risk for stasis dermatitis. (**c**) Stasis dermatitis associated with varicose veins. In this patient, eczematous changes occurred over varicose veins. (**d**) The leg on the left shows active disease, whereas the one on the right shows chronic changes.

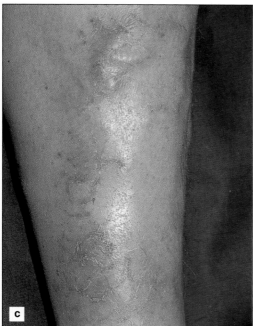

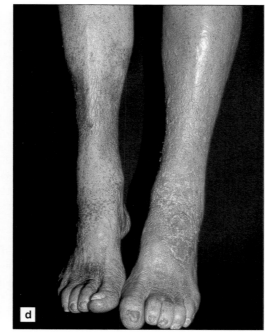

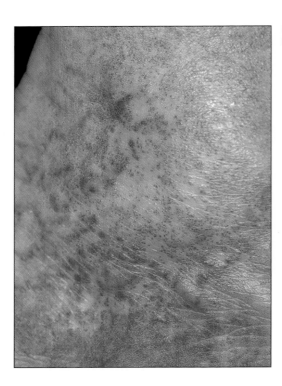

Figure 15.53 Atrophie blanche.

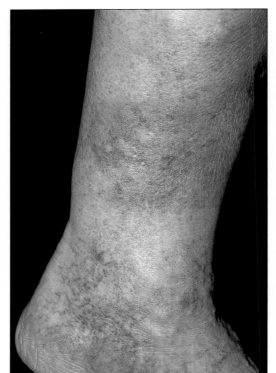

Figure 15.54 Lipodermatosclerosis. This patient showed three manifestations of venous insufficiency: lipodermatosclerosis, atrophie blanche, and an ankle flare.

Lipodermatosclerosis

Lipodermatosclerosis, also known as sclerosing panniculitis, represents deep stasis; that is, the dermis and fat develop inflammation and sclerosis in the setting of venous insufficiency. In the acute phase, the skin of the medial lower leg, just above the ankle, is tender, warm, and erythematous. Ulceration is uncommon. As the condition becomes chronic, the skin becomes indurated and adherent. Other signs of chronic venous insufficiency may be noted (Fig. 15.54). A biopsy should be avoided if possible, as healing will invariably be difficult. Large series associate lipodermatosclerosis with female gender, high body mass index, venous disease, and middle age.

The usual measures to diagnose and treat chronic venous insufficiency should be followed, with emphasis on the faithful use of compression stockings. Stanozolol (2 mg twice a day) has been recommended for the acute phase, although it may cause significant side effects and should be used only by those familiar with it. It is also helpful to reduce the chronic signs of lipodermatosclerosis, but not to heal any ulcers that have developed. Pentoxifylline (400 mg three times a day) has been suggested.

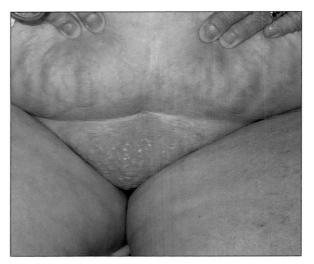

Figure 15.55 Lymphedema from cardiomyopathy causing lymphangiomas of the pubic area. This may also occur on the scrotum.

PRACTICE POINTS

- In the management of venous ulcers, leg edema must be controlled or prevented. Compression bandages from the mid-foot (including the heel) to just below the knee are more effective than any topical medicament or dressing.
- Patients with venous eczema are particularly prone to development of contact dermatitis; this may be due to the contents of emollients (fragrances and preservatives) or topical medications (antibiotics such as aminoglycosides, corticosteroids, and preservatives), or may be due to rubber chemicals in elasticated support bandages.
- Bacterial evaluation of leg ulcers needs the results to be evaluated in the clinical context; colonization of ulcers needs to be distinguished from local cellulitis.

In developed countries, a minority of cases are due to an inherited predisposition with onset expected at various ages in childhood or young adult life (e.g. Milroy disease); such cases are often severe, due to anatomic abnormalities of the lymphatics. It is also an early feature in Turner syndrome.

More commonly, lymphedema of the legs is the end result of chronic edema (of various causes) combined with poor mobility in older patients, especially in women; the classic pattern has been termed 'armchair legs'. Many now feel that any chronic edema state, even if primarily cardiac, will involve at least some component of lymphedema (Fig. 15.55).

Other causes include lymphatic obstruction of a limb (arm or leg) due to tumor, lymphadenectomy, or radiation therapy to lymph nodes.

Clinical

Mild lymphedema of the legs may be indistinguishable from edema of cardiac causation but is refractory to diuretic therapy. With chronicity, redness of the legs may become prominent, and warty or nodular lesions develop (Fig. 15.56). A chronically enlarged, edematous leg or legs with a verrucous or cobblestoned surface is characteristic (Fig. 15.57). Stemmer sign, thickening of the skin over the dorsal toes, is highly characteristic.

LYMPHATIC DISEASE

Lymphedema and chronic edema
Etiology and pathogenesis

Lymphedema occurs in several situations. In many tropical countries, the commonest cause is infection by filariae, which cause lymphatic obstruction leading to elephantiasis of the legs, scrotum, penis, and vulva.

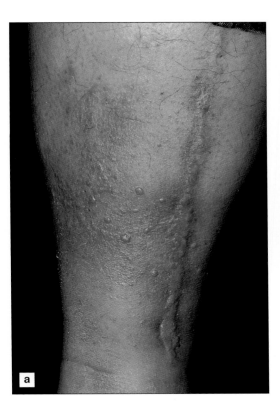

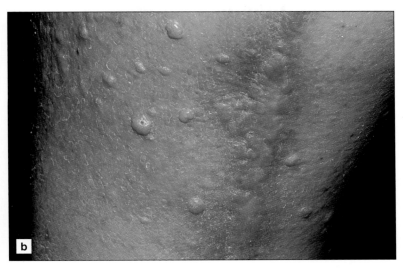

Figure 15.56 Stasis dermatitis aggravated by saphenous vein grafting. (**a**,**b**) Note the edematous leg, papillomatous thickening, and the vein graft scar.

Figure 15.58 Bulla formation in the setting of stasis dermatitis. The rapid onset or exacerbation of leg edema may induce bulla formation.

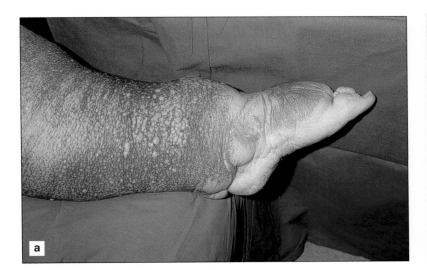

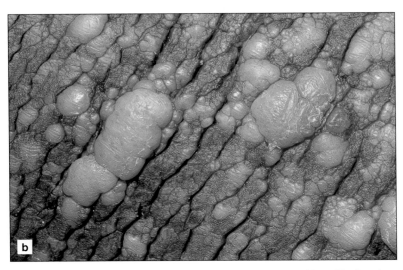

Figure 15.57 Elephantiasis nostras. (**a**) Note greatly thickened leg with distortion of features. (**b**) Close-up view shows multiple papules and nodules.

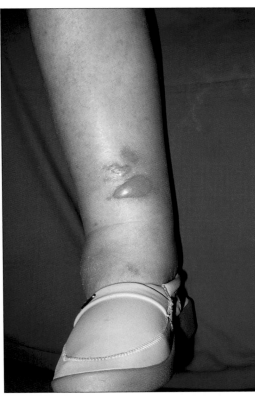

In its most advanced chronic stages, the skin of the leg is 'mossy', cobblestoned, or verrucous, a pattern termed elephantiasis nostras verrucosa.

Bullae may occur (Fig. 15.58) and are more likely to form if the edema develops or increases in severity acutely. A reticulate pattern of ridges on the lower leg in lymphedema appears to follow thermal damage, similar to the patterning in EAI, and has been termed lymphedema ab igne.

Recurrent streptococcal cellulitis is a frequent and important complication of chronic edema or lymphedema, and requires aggressive therapy (Fig. 15.59).

Ulceration may occur, and chronic weeping from such areas is difficult to manage.

315

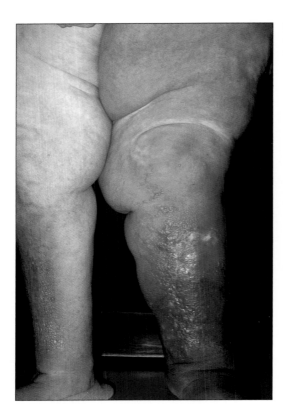

Figure 15.59 Bacterial cellulitis in the setting of chronic lymphedema.

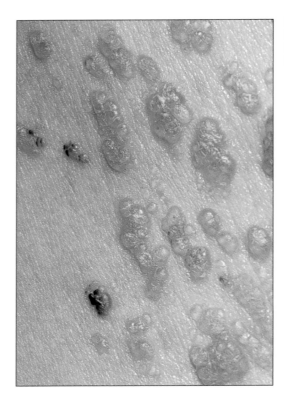

Figure 15.60 Lymphangioma. These lesions represent dilated lymphatic vessels.

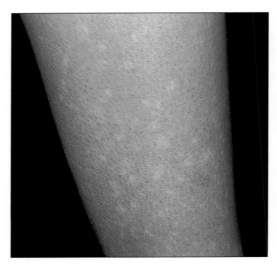

Figure 15.61 White avascular spots. These white spots are most commonly seen on the arms of young women. They represent a relative decrease in blood content and are entirely benign.

Differential diagnosis

This includes pure cardiac edema and pretibial myxedema, plus rare disorders such as lichen myxedematosus; the main diagnostic issue is between the different causes of lymphedema.

The redness of chronic edema may be confused with cellulitis but is typically bilateral and is not associated with pyrexia or malaise; it commonly causes diagnostic difficulty in determining whether a true episode of cellulitis has settled.

Treatment

Elevation of the legs, support hose, and antibiotics for infection (aggressive treatment with intravenous penicillin) are all helpful. Daily compression may be useful for severe cases. A 'short stretch' bandage is best in lymphedema, as compression is only effective during activity, as this stimulates lymph flow. A high-potency topical steroid may decrease the pebbly thickening. Acitretin, an oral retinoid, may be tried for the verrucous change.

For those with upper limb lymphedema, and to a lesser extent for the legs, massage treatments to each quadrant of the trunk in turn (the area adjacent to the affected limb last) can be helpful.

PRACTICE POINTS

- It is often stated that cardiac edema can be pitted by pressure but that lymphedema cannot; this is not correct. Pitting occurs in early lymphedema but becomes less possible with chronicity as fibrosis occurs.
- The redness of chronic edema may be confused with cellulitis but is typically bilateral and is not per se associated with pyrexia or malaise; cellulitis is a common complication of lymphedema but is rarely symmetric.

Lymphangioma

Just as blood vessels may dilate, forming hemangiomas, lymphatic vessels may dilate, forming lymphangiomas. Grouped vesicles, with onset from birth to adulthood, are characteristic of lymphangioma circumscriptum (Fig. 15.60). The fluid may be blood-tinged or show a blood–fluid line. These lesions often communicate with deeper lymphatics, which may explain why therapy involving simple destruction commonly leads to recurrence.

No treatment is necessary. Simple destruction or surgical excision may be tried. The CO_2 laser or, if the fluid is blood-tinged, the tunable dye laser, can be used.

VASCULAR STEAL

White avascular spots

White, avascular macules approximately 5 mm in size (Fig. 15.61) may occasionally be seen on the arms and legs of white people, usually in children or in women. Occasionally, they are numerous enough to prompt a patient to seek medical attention. The white macules are due to decreased blood content, probably secondary to local arteriolar vasoconstriction. There is often a centrally placed prominent red arteriole if the lesions are examined carefully. Compression of this restores the normal color (by contrast to idiopathic guttate hypomelanosis, which is unaffected by pressure). No treatment is needed or known to be effective.

Nevus anemicus

The white appearance of the nevus anemicus results from a paucity of blood within the lesion, secondary to permanent vasoconstriction. This vasoconstriction is a result of hyperreactivity to normal levels of circulating catecholamines. Vitiligo may look similar, but is whiter than nevus anemicus, and the edges cannot be obliterated with pressure. In addition, Wood's light accentuates vitiligo but makes the nevus anemicus invisible (as the epidermal pigment is normal).

This uncommon, congenital, white patch occurs most commonly on the trunk. The border is irregular and sharply demarcated, but can be obliterated by blanching the surrounding skin (Fig. 15.62). It seems to be more common in females and may be seen in association with a PWS.

There is no known effective treatment.

RADIATION THERAPY

Radiation dermatitis
Etiology and pathogenesis
Radiation therapy, if given in sufficient quantity, causes irreversible damage to the skin. The acute phase of radiation dermatitis may be likened to a sunburn. Chronic radiation dermatitis, which develops years to decades after the exposure, leads to fibrosis and, potentially, the development of

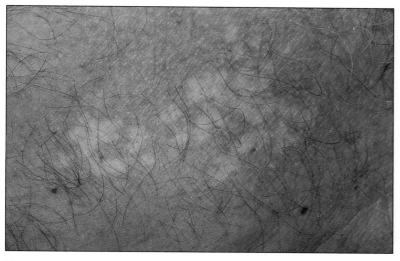

Figure 15.62 Nevus anemicus. The edges can be obliterated with pressure, verifying that this white lesion is caused by decreased blood content, not decreased pigment.

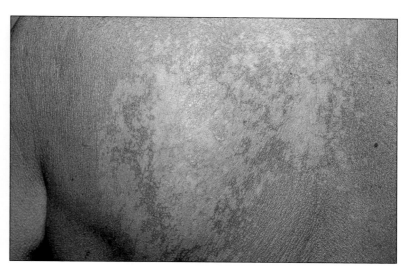

Figure 15.63 Acute radiation dermatitis. The skin is red and inflamed in this radiation port.

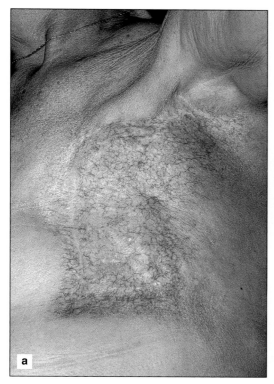

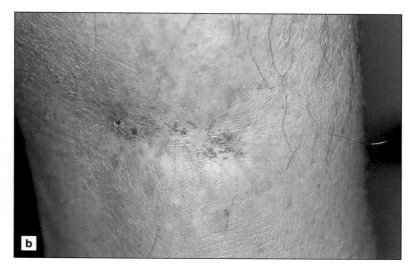

Figure 15.64 Radiation damage. (**a**) Multiple telangiectases years after mastectomy and radiation therapy for breast cancer. (**b**) Atrophy, scarring, and telangiectases years after X-ray treatment for a childhood hemangioma. (**c**) Multiple comedones developing in a radiation port. The development of comedones after UV damage is analogous to that seen in Favre–Racouchot syndrome.

malignant skin tumors. Typical sources of radiation damage are treatment for breast cancer (mastectomy site), cardiac catheterization (axilla), or X-ray epilation (scalp).

Clinical

In acute radiation dermatitis, the skin is bright red in the areas exposed to X-rays (Fig. 15.63). Months to years after radiation therapy, patients may develop atrophy, induration, fibrosis, prominent telangiectases, and hypo- or hyperpigmentation (Fig. 15.64). Rarely, comedones may develop. The affected skin is more likely than normal skin to develop basal or squamous cell carcinomas.

Differential diagnosis

The main issue is in those whose radiotherapy was for a skin neoplasm, as distinguishing recurrent tumor from ulcerated radionecrosis may be clinically difficult. Significant pain favors radionecrosis.

Treatment

Acute radiation dermatitis may be treated with topical steroids. There is no good treatment for chronic radiation dermatitis other than monitoring for malignancy, but if ulceration occurs it is worth considering the role of secondary infection by obtaining bacteriology swab results before embarking on a biopsy.

FURTHER READING

Boon LM, Mulliken JB, Enjolras O, et al. Glomuvenous malformation (glomangioma) and venous malformation. Distinct clinicopathologic and genetic entities. Arch Dermatol 2004; 140: 971–6

Enjolras O, Mulliken JB. Vascular tumors and vascular malformations (new issues). Adv Dermatol 1997; 13: 375–422

Esterly NB. Cutaneous hemangiomas, vascular stains and malformations, and associated syndromes. Curr Probl Dermatol 1995; 7: 65–108

Mekkes JR, Loots MAM, van der Waal AC, et al. Causes, investigation and treatment of leg ulceration. Br J Dermatol 2003; 148: 388–401

Mortimer PS, Levick JR. Chronic peripheral oedema: the critical role of the lymphatic system. Clin Med 204; 4: 448–53

Page EH, Shear NH. Temperature dependent skin disorders. J Am Acad Dermatol 1988; 18: 1003–19

16 Blistering Disorders

INTRODUCTION

Blisters are formed when a potential space within or beneath the epidermis fills with fluid. Depending on the thickness and structural integrity of the blister roof, there may be an obvious tense blister or just an erosion with wrinkled epidermis at the margin. Blisters occur for reasons as trivial as frictional injury, while at the opposite end of the spectrum there are potentially lethal immunobullous disorders and drug-induced blistering. It is therefore important to understand an approach to diagnosis of blistering eruptions.

APPROACH TO BLISTERING ERUPTIONS

Classification, patterns, and causes of blistering

Blisters may be classified according to:
- aetiology, for example immunobullous, mechanobullous, infective, or inflammatory (Table 16.1); and
- pathologic features, such as the part of the skin where blister formation occurs (e.g. intraepidermal or subepidermal).

Each of these classifications has clinical relevance. It is important to interpret the clinical morphology, as this helps in identification of the level of blistering within the skin, which in turn narrows the diagnostic possibilities. For example, subepidermal blisters with a normal epidermis over the blister split are typically tense, unilocular blisters (e.g. bullous pemphigoid), intraepidermal blisters may present as crusts rather than intact blisters (e.g. pemphigus), and blisters with epidermal necrosis look gray even if they actually have clear fluid content (e.g. erythema multiforme). Associated clinical history such as duration, features such as inflammation, and investigations such as immunopathology all help to refine the diagnosis.

Investigation of blistering disorders

The investigation of blisters will, in general, fall into three categories.
- History and examination—clinical history, family history, antecedent events including possible contact allergens, medications, pattern and morphology of the blisters and of any associated rash, mucous membrane involvement, etc.
- Investigations to establish the cause or diagnosis—skin biopsy is usually the most important, but tests such as swabs for bacteriology or virology may be important if infection is suspected, and others such as antibodies for vasculitis, porphyrin levels, etc. may be dictated by the likely diagnosis in individual cases. To diagnose the immunobullous disorders, skin biopsies generally require some tissue to be frozen for direct immunofluorescence (see later). It is helpful to appreciate important structures in the skin of relevance to blistering disorders (Fig. 16.1).
- Investigations needed as a therapeutic baseline—especially for immuno-bullous disorders, where corticosteroids or immunosuppressive therapy may be required (check blood pressure, glucose, full blood count, and renal and hepatic function); see Chapter 4 for more detail.

MECHANICAL AND PHYSICAL CAUSES OF BLISTERING

Traumatic causes of blistering

The commonest causes of blistering are those due to simple physical, chemical, or thermal trauma. Blisters due to friction or burn injury (Fig. 16.2) are most common in the community but are generally not seen by dermatologists. Cold injury (including therapeutic cryotherapy) and pressure are less common causes.

Edema of the lower leg (Fig. 16.3) is a very under-recognized cause of blistering, which is most apparent in the elderly. It typically occurs when the edema has developed rapidly, for example as a result of stopping diuretic therapy. Blisters are confined to the lower leg and have clear fluid content (at least initially). The main differential diagnosis is from bullous pemphigoid.

Epidermolysis bullosa

The major mechanobullous disorders are those in which there is an inherited defect in structures such as hemidesmosomes or anchoring fibrils, making the skin more fragile and susceptible to mechanical stimuli that produce blisters, notably friction and other direct trauma (Fig. 16.4). This group of disorders, collectively known as epidermolysis bullosa, is discussed in Chapter 19.

Table 16.1   CAUSES OF BLISTERING

Category	Cause
Physical	Friction, burns, pressure, edema (Figs 16.2–16.5) Miliaria (Ch. 23)
Inherited	Epidermolysis bullosa (mild physical damage, inherited predisposition to blistering) Hailey–Hailey disease (Fig. 16.39 and Ch. 19)
Inflammatory	Eczemas, pompholyx (Ch. 6), drug and plant phototoxicity (Ch. 17) Erythema multiforme and Stevens–Johnson syndrome (Ch. 11), toxic epidermal necrolysis (Ch. 18) Fixed drug eruption (Ch. 18) Vasculitis (Ch. 14) Neutrophilic dermatoses (Sweet disease, pyoderma gangrenosum, subcorneal pustular dermatosis; Ch. 14) Rare variants of systemic lupus erythematosus (Ch. 13), lichen planus (Ch. 8), lichen sclerosus (see Fig. 16.13)
Infections	Bacterial (Ch. 24): staphylococci (impetigo, staphylococcal scalded skin, blistering distal dactylitis), streptococci (impetigo, cellulitis, blistering distal dactylitis) Viral (Ch. 25): herpesviruses (herpes simplex, varicella, herpes zoster), hand foot and mouth disease, orf
Bites and infestations	Insect bites or papular urticaria Scabies (Fig. 16.10 and Ch. 27)
Immunobullous	Pemphigus, pemphigoid, cicatricial pemphigoid, dermatitis herpetiformis, linear IgA disease or chronic bullous dermatosis of childhood, epidermolysis bullosa acquisita, paraneoplastic pemphigus (all this chapter), pemphigoid gestationis (Ch. 12)
Metabolic	Porphyria, pseudoporphyria (Ch. 17), cutaneous amyloidosis (Ch. 11)

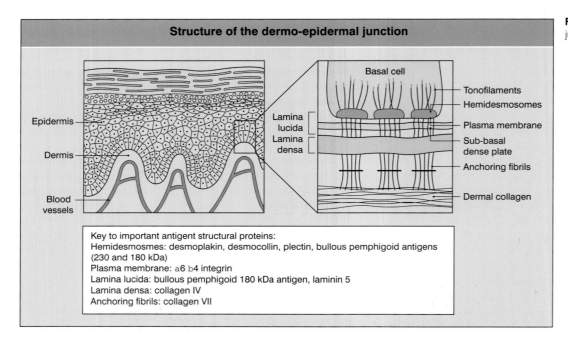

Structure of the dermo-epidermal junction

Basal cell

Tonofilaments
Hemidesmosomes
Plasma membrane
Sub-basal dense plate
Anchoring fibrils
Dermal collagen

Lamina lucida
Lamina densa

Epidermis
Dermis
Blood vessels

Key to important antigent structural proteins:
Hemidesmosmes: desmoplakin, desmocollin, plectin, bullous pemphigoid antigens (230 and 180 kDa)
Plasma membrane: a6 b4 integrin
Lamina lucida: bullous pemphigoid 180 kDa antigen, laminin 5
Lamina densa: collagen IV
Anchoring fibrils: collagen VII

Figure 16.1   Structures of the dermo–epidermal junction (basement membrane zone).

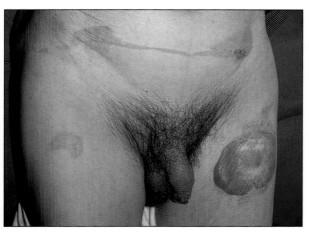

Figure 16.2   Thermal burn on the abdomen due to boiling water spilt from a kettle. The linear shape at the site of constriction of the waistband suggests an external cause, and there was sparing in the area of the patient's underclothing due to the protection given by the additional layer of thicker material.

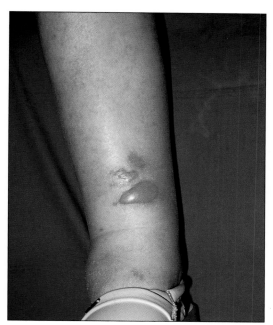

Figure 16.3 A tense unilocular blister with clear fluid content and featureless background on the lower leg due to rapid development of edema of the leg. In some such instances, there may be an asteatotic eczema appearance; in longstanding edema, there may be marked redness as well.

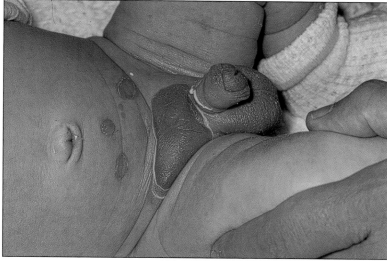

Figure 16.5 Localized impetigo in the groin of an infant. Blisters in impetigo are superficial and rupture easily, but a rim of old blister is clearly visible.

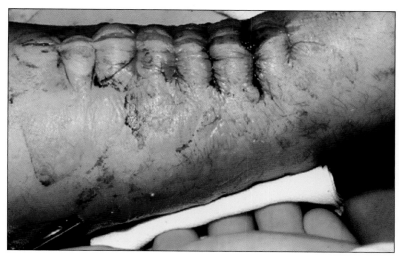

Figure 16.4 Patients with epidermolysis bullosa blister easily as a result of injury, in this case the combination of trauma and the handling required during orthopedic surgery.

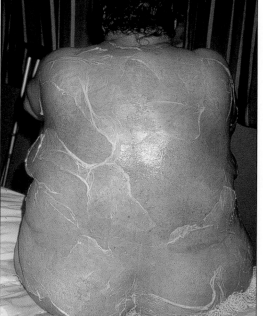

Figure 16.6 Staphylococcal scalded skin syndrome (SSSS) is an exotoxin-mediated blistering eruption due to staphylococcal infection. It usually occurs in children, but may occur in adults who have impaired renal function (the toxin is excreted in urine) or who are immunosuppressed. This patient was a rare example of adult SSSS with neither of these background factors, but with a severely infected hip wound. See also Chapter 24.

Epidermolysis bullosa acquisita is an unrelated immunologically mediated disease in which skin fragility is a prominent feature, discussed later in this chapter.

INFECTIVE CAUSES OF BLISTERING

Bacterial infections

Infections that may cause blisters or pustules are numerous; see Chapter 24. The most common are staphylococcal infections (local blistering in impetigo, more widespread toxin-mediated blistering in staphylococcal scalded skin syndrome (SSSS), Figs 16.5 and 16.6) and streptococcal infections causing erysipelas or cellulitis.

Staphylococcal scalded skin syndrome is due to toxin-producing staphylococci. It is usually manifest only in children or in immuno-suppressed or renally impaired adults, but occurs occasionally in healthy adults. The main differential diagnosis is toxic epidermal necrolysis.

Viral infections

These are discussed in more detail in Chapter 25. Herpes infections such as herpes simplex or varicella zoster typically produce vesicles or blisters (Figs 16.7 and 16.8).

Bites and infestations

A number of venomous bites from spiders and insects may cause blisters, some of which may be necrotic. Several biting insects cause an eruption known as papular urticaria, which generally occurs on the legs (Fig. 16.9).

Pustules or blisters on the soles of the feet in infants are strongly suspicious of scabies (Fig. 16.10), which is discussed in Chapter 27.

PRACTICE POINTS

- Lower leg edema is a common and under-recognized cause of blistering, usually in elderly patients and usually occurring when the edema has developed rapidly.
- Extensive superficial blistering in an unwell child with no previous blistering problem is likely to be staphylococcal scalded skin; prompt antistaphylococcal antibiotic therapy is required.
- Blisters on the soles of the feet of an infant are strongly suggestive of scabies.

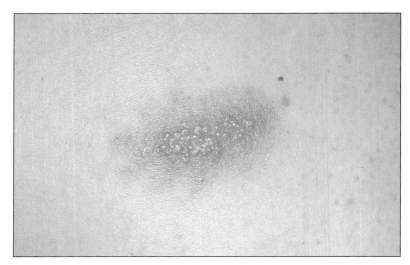

Figure 16.7 Herpes simplex: a localized area of erythema with closely clustered, uniformly sized vesicles.

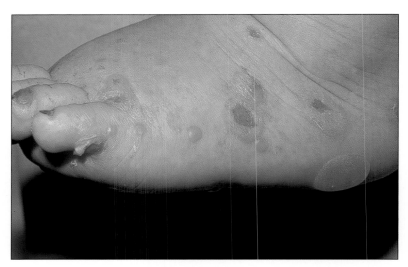

Figure 16.10 Scabies infestation in infants often causes vesicopustules on the feet. Sometimes larger blisters are seen, as shown here. The presence of larger blisters on the hands in scabies affecting older children usually represents secondary impetigo.

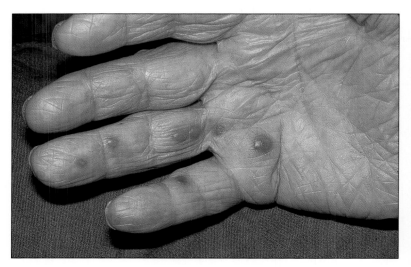

Figure 16.8 Herpes zoster affecting the C8 distribution of the hand. The blisters are often larger than in varicella.

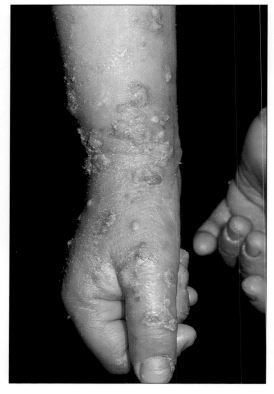

Figure 16.11 Streptococcal infection in a child with atopic eczema: large blisters with cloudy fluid content.

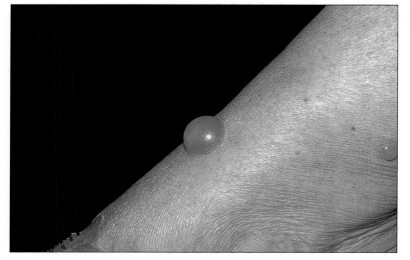

Figure 16.9 Papular urticaria may have a mixed morphology, with papules, crusted lesions, and blisters. In this case, the blisters do not have apparent background inflammatory changes. A typical pattern is one of scattered lesions on the lower legs, and most cases occur in the summer months (sometimes recurring annually).

INFLAMMATORY CAUSES OF BLISTERING

Eczemas and related disorders

Eczemas often cause vesicles or frank blisters, especially the pompholyx pattern on the hands and feet (Ch. 6). Blistering in eczema is sometimes due to secondary infection, in which case there is usually a cloudy fluid content (Fig. 16.11). Acute allergic contact eczemas also tend to cause blistering, particularly the types due to plants (Fig. 16.12). Many other inflammatory dermatoses may occasionally cause blistering (Fig. 16.13).

Phototoxic reactions (Fig. 16.14) due to psoralens in plants and fruits are a cause of blistering that often leaves residual pigmentation. This is discussed further in Chapter 17.

Erythema multiforme and Stevens–Johnson syndrome

These conditions are discussed in more detail in Chapter 11. Erythema multiforme produces skin lesions; Stevens–Johnson syndrome also affects mucous membranes (Fig. 16.15).

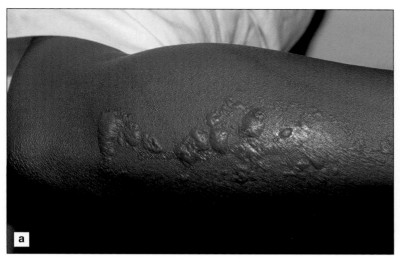

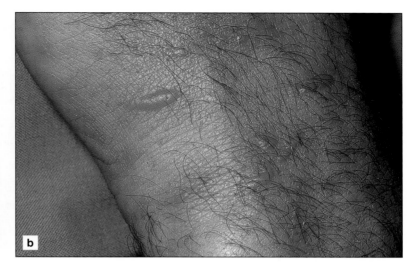

Figure 16.12 Contact allergy. (**a**) Contact allergy appearing on the forearm. Blistering is unusual in endogenous eczema at this site. (**b**) Allergy to an ivy plant. The lesions are often linear in shape, as the limb has brushed against the culprit foliage.

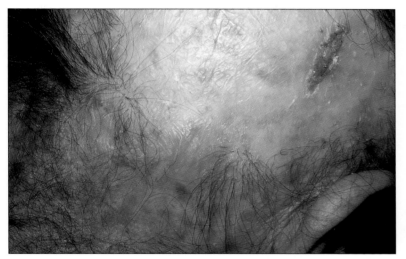

Figure 16.13 Bullous lichen sclerosus is very unusual. It may cause significant scarring, as shown here with a large blister on the posterior scalp.

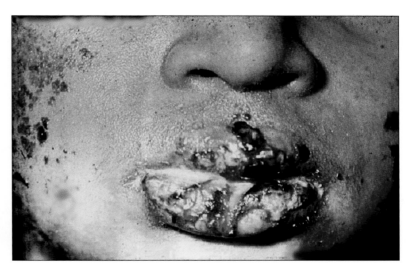

Figure 16.15 Stevens–Johnson syndrome, showing mucosal blistering and crusting (see also Ch. 11). (Courtesy of Dr. G. Dawn.)

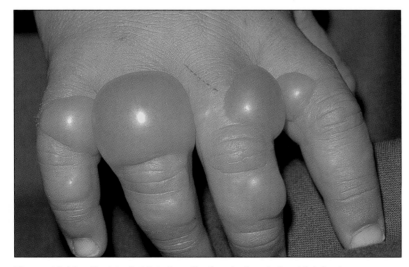

Figure 16.14 Phototoxic blistering affecting the hand of a child. Such cases are often due to fruit juices, such as lemon or lime, or from contact with common hedgerow plants of the Umbelliferae family. (Courtesy of Dr. W. D. Paterson.)

Drugs

Drugs may cause blistering of several types (Table 16.2; see also Ch. 18). The most severe is toxic epidermal necrolysis (Fig. 16.16).

Subcorneal pustular dermatosis (Sneddon–Wilkinson disease)

Etiology and pathogenesis

Most cases are of unknown etiology, but a significant minority have an underlying monoclonal gammopathy (usually IgA type) or myeloma.

Clinical

Most patients are adult, and there is a female predominance. The lesions are bullous or pustular, and may consist of clear fluid with a 'pus level' as occurs also in bullous pemphigoid (Fig. 16.17). In subcorneal pustular dermatosis, they are often grouped lesions with an annular polycyclic arrangement (Fig. 16.18). The trunk and flexures are the main sites. Biopsy shows an extremely superficial (subcorneal) pustule with neutrophil content; some cases have positive intercellular direct immunofluorescence for IgA. Pyoderma gangrenosum may occasionally coexist, usually, but not invariably, in patients with a paraproteinemia.

Differential diagnosis

The blisters in this condition may resemble those of pemphigoid or of impetigo, although other bullous eruptions may also be considered.

Table 16.2   DIFFERENT MECHANISMS OR PATTERNS OF DRUG ERUPTION THAT MAY CAUSE BLISTERS

Mechanism or pattern	Comments
Fixed drug eruption	Usually solitary, localized; may be bullous, heal with pigmentation
Erythema multiforme or toxic epidermal necrolysis	Associated with isolated or semiconfluent background inflammation; see Chapter 18 for likely causes (also Fig. 16.15)
Photosensitivity	Blisters on a background of eczematous rash in photosensitive distribution
Porphyria and pseudoporphyria	Porphyria cutanea tarda (PCT) pattern of blisters and skin fragility, mainly hands and face; PCT may be provoked by estrogens, pseudoporphyria especially by furosemide and naproxen
Blistering at pressure areas	Classically due to barbiturate-induced coma
Eruptions that resemble idiopathic immunobullous disorders	Some are provocation of immunobullous disease (e.g. penicillamine-induced pemphigus, vancomycin-induced linear IgA disease, progesterone dermatitis), others are non-specific or resemble other inflammatory disease patterns (see also Ch. 18)

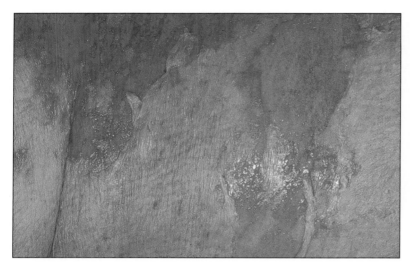

Figure 16.16   Toxic epidermal necrolysis. The fragile sheared blisters and resulting erosions cannot be distinguished clinically from staphylococcal scalded skin syndrome, but the level of blister splitting is different and most cases of toxic epidermal necrolysis are in adults.

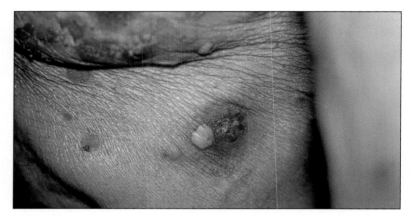

Figure 16.18   Subcorneal pustular dermatosis, demonstrating typical grouped crusting and large pustules. Pemphigoid may be considered clinically, but biopsy shows an extremely superficial (subcorneal) pustule with neutrophil content. (Courtesy of Gary W. Cole, M.D.)

Treatment

The disorder usually responds to sulfones such as dapsone (see Ch. 4). Any associated gammopathy must also be treated. Phototherapy has also been used.

Other disorders

Many other disorders can on occasion cause pustules, vesicles, or bullae, but are described in other chapters. For example, fungal infections (especially of the foot) may cause blisters.

IMMUNOBULLOUS DISORDERS

Introduction

This is an uncommon but important group of disorders, in which there are circulating and tissue antibodies against normal skin structures (Table 16.3). It is important to have some concept of the relevant immunofluorescence testing that confirms these diagnoses, each of which has typical immunopathology features. Two types of test are routinely performed, detailed here; more specialized techniques, such as immuno-blotting, are used to confirm the molecular weight of target antigens.

Immunofluorescence tests
Direct immunofluorescence testing

Direct immunofluorescence (DIF) testing (Fig. 19.19) is performed on a biopsy of perilesional skin or, in the case of dermatitis herpetiformis, from sites of predilection. The rationale for using perilesional skin is that this is

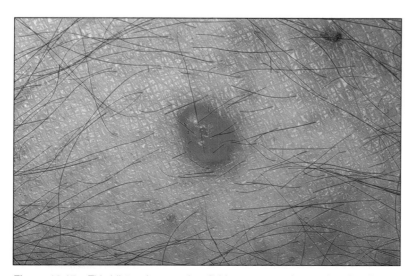

Figure 16.17   This blister shows a clear fluid component above a 'pus level' determined by gravity, in this instance in a case of bullous pemphigoid. This may also occur in subcorneal pustular dermatosis and in impetigo.

Table 16.3   THE IMMUNOBULLOUS DISORDERS AND THEIR TARGET ANTIGENS

Disease	Antigen(s)	Location of direct immunofluorescence
Bullous pemphigoid (BP)	BP230 (BPAg1; 230 kDa) BP180 (BPAg2; 180 kDa)	Basement membrane zone; both are in basal cells and lamina lucida
Pemphigus foliaceous (PF)	Desmoglein 1 (Dg1; 160 kDa)	Epidermal intercellular – a component of keratinocyte desmosomes

Pemphigus vulgaris (PV)
  Mucosal only
  Mucosal and skin
	Desmoglein 3 (Dg3; 130 kDa)
	Dg1 and Dg3
		As Dg1

Cicatricial pemphigoid (CP)	Laminin 5 Type XVII collagen β4-integrin (205 kDa) BP230	Lamina densa of basement membrane zone Lamina lucida of basement membrane zone Lamina lucida of basement membrane zone Lamina lucida of basement membrane zone
Paraneoplastic pemphigus (PNP)	Desmoplakin I (250 kDa) Desmoplakin II (210 kDa) Envoplakin (210 kDa) BP230 Periplakin (190 kDa, 170 kDa and (= plakglobin) 83 kDa)	Direct immunofluorescence in PNP is positive between epidermal cells and at the basement membrane zone
Epidermolysis bullosa acquisita (EBA)	α chain of type VII collagen (290 kDa) (also 145-kDa antigen)	Lamina densa and sublamina densa of basement membrane zone
Linear IgA disease (LAD)	Various proteins, including parts of type XVII collagen (97, 120, 285 kDa) and BP230	Lamina lucida of basement membrane zone
Dermatitis herpetiformis (DH)	Tissue transglutaminase	Basement membrane zone, sublamina densa

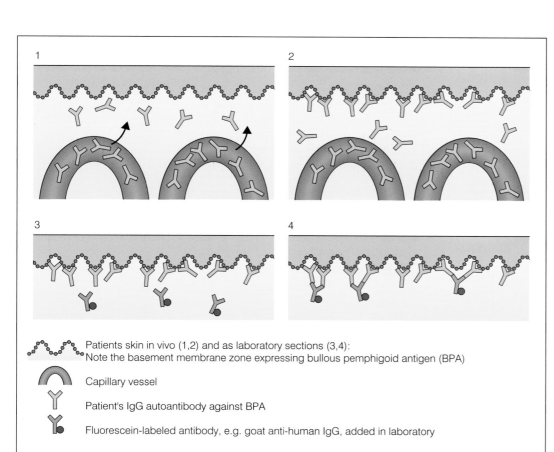

Patients skin in vivo (1,2) and as laboratory sections (3,4):
Note the basement membrane zone expressing bullous pemphigoid antigen (BPA)

Capillary vessel

Patient's IgG autoantibody against BPA

Fluorescein-labeled antibody, e.g. goat anti-human IgG, added in laboratory

Figure 16.19 Direct immunofluorescence testing. This test detects the patient's own autoantibodies to a normal structure, shown here using bullous pemphigoid antigen as an example. The circulating autoantibody (1) has passed from the vessels and has bound to the basement membrane zone *in vitro* (2), and can be identified in the laboratory using an appropriate fluorescein-labeled anti-human antibody (in this case, anti-IgG but other immunoglobulin types or antibodies to detect complement or fibrin may be relevant). This antibody is applied to the histology slide of lesional skin (3) and binds to the autoantibody that has already bound to the bullous pemphigoid antigen (4). Thus the agent that is bound or deposited, and the site binding, can be determined by fluorescence microscopy. (After an original drawing by Dr. N. H. Cox.)

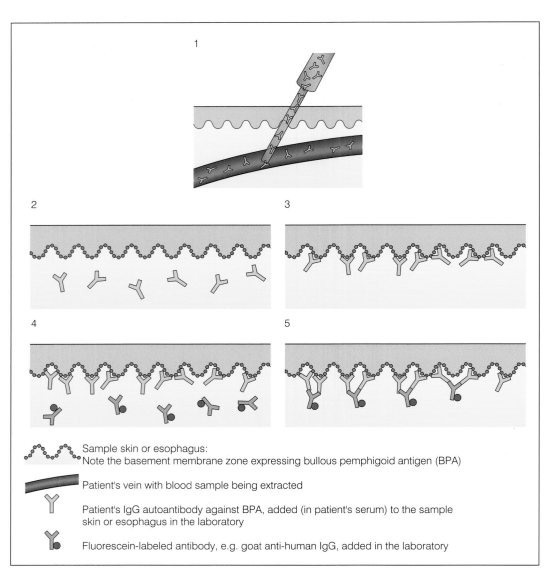

Figure 16.20 Indirect immunofluorescence testing. This test demonstrates that the patient has circulating autoantibodies to a normal structure, shown here using bullous pemphigoid antigen (BPA, a normal component of the basement membrane zone) as an example. The patient's serum, containing autoantibodies against BPA, is removed as a standard blood sample (1), and is incubated with an appropriate epithelial tissue (human, rodent or monkey skin, esophagus or bladder are all possible substrates depending on the likely diagnosis) (2). The antibodies will bind to the relevant antigens, in this case to BPA in the basement membrane zone (3). The binding can then be identified in the laboratory using an appropriate fluorescein-labeled anti-human antibody, as described for the latter part of the direct immunofluorescence test (4, 5). (After an original drawing by Dr. N. H. Cox.)

Sample skin or esophagus:
Note the basement membrane zone expressing bullous pemphigoid antigen (BPA)

Patient's vein with blood sample being extracted

Patient's IgG autoantibody against BPA, added (in patient's serum) to the sample skin or esophagus in the laboratory

Fluorescein-labeled antibody, e.g. goat anti-human IgG, added in the laboratory

intact, with the normal structures identifiable; blistered skin is more confusing due to the potential for loss of blister roof during processing, and because regeneration changes alter the perceived level of splitting within the skin. In DIF, the biopsy is frozen without chemical fixation and cut into thin tissue sections. These are then incubated with fluorescein-labeled antibodies to detect parts of the section where there has been deposition of immunoreactants such as IgG, IgA, IgM, complement C3, or fibrinogen. In standard use, to increase specificity, two antibodies are applied in sequence, for example rabbit–antihuman IgG followed by a fluorescein-labeled antirabbit immunoglobulin. The specimen is viewed with a fluorescence microscope to localize the region of antibody deposition. Thus, for example, the test may demonstrate that there has been deposition of IgG between epidermal cells (pemphigus) or of IgA at the dermal papillae (dermatitis herpetiformis).

Direct immunofluorescence is relatively crude, as immunoreactants deposited at the dermo–epidermal junction may be targeted at numerous closely adjacent antigens, which cannot be distinguished on routine samples. The technique is therefore often further refined by splitting the skin using saline. 'Salt-split skin' is cleaved through the lamina lucida of the dermo–epidermal junction, such that the epidermal part has part of the lamina lucida attached, while the dermal part has the lamina densa and part of the lamina lucida (see Fig. 16.1). DIF testing on these two parts of the skin will identify the localization of the antibody more accurately. For example, IgG and C3 are deposited at the dermo–epidermal junction in both bullous pemphigoid and epidermolysis bullosa acquisita; in bullous pemphigoid, the deposition is in the lamina lucida and hemidesmosome region (epidermal side of salt-split skin), but in epidermolysis bullosa acquisita the antigen is the anchoring fibrils below the lamina densa (dermal side of salt-split skin).

Indirect immunofluorescence testing

Indirect immunofluorescence (IIF) testing (Fig. 16.20) uses much the same technique, but is designed to detect circulating antibodies rather than those that have bound to tissues, and is therefore performed using a blood sample. The substrate may be human skin, but other species and organs (such as esophagus) can also be used. This is incubated with the patient serum, then with a labeled antihuman immunoglobulin. Positive immunofluorescence identifies that a circulating antibody is present, and also determines the site of binding as already described. This test is, in general, less useful, but in some disorders, such as pemphigus, the titer of positive results may correlate with clinical assessment of disease severity.

Bullous pemphigoid
Etiology and pathogenesis
Bullous pemphigoid (BP) is the most common of the immunobullous disorders but is still rare, with an incidence of about 10 per million per year. The targets for immunologic attack are hemidesmosome proteins known as the BP antigens (Table 16.3). These are derived from keratinocytes, and are mainly found within the basal pole of the basal cells, with a small amount extracellularly in the lamina lucida. A rare 200-kDa target antigen has also been reported. Binding of antibodies, activation of complement, and chemoattraction of neutrophils and eosinophils all contribute to the blistering process.

Clinical
Bullous pemphigoid is primarily a disorder of elderly individuals. Most develop a widespread rash with tense, unilocular blisters of diameter 1–2 cm, which contain clear, straw-colored fluid, or are hemorrhagic (Figs 16.21–16.26). A pompholyx pattern of vesicles occurs on the palms

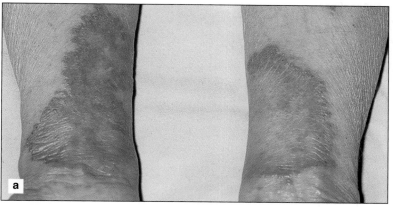

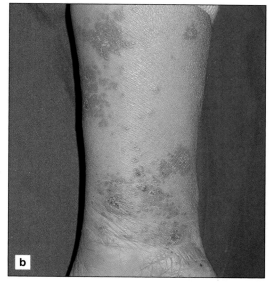

Figure 16.21 Eczematous lesions are a precursor phase in many patients, but will demonstrate positive immunofluorescence if the diagnosis is suspected and appropriate samples are taken. Clues include an annular morphology (**a**) and small blisters (**b**).

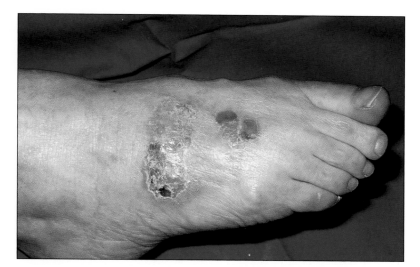

Figure 16.22 Localized bullous pemphigoid. This patient had a small crop of blisters on the foot, with positive direct immunofluorescence for IgG and C3. She was treated with topical steroids only and never developed more widespread disease.

and soles in 25% of patients (Fig. 16.26). A preceding urticated eczematous phase, often with rather annular lesions, is common and may precede blistering by several months. Oral lesions are uncommon, occurring in about 10–20% of patients, and usually mild if they do occur.

In about 10–20% of cases, pemphigoid may be localized, for example to a lower leg or around the umbilicus. This causes diagnostic difficulty but may respond to topical treatment alone. A nodular variant also causes diagnostic difficulty.

Differential diagnosis
This includes the following.
- Other immunobullous diseases—epidermolysis bullosa acquisita, pemphigus vulgaris (see comparison in Table 16.4), cicatricial pemphigoid, and pemphigoid gestationis.
- Inflammatory diseases
  Differential in prebullous phase—eczemas, drug eruptions, and urticaria.
  Differential in blistering phase—papular urticaria and blistering due to lower leg cellulitis (Fig. 16.27).
- Non-inflammatory blisters—blistering due to lower leg edema (a common disorder, discussed earlier).
- Bullous drug eruption—especially furosemide, ibuprofen, captopril, and some antibiotics.

The diagnosis is established by skin biopsy with DIF: there is a subepidermal blister and deposition of IgG and C3. IIF is less useful, as it is not routinely positive and titers do not correlate with disease activity.

Treatment
Localized BP may be adequately treated with topical corticosteroids, but most patients with generalized disease require systemic corticosteroids. Typically, a dose of about 1 mg/kg per day of prednisolone or prednisone is used initially until new blisters cease to develop, and then reduced every few days in the absence of significant new blisters. The usual risks of these agents, such as fluid retention, hypertension, diabetes, and osteoporosis, are often of particular importance in patients with pemphigoid, who are typically elderly and may have other concurrent illnesses. It is common for additional immunosuppressive therapy to be used, sometimes as monotherapy but more commonly added for its steroid-sparing effect; the usual choice is azathioprine or dapsone, but cyclophosphamide, ciclosporin, mycophenolate mofetil, methotrexate, or intravenous immunoglobulins (IVIG) are also used (see Ch. 4 for monitoring details). A combination regimen of a tetracycline with nicotinamide may also be helpful and less toxic.

Cicatricial pemphigoid

Etiology and pathogenesis
Cicatricial pemphigoid (CP) is due to antibodies that target several potential antigens (Table 16.3).

Clinical
This disorder is twice as common in women as in men. It affects the oral mucosa in 90%, presenting either with blisters and erosions or, commonly, with gingivitis (Figs 16.28–16.32). Conjunctivae are affected in 70%, and are of particular importance due to the development of scarring between bulbar and tarsal surfaces (symblepharon). The skin may be affected in about 20% of patients, often around the scalp, head, and neck; genital mucosa is involved in a similar proportion. Larynx, pharynx, and nasal mucosa may also be affected.

Differential diagnosis
This includes the following.
- Other immunobullous disorders—especially linear IgA disease (mucosal lesions) and BP (truncal involvement).
- Mouth—lichen planus.

Routine histology and DIF will help to distinguish lichen planus and other mucosal lesions; most patients with CP have positive DIF for IgG but may require oral or conjunctival biopsies to demonstrate this.

Treatment
Local measures are used for affected sites, such as steroid mouthwashes and eyedrops. In cases that require systemic therapy, this is as for BP. Ophthalmologic follow-up is recommended. Surgical treatment may be needed to treat ocular or laryngeal scarring.

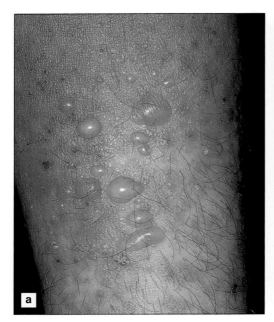
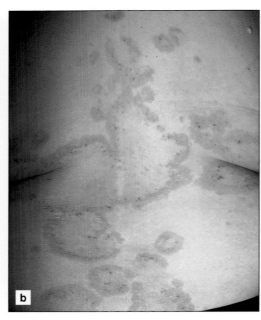
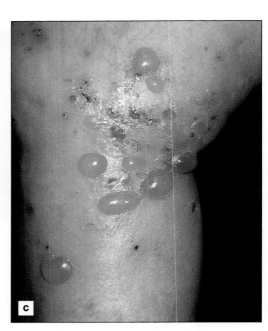

Figure 16.23 Established bullous pemphigoid involves a mixture of tense clear or hemorrhagic blisters and a variable eczematous background (**a–c**). (Panel c courtesy of Dr. G. Dawn.)

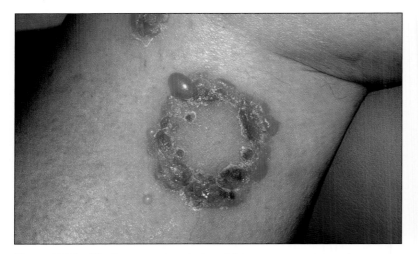
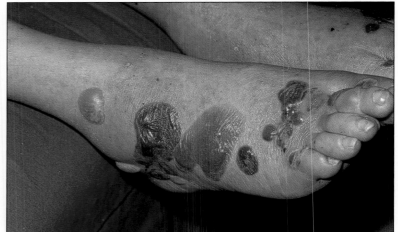

Figure 16.24 Like the eczematous lesions, blisters may occur in annular arrangements in bullous pemphigoid.

Figure 16.25 Hemorrhagic blisters are a common feature in pemphigoid, shown here on the dorsum of the foot in an elderly man. This is a variant with minimal inflammatory component. In this case, there are tense unilocular blisters but no erythema or eczematous component, a pattern termed cell-poor pemphigoid, as the clinical lack of inflammation is paralleled by a histologic lack of infiltrate. More commonly, as in Fig. 16.23, there is a mixture of inflamed and non-inflamed lesions.

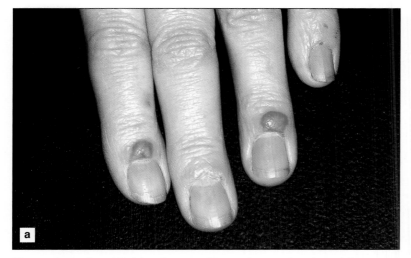
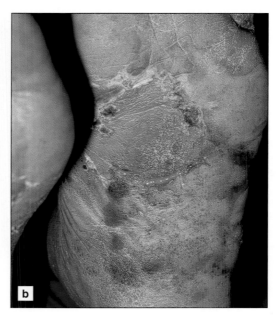

Figure 16.26 Pemphigoid on the extremities tends to produce larger blisters on the dorsa of hands or feet (**a**), but pompholyx-like lesions on the palmoplantar surfaces (**b**). Pompholyx-like lesions occur in about 25% of patients, but usually there is relatively extensive pemphigoid blistering at more typical sites. (Panel a courtesy of Dr. G. Dawn.)

Table 16.4   COMPARISON BETWEEN BULLOUS PEMPHIGOID AND PEMPHIGUS VULGARIS

Characteristic	Bullous pemphigoid	Pemphigus vulgaris
Frequency	Uncommon	Rare
Age group	Most > 70 years	Often 50–60 years
Blister morphology	Tense, clear fluid content May be pompholyx changes on palms or soles	Fragile, may just be blister remnants at the margin of erosions
Adjacent skin	May be urticated or eczematous	Normal, but may be able to induce blister by shearing force (Nikolsky sign)
Mucous membrane involvement	About 25%, usually minor	Present in 80%, typically precedes skin involvement by several months
Direct immunofluorescence	Positive at basement membrane zone	Positive epidermal intercellular
Response to treatment	Usually good	Often refractory

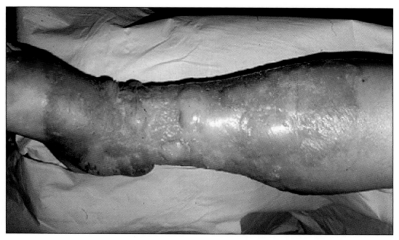

Figure 16.27   Blisters due to cellulitis. The elderly lower leg is the commonest site, so pemphigoid is often erroneously considered to be the likely diagnosis.

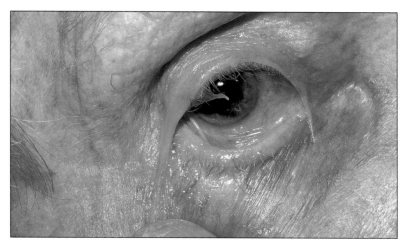

Figure 16.28   Cicatricial pemphigoid affecting the eye, causing scarring (symblepharon) and severe visual impairment. For this reason, the name benign mucous membrane pemphigoid is something of a misnomer.

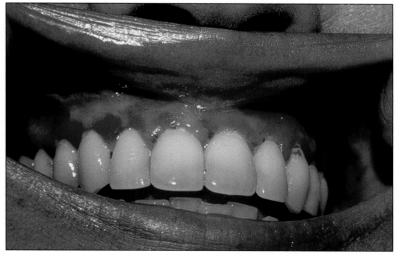

Figure 16.29   Gingivitis in a patient with cicatricial pemphigoid. This pattern of periodontal, chronic, red, velvety gingivitis is very suggestive of this disorder but may occur in other blistering diseases (see Figs. 16.38b and 16.59).

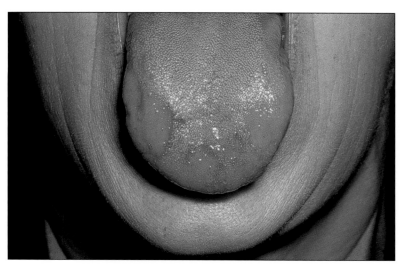

Figure 16.30   Cicatricial pemphigoid affecting the tongue. The lesions are rather annular, and may be mistaken for migratory glossitis (geographic tongue, Ch. 20) unless there are other associated features.

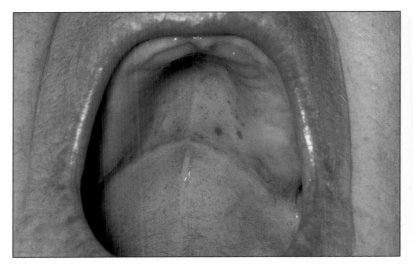

Figure 16.31 Involvement of the palate in cicatricial pemphigoid, manifest as purpuric spots. Intraoral lesions of dermatitis herpetiformis may also produce similar purpuric lesions.

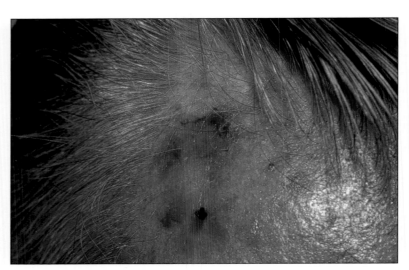

Figure 16.32 Cicatricial pemphigoid may affect skin as well as the mucous membranes, usually on the head and neck (termed the Brunsting–Perry type).

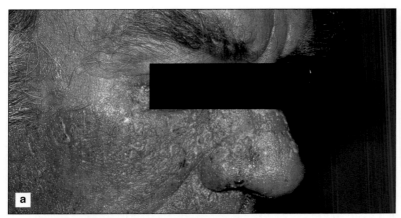

Figure 16.33 Pemphigus foliaceus. This typically causes a rather seborrheic eczema–like eruption (**a**) with some crusting or erosions, rather than frank blisters. However, it is usually more extensive on the face and trunk than would be the case in seborrheic eczema. Some cases of pemphigus foliaceus have a more actively crusted and bullous morphology (**b**).

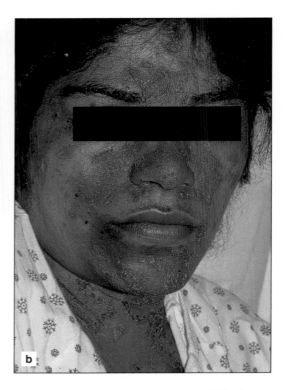

Table 16.5	TYPES OF PEMPHIGUS AND THEIR CLINICAL ASPECTS
Type of pemphigus	**Clinical aspects**
Pemphigus vulgaris (PV)	Causes blistering above the basal cell region of the epidermis. It usually presents as oral erosions some months prior to skin involvement, and may affect other mucosae. Intact blisters are relatively uncommon, as the epidermis is fragile; large erosions and crusted areas are more typical.
Pemphigus foliaceus (PF)	This has a more superficial epidermal split, and usually presents as a facial and upper trunk eruption that is red and crusted. It often resembles either seborrheic dermatitis or lupus erythematosus.
Pemphigus vegetans	A variant of PV that mainly affects the tongue and major flexures.
Pemphigus erythematosus	A variant of PF that resembles lupus erythematosus and is associated with positive antinuclear antibodies.
Fogo selvagem	A variant of PF that occurs as an endemic disorder in Brazil (also known as Brazilian pemphigus), typically affecting younger individuals. It is probably provoked by an infectious process.
Neonatal pemphigus	This occurs in children born to a mother with active pemphigus. It is due to transplacental transfer of circulating autoantibodies, and is a transient disorder, as it is due to maternal rather than fetal antibody.
Drug-induced pemphigus	Some drugs with sulfhydryl groups, typically penicillamine but also several others (Table 16.6), may cause pemphigus foliaceus (see also Ch. 18).

Table 16.6   DRUGS THAT MAY CAUSE PEMPHIGUS

Category	Drug(s)
Rheumatologic	Penicillamine
Cardiac	Captopril, beta-blockers
Antibiotics	Ceftazidime, penicillin, rifampin
Miscellaneous	Progesterone, heroin, pyrazoles

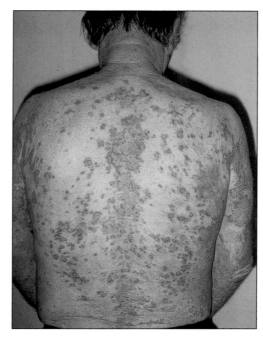

Figure 16.34 Pemphigus foliaceus, showing a typical pattern of scattered, crusted patches on the trunk. This variant of pemphigus is often said to respond well to therapy, but personal experience is that it can be a prolonged and difficult condition to manage.

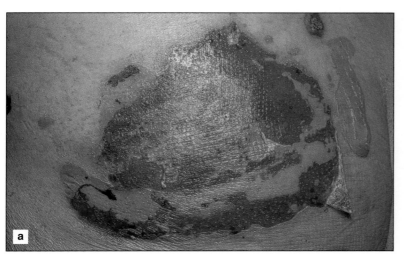

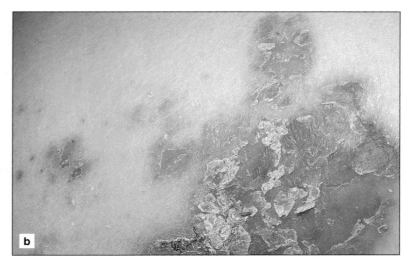

Figure 16.35 Blisters in pemphigus are fragile, as they are due to separation between epidermal cells. Often, the presenting feature is erosions rather than clinically apparent blisters (**a**). Close-up inspection of pemphigus foliaceous may often reveal similar peeled remnants of blisters among the secondary crusting (**b**).

Pemphigus

Etiology and pathogenesis

Most pemphigus occurs as an autoimmune phenomenon, with circulating antibodies against desmosomal proteins of the epidermis (Table 16.2). Damage to the desmosomal intercellular attachment causes separation between the keratinocytes, with intraepidermal blistering. It has recently been documented that the same molecule, desmoglein 1, is targeted by auto-antibodies in pemphigus foliaceous and by circulating toxin in the SSSS.

Clinical

The main types of pemphigus are listed in Tables 16.5 and 16.6; see also Figs 16.33–16.43.

Familial benign pemphigus (Hailey–Hailey disease) is confusingly named; it is a totally different disorder, which is not immunobullous but due to an inherited defect in keratinocyte adhesion by desmosomes (Fig. 16.44 and Ch. 19).

Differential diagnosis

This includes the following.

- Other cutaneous bullous diseases—especially BP (Table 16.4), epidermolysis bullosa acquisita, paraneoplastic pemphigus, toxic epidermal necrolysis and bullous drug eruptions, and porphyria cutanea tarda.
- Erosive or bullous oral disease—CP and lichen planus (less commonly hand, foot, and mouth disease).
- Major flexures—pemphigus vegetans may resemble contact dermatitis, Hailey–Hailey disease (Fig. 16.44), or granular parakeratosis (see Fig. 2.32).

Treatment

Most cases require systemic corticosteroids, usually under a fairly aggressive regimen to achieve disease control; initial corticosteroid doses are usually 1–1.5 mg/kg per day. In some cases, pulsed doses of intravenous methylprednisolone may be necessary to achieve control of pemphigus. Plasmapheresis may remove circulating antibodies and achieve control, but needs to be used with other therapies to prevent relapse. Many patients will require additional immunosuppressive agents, either to achieve disease control or because the daily steroid dose cannot be reduced to a level appropriate for long-term maintenance. The usual immunosuppressive agents likely to be used are azathioprine, cyclophosphamide, gold, and ciclosporin. IVIG appears to be useful in some cases; other agents that have been used include mycophenolate mofetil, methotrexate, gold, and dapsone. Pemphigus foliaceus is often felt to respond well but can be extremely refractory in some instances.

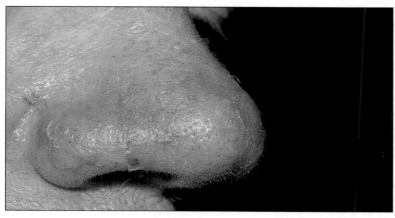

Figure 16.36 An uncommon, but probably underestimated, variant of pemphigus foliaceus is a type confined to the tip of the nose. As this may respond to topical therapy, and may resolve without recurrence or worsening in some patients, it may be treated more often than it is diagnosed.

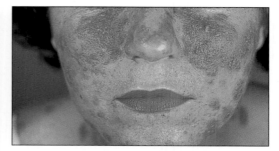

Figure 16.37 Pemphigus erythematosus is a rare variant of pemphigus with a very superficial level of blistering and positive antinuclear antibody tests. Extensive facial lesions may occur, with crusting rather than obvious blistering, a pattern that may resemble pemphigus foliaceus, lupus erythematosus (as shown), or seborrheic dermatitis. (Courtesy of James Steger, M.D.)

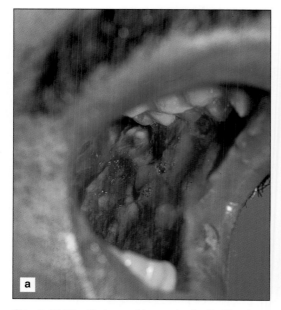

a

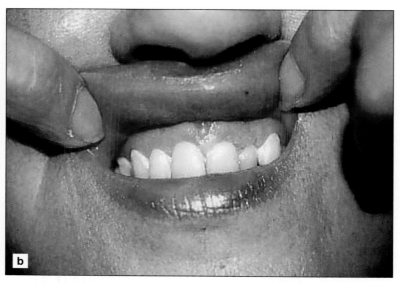

b

Figure 16.38 Oral pemphigus vulgaris. Oral involvement commonly precedes skin involvement at other sites, often by several months, and may be misdiagnosed as aphthous, herpetic, or non-specific ulceration initially, as shown in (**a**), affecting the mouth and lip. However, it is usually severe and progressive, which should arouse suspicion about the diagnosis. In some patients, the appearance of oral lesions is that of gingivitis, which may mimic cicatricial pemphigoid, epidermolysis bullosa acquisita, or even lichen planus (see also Figs 16.29 and 16.59). (Panel b courtesy of Dr. G. Dawn.)

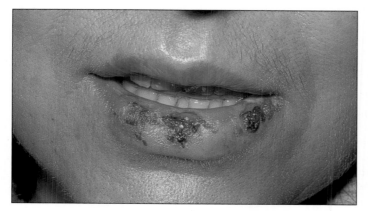

Figure 16.39 Pemphigus vulgaris affecting the lip. This eruption followed herpes simplex infection, and Stevens–Johnson syndrome was considered, but biopsy confirmed the diagnosis of pemphigus. Unusually, no other sites were affected over 1 year of follow-up. In this patient, relapses to date have responded to strong topical steroids and have not required any systemic therapy.

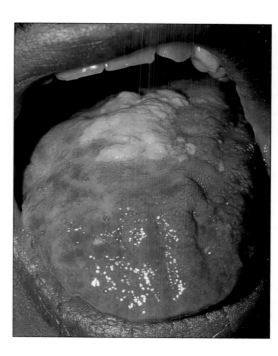

Figure 16.40 Pemphigus affecting the tongue. Candidiasis may be difficult to exclude, and is of importance if the patient is already taking steroids or other immunosuppressive therapy.

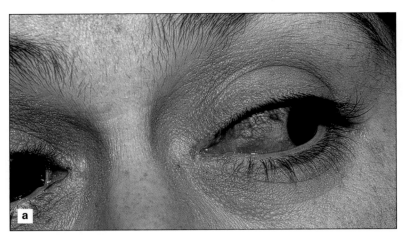

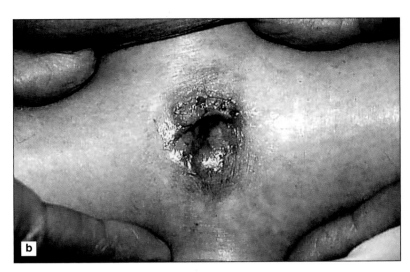

Figure 16.41 Pemphigus at unusual sites. (**a**) Mucosae other than that of the mouth may be affected, in this case the eyes ocular conjunctivae . (**b**) Pemphigus affecting the umbillicus; at this site, unless there is extensive disease elsewhere, it may mimic cicatricial pemphigoid. (Panel b courtesy of Dr. G. Dawn.)

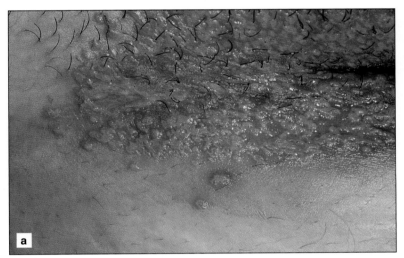

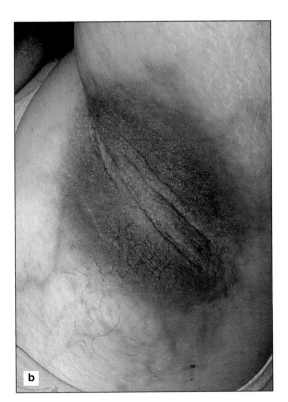

Figure 16.42 Pemphigus vegetans. This affects the major creases such as groins or axillae, and may present as eroded (**a**) or thickly crusted (**b**) plaques.

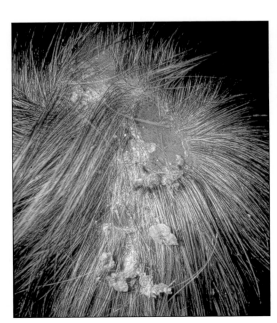

Figure 16.43 The scalp is relatively commonly involved in pemphigus vulgaris, erosions at this site often developing prominent crusting. (Courtesy of Bob Butler, M.D.)

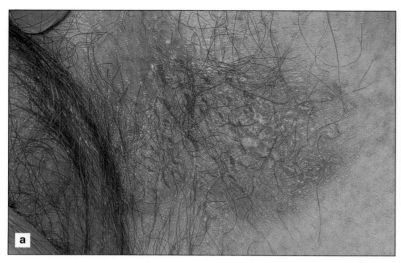

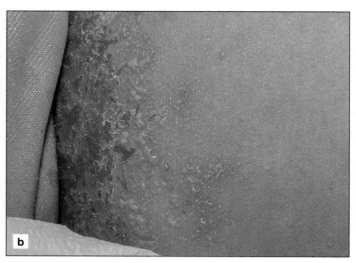

Figure 16.44 Familial benign pemphigus (Hailey–Hailey disease) shares with pemphigus the fact that there is dyscohesion between keratinocytes. However, the mechanism involves an inherently abnormal desmosome rather than an immunologically mediated process. Clinically, the lesions affect mainly the major flexures, and have small surface tears (**a**) rather than blisters, although the latter are sometimes apparent (**b**); the disorder is more likely to be confused with eczema than with immunobullous diseases.

PRACTICE POINTS

- Bullous pemphigoid (BP) is rare, but is the most likely cause of widespread blistering in the elderly.
- Blisters on the lower leg in the elderly are more commonly due to edema than to BP.
- A preceding therapeutically refractory 'urticated' eczematous rash often precedes blistering in BP.
- Pemphigus vulgaris is much rarer than BP and is usually manifest as skin and mucous membrane erosions; it does not have the widespread intact and sometimes hemorrhagic blisters that occur in BP.
- If biopsy is performed from any blistering eruption, frozen tissue for immunofluorescence should be submitted as well as a routine histology sample.

Paraneoplastic pemphigus
Etiology and pathogenesis

Paraneoplastic pemphigus (PNP) is particularly associated with lymphoreticular tumors. Castleman tumor is disproportionately associated with this disorder, and thymomas may also be found.

Clinical

Paraneoplastic pemphigus may not cause overt blistering. The clinical picture typically includes troublesome cheilitis and conjunctivitis, with an itchy and rather lichenoid papulosquamous eruption at other sites. Palmoplantar lesions occur, and there may be nail dystrophy (Figs 16.45–16.47). Biopsy features include necrosis of keratinocytes as well as the acantholysis and bulla formation anticipated in pemphigus; immunofluorescence studies are positive, but immunoblotting demonstrates different antigens from those in pemphigus vulgaris or pemphigus foliaceous (Table 16.2).

Differential diagnosis

This includes the following.

- Other immunobullous disorders—especially pemphigus vulgaris and epidermolysis bullosa acquisita.
- Inflammatory disorders—lichen planus (cutaneous or mucosal), and erythema multiforme major or toxic epidermal necrolysis.
- Oral—infective gingivostomatitis, candidiasis, and herpetic stomatitis.
- Drug reactions—especially rash or stomatitis due to chemotherapy or antibiotics.

Treatment

Treatment of the underlying disorder is the priority, but the disorder may occur as a consequence of advanced lymphomas where previous

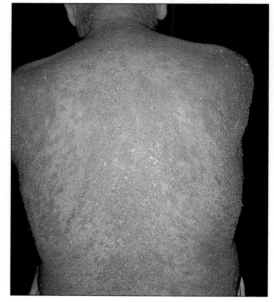

Figure 16.45 Paraneoplastic pemphigus. Diffuse rash on the trunk, with a rather purple color. Blistering was not a feature in this patient, and lichenoid drug eruption was initially suspected. He was taking various medications for a known lymphoma.

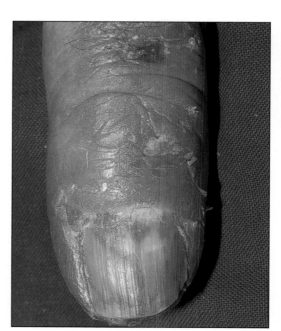

Figure 16.46 Paraneoplastic pemphigus. Acral rash with rather lichenoid or eczematous morphology, and associated nail dystrophy (same patient as in Fig. 16.45).

treatments have failed. In such cases, treatments with systemic steroids as for pemphigus are used, but this is a therapeutically refractory variant of pemphigus.

Dermatitis herpetiformis
Etiology and pathogenesis
Dermatitis herpetiformis (DH) is essentially always associated with the presence of gluten enteropathy, although few patients actually have gastrointestinal symptoms. IgA (of IgA1 type) is deposited in the skin at the papillary tips or in a linear granular pattern at the dermo–epidermal junction at sites of predilection (see later), but the mechanism of its effect is uncertain, as it is demonstrated in non-lesional as well as in lesional skin. Persistence of IgA in the skin for many months after establishing a gluten-free diet may explain the slow response to this treatment, but it is less easy to explain the immediate recurrence of symptoms on inadvertent gluten rechallenge. Nonetheless, the presence of IgA with this distribution pattern on DIF testing is diagnostic.

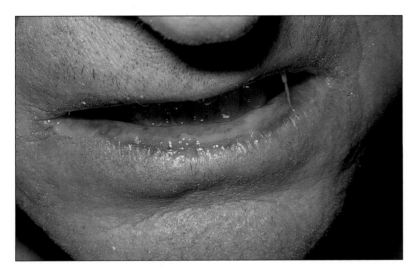

Figure 16.47 Paraneoplastic pemphigus (PNP) demonstrating an erosive cheilitis. This is a frequent feature in PNP and often responds very poorly to treatment.

Other autoimmune disorders may be associated, such as thyroid disease; one study has shown an increased frequency of diabetes.

Clinical
Dermatitis herpetiformis usually affects older children or young adults. Lesions typically occur on extensor elbows and knees, over scapulae, and on the sacrum or buttock. Involvement of scalp, ears, and face are often underestimated, but these are not uncommon sites of lesions. The individual lesions are small and intensely itchy vesicles of a few millimeters in diameter, usually excoriated, and sometimes with a mildly eczematous or urticated background (Figs 16.48–16.50). Oral and palmar lesions are both uncommon, but both may be purpuric if they occur. Biopsies for DIF can be taken from sites of predilection for that individual (usually extensor aspect of the forearm near the elbow) even in the absence of active rash at the time; complement C3 is often present in addition to the typical IgA deposits.

Blood tests in DH may be performed for various reasons.
- For diagnostic support—antigliaden antibodies and antireticulin antibodies.
- As screening tests for underlying malabsorption—full blood count, ferritin, and folate.
- To search for associated thyroid autoimmunity or pernicious anemia—antibody tests.
- As a baseline or monitoring for dapsone therapy—full blood count, reticulocyte count, and glucose-6-phosphate dehydrogenase.

Frank malabsorption is uncommon, even though partial villus atrophy is usual. There is an association between DH and lymphoma, especially of the small intestine.

Differential diagnosis
Dermatitis herpetiformis may be difficult to diagnose, as the blisters it causes are small, very itchy, and frequently destroyed by scratching. The sites of predilection are diagnostically helpful, but it should be noted that lesions of scabies are also very itchy and are common at the elbow region. The main differentials are as follows.
- Other itchy conditions—scabies (note that rash on the elbows is common in scabies) and simple excoriations (secondary to eczema, dry skin, or systemic causes of pruritus).
- Other immunobullous disorders—especially linear IgA disease.

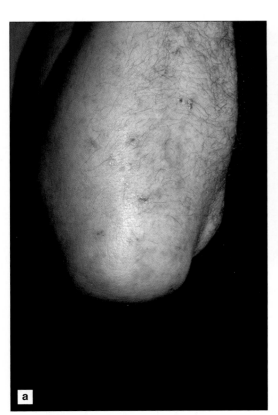

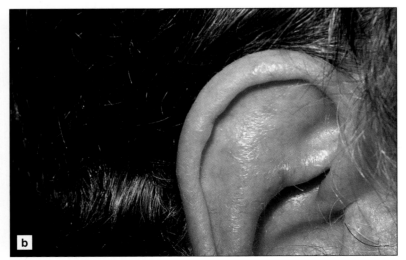

Figure 16.48 Typical sites for dermatitis herpetiformis. (**a**) The extensor aspect of the forearm near the elbow is classic; note that scabies may produce an almost identical picture at this body site. (**b**) The ear is an underestimated site; two small intact blisters are present.

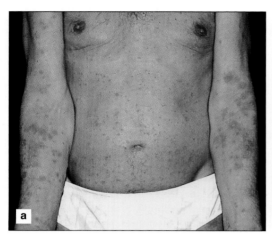

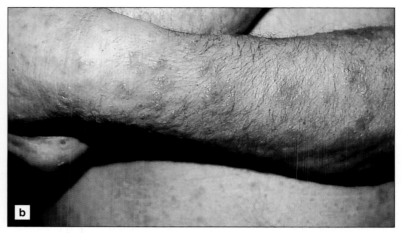

Figure 16.49   More florid dermatitis herpetiformis affecting the arms and trunk. At a distance, the lesions suggest eczema or scabies (**a**), but closer examination (**b**) shows blistering with an annular morphology. (Courtesy of Dr. G. Dawn.)

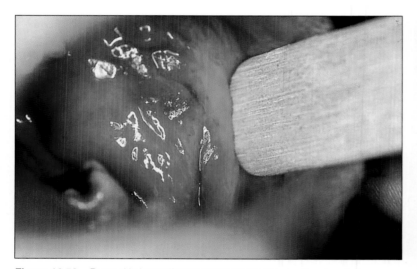

Figure 16.50   Dermatitis herpetiformis rarely affects the mouth; when it does, lesions are generally purpuric. (Courtesy of Dr. G. Dawn.)

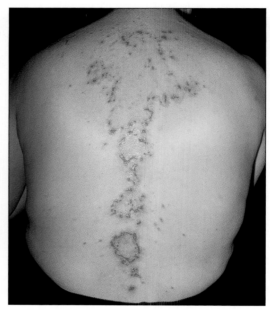

Figure 16.51   Linear IgA disease on the back, an example with a strikingly annular pattern of involvement.

- Other causes of small blisters—herpes infection and staphylococcal impetigo.

Treatment

Dapsone is the initial treatment of choice, and has sufficiently dramatic effect on itch within 24 h that it is diagnostically useful. Side effects and monitoring are discussed in Chapter 4. Other sulfones, such as sulfa-pyridine or sulfamethoxypyridazine, may be alternatives to dapsone in some cases.

A gluten-free diet is also important but takes 6 months or so to work. It is of particular value in patients who require only low doses of dapsone (who may be able to stop all drug treatment), or those in whom adequate dosage is limited by hematologic side effects, but patients in between these extremes often find the diet more difficult than taking dapsone. Strict gluten-free diet reduces the risk of lymphoma.

Linear IgA disease
Etiology and pathogenesis

In linear IgA disease (LAD), there is deposition of IgA (mainly IgA1) at the dermo–epidermal junction, both within the lamina lucida and in the region of the sublamina densa anchoring fibrils. On DIF, it has a linear distribution that is distinct from DH, and there is no association with gluten-sensitive enteropathy. Most cases are of unknown etiology, but drugs are implicated in some cases (vancomycin, diclofenac, and lithium), and associations have been reported with autoimmune diseases (ulcerative

colitis, rheumatoid arthritis, and systemic lupus erythematosus) and with various malignancies.

Clinical

Blisters may resemble DH or BP, and often have an annular arrangement (Figs 16.51 and 16.52). The trunk and limbs are the most common sites. Mucosal involvement is relatively common; the eyes and mouth are each involved in about 50% of cases, occasionally very severely, with scarring and visual impairment (Fig. 16.53).

Differential diagnosis

This can usefully be considered according to blister size and presence of mucosal disease.
- Small blisters—DH and herpes infections.
- Larger blisters—BP and impetigo.
- Mucosal—CP and erosive LP.

Treatment

Treatment of LAD is usually similar to DH initially, with dapsone or other sulfones. Topical corticosteroids may be useful, and some patients require systemic steroids or other immunosuppressive agents such as cyclo-phosphamide or azathioprine.

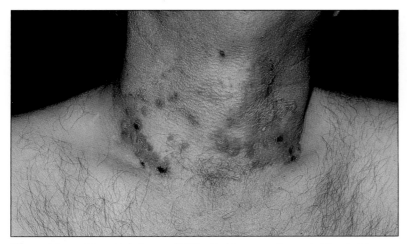

Figure 16.52 Linear IgA disease (LAD) with blisters on the neck. The slightly annular appearance shown here is suspicious of LAD.

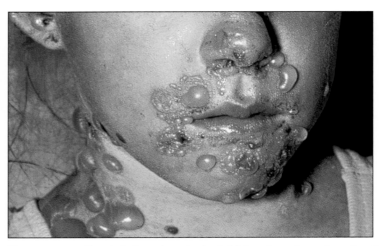

Figure 16.54 Chronic bullous dermatosis of childhood causing an impetigo-like blistering eruption on the face. The blisters of impetigo are generally more fragile and cause yellow crusting rather than tense, clear blisters. (Courtesy of Charlie Rosenberg, M.D.)

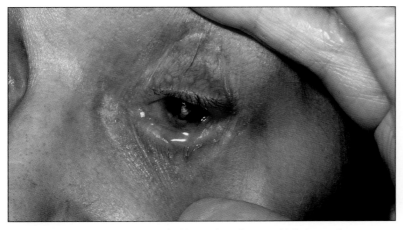

Figure 16.53 Linear IgA disease with scarring of eye and blindness; there was also marked scarring of hands (Fig. 4.15).

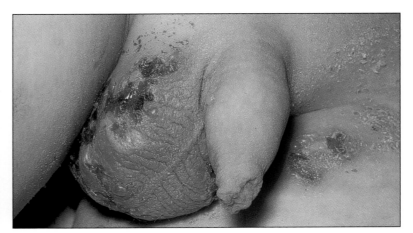

Figure 16.55 Genital involvement and pubic lesions are typical in chronic bullous dermatosis of childhood, shown here in a child who had been treated for several months for herpes simplex and impetigo. There was a dramatic response to sulfapyridine, with no recurrences after 12 months.

Chronic bullous dermatosis of childhood

Etiology and pathogenesis
Chronic bullous dermatosis of childhood (CBDC) is probably the child-hood version of LAD, typically occurring in the first decade of life.

Clinical
Clusters of blisters occur, especially in the genital area and around the mouth, where they may be confused with impetigo (Figs 16.54 and 16.55). In older children, they may be more widespread. Mucous membranes may be affected.

Differential diagnosis
This is the same as for LAD, although it is common for infective causes (impetigo and herpes infection) to head the differential diagnosis list in children; CBDC is rare, and many children are erroneously treated for infection for long periods. Childhood BP (Fig. 16.56) may also need to be considered.

Treatment
Treatment of CBDC is similar to that of DH or LAD, but sulfapyridine is probably the treatment of choice. Dapsone is also effective, but it may be difficult to obtain formulations suitable for young children. Cortico-steroids and colchicine have also been used with benefit. Remission over a period of a few years is frequent, and the disorder usually remits by puberty.

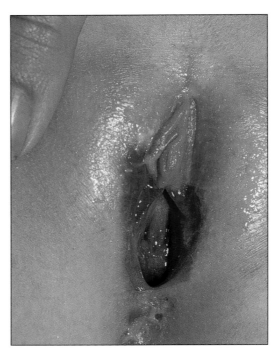

Figure 16.56 Bullous pemphigoid is rare in children, but can occur and may resemble chronic bullous dermatosis of childhood in having genital involvement, as shown here.

- Dermatitis herpetiformis (DH) often escapes diagnosis for long periods, as it may be subtle and intermittent, but it is important to diagnose, as gluten-free diet may be curative and addresses associated malabsorption and small-bowel lymphoma risk.
- Itchy papules or vesicles on the elbows are more commonly due to scabies than to DH.
- Dapsone has such dramatic effect in DH and related disorders that it is diagnostically useful; however, it does have potentially significant side effects, and is generally reserved for cases with a proven diagnosis or with convincing clinical features.
- It is important to perform immunofluorescence when submitting a skin biopsy from a patient with suspected DH; not only may the histology of lesions be non-specific due to scratching, but the treatment involves lifelong dietary alteration and warrants a proven diagnosis.

Epidermolysis bullosa acquisita
Etiology and pathogenesis
Epidermolysis bullosa acquisita (EBA) is a rare immunobullous disorder that is due to antibodies against a lamina densa or sublamina densa antigen, identified as 290-kDa and 145-kDa proteins by immunoblotting, and now known to be the C terminus of type VII procollagen that forms part of the anchoring fibrils. Antibody (IgG) and complement C3 deposition is associated with neutrophil-mediated tissue damage.

Epidermolysis bullosa acquisita is associated with a wide range of other disorders, including the following.
- Inflammatory diseases—inflammatory bowel disease, rheumatoid arthritis, and psoriasis.
- Endocrine disorders—thyroiditis, diabetes, and multiple endocrinopathy syndrome.
- Amyloidosis.
- Neoplasia—myeloma, lymphoma, lung carcinoma, and monoclonal cryoglobulinemia.

Clinical
Epidermolysis bullosa acquisita may present in two main forms. One is reminiscent of porphyria cutanea tarda, with blisters over trauma sites such as knuckles, skin fragility, and healing with milia. The other pattern, in which skin fragility may also be prominent, is much more suggestive of BP (Figs 16.57–16.59).

Differential diagnosis
This depends on the clinical pattern.
- Porphyria cutanea tarda-like pattern—true porphyria cutanea tarda and pseudoporphyria (Ch. 17) are the main differentials.

- Bullous pemphigoid-like pattern—BP, pemphigus vulgaris, PNP, erythema multiforme major or toxic epidermal necrolysis, and SSSS.
- Oral lesions—pemphigus vulgaris and CP.

The differential from PNP or SSSS is particularly important in patients with tumor-associated EBA, who may be immunosuppressed by their disease or its treatment, and in whom blistering eruptions may be linked with chemotherapy or infection.

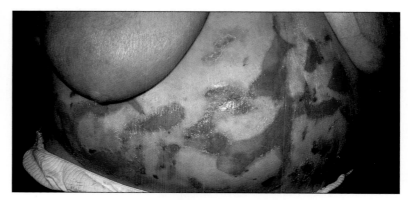

Figure 16.58 Epidermolysis bullosa acquisita, in this case occurring as a paraneoplastic phenomenon. Fragility of the skin is a typical feature, whatever the cause, and may be very difficult to control. Minor trauma with subsequent shearing of the skin accounted for the bizarre shapes seen here.

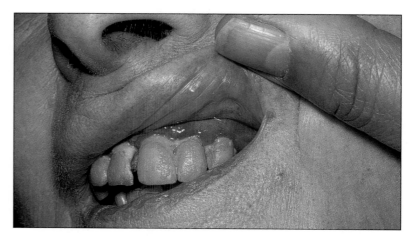

Figure 16.59 Erosive gingivitis in a patient with epidermolysis bullosa acquisita. This is clinically indistinguishable from the gingivitis that may occur in cicatricial pemphigoid (Fig. 16.29).

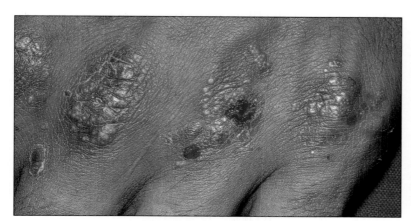

Figure 16.57 Epidermolysis bullosa acquisita resembling porphyria cutanea tarda, in a patient with Crohn disease. There is scarring and milia formation within the lesions.

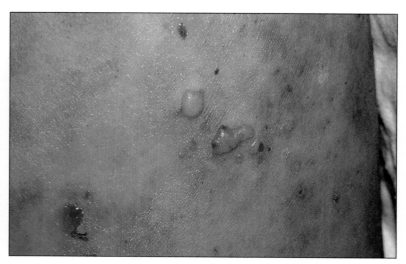

Figure 16.60 Blisters are rare in lupus erythematosus but may cause diagnostic difficulty, particularly in children, as in this case.

Treatment

Epidermolysis bullosa acquisita is relatively resistant to therapy, and may be very troublesome in patients with significant fragility of the skin. High-dose prednisolone, cyclophosphamide, azathioprine, methotrexate, and ciclosporin are all possible treatment options.

Other autoimmune diseases

Blisters may occur in other inflammatory autoimmune conditions, such as lichen planus (see Fig. 8.20) or lupus erythematosus (Fig. 16.60).

FURTHER READING

Anhalt GJ. Paraneoplastic pemphigus. Adv Dermatol 1997; 12: 75–96

Bhushan M, Cox NH, Chalmers R. Acute oedema blisters: a report of 13 cases. Br J Dermatol 2001; 144: 580–2

Harman KE, Albert S, Black MM. Guidelines for the management of pemphigus vulgaris. Br J Dermatol 2003; 149: 926–37

Mutasim DF, Adams BB. Immunofluorescence in dermatology. J Am Acad Dermatol 2001; 45: 803–22

Robinson ND, Hashimoto T, Amagai M, et al. The new pemphigus variants. J Am Acad Dermatol 1999; 40: 649–71

Wojnarowska F, Briggaman RA (eds) Management of Blistering Disorders. London: Chapman and Hall, 1990

Wojnarowska F, Kirtschig G, Highet AS, et al. Guidelines for the management of bullous pemphigoid. Br J Dermatol 2002; 147: 214–221

17 Photodermatology and Photodermatoses

BASIC PHOTOBIOLOGY

Photodermatology is the study of photobiology as it relates to the skin. The emphasis in this chapter will be on abnormal responses to ultraviolet radiation (UVR), the photodermatoses. To help in understanding these disorders and aspects of therapeutic photodermatology, some basic science knowledge is required.

Dermatologically relevant non-ionizing radiation

The non-ionizing radiation in sunlight that is of dermatologic relevance (Fig. 17.1) lies between the ultraviolet (UV) and the infrared areas of the electromagnetic spectrum, a region that includes:
- UVR of wavelengths 200–400 nm (subdivided into UVC, 200–280 nm; UVB, 280–315 nm; and UVA, 315–400 nm);
- visible radiation (light) of wavelengths 400–700 nm; and
- infrared radiation above 700 nm.

Each of these different wavelengths of radiation has different effects on the skin, and for any wavelength the effect depends on the intensity and duration of exposure.

Short-wavelength UVR (UVC) is used in investigative photobiology and in germicidal lamps, but is absorbed by the ozone layer and is therefore of little relevance in biologic terms. Some lasers therapeutically utilize longer wavelengths (Ch. 5) but are not discussed here.

Infrared radiation produces heat; is probably important in the causation of some skin disorders, such as erythema ab igne (see Ch. 15); and is used therapeutically to eradicate some cutaneous vascular lesions (infrared coagulator); but it is not relevant in the major photodermatoses.

The wavelengths of main dermatologic relevance are the UVA and UVB regions of the UV spectrum, and, to a lesser extent, visible light.

Effects of radiation of different wavelengths

Within the UV and visible parts of the spectrum, penetration to deeper parts of the skin increases with wavelength. The fall-off in penetration that occurs with each wavelength is in part due to scatter and reflection from different parts of the skin, but the major factor is absorption of radiation by various chemicals in the skin, known as chromophores. Some of the most relevant chromophores and their biologic effects include:
- DNA, RNA, urocanic acid, keratin, and other proteins in the epidermis;
- dehydrocholesterol;
- melanin; and
- oxyhemoglobin.

DNA, RNA, urocanic acid, keratin, and other proteins in the epidermis largely absorb shorter wavelengths below 300 nm. As a result of this absorption process, UVB is about 90% absorbed within the epidermis and essentially no UVB penetrates deeper than the upper dermis, whereas about 30% of UVA at 400 nm and 85% of red light penetrates into the dermis. At least some aspects of photoaging, such as wrinkles, must therefore be primarily due to longer wavelengths, as the shorter wavelengths do not penetrate significantly to the majority of the collagen of the skin. As currently available sunscreen chemicals are much more effective at blocking shorter-wavelength UVB than UVA, they will inevitably provide better protection against burning than against the development of wrinkles.

Dehydrocholesterol absorbs maximally around 270–280 nm to form vitamin D.

Melanin absorbs maximally below 300 nm, with gradually decreasing absorption throughout the visible light spectrum and into the near infrared. This explains the greater penetration of UVR into pale skin than into more pigmented skin (Fig. 17.2).

Oxygenated hemoglobin has a major absorption peak at 418 nm, and less marked peaks at 542 and 577 nm. Knowledge of absorption spectra is important in laser therapy, where the ability to target a specific skin structure depends not only on the absorption characteristics of that structure, but also on whether the laser wavelength will penetrate to the correct depth and whether there is absorption by other chromophores. In the case of hemoglobin (which is a potential laser target within blood vessels), the ideal laser wavelength appears to be at the major absorption peak of 418 nm. However, laser light at this wavelength is therapeutically ineffective, because it is significantly absorbed by melanin and does not penetrate adequately to the dermis; wavelengths between 540 and 580 nm are more effective.

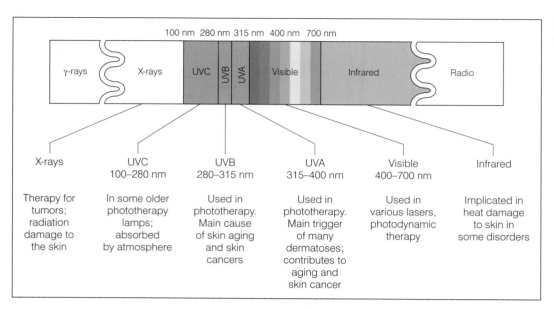

Figure 17.1 The electromagnetic spectrum in relation to the skin.

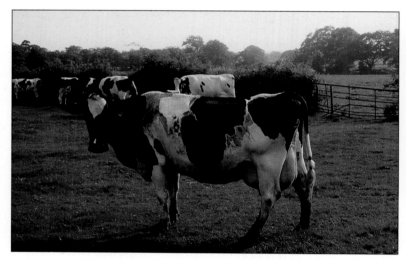

Figure 17.2 A dramatic demonstration of the different penetration into white skin (badly burned) compared with black skin (unburned) despite the same UV dose to each area. Photosensitivity in cattle is usually the result of ingested plants that are either photosensitizers or cause liver toxicity.

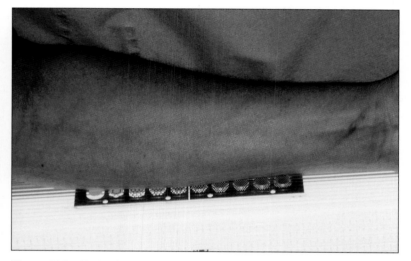

Figure 17.3 Testing for minimal erythema dose (MED). The machine shown is for testing the MED to TL01 (311 nm) UVR. The fluorescent tube producing UVR is in the cabinet that does not transmit this wavelength (although blue-visible light can be seen). A series of graded metal grids allow a series of doses to be transmitted, with $\sqrt{2}$ increments. With knowledge of the highest dose transmitted, and by observing the number of sites that develop erythema after 24 h, the MED can be determined. Note the the arm would actually be flat over the grid apertures during testing but has been tilted to demonstrate the apparatus.

Action spectrum

This is the efficacy of radiation of different wavelengths in producing a specific effect, assuming that the same dose at each wavelength is administered. The results for each wavelength are usually expressed relative to the most effective wavelength. This can be applied to clinical effects such as efficacy in producing erythema, treatment of dermatoses, treatment of neonatal jaundice, and prevention of rickets.

Maximum erythema occurs following exposure to UVR of 300–305 nm (in the UVB range), whereas the dose of UVA required to produce the same degree of erythema is at least 1000-fold greater. The dose of UVA in natural sunlight is about 100 times higher than that of UVB, due to the absorption of shorter wavelengths by the ozone layer. The net result is that UVB accounts for about 90% of erythema due to sunlight, and UVA erythema is less important.

Similarly, the action spectrum for the treatment of many common dermatoses, such as psoriasis, demonstrates that the main effective wavelengths are in the UVB part of the spectrum. Patients with these dermatoses therefore often improve in natural sunlight or after UVB therapy, but derive limited benefit from UVA-producing sunbeds (tanning beds), which are designed to have minimal UVB output. However, burning due to UVB therapy may be a limiting factor. The TL01 lamp, which has become popular in dermatology, achieves a useful compromise: it emits a narrow band of radiation at 311 nm, which is less erythemogenic than shorter wavelengths but still therapeutically active.

Minimal erythema doses

The minimal erythema dose (MED) is the smallest dose of UVR that produces visible erythema. The minimal phototoxicity dose (MPD) is exactly the same thing, but is the term used when the production of erythema also involves a photosensitizing drug, including therapeutic use in photochemotherapy. This type of assessment is used to determine UV sensitivity before therapeutic UVR, and typically involves performing a sequence of doses to 1-cm diameter areas of skin (Figs 17.3–17.5). It is also used in diagnostic phototesting to identify individuals who have abnormal degrees of photosensitivity (discussed in more detail later).

Visual assessment of minimal erythema of small test sites is inexact and varies at different body sites. When MED tests are performed prior to UV therapy, it is common to use a therapeutic dose of 50–70% of the recorded MED to ensure that more sensitive areas than the test site do not receive significantly erythemogenic doses. Erythema due to UVR has a different time course at different wavelengths, so the timing of the assessment is important:
- UVB-induced erythema is usually assessed at 24 h after exposure; and
- psoralen-induced photosensitivity, used in psoralen plus UVA (PUVA) photochemotherapy, has a broader and more individually variable peak of erythema at 48–120 h after exposure.

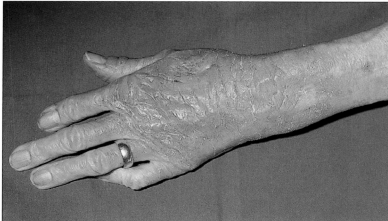

Figure 17.4 Chlorpromazine photosensitivity. This affects the dorsum of the hand and exposed area of the wrist. The distal part of the fingers is often less affected, as shown here.

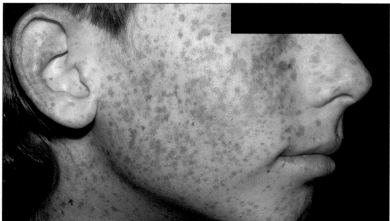

Figure 17.6 Freckles on the cheek in a patient of skin type I–II, who also has red hair.

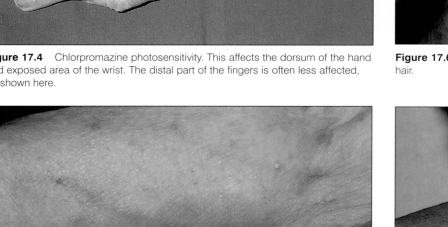

Figure 17.5 Phototests for the patient shown in Figure 17.3. Four square sites were irradiated, and all have produced spreading erythema, down to a dose of about a 50th of that which would cause erythema in an average person in the absence of photosensitizing medication.

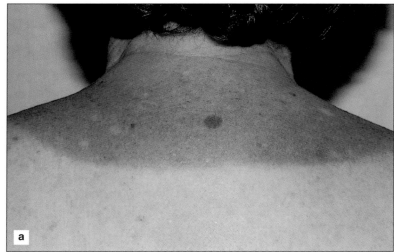

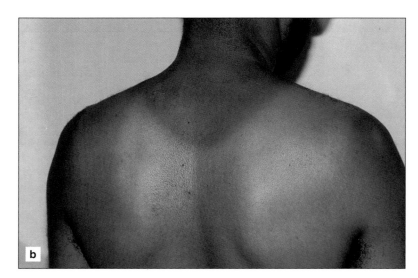

Figure 17.7 (**a**,**b**) Sunburn on the upper back. Note the sharp cut-off at the line of clothing, and also the relative sparing further up the neck due to shielding by the hair.

Table 17.1	SUN-REACTIVE SKIN TYPES	
Skin type	**Definition**	**Description**
I	Always burns, never tans	Pale skin, red hair, freckles
II	Always burns, some tanning	Fair skin
III	May burn, tans gradually	Darker-skinned white races
IV	Rarely burns, always tans	Mediterranean
V	Rarely burns, dark tan	Latin American, Mid-Eastern
VI	Never burns, deep pigmentation	Black

Skin type

The sun–reactive skin type is an inexact but useful tool for estimating individual sensitivity to sunlight. Six types are described (Table 17.1), which take into account the susceptibility to sunburn and ability to tan; some types may correlate with racial phenotype, such as the olive skin and easy tanning of Mediterranean individuals, or the pale skin, freckles, red hair, and easy burning of Celts (Fig. 17.6). The skin type assessment is used by sunscreen manufacturers to advise on the potency of sunscreen required for different skin types. However, when extrapolated for the

therapeutic use of UVR, this method for assessing the risk of undue erythema is limited, because there is an approximately fourfold variation in the range of MEDs within any group of individuals who have the same self-reported skin type.

ADVERSE EFFECTS OF UV RADIATION

The UV part of the spectrum from 280 to 400 nm is the most important wavelength range in dermatology. It has important physiologic effects on

Table 17.2   EFFECTS OF ULTRAVIOLET RADIATION

Beneficial effects	Adverse effects
Physiologic	**Short-term dose-related**
Production of vitamin D	Erythema (sunburn)
Feeling of well-being	Tanning*
Protective	**Long-term dose-related**
Tanning*	Carcinogenesis
Production and dispersal of melanins (tanning)	Wrinkling and other photodamage
Epidermal proliferation	**Photodermatoses**
Production of urocanic acid	Drug-related
Therapeutic	Idiopathic
Beneficial for several dermatoses	Photoaggravation of other dermatoses
Therapeutic photosensitization, for	
example psoralen plus UVA (PUVA)	

*tanning is included both as beneficial and adverse. It does have some (beneficial) protective effect but this is very minor, and others would view any tanning as being a marker of (damaging) sun exposure.

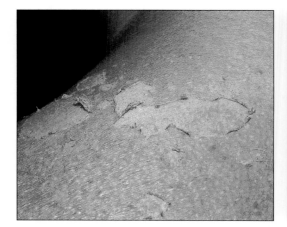

Figure 17.8   Sunburn producing superficial blistering. Sunburn typically causes peeling and patchy pigmentation as it resolves, even if frank blistering has not been an early feature.

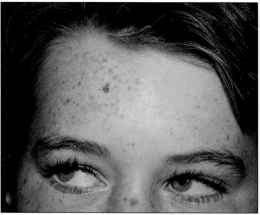

Figure 17.9   Skin type I–II (red hair and freckles). Freckling affecting predominantly the right side of the forehead, provoked by an episode of sunburn.

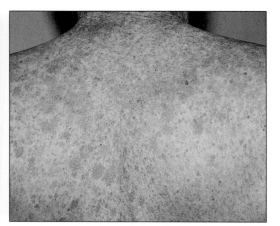

Figure 17.10   Stellate freckles on the upper back. This pattern is common in young men after episodes of sunburn, and is common in pale-skinned individuals who live in sunny climates.

the skin and useful therapeutic effects for some dermatoses, but also has adverse effects, including carcinogenesis and provocation of several specific dermatoses. These effects are summarized in Table 17.2. Aspects of carcinogenesis are discussed in Chapter 32.

Short-term (sunburn and tanning)

Excessive exposure to UVB causes erythema, which is initially visible about 4–6 h after exposure, peaks at about 24 h, and fades over a few days unless there is further exposure (Figs 17.7 and 17.8). At higher doses, the erythema is accompanied by edema and pain. A dose of several times the MED can be obtained from natural sunlight before erythema becomes visible or any discomfort is felt. This is particularly likely if there is cloud cover, which induces a false sense of security, because it reduces infrared radiation (heat) and visible sunlight but is not an effective barrier against UVB or UVA.

The inflammatory mediators that are most important in sunburn and UVB-induced erythema are arachidonic acid metabolites, particularly prostaglandins PGD_2, PGE_2, $PGF_{2\alpha}$, and PGI_2, and the monohydroxy-eicosatetraenoic acid 12-HETE. The clinical importance of this is that inhibitors of these chemicals, such as indomethacin, are therapeutically useful in reducing the intensity of sunburn. The best results are obtained by early treatment within about the first 12 h after exposure.

Tanning is viewed by many as a desired effect of sun exposure. Melanin dispersal is an early effect after UV exposure, before new melanin production is clinically manifest. It has a protective effect but must nonetheless be viewed as an indicator that solar exposure (and therefore solar damage) has occurred. Darkening of freckles occurs (Fig. 17.9) and is seasonal; new freckle-like lesions on the trunk after sunburn are often permanent (Fig. 17.10).

(Long-term) photoaging

The chronic effects of photodamage are well known and include atrophy and elastic tissue damage (solar elastosis), which are manifest in the skin as wrinkling, cutis rhomboidalis nuchae, solar purpura, pseudoscars, and colloid milium (Figs 17.11–17.18). Therapeutic aspects of photoaging are discussed in Chapter 5.

Photodermatoses and photosensitivity reactions

A classification of photodermatoses is given in Table 17.3. These constitute the remainder of the discussion in this chapter.

APPROACH TO A PATIENT WHO HAS APPARENT PHOTOSENSITIVITY

In addition to a number of standard questions, which are applicable for any dermatosis, there are specific questions that have diagnostic importance in photodermatoses (summarized in Table 17.4). Some of these are aimed at distinguishing between specific photosensitivity disorders, but others aim to identify eruptions that may be confused with photosensitivity. For example, airborne contact dermatitis (i.e. contact dermatitis to an airborne allergen) may affect exposed skin and therefore mimic photosensitivity; in chronic actinic dermatitis, patients may have both photosensitivity and contact allergies.

History and examination

Specific attention should be paid to the following.
- Age and sex of the patient. The genodermatoses with photosensitivity are usually apparent in children; polymorphic light eruption usually has

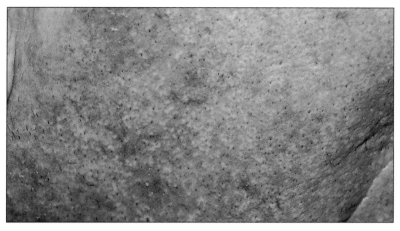

Figure 17.11   Elastosis, a form of solar aging, is clinically apparent as semiconfluent yellowish papules that are usually most prominent on the lateral aspects of the forehead, cheeks, and nape of neck.

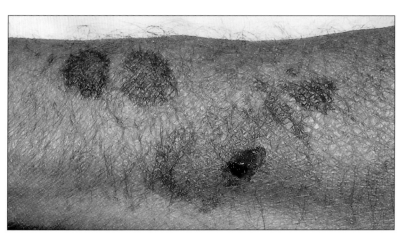

Figure 17.13   Solar aging on the exposed dorsal forearms causes skin atrophy and flattening of the rete ridges. Minor shearing injuries in this thinned skin commonly cause macular areas of purpura.

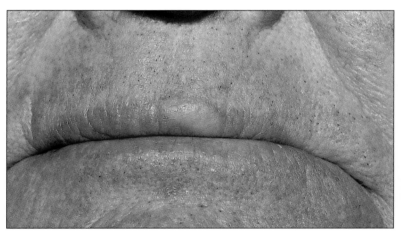

Figure 17.12   Elastoma, a localized nodule of solar-induced elastotic material.

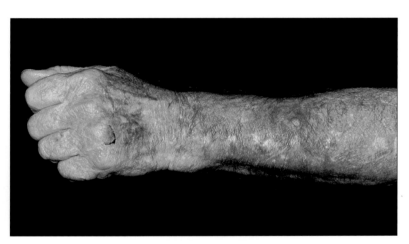

Figure 17.14   Solar aging may cause easy tearing and stellate-shaped 'solar pseudoscars', as well as purpuric areas; all are shown here.

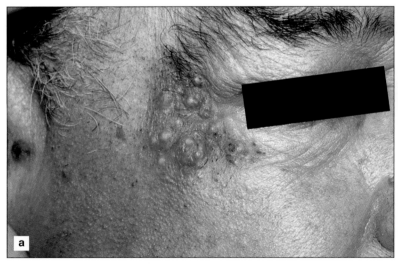

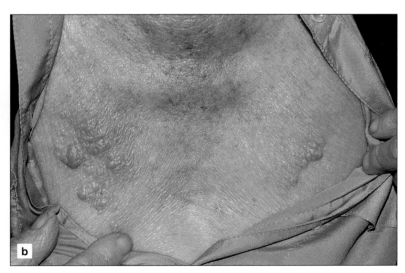

Figure 17.15   Nodular elastosis is a photoaging disorder that is most apparent around the eyes (**a**), although it may also occur at other sites (**b**). The elastotic nodules may be accompanied by comedones and cysts (also termed the Favre–Racouchot syndrome), and are occasionally confused with skin malignancies.

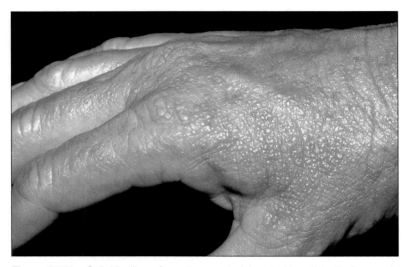

Figure 17.16 Colloid milium. Amorphous material, probably actinically damaged elastic fibers, is deposited in the dermis to produce translucent papules on sun-exposed skin. There are also juvenile and nodular forms of this disorder, and a type that is induced by topical hydroquinone (a depigmenting agent).

an onset in later childhood and is predominantly a disorder that occurs in women; actinic reticuloid is mainly (but not exclusively) a disorder of older men.

- Timing of the eruption in relation to exposure. Solar urticaria occurs within seconds or minutes, whereas polymorphic light eruption typically occurs many hours after exposure.
- Timing of the eruption in relation to the season. Polymorphic light eruption is typically prominent in the spring and improves later in the summer, recurring from year to year.
- Type and severity of symptoms. Burning pain is typical of erythropoietic protoporphyria, while itch is more typical of most photosensitivity eruptions. This also needs to be put into context in terms of the previous 'normal' sunlight response for the individual.
- Type and amount of exposure required to provoke symptoms and response to photoprotection. This gives some indication of severity and may also be useful for determining the causative wavelengths (e.g. triggering by tanning beds implies that UVA is responsible).
- Effect of window glass. This blocks UVB but not UVA, so development of the eruption when protected by window glass implies that UVA is responsible.
- Medications. This should include a specific enquiry about systemic medications, topical agents (including sunscreens), and anything that the patient has purchased without specific medical advice. Some drugs, such as quinine for nocturnal cramps, are important photosensitizers but are often not viewed as medicines by patients.

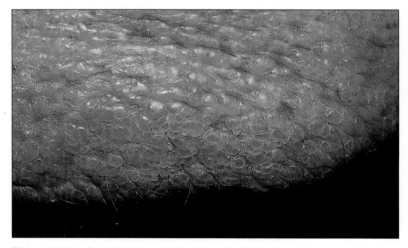

Figure 17.17 Colloid milium: another example of this unusual form of actinic damage.

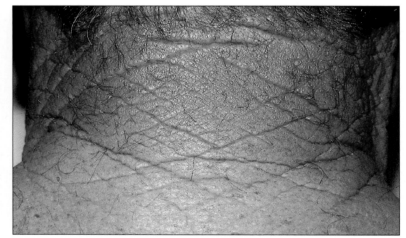

Figure 17.18 Cutis rhomboidalis nuchae. A pattern of photoaging that is apparent at the nape of the neck, usually in men who have worked outdoors. The diamond-shaped (rhomboid) patterning of skin creases is characteristic.

Table 17.3 CLASSIFICATION OF PHOTODERMATOSES AND PHOTOSENSITIVITY DISORDERS	
Classification	**Disorder**
Genetic or inherited	Xeroderma pigmentosum Bloom syndrome, Rothmund–Thomson syndrome Albinism Porphyrias
Reactions to exogenous agents	Drug phototoxicity or photoallergy (internal) Reactions to external photosensitizers or plants Porphyria cutanea tarda, (many cases are caused by alcohol, less commonly, estrogen intake); pseudoporphyria (diuretics, naproxen, high dose UVB)
Idiopathic photodermatoses	Solar urticaria Polymorphic light eruption and variants Hydroa vacciniforme Actinic prurigo Photosensitivity dermatitis or actinic reticuloid
Dermatoses associated with photoaggravation	See Table 17.10

Table 17.4   QUESTIONS AND CLINICAL SIGNS OF PARTICULAR RELEVANCE IN PHOTODERMATOSES AND ABNORMAL LIGHT SENSITIVITY

Age and sex of patient
How soon does the eruption occur after exposure to sun?
What time of year does the problem occur? (Mainly spring, mainly summer, all year?)
Type of and severity of symptoms (burning, itch, etc.)
Normal response to light (skin type) and relative amount required to produce the problem compared with 'ordinary' sunburn
Type of light that produces the problem (sunlight, sunbed, both)
Effect of window glass: does the eruption still occur?
Medications (oral and topical) and alcohol intake (relevant in porphyria)
Other topical agents that may be implicated as photosensitizers
Family history of a similar problem
Other systemic symptoms
Sites affected by the eruption, and areas of sparing
Morphology of the eruption (erythema, urticarial, papular, blisters, etc.)

- External agents that may be applied. Several external agents may provoke photosensitivity, including some topical medications, sunscreens, perfumed agents (e.g. bath oils, perfumes, and perfumed moisturizers), and plants. It may also be important to know what type of sunscreen the patient has tried, as it may or may not be appropriate to prevent the problem (sunscreens are discussed in more detail at the end of this chapter).
- Family history. This may be important for porphyrias and rarer genodermatoses, and is often positive in polymorphic light eruption.
- Other symptoms and previous history. These may reveal preexisting dermatoses or symptoms suggestive of, for example, lupus erythematosus or variegate porphyria.
- Pattern of involvement and sites of sparing. In the differential diagnosis between photosensitivity and airborne contact dermatitis, sparing of shielded areas (lower eyelids, beneath the nose, behind ears, and neck and face creases) is a useful indicator of photosensitivity (Figs 17.19–17.21). However, these areas of sparing are lost in more chronic photosensitivity, and lack of sparing does not exclude photosensitivity. Similarly, acute photosensitivity is usually confined to exposed skin, but extension of the rash to shielded areas occurs with chronicity.
- Morphology of the eruption. Sheet-like erythema is suggestive of drug-induced phototoxicity, pure wheals occur in solar urticaria, polymorphic light eruption may have early urticarial features but eczematous morphology later, photoallergic eruptions tend to be more papular than those with phototoxic mechanisms, and blisters may occur in any severe photosensitivity but are a typical feature of porphyria cutanea tarda and reactions to plants (Fig. 17.22).

Phototests, patch tests, and photopatch tests
Provocation testing
Although this would appear to be a simple test, most photodermatoses cannot be easily provoked using small test areas under artificial conditions. One reason for this is that most photodermatoses are UVA-triggered, and routinely available UVA lamps require long exposures to achieve the required stimulus. Additionally, under test conditions, irradiation of relatively wide areas of skin is required on 2 or 3 consecutive days. Provocation tests:
- are almost always positive in solar urticaria using small doses of UVR (usually UVA) and readings after a few minutes;
- are variably positive in polymorphic light eruption (up to 90% positive using consecutive daily exposures with a solar simulator source) and

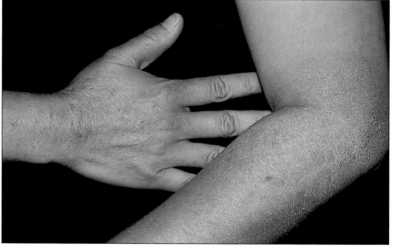

Figure 17.19   Photodermatitis showing a typical distribution pattern. There is a cut-off from short sleeves, and relative sparing of the ulnar border of the hand, finger webs, and distal fingers.

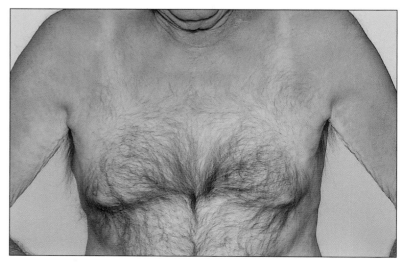

Figure 17.20   Photosensitivity due to a thiazide diuretic, showing sparing under clothing.

347

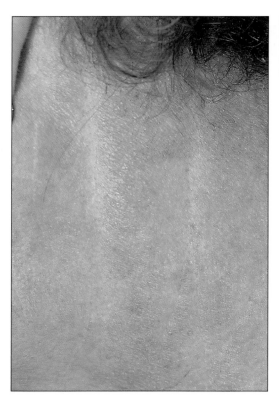

Figure 17.21 Photosensitivity due to a thiazide diuretic, showing sparing of skin creases on the neck.

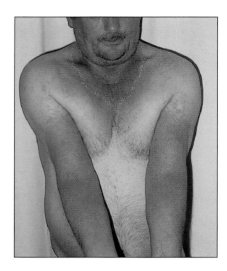

Figure 17.23 Airborne contact dermatitis (to balsams, probably in sawdust) affecting the face, V of the neck, and exposed areas of the arms. This can mimic photosensitivity.

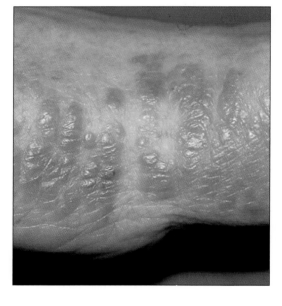

Figure 17.22 Papules and blisters on the wrist due to contact and subsequent phototoxic reaction to plant sap; note the streaky pattern.

wavelengths producing abnormal results may correlate with the known pattern for a photosensitizing drug).

Other test techniques include the use of metal halide lamps, solar simulators (optically filtered xenon arc lamps, which emit a spectrum of UVR similar to that of natural sunlight), phototherapy equipment (which is available in most dermatology departments), and other fluorescent tube lamps.

Patch testing

Patch testing is potentially helpful in patients for whom there is diagnostic uncertainty between photosensitivity and an airborne contact dermatitis (Fig. 17.23). Allergies to balsams and perfume agents are particularly relevant in this differential diagnosis. Some allergens, notably the Compositae mix (an extract of plants in the daisy family), are of importance because positive results are common in chronic actinic dermatitis. Allergy to sunscreens may cause confusion in a small proportion of patients, and a sunscreen series is often tested in photosensitive patients. Most sunscreen allergy is due to fragrances or antimicrobials; allergy (or photoallergy, see later) to the sunscreen ingredient itself is much less common.

Photopatch testing

Photopatch tests are used in investigation because some topically applied agents cause a contact dermatitis only when they are on the skin and are also exposed to light (i.e. they cause a photocontact allergic reaction). Sunscreens, balsams, and perfumes (Figs 17.24–17.26), and some reactions to plants, are particularly likely to do this. The technique of investigation involves applying a duplicate set of relevant patch tests. After 24 h, one set of tests is removed, irradiated with UVA at a dose that is insufficient to cause erythema in itself (determined by previous phototesting), and reapplied for a further 24 h before reading. Comparison of corresponding tests may indicate:

- a standard contact reaction (both tests positive and equivalent);
- a pure photocontact reaction (irradiated test positive, non-irradiated test negative); or
- both contact and photocontact reactions (both tests positive, but greater reaction in the irradiated series).

systemic drug-induced phototoxicity (single exposure read at 24 h, repeated on and off the drug); and
- may be positive in lupus erythematosus using a UVB source.

Phototesting

Phototesting involves exposure of the skin to a series of doses of UVR to determine the MED. By comparison with the range of results for the normal population, it can be determined whether the patient has abnormal photosensitivity (i.e. an MED below the lower limit of normal).

The readily available fluorescent lamps are of limited value for testing, however: UVB-producing sources can achieve sufficient doses in a short time, but most photosensitivity is in the UVA range and standard UVA lamps require long exposure times to administer appropriate doses. Monochromator testing is the most accurate technique, using a series of narrow bands centered at specific wavelengths. This can be important, as some individuals are abnormally sensitive to a relatively narrow range of wavelengths. Monochromator testing also allows accurate repeat testing to monitor progression. The pattern of abnormal results in any individual may also be important in determining the likely cause (e.g. the

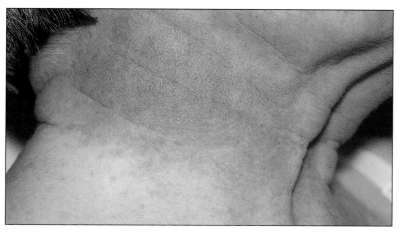

Figure 17.24 Photocontact reaction to a fragranced bath additive. This demonstrates the typical cut-off at the neck where the light exposure is shielded, although the whole body was exposed to the fragrance material.

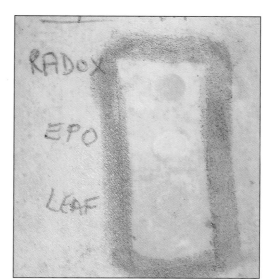

Figure 17.26
Photocontact reaction to a fragranced bath additive, showing a positive photopatch test (labeled 'Radox'). This was in the same patient as shown in Figures 17.24 and 17.25. The other (negative) tests were to a topical evening primrose oil preparation ('EPO') and a plant leaf with which the patient had been in contact.

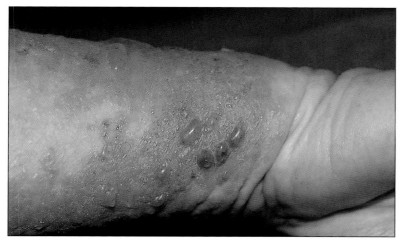

Figure 17.25 Photocontact reaction to a fragranced bath additive. This demonstrates the severity of the blistering in the patient shown in Figure 17.24.

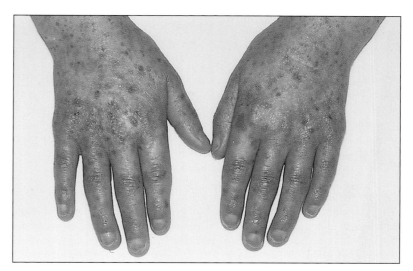

Figure 17.27 Xeroderma pigmentosum. This shows freckling and wrinkling of the dorsa of the hands in a child. These changes are similar to those normally seen in much older patients. See also Fig. 19.67.

GENODERMATOSES WITH PHOTOSENSITIVITY

This category includes several very rare disorders, which will not be discussed in detail, such as Rothmund–Thomson syndrome (poikiloderma congenitale), Bloom syndrome, Cockayne syndrome, trichothiodystrophy, and Hartnup disease (which causes a pellagra-like eruption). Porphyrias are discussed later. Xeroderma pigmentosum is considered separately here.

Xeroderma pigmentosum
Etiology and pathogenesis
Xeroderma pigmentosum (XP) is the term used for eight clinically similar autosomal recessive diseases in which there are different defects of DNA repair.

Ultraviolet B causes pyrimidine dimer production within the DNA molecule, especially thymidine dimers. Normally, these are excised and replaced by thymine, a process known as excision repair. This causes 'unscheduled' DNA synthesis (i.e. DNA is synthesized at times other than for cell replication), which can be detected by autoradiography. In seven of the XP types, the defect involves defective endonuclease-mediated excision repair, manifested as low levels of unscheduled DNA synthesis following exposure to UVR.

Fusion of fibroblasts from different XP strains can normalize the level of unscheduled DNA repair in UV-exposed cell cultures, so cells from patients with XP can be assigned to different types. These are known as complementation groups, as they depend on which cell strain is complementary and corrects the defect, and are labeled groups A–G. The most frequent are XP-A and XP-C.

The final type of XP, known as XP variant, accounts for about 30% of patients who have XP. It is characterized by normal levels of unscheduled DNA repair and may be due to a defect of postreplication repair.

Clinical features
All types share some common features that are perennial and progressive; they may also be apparent to a minor degree in heterozygotes. Features may vary in severity within groups, but are typically severe in the commonest (XP-A) type.

Age of onset may be from the first few months of life, usually in the first few years, but is occasionally in the second decade. There may be episodes resembling prolonged sunburn, with associated freckling and dryness of exposed skin (Fig. 17.27). Skin tumors develop subsequently, usually in large numbers, and include basal cell carcinomas, squamous cell carcinomas, and melanomas. Mucous membranes, especially the conjunctivae and lower lip, are also affected; photophobia is common. In some of the subtypes, particularly XP-A and XP-D, progressive neurologic abnormalities are a significant feature, with an onset in the first two decades. These may be mild, especially sensorineural deafness, but a severe disorder of mental retardation, peripheral neuropathy, and cerebellar abnormalities may occur (De Sanctis–Cacchione syndrome).

Phototesting is characterized by abnormal photosensitivity, which produces prolonged erythema compared with the usual 24-h peak of erythema. Complementation group is determined by cell culture and may be prognostically important (e.g. neurologic disease is not a feature of XP variant but is often severe in XP-A).

Differential diagnosis

In most instances, where there are established skin changes, the differential diagnosis is between the different types of XP rather than from other disorders. The rare photosensitivity genodermatoses may also need to be considered. Early or milder cases, especially in patients who have freckles but no gross photosensitivity, may be difficult to distinguish from those with prominent ordinary freckles or with various disorders featuring facial lentiginosis (all rare).

Treatment

Once the diagnosis has been established, strict sun avoidance and high protection factor sunscreens are essential to delay the development of tumors. Antenatal diagnosis is possible by culturing amniotic fluid cells. Topical endonucleases to replace the deficient repair enzymes are being investigated. Tumors are treated by excision. Systemic retinoids reduce the frequency of epidermal tumors.

IDIOPATHIC PHOTODERMATOSES

Polymorphic light eruption

Etiology and pathogenesis

Polymorphic light eruption (PLE) is the commonest of the idiopathic photodermatoses. The true incidence is uncertain, as minor versions are often misinterpreted as sunburn or as prickly heat. In most series, it is commonest in women, and may occur in up to 30% of young women using tanning beds. It is familial in about 10% of cases. The onset is typically in the second decade, but earlier in 25%. About 10% of young women with this disorder may have a low-titer positive antinuclear antibody (ANA), but long-term follow-up does not suggest a progression to lupus erythematosus.

Clinical features

The eruption has mixed features, but generally follows a reproducible pattern in any individual. Some patients have predominantly papules (Fig. 17.28), vesicles, urticated plaques, eczematous areas, or (less commonly) erythema multiforme-like lesions. Solar purpura may be a variant of PLE. Onset is usually from a few hours to a few days after exposure (typically 6–12 h), and the eruption predominantly affects exposed sites; it fades after a few days without further exposure.

In most patients, the disorder is seasonal, with springtime predominance. The eruption typically appears during the first sunny days of the year and improves as the summer progresses. This process, known as 'hardening', may involve increased UVB-induced tanning and thickening of the stratum corneum. Provocation may be by UVB, UVA, or both. This may be a reason why the condition in some individuals improves as the summer progresses, but in some (usually those more severely affected) continues to deteriorate. Patients who have significant UVB provocation are likely to have more episodes of skin eruption in later summer.

The histologic features of PLE are a dense perivascular lymphocytic infiltrate in the upper and mid-dermis, and upper dermal edema. The edema may be prominent in the erythema multiforme-like pattern. There may be extravasation of erythrocytes. Mild vascular deposition of complement C3 has been reported in some patients. Lesions produced by provocation testing have this same histology, and biopsy of provoked lesions may be necessary in some individuals. Jessner lymphocytic infiltrate has similar histology, but edema is rarely marked. Lupus erythematosus may also have a similar appearance, but usually there is less perivascular infiltrate, and the abnormalities are predominantly at the dermo–epidermal junction; these include a lymphocytic infiltrate, basal epidermal liquefaction, thickened basement membrane, and deposition of complement C3 and immunoglobulin IgG, IgA, or IgM.

Other tests that may be useful include serologic tests for lupus erythematosus, especially ANA and anti-SSA (anti-Ro). Although ANA may be positive in PLE, this is of low titer and occurs in only about 10% of patients. By contrast, about 90% of patients who have systemic lupus erythematosus have positive ANA, and most who have subacute cutaneous lupus erythematosus have positive anti-SSA.

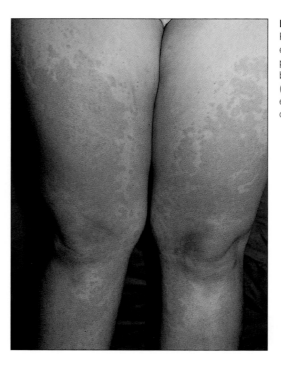

Figure 17.28
Polymorphic light eruption on the legs. The pattern of eruption may be of urticarial pattern (as in this case), eczematous, or a mixture of the two.

Table 17.5 DIFFERENTIAL DIAGNOSIS OF POLYMORPHIC LIGHT ERUPTION

Type of disorder	Examples
Other photosensitivity disorders	Solar urticaria Hydroa vacciniforme Actinic prurigo Reactions to external photosensitizers
Non-photosensitive disorders	Prickly heat ('heat rash', miliaria rubra) Eczemas, especially airborne contact Rosacea
Photoaggravated dermatoses	Lupus erythematosus Psoriasis Jessner lymphocytic infiltrate

Differential diagnosis

Polymorphic light eruption is virtually always a clinical diagnosis, but investigations may be required to distinguish it from other photodermatoses; from some non-photosensitive disorders; and (of greatest importance and difficulty) from photoaggravated disorders, especially lupus erythematosus (Table 17.5). Provocation tests can be useful, as can additional phototesting or photopatch testing if other photodermatoses are suspected.

A particular difficulty for the physician is proving the diagnosis in retrospect in a patient who developed rash after their first day on holiday. Patients generally blame such rashes on heat (causing 'prickly heat' or 'heat rash', more accurately termed miliaria rubra) rather than blaming light; it is likely that PLE is underestimated. Both eruptions are likely to respond to avoidance of sun, as this usually parallels avoidance of heat. If the eruption affects covered sites mainly, then the diagnosis of miliaria may be confirmed, but often there are few covered sites to judge this. Another possible diagnosis in this situation is sunscreen allergy, but this usually becomes apparent with repeated exposure.

Treatment

This comprises topical corticosteroids, oral antihistamines, sunscreens, and sun avoidance. Low-dose PUVA or narrow-band UVB in early spring may produce hardening. Azathioprine is used for severe disease.

Juvenile spring eruption

Etiology and pathogenesis

This eruption may be a variant of PLE, but is clinically distinct.

Clinical features

The lesions consist of tiny blisters on the rim of the ears, typically in boys aged between 5 and 14 years (Fig. 17.29). They cause itch or pain, but are transient and usually last about 2 weeks. This is typically a disorder of early spring, but may occur throughout the summer and may recur on an annual basis throughout childhood. It typically starts 1–2 h after exposure to intense sunlight, but phototests are normal and provocation tests are negative.

Differential diagnosis

Juvenile spring eruption is a clinical diagnosis, but some children are erroneously thought to have prolonged sunburn, herpes simplex, impetigo, porphyria or pseudoporphyria (usually due to naproxen in this age group), or dermatitis.

Treatment

Topical corticosteroids may be used. The important aspect is a broad-spectrum sunscreen to prevent the eruption, but benefit is variable. Physical barriers are most effective.

Solar urticaria

Etiology and pathogenesis

This is an idiopathic non-familial condition. Like other urticarias, it involves degranulation of mast cells to release histamine and other inflammatory mediators. It appears to involve IgE, but the involvement of other photoactive molecules is less clear. Passive transfer has been demonstrated, as the serum from some affected individuals causes the reaction when injected into non-photosensitive recipients.

Most patients have sensitivity in the UVA range, but some also have sensitivity in the visible range, and a few in the UVB range. Some react only to visible light.

Clinical features

Lesions have the typical morphology of urticaria (Fig. 17.30). They occur on exposed sites (some may occur due to transmission of light through thin clothing). Onset is within minutes of exposure to light, and lesions last minutes to a few hours. As can be anticipated from the spectrum to which patients are sensitive, window glass rarely provides photoprotection. Artificial light sources, notably fluorescent lamps, are occasionally sufficient to provoke lesions. The condition is typically troublesome and often symptomatic throughout the year, significantly limiting normal activities. However, it may remit spontaneously after a few years in some patients.

Differential diagnosis

The disorder is so characteristic in its onset within a minute or so of sunlight exposure that it is difficult for it to be mistaken for anything else. It may occasionally be confused with PLE if an accurate history of timing of onset is not obtained. It may also be confused with other urticarias in which symptoms may be restricted to outdoor activities, such as cholinergic urticaria (due to heat or exercise, which provoke sweating), exercise-induced urticaria, food-dependent exercise-induced urticaria, and heat urticaria (temperature-dependent rather than sunlight-provoked). Provocation tests are positive, usually to UVA (Fig. 17.31). In young children, especially if the urticaria is not apparent for examination, it may be necessary to exclude erythropoietic protoporphyria.

Treatment

Avoidance and sunscreens are important. Physical methods to block UVR, such as special films applied to house and car window glass, may be necessary. Sunscreens may be useful, but most commercial preparations have a relatively poor UVA-blocking effect (up to about eightfold protection) and block very little visible light.

Systemic antihistamines may produce an up to about 10-fold reduction in wheals and itch.

Therapeutic UVB may produce useful tanning, epidermal thickening, and tolerance in individuals with UVA or visible light provocation, but will provoke urticaria in the 25–50% of patients whose sensitivity extends into the UVB range. Those patients who respond to UVB usually need maintenance treatments every few days (even daily) to achieve ongoing benefit. PUVA may also be useful, and can produce prolonged benefit. It may have immunologic effects in addition to tanning and skin thickening,

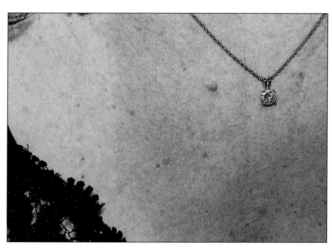

Figure 17.30 Solar urticaria, occurring as a confluent sheet on the exposed V of the neck.

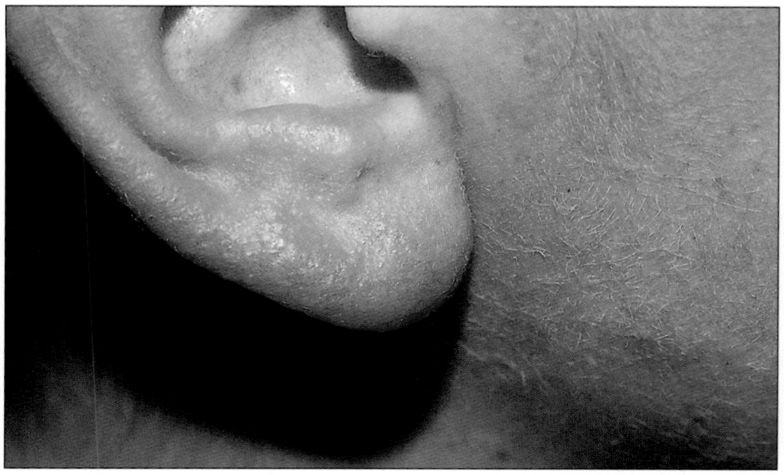

Figure 17.29 Juvenile spring eruption at the typical site on the helix of a young boy.

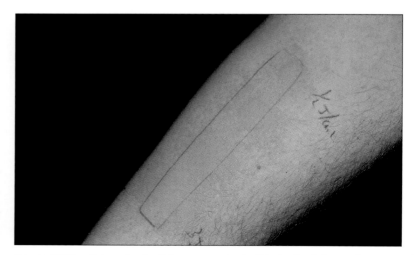

Figure 17.31 Solar urticaria. This was provoked within 1 min of diagnostic phototesting, at all the doses administered.

but is often difficult to administer in patients with a high degree of UVA provocation.

Immunosuppressive agents such as ciclosporin have been used with benefit, but in the author's experience have not proved helpful.

Hydroa vacciniforme
Etiology and pathogenesis
The etiology of this rare sporadic condition is uncertain. It is a clinically characteristic eruption in which histology shows epidermal degeneration, perivascular inflammation, vascular thrombosis, and necrosis. It is most common in boys, and is a recurrent problem in the summer months, but usually resolves in adolescence.

Clinical features
There is a papular and vesicular eruption of discrete lesions, which are predominantly at photoexposed sites on the face and hands or forearms (Figs 17.32 and 17.33). Milder cases heal with little residue (hydroa estivale), but the typical pattern is necrosis of the lesions with a varioliform appearance and scarring.

Differential diagnosis
The differential diagnosis includes herpes simplex, varicella, impetigo, erythropoietic protoporphyria, PLE, lupus erythematosus, and actinic prurigo. Investigations include phototests and provocation tests (which are sometimes positive with UVA), porphyrins, ANA, and anti-SSA.

Treatment
Sunscreens are of limited benefit. Antimalarials (discussed in the treatment of lupus erythematosus, see Ch. 13) and β-carotene may be helpful.

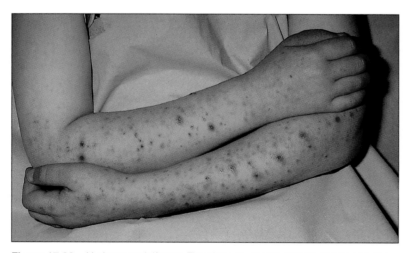

Figure 17.32 Hydroa vacciniforme. The close-up morphology is of non-specific papules, vesicles, and scabbed lesions, but with localization to photoexposed skin, as shown here on the arms.

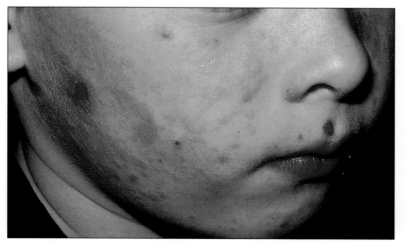

Figure 17.33 Hydroa vacciniforme. Lesions on the cheek of the patient shown in Figure 17.32.

Actinic prurigo
Etiology and pathogenesis
This disorder is rare in Europe, but has a strong familial tendency in native North and South American peoples. It is most common in girls. The histologic features are those of eczema (Ch. 6).

Clinical features
Initially, papules and vesicles develop in sun-exposed areas (Fig. 17.34). It is most apparent in the summer, but often fails to clear completely in winter months, and generally progresses to a more eczematous morphology with plaques, lichenification, and crusting. It may clear in some patients in their late teens, but some cases are chronic.

Differential diagnosis
This includes other photodermatoses, especially PLE and hydroa vacciniforme, and dermatitis of other causes, especially photoaggravated atopic disease. Phototests may be abnormal, and patch tests may be required to exclude contact dermatitis.

Treatment
This condition is generally refractory to treatment. Sunscreens are of limited benefit. Treatments for dermatitis (see Ch. 6) are used, and severe cases may require immunosuppressive medication.

Chronic actinic dermatitis (photosensitivity dermatitis, actinic reticuloid)
Etiology and pathogenesis
This is a spectrum of disease that may progress from a chronic eczematous pattern of photosensitivity to a more infiltrated skin eruption (termed actinic reticuloid), which is difficult to distinguish histologically from mycosis fungoides. Some patients are those who have previously been diagnosed as having a photoallergy (see later) that has not resolved (also known as 'persistent light reactors').

In addition to abnormal phototest sensitivity (which usually spans UVB, UVA, and visible light), patients often have multiple contact allergies. Some of these appear logical (e.g. reactions to oleoresins of the Compositae plant family, fragrances, or lichens, which may all cause an airborne contact allergy), but others are less easy to explain (e.g. high frequency of reactions to chromate and rubber). There is also a high frequency of reactions to sunscreens, which may reflect many years of using these chemicals. The precise mechanism of chronic actinic dermatitis remains uncertain, and it is not known why some patients progress to develop a more lymphomatous pattern.

The disorder typically occurs in the elderly, and there is a strong male predominance.

Clinical features
A diffuse eruption with eczematous morphology and severe itch initially affects the photoexposed areas of the body, but gradually spreads to

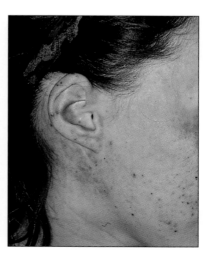

Figure 17.34 Actinic prurigo. This disorder appears eczematous but occurs at exposed sites, typically in girls.

covered sites (Figs 17.35 and 17.36). Some patients develop increasingly lichenified and indurated skin, which may produce a leonine facies and may have histologic features strongly suggestive of lymphoma. The problem is initially most apparent in summer, but the duration of symptoms gradually extends into winter months, and eventually the condition becomes perennial. Minor sunlight exposure, light through glass, and even fluorescent lamps may provoke symptoms.

Differential diagnosis

This includes drug-induced photosensitivity, photosensitivity due to external agents, eczemas (especially airborne contact dermatitis and late-onset atopy), drug eruptions, and (in its earlier stages) other photosensitivity disorders such as PLE. Patch tests, phototests, and photopatch tests are all indicated. Tests to plant extracts may be necessary, although a commercially available Compositae extract has simplified this test procedure; in Europe, this is a routine component of the Extended European Standard Battery of patch test agents.

Treatment

Patients who have positive contact reactions need to avoid the relevant agents. In particular, those who react to Compositae need to be warned about plants that may cause reactions, which vary in different parts of the world. This family includes chrysanthemum, dahlia, sunflower, cornflower, lettuce, chicory, feverfew, ragweed, and some other weeds; they may cross-react with colophony (a resin).

Interventions include use of broad-spectrum sunscreens and physical protection from sunlight. UV-blocking museum film may be needed on house and vehicle windows. However, in some patients, the photosensitivity includes visible light, which is poorly blocked by sunscreens or window films.

Topical and systemic corticosteroids may be helpful. Some patients respond to PUVA photochemotherapy. Azathioprine often gives good control, while other immunosuppressive agents such as ciclosporin have been used more recently.

PHOTOSENSITIVITY DUE TO DRUGS AND EXTERNAL AGENTS

Photosensitivity due to systemic drugs
Etiology and pathogenesis

Many drugs can cause photosensitivity (Figs 17.37–17.40). In most cases, the mechanism is phototoxicity, which is not immunologically mediated, but other drugs cause photoallergy. For some drugs, the mechanism is either uncertain, or both major mechanisms may be involved. Some of the commoner drugs and their mechanisms of photodamage are listed in Table 17.6.

The main mechanism of phototoxicity is absorption of UVR by the drug or its metabolite(s) *in vivo,* to produce an 'excited state' molecule. Return to the ground state releases various forms of energy, which damage cellular organelles and may create proinflammatory reactive oxygen molecules. Some drugs typically cause damage to cell nuclei, notably the psoralens, which intercalate between DNA strands to form photoadducts.

Photoallergy occurs in a minority of exposed individuals and involves immunologic mechanisms. The first step is UVR conversion of the photoallergic drug or metabolite to create either a hapten or an excited state. This then binds to a carrier protein to produce the antigen, which causes a type IV hypersensitivity reaction. The clinical features of phototoxicity and photoallergy are therefore different.

Clinical features

The main clinical aspects of the two different types of reaction are listed in Table 17.7. Acute drug-induced photosensitivity, especially of the phototoxic type, is usually manifest as very discrete erythema with characteristic areas of sparing (see Figs 17.19–17.21). This sparing may be lost if the cause is not recognized and the eruption becomes more chronic.

Associated photoonycholysis may occur, and appears to be particularly frequent with tetracyclines and the (now withdrawn) non-steroidal antiinflammatory drug benoxaprofen.

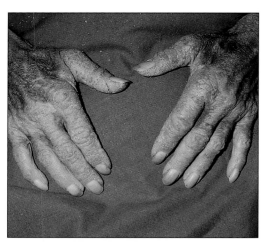

Figure 17.35 Chronic actinic dermatitis. This is typically seen in elderly men. The close-up morphology is that of chronic dermatitis.

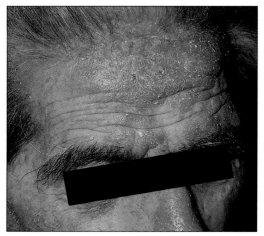

Figure 17.36 Chronic actinic dermatitis. (Same patient as in Fig. 17.35.)

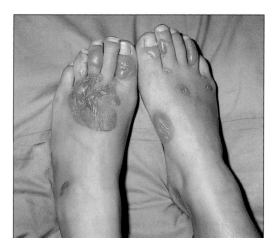

Figure 17.37 Drug-induced photosensitivity due to nalidixic acid. There is a large bullous reaction.

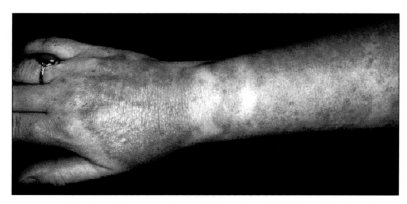

Figure 17.38 Drug-induced photosensitivity with a rather lichenoid pattern, due to a proton pump inhibitor. Sparing of sun-shielded areas is often lost in chronic photosensitivity, but sparing of the relatively shielded fingers and sparing under a watch can be discerned in this case.

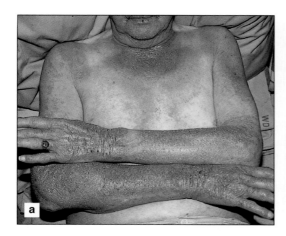
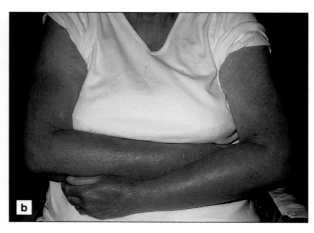

Figure 17.39 (**a,b**) Two examples of drug-induced photosensitivity due to quinine. This is often a chronic condition that takes months to resolve. As in Figure 17.38, (a) shows sparing of the watch strap area and more obvious sparing under clothing.

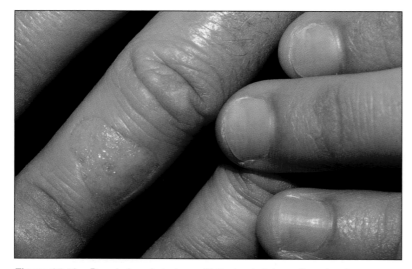

Figure 17.40 Drug-induced photosensitivity due to tetracycline, showing a recently ruptured blister and photoonycholysis (nails of the same patient are shown in Fig. 18.42).

Pigmentation may be a prominent feature with some photosensitizers; for example, tanning is inevitable with the therapeutic use of psoralens in PUVA. A grayish pigmentation with a photodistribution may occur without overt photosensitivity in some instances, and is usually related to long-term administration of medication. Drugs that cause pigmentation of this type include phenothiazines, amiodarone, and occasionally tetracyclines. It is also a feature of photolichenoid eruptions.

Patients who have severe photosensitivity due to a drug develop a rash regardless of the season, but some who have milder photosensitivity may have been on the drug for many months before symptoms develop in the summer months; this is important, as it may erroneously suggest that the drug is not relevant. Some drug photosensitivity is inadvertently revealed by the therapeutic use of UVR if patients are on drugs that are uncommon photosensitizers.

Phototests are generally positive, as most common drug photosensitivity occurs in the UVA range, and can be useful for rechallenge or for monitoring progress when the relevant drug is withdrawn. Photopatch tests may be positive if there is a photoallergic mechanism.

Differential diagnosis
This includes the following.
* Simple sunburn—in acute cases.
* Polymorphic light eruption—usually more scattered and papular in morphology.

Table 17.6 SYSTEMIC DRUGS THAT CAUSE PHOTOSENSITIVITY			
Group	**Examples**	**Mechanism**	**Wavelength**
Non-steroidal antiinflammatory drugs	Tiaprofenic acid, piroxicam, azapropazone	Mostly phototoxicity, some photoallergy	Mostly UVA
Hypoglycemics	Tolbutamide, sulfonylureas	Phototoxicity or photoallergy	UVB
Diuretics	Thiazides Furosemide	Phototoxicity (mostly) or photoallergy Phototoxicity	UVA (most) or UVB UVA
Psychiatric	Chlorpromazine Promethazine Tricyclics	Phototherapy or photoallergy Phototoxicity Phototoxicity	UVA or UVB UVA or UVB UVB
Antimicrobials	Nalidixic acid Ciprofloxacin, ofloxacin Tetracyclines Sulfonamides Griseofulvin	Phototoxicity Phototoxicity Phototoxicity Photoallergy Phototoxicity	UVA UVA Mostly UVA UVA or UVB UVA or UVB
Others	Amiodarone Cytotoxics Quinine Psoralens Porphyrins	Phototoxicity Mostly phototoxicity Photoallergy Phototoxicity Phototoxicity	UVA Mostly UVA UVA UVA Visible

Table 17.7 COMPARISON BETWEEN PHOTOTOXICITY AND PHOTOALLERGY

Characteristic	Phototoxicity	Photoallergy
Frequency	High	Low
Relationship to starting drug	May occur shortly after medication started	Requires at least 24 h, usually longer
Morphology	Usually diffuse erythema of exposed skin, resembles an exaggerated sunburn	Usually more papular or eczematous, may be scattered distribution, may be lichenoid morphology
Response to withdrawal of causative drug	Usually significantly improved within 1–2 weeks	May be prolonged symptoms and rash, with abnormal phototest results
Cross-reaction to related agents	Non-specific	Yes, including after phototoxicity occasionally
Concentration of drug required	High	Low

Table 17.8 EXTERNAL AGENTS THAT CAUSE PHOTOSENSITIVITY

Category	Examples	Mechanism	Wavelength
Plants	Psoralens (5-methoxypsoralen, 8-methoxypsoralen) in Umbelliferae and Rutaceae	Phototoxicity	UVA
	Oleoresins in Compositae (e.g. daisy, ragweed, tansy)	Photoallergy	UVA
Fragrances	6-methylcoumarin, musk ambrette	Photoallergy	UVA or UVB
Sunscreen ingredients	Fragrances, *para*-aminobenzoic acid (PABA) and esters, benzophenones, cinnamates	Mostly photoallergy	UVA
Topical medications	Phenothiazine antihistamines	Photoallergy or phototoxicity	UVA
	Tars	Phototoxicity	UVB
	Psoralens	Phototoxicity	UVA
	Antiseptic vital dyes	Phototoxicity	Visible
	Benzoyl peroxide	Phototoxicity	UVA or UVB
Antimicrobials (e.g. soaps)	Chloro- and bromo-salicylanilides	Photoallergy	UVA
	Bithionol	Photoallergy	UVA

- Contact dermatitis—especially due to airborne allergens.
- Photosensitivity dermatitis or actinic reticuloid—which may be very difficult to distinguish from chronic drug-induced photosensitivity.
- Photoaggravated dermatoses.
- Atopic dermatitis—especially in older patients.

Treatment

The mainstay of treatment is withdrawal of the relevant drug, with physical protection, avoidance of sunlight, and use of sunscreens until symptoms remit. Topical corticosteroids and oral antihistamines have symptomatic benefit. Some photoallergic eruptions, such as those due to quinine, may persist for several months.

Photosensitivity due to external agents
Etiology and pathogenesis

A list of external photosensitizers is given in Table 17.8. As with medications used internally, these can be divided into phototoxic and photoallergic types.

Clinical features

The morphology depends to some extent on the mechanism, as for systemic phototoxicity and photoallergy. The site of application of the agent also alters the pattern. For example, the pattern caused by plants (Figs 17.41–17.44) may vary depending on the type of exposure. The typical morphology is a streaky distribution on limbs that have rubbed against a plant; sap or juices of plants and fruits may create trickles, and the spatter of psoralens on to the exposed trunk when using high-speed garden tools to cut hedgerow plants is known as strimmer (or weed whacker) dermatitis (Fig. 17.45). The psoralens produced by the Umbelliferae (such as hogweeds and cow parsley, Fig. 17.46) typically cause an intense phototoxicity with large blisters and significant pigmentation. Therapeutic use for PUVA may also cause unusual reactions (Fig. 17.44b). Compositae are discussed in the section on photosensitivity dermatitis.

These eruptions typically occur during the summer, but some plant reactions are influenced by the growing season. Some reactions, such as those to perfume agents, may occur at other times of the year as well. Sunscreen ingredients cause particular problems, as patients expect these to be photoprotective. Except for the psoralen type, most of these reactions are photoallergic in mechanism and can be identified by photopatch testing.

Differential diagnosis

External causes of photosensitivity may be more difficult to diagnose, as the pattern will depend on both the site of application and the site exposed to light; additionally, some of the causes are airborne rather than deliberately applied to the skin, and others may be assumed to be protective (sunscreens). It is impossible to list all differential diagnoses that might apply, but other photodermatoses clearly need to be excluded. As the most likely sites to be affected are the face and hands, various forms of dermatitis (especially contact dermatitis), as well as photoaggravated facial dermatoses such as lupus erythematosus, may be in the differential.

Treatment

This comprises identification and avoidance of the trigger. The choice of sunscreen may be difficult for those who react to fragrances, benzophenones, or cinnamates, and may require photopatch testing the individual constituents.

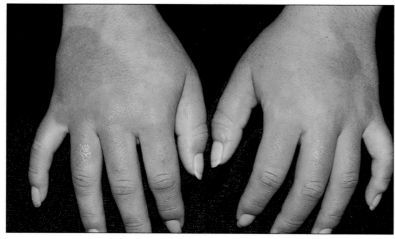

Figure 17.41 Phytophotodermatitis due to psoralen in lime juice. This is a common cause of phototoxicity in warm climates where these fruit are grown.

PRACTICE POINTS

- Polymorphic light eruption (PLE) is common, especially in women; it is the most likely cause of rash in individuals using sunbeds (tanning beds), and may well explain many cases of supposed prickly heat (heat rash) occurring early on sunny vacations.
- Several photodermatoses, including common problems such as PLE and reasonably common drug-induced photosensitivity, are provoked by long-wavelength ultraviolet radiation (UVA) and may therefore occur through glass when the individual expects to be protected.
- Patients with solar urticaria or chronic photosensitivity dermatitis may experience provocation by visible light, which is very difficult to block using standard measures.
- In a patient with presumed porphyria cutanea tarda, it is important to consider and exclude variegate porphyria and drug-induced pseudoporphyria.
- Very few disorders produce symptoms within minutes of sun exposure; if this occurs, consider solar urticaria (any age) or erythropoietic protoporphyria (usually apparent in very young children).

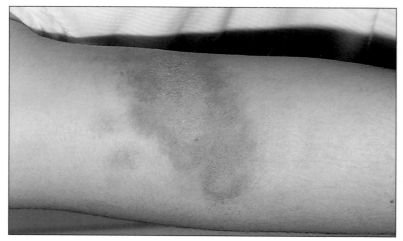

Figure 17.42 Phytophotodermatitis. Residual pigmentation is a characteristic feature of this eruption, although blistering may cause a paler area, as shown here.

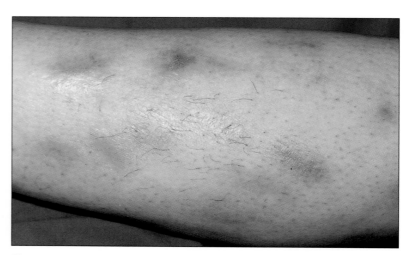

Figure 17.43 Phytophotodermatitis on the leg. The pigmentation is often in a streaky pattern where limbs have brushed against vegetation.

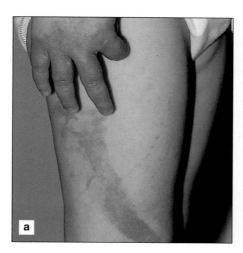

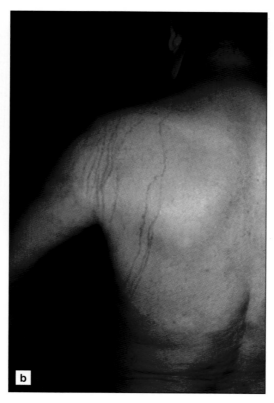

Figure 17.44 Pigmentation in trickles. (**a**) Fruit juice has trickled down the child's fingers and leg and caused a phototoxic reaction. (**b**) During bath PUVA, the patient lies in a bath of dilute psoralen solution, and then has UVA exposure. This patient, unknown to nursing staff, sat in the bath and splashed the water (not very effectively) on to his back. He therefore has even pigmentation up to lower thoracic level, but trickles of pigmentation down his upper back.

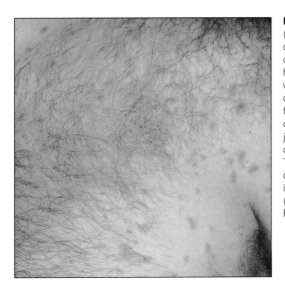

Figure 17.45 Strimmer (weed whacker) dermatitis on the chest, due to psoralens in hedgerow and garden weeds. These tools create a spray of plant fragments, which leave drops of photosensitizing juice on the exposed skin of the person using them. The brown colour is characteristic, as shown in Figures 17.41–17.44. (Courtesy of Prof. N. Reynolds.)

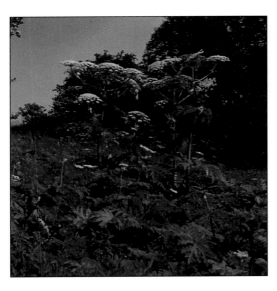

Figure 17.46 Giant hogweed. This member of the Umbelliferae contains psoralens and has a particular tendency to cause phototoxic reactions.

PORPHYRIAS

These disorders result from altered metabolism in the heme biosynthesis pathway, leading to an accumulation of porphyrins. In the types that affect the skin, the relevant porphyrins are changed to an 'excited' state after exposure to light. Their energy is then transferred to oxygen to produce reactive oxygen species, which in turn interfere with the membranes of intracellular organelles and so produce cellular damage. Maximal absorption is at 400–410 nm (the Soret band), which is at the violet end of the visible light spectrum and is difficult to block well with commercially available sunscreens. A summary of porphyrias that have cutaneous features is provided in Table 17.9. The most important to dermatologists are discussed here.

Erythropoietic protoporphyria
Etiology and pathogenesis
Erythropoietic protoporphyria (EPP) is an autosomal dominant disease that results from an accumulation of protoporphyrin due to a deficiency of ferrochelatase.

Clinical features
Symptoms start in young children. Severe burning pain occurs soon after sun exposure (usually within minutes, but up to within 1 h), with subsequent edema and petechial hemorrhages. EPP may also be exacerbated by high-intensity artificial light sources. Significant blisters are uncommon, and diagnosis may be difficult in young children, who scream due to the pain but for whom the relationship to sunlight exposure may not be apparent. Occasionally, the diagnosis may not be made for many years; the oldest patient diagnosed by the author was in her twenties.

Long-term changes may be relatively subtle; they include pitted and linear scarring, and a cobblestoned pattern of skin thickening on hands and face (Figs 17.47 and 17.48). Cholelithiasis and eventual hepatic failure may occur in some individuals.

Porphyrin assays should be performed, including erythrocyte fluorescence and plasma porphyrin measurement. Liver function tests are indicated at intervals, and family members should be screened.

Table 17.9 FEATURES OF THE DERMATOLOGICALLY RELEVANT PORPHYRIAS

Type (and enzyme deficiency)	Age of onset	Skin signs	Neurologic disease	Skin		
				Urine	Stool	Blood
Congenital erythropoietic porphyria (Günther) (UROGEN cosynthetase)	First month (very rare)	Severe photosensitivity, blisters, erosions, skin and eye scarring; hypertrichosis; teeth fluorescence	No	UP-1	CP	RBC fluorescence and plasma UP-1, CP
Erythropoietic protoporphyria (ferrochelatase = heme synthetase)	First few years	Burning, scarring	No	–	PP	RBC fluorescence and plasma PP-1
Porphyria cutanea tarda (UROGEN synthetase)	Most over 50 years (inherited type presents earlier)	Blisters, fragility, scarring, milia, pigmentation, hypertrichosis	No	UP-1 > UP-III	CP	–
Variegate porphyria (PROTOGEN oxidase)	Child or young adult	As for porphyria cutanea tarda	Yes	PP, CP	PP, CP	–
Hereditary coproporphyria (COPROGEN oxidase)	Adult	As for porphyria cutanea tarda in 30%, at times of neurologic symptoms	Yes	CP	CP	–
Hepatoerythropoietic porphyria (UROGEN decarboxylase)	First 2 years (very rare)	Blisters, burning; as for Günther disease	No	UP	CP	RBC, PP, isoCP

COPROGEN, coproporphyrinogen; CP, coproporphyrin; isoCP, isocoproporphyrin; PP, protoporphyrin; PROTOGEN, protoporphyrinogen; RBC, red blood cells; UP, uroporphyrin; UROGEN, uroporphyrinogen

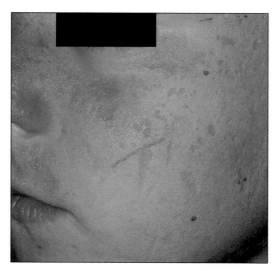

Figure 17.47 Erythropoietic protoporphyria. This causes burning pain in early childhood, but later gives rise to small depressed scars at exposed sites. Linear scars, as shown here, are relatively common and possibly represent scratches.

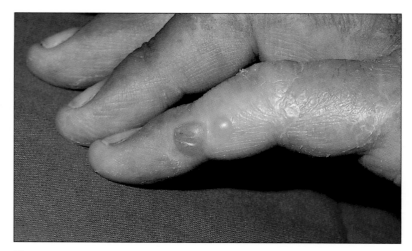

Figure 17.49 Porphyria cutanea tarda. Blisters are typically unilocular, up to about 1 cm in diameter, and have clear fluid content, as shown here.

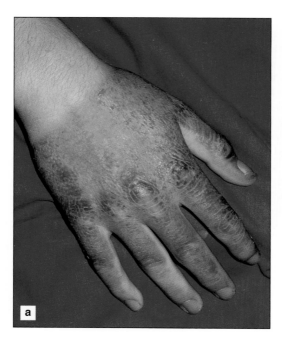

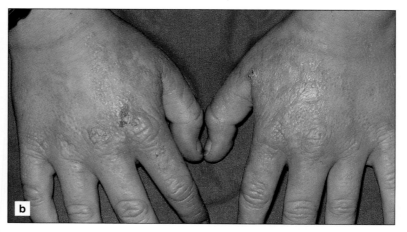

Figure 17.48 Erythropoietic protoporphyia. (**a**) Acute phase: many patients experience burning pain without visible signs, but significant edema or purpura may occur. (**b**) Longstanding scar-like lesions. Note the predominant involvement of the radial aspect of the hand, which is exposed to more sunlight than the ulnar aspect.

Differential diagnosis

Sunburn may be considered in young children, but the rapidity of developing symptoms after sun exposure is totally dissimilar to sunburn. Solar urticaria has early onset after sun exposure and can be distinguished by the occurrence of whealing, but this may not be apparent from the history. Some rare pediatric photosensitivity disorders may need to be excluded. In patients with skin thickening, various cutaneous infiltrates may need to be considered (Ch. 11), but this is not usually a feature until well after the diagnosis has been made.

Treatment

This includes sunscreens and sun avoidance. β-Carotene may be beneficial, and antihistamines may reduce symptoms.

Porphyria cutanea tarda
Etiology and pathogenesis

Type I porphyria cutanea tarda (PCT) is sporadic, whereas type II is rare and is an autosomal dominant condition. The major etiologic factor of the sporadic type is alcohol ingestion, although high-dose estrogens (used to treat prostatic cancer) used to be a common trigger before the use of more specific antiandrogens. It can be provoked by estrogens in oral contraceptives, but this is less common as doses are now typically low. Hepatic damage from other causes may also provoke PCT, including hepatitis B. Patients who have HIV infection and hepatitis B often have elevated porphyrin levels but do not necessarily develop clinical PCT.

Clinical features

Porphyria cutanea tarda is typically apparent in middle-aged men who have a history of excessive alcohol intake, but is increasingly common in women. Manifestations include skin fragility, blisters (typically about 1 cm in diameter), scarring, and pigmentation (Figs 17.49 and 17.50). Milia are common. Hypertrichosis occurs mainly on the cheeks, but the blisters and fragility occur mainly on the dorsum of the hands (presumably due to the greater degree of minor trauma at this site). Sclerodermoid changes and dystrophic calcification are later features.

The evolution is often indolent but more apparent in summer months, and mild cases may be difficult to diagnose, especially in patients who have a manual occupation. Pseudoporphyria (see later) is clinically identical, as is bullous dermatosis of hemodialysis. The differential diagnosis includes dermatitis, scabies, and other photosensitivity disorders. Variegate porphyria should be excluded by porphyrin assay.

Examination of urine with a Wood's lamp may show characteristic pink fluorescence (Figs 17.51 and 17.52). This can be accentuated by acidification and extraction of porphyrins into a layer of amyl alcohol. Formal porphyrin assays are important, and characteristically demonstrate elevated urinary uroporphyrin levels. Skin biopsy shows thickened basement membrane at the dermo–epidermal junction, and dermal papillae project into the blister space (a pattern known as festooning). Abnormalities of liver function tests, elevated serum glucose levels, and iron overload are all common.

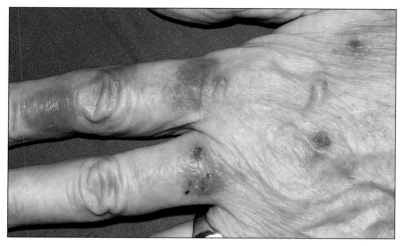

Figure 17.50 Porphyria cutanea tarda. This demonstrates fragile skin and scars on the dorsum of the hand; milia and pigmentation at the sites of pervious blisters are common.

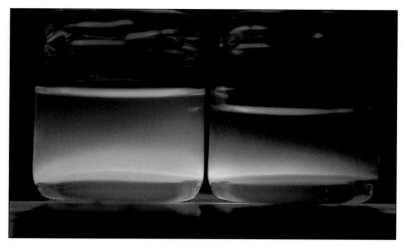

Figure 17.52 Porphyria cutanea tarda (PCT): urine sample. Same urine samples as shown in Figure 17.51, demonstrating pink fluorescence of the PCT urine sample under Wood's light.

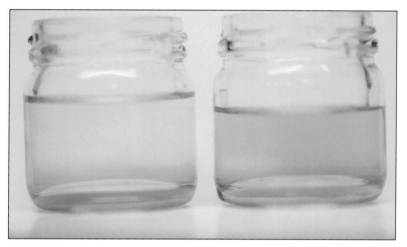

Figure 17.51 Porphyria cutanea tarda: urine sample. This has a slightly darker color compared with that of the control urine.

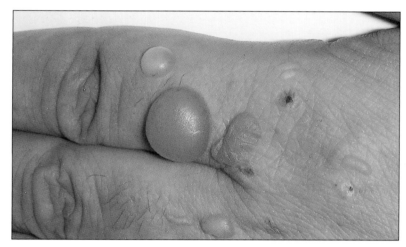

Figure 17.53 Porphyria cutanea tarda in a patient having dialysis. This is a difficult management problem.

Differential diagnosis

Blisters occurring mainly on the dorsum of the hands are rare in any other disorder, but simple burns or trauma may be blamed (especially as there is associated skin fragility), and occasionally drug reactions. A lot of patients with PCT have been treated for presumed 'eczema' prior to referral. Other forms of porphyria (notably variegate porphyria, discussed later) and the pseudoporphyrias (see later), especially drug-induced forms, are important considerations.

Treatment

Identified triggers such as excessive alcohol intake should be avoided, but improvement is typically slow. Venesection is usually effective, probably by mobilizing and depleting the iron overload: 500 mL of blood is removed every week or fortnight until the hemoglobin level falls to about 11 g/dL.

Chloroquine or hydroxychloroquine bind porphyrins, and are then excreted in the urine. Twice-weekly, low-dose administration is safer than higher-dose regimens.

Deferoxamine (desferrioxamine) has also been used to decrease iron levels but is probably not as effective as venesection.

Patients who have porphyria and chronic renal failure and are on dialysis pose a particular problem (Fig. 17.53). Venesection is contra-indicated, as they may already be anemic, and chloroquine–porphyrin complexes do not dialyze out. Erythropoietin can increase heme synthesis and reduce porphyrin levels in some of these patients.

Variegate porphyria

Variegate porphyria (VP) is most simply viewed as a hybrid of PCT and acute intermittent porphyria (AIP); it has cutaneous features similar to those of PCT, but the same neurologic features that characterize AIP. Additionally, numerous drugs may provoke AIP symptoms, so the patient with VP will need advice on avoidance of these. It is therefore important to differentiate VP from PCT by appropriate blood, urine, and stool samples (especially in younger patients without an obvious PCT trigger such as alcohol, or in those with a personal or family history of unexplained internal symptoms). It is particularly common in South Africa.

Pseudoporphyrias

Etiology and pathogenesis

These disorders fall into three main groups.

- Drug-induced pseudoporphyria. Some drugs can produce a PCT-like picture, but with normal porphyrin levels. The most frequent are nalidixic acid, naproxen, and high-dose furosemide. Pyridoxine, tetracyclines, dapsone, and ciclosporin can also cause this reaction. In children, naproxen is the most likely culprit.
- Hemodialysis pseudoporphyria. A bullous disorder of dialysis can occur that is identical to PCT. Some cases may actually be due to drugs (especially furosemide), and true PCT can also occur in dialysis patients.
- Sunbed pseudoporphyria. A PCT-like eruption can occur in fair-skinned individuals who frequently use sunbeds (Fig. 17.54).

Clinical features and differential diagnosis

All features are as for PCT, except for the porphyrin tests, which are negative.

Treatment

This comprises withdrawal of the trigger.

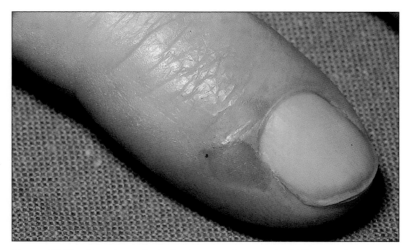

Figure 17.54 Pseudoporphyria due to excessive use of a UVA-producing tanning sunbed. Most cases of pseudoporphyria are drug-induced, especially due to non-steroidal antiinflammatory drugs.

DERMATOSES THAT MAY BE AGGRAVATED BY SUNLIGHT

Examples of dermatoses that may be aggravated by sunlight are listed in Table 17.10. Some of these are characteristically provoked by sunlight, and the relationship is usually apparent, such as lupus erythematosus and pellagra. Similarly, some patients who have dermatomyositis have a striking cut-off of lesional skin at areas such as the nape or V of the neck. Other conditions, such as disseminated superficial actinic porokeratosis, may be much less clearly related to sunlight or may be related to heat and humidity rather than to sunlight (e.g. Hailey–Hailey disease).

Several of the disorders that may be sunlight-aggravated can also demonstrate a Koebner (isomorphic) reaction to minor injury, for example psoriasis (Fig. 17.55) and pemphigus.

In most examples, other than documenting the patient's experience and the distribution of the skin eruption, there are no useful tests to distinguish which individuals will have problems with photoaggravation. However, in lupus erythematosus, it can be predicted that some individuals, notably those who have subacute cutaneous lupus erythematosus and other anti-SSA (anti-Ro)-positive patients, will have a more obvious sunlight aggravation of their disease.

Disorders that are typically improved by sunlight, but may worsen in some individuals, are of interest. They include disorders such as psoriasis, atopic dermatitis, and acne. The mechanisms involved are uncertain, but the type and timescale of provocation are often consistent for any individual. The tendency for photoaggravated psoriasis to be a problem in women rather than in men suggests that it may represent a Koebner reaction in PLE in some cases. Some patients who have psoriasis of this type respond well to PUVA, or even to narrow-band (311-nm) UVB if the reaction is triggered by UVA.

In general, other than sun protection, the treatments are standard for each of the different disorders and are discussed in the relevant chapters of this book.

PHOTOTHERAPY AND PHOTOCHEMOTHERAPY

These topics are discussed in more detail in Chapters 4 (*Systemic therapies*) and 7 (*Psoriasis and related disorders*).

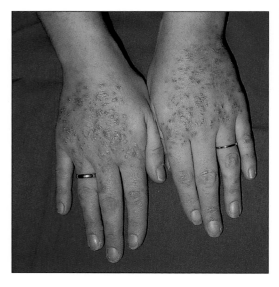

Figure 17.55 Psoriasis aggravated by sunlight. This is a seasonally recurrent problem, which occurs mainly in women. Note the relative sparing of the wrists.

Table 17.10 DERMATOSES THAT MAY BE AGGRAVATED BY SUNLIGHT	
Association with sunlight	**Dermatosis**
Frequently sunlight-provoked	Lupus erythematosus Dermatomyositis Reticulate erythematous mucinosis (REM) syndrome Darier disease Pellagra Herpes simplex
Variably sunlight-provoked	Transient acantholytic dermatosis (Grover disease) Pemphigus (especially foliaceous and erythematosus types) Rosacea Disseminated superficial actinic porokeratosis Hailey–Hailey disease
Usually unrelated to sunlight, but provoked in occasional cases	Lichen planus Erythema multiforme Granuloma annulare
Usually improve in sunlight, but aggravated in some cases	Psoriasis Atopic dermatitis Acne Cutaneous T-cell lymphoma

SUN PROTECTION

Sun avoidance and clothing

Physical avoidance of sunlight is important in everybody, but is of critical importance in treatment of patients with photodermatoses. Patients should be advised:

- to avoid sunlight, especially between 10 a.m. and 4 p.m.;
- to sit in shade;
- to wear protective clothing, such as long-sleeved shirts with a close weave and wide-brimmed hats;
- to be aware that many photodermatoses are UVA-triggered and may therefore be provoked even on dull days, and that UVA tanning beds are contraindicated;
- to use sunscreens (see later); and
- in severe cases, to consider UVA-blocking adhesive film on house and vehicle windows.

Sunscreens

Therapeutically relevant points regarding sunscreens that may influence choice, or that may need to be explained to patients, include the following.

- Chemicals used in sunscreens may be divided into absorbent and reflective types (many modern sunscreens contain a mixture of both).
- Most of the absorbing chemicals block UVB wavelengths well, but UVA wavelengths poorly, although the benzones block UVA. Reflective agents will give protection more broadly across the spectrum. This is important, as most photodermatoses are triggered by UVA.
- Sun protection factor (SPF) ratios refer to the UVB sunburn-blocking activity of the sunscreen; however high the quoted UVB SPF, UVA can generally be blocked only about eightfold, even with reflective-type sunscreens.

- The SPF achieved depends on the thickness of application; most people apply less than the amount used by manufacturers when determining the SPF.
- For most photodermatoses, a reflective sunscreen (usually titanium dioxide), or one containing a combination of high-potency UVA- and UVB-absorbing chemicals, is required.
- Most commercial sunscreens contain fragrances and often other potential sensitizers (especially hydroxybenzoates), which it may be important to avoid.
- Patients who are allergic to sunscreens need to be aware that these are often incorporated into cosmetics, emollients, lip salves, and antiaging creams.
- Artificial tanning agents do not in themselves give any UV protection; some contain added sunscreen but usually at low SPF, so patients with light sensitivity should also use a reliable sunscreen.

PRACTICE POINTS

- Sunscreens are much better at blocking the burning effects of UVB than they are at blocking UVA, which is more important for aging changes and for provocation of many photodermatoses.
- In patients with photosensitivity, especially chronic photosensitivity dermatitis, who continue to have problems despite use of an appropriate sunscreen, it is important to consider sunscreen allergy or photocontact allergy.
- Artificial tanning agents do not block UV radiation, and thus do not prevent sunburn.
- Physical protection from sunlight by avoidance or using suitable clothing gives much better protection than any sunscreen can achieve.

FURTHER READING

Chung JH, Nanft VN, Kang S. Aging and photoaging. J Am Acad Dermatol 2003; 49: 690–7

DeLeo VA (ed) Photosensitivity Diseases. Dermatologic Clinics. Philadelphia: Saunders, 1986

Frain-Bell W, Hetherington A, Johnson BE. Contact allergic sensitivity to chrysanthesum and the photosensitivity dermatitis and actinic reticuloid syndrome. Br J Dermatol 1979; 101: 491–501

Garzon MC, DeoLeo VA. Photosensitivity disorders in childhood. Adv Dermatol 1997; 13: 307–51

Hawk JLM. Cutaneous photobiology. In: Champion RH, Burton JL, Durns DA, et al (eds) Textbook of Dermatology, 7th edn. Oxford: Blackwell Science, 2004

Lambert WC, Kuo H-R, Lambert M. Xeroderma pigmentosum and other disorders of DNA and chromosomal instability. Curr Opin Dermatol 1997; 4: 79–92

Todd DJ. Erythropoietic protoporphyria. Br J Dermatol 1994; 131: 751–66

18 Drug Eruptions

INTRODUCTION TO DRUG ERUPTIONS

Adverse drug reactions are common, and a skin eruption is a feature in about 30% of cases. About 2% of hospital inpatients may develop a drug rash (also termed toxicoderma in some countries). Unfortunately, most cutaneous drug eruptions are of a non-specific morphology (Fig. 18.1); additionally, most of those that occur in a hospital setting are in individuals who are ill and taking many drugs. Diagnosis can therefore be difficult, especially as few drug eruptions are amenable to any form of testing other than the response to drug withdrawal (and sometimes to rechallenge). However, the diagnosis and identification of the likely cause can often be made with reasonable confidence based on a few basic principles.

- Is the morphology of the eruption consistent with a previously documented morphology of rash ascribed to the suspect drug? (Bear in mind that a non-specific maculopapular eruption is the commonest pattern.)
- Is the timing in relation to administration of the drug consistent? (Usually within 10 days.)

- Have other possible causes of rash been reasonably excluded? (Especially viral exanthems that may look similar to drug eruptions, but also reactions to food or to 'natural' remedies.)
- Is the suspect drug likely to cause rash? (A relatively small list of drugs are most likely to cause rashes, either because rash is common with the drug in question and/or because the drug is commonly used, such as antibiotics.)

Mechanisms of drug eruption

There are several mechanisms of drug eruption, some of which correlate with particular patterns of reaction. Some of these are listed with examples in Table 18.1. Recent research has identified the fact that some clinical patterns may relate to specific patterns of T-cell or cytokine activation; for example, a high proportion of CD8$^+$ cells in the epidermis tend to correlate with development of blistering. This has allowed the type IV immunologic reactions to be divided into those that tend to activate monocytes (type IVa), eosinophils (type IVb), or neutrophils (type IVd); type IVc, involving cytotoxic functions, takes part in all type IV reactions.

Host factors may also influence the risk or the severity of drug eruptions. These include the following.

- Genetic polymorphisms. The best known is the acetylator polymorphism, in which the population can be divided into slow and fast acetylators; slow acetylators have a higher risk of drug-induced lupus erythematosus related to hydralazine, and also of pellagra due to isoniazid. A more important metabolic defect, as it may be associated with severe rash and systemic symptoms, is implicated in the anticonvulsant hypersensitivity syndrome (Fig. 18.2), in which patients may develop rash due to several aromatic anticonvulsants (such as phenytoin, carbamazepine, and phenobarbital); such patients may have a deficiency of epoxide hydrolases, which would normally metabolize toxic arene oxide drug metabolites.
- Human leukocyte antigen (HLA) type. For example, HLA-B22 is associated with development of fixed drug eruptions, and HLA Bw35 with reactions to gold. HLA haplotype A30 B13 Cw6 seems to be particularly linked with fixed drug eruptions to co-trimoxazole and may explain some familial cases.

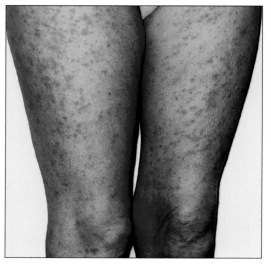

Figure 18.1 A typical non-specific acute maculopapular drug eruption. In this case, the cause was cimetidine, but numerous drugs cause the same reaction pattern. (Courtesy of Dr. G. Dawn.)

Table 18.1   SOME MECHANISMS OF SKIN REACTIONS TO SYSTEMIC DRUGS

	Description	Mechanism	Morphology	Example
Immunologic	Type I, hypersensitivity	IgE binding to mast cells	Urticaria	Penicillin
	Type II, cytotoxic	Antibodies activating complement	Purpura	Quinidine
	Type III, immune complex	Immune complex	Vasculitis, serum sickness	Penicillin
	Type IV, cell-mediated (divided into four subtypes: see text)	Lymphocyte- and cytokine-mediated	Maculopapular, eczematous, granulomatous	Penicillin
Non-immunologic	Binding to mast cells	Releases inflammatory mediators	Urticaria	Opiates
	Unwanted pharmacologic effect	Related to anticipated mode of action	Various	Ichthyosis due to lipid-lowering drugs, alopecia due to cytotoxics, retinoid dry lips and eczema craquelée (Figs 18.5 and 18.6)
	Overdose	Related to anticipated mode of action	Various	Easy bruising due to over-anticoagulation
	Relative overdosage	Genetic polymorphisms, renal or hepatic disease, drug interactions (e.g. competitive protein binding) may all cause overdosing	Various	Methotrexate toxicity due to renal disease or concurrent medication
	Chronic toxicity	Accumulation of drug or metabolites	Pigmentation	Minocycline, amiodarone, phenothiazines
	Exacerbation of preexisting disease	Various, for example effects on neutrophil function	Various	Psoriasis or lithium

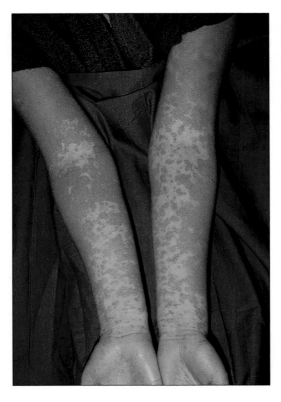

Figure 18.2 Semiconfluent rash on the arms due to phenytoin, associated with fever and malaise. Anticonvulsant reactions are commonly relatively severe.

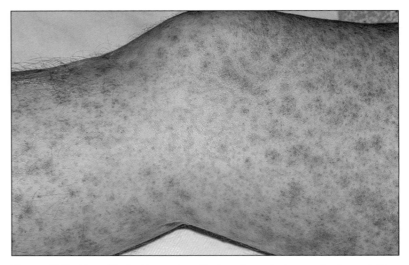

Figure 18.3 Vasculitic-looking rash on the leg of a patient prescribed amoxicillin for a viral infection. Many such patients do not have rash related to other penicillins, and they may subsequently tolerate ampicillin derivatives without any adverse effect.

- Age. Increased age may increase the risk of drug eruptions, but this may simply reflect the higher frequency of medications prescribed in older patients, especially multiple medications.
- Sex. For example, drug rashes due to imatinib (a signal transduction inhibitor used in leukaemia treatment) are much more common in women.
- Associated diseases. Examples include the following.

Infectious mononucleosis—ampicillin and derivatives are a common cause of drug rash (Figs 18.3 and 18.4). However, if given to patients with infectious mononucleosis, the likelihood of rash increases to over 90%. A similar but less dramatic increase applies if ampicillin is used in the context of other viral infections (especially cytomegalovirus), compared with use of the same drug for bacterial infection.

HIV infection—there is an increased risk of severe adverse reactions to sulfonamides and some other antibiotics in patients with HIV infection. A deficiency of glutathione allows increased levels of a toxic hydroxylamine derivative of sulfamethoxazole, a drug that patients with AIDS may take on a prolonged basis for prophylaxis against pneumocystis pneumonia. Drug-induced lichenoid photo-reactions in patients with HIV infection may be more common in black patients.

Hepatitis B infection may predispose to the dapsone hypersensitivity syndrome.

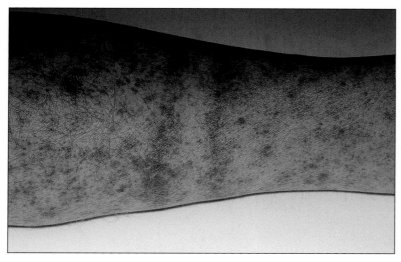

Figure 18.4 A similar eruption to that in Figure 18.3, demonstrating accentuation at a pressure area under the elastic of a sock.

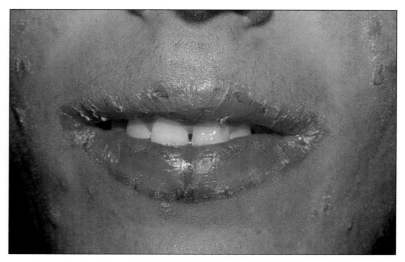

Figure 18.5 Some adverse drug reactions are predictable and dose-related, such as cheilitis due to systemic retinoids for acne.

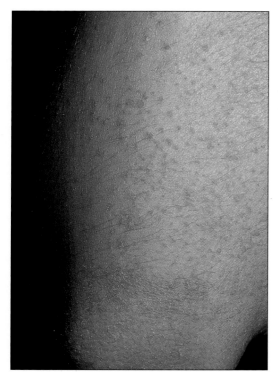

Figure 18.6 Mild eczematous changes may also occur due to retinoids, usually on the dorsum of the hands and forearms, but are less well recognized than the cheilitis shown in Figure 18.5.

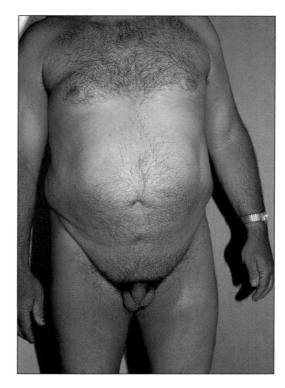

Figure 18.7 Inverse pattern of drug eruption. Rarely does a drug eruption affect the body folds preferentially. Here the bathing trunk area and axilla are affected.

Mastocytosis—several drugs non-specifically lead to mast cell degranulation and may trigger systemic symptoms in patients with significant mastocytosis (see list in Ch. 11).

Collagen vascular disease—a papular eruption closely linked to use of methotrexate has been reported. Griseofulvin-triggered lupus erythematosus has been suggested to be more frequent in patients who have anti-SSA or anti-SSB antibodies.

Atopy—reactions to gold may possibly be more common.

- Other medications. For example, ampicillin is more likely to cause rash if given to patients taking allopurinol.
- Smoking. Reactions to gold are more common in smokers.
- Others. Although the mechanism is uncertain, it has been suggested that patients with multiple drug allergy syndrome (MDAS) have a much higher frequency of detectable β-lactam-specific IgE and also of circulating serum factors that cause histamine release from donor basophils, by comparison with patients with single antibiotic allergies. Such patients clinically have reactions to several chemically unrelated antibacterial agents.

Approach to making the diagnosis

Most drug eruptions have a maculopapular or 'urticated' morphology, and start within a few days up to about 2 weeks after taking the relevant drug.

Thus most drug eruptions are relatively simple to diagnose (Figs 18.5 and 18.6). The more acute-onset urticarial eruptions are even simpler to suspect. However, there are several confounding problems.

- Multiple medications, especially if several have been started on a similar timescale.
- Rash resembling idiopathic eruptions, such as pemphigus due to penicillamine.
- Rash due to underlying disease, such as rash due to viral illness for which an antibiotic has been prescribed, to which the patient may erroneously be assumed to have a drug allergy.
- Forgotten or unapparent drug triggers, such as over-the-counter medications, herbal medicines, and food additives.
- Onset or worsening after a drug has been stopped; this is particularly common after short courses of antibiotics.
- Unusual timing; for example, vasculitis due to furosemide may occur months after the drug is started, and pemphigus due to penicillamine typically requires over 6 months of treatment before the rash occurs.
- Unusual morphology; patterns of eruption are discussed later (see also Figs 18.7 and 18.8).
- New drugs, for which the likely patterns of drug eruption may not be well known.

365

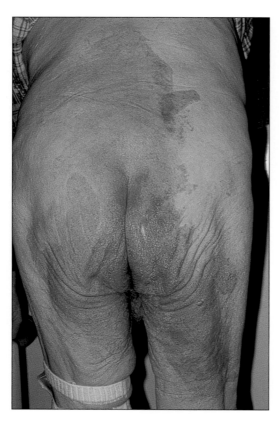

Figure 18.8 A classic pattern but often not recognized. This eruption is due to co-danthramer, a laxative that is metabolized to dithranol (anthralin) in the bowel. It therefore causes irritation (red) and staining (orange-brown) of the skin of the buttocks and posterior thighs, typically in immobile patients.

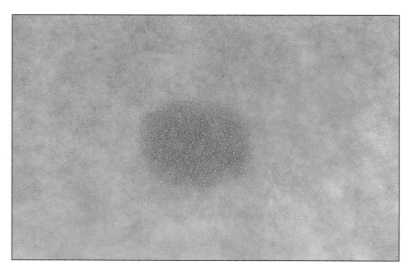

Figure 18.9 Occasionally, replacing a drug that has caused a skin reaction may be followed by a reaction to the second drug. This example shows a fixed drug eruption due to carbamazepine, with a background exanthem pattern due to phenytoin.

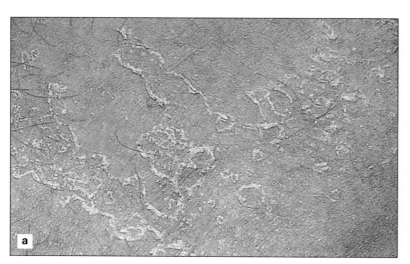

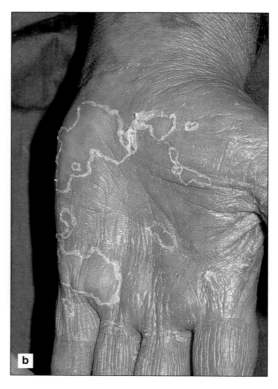

Figure 18.10 Withdrawal of a suspect drug is usually followed by resolution of the eruption within a few days or weeks. A sunburn-like desquamation is common during this phase, and may be generalized (**a**), although it is most obvious on palms and soles, where the skin is thicker (**b**). (Panel a from Lawrence CM, Cox NH. Physical Signs in Dermatology, 2nd edn. London: Mosby, 2002.)

- Drugs that rarely cause rashes, in which the diagnosis may not be suspected.
- Cross-reactions between drugs; for example, between cephalosporins and penicillins.
- More than one eruption; this is not uncommon with use of antibiotics or anticonvulsants, when a substitute is required following an adverse reaction to the first treatment choice (Fig. 18.9).

The basic questions listed in the introduction should therefore be applied. In patients who have started several drugs in close temporal proximity, and who have a non-specific morphology of eruption, it is helpful to have an idea of the relative risk of rash due to the various implicated drugs. It is essential to document timing of the eruption in relation to any suspect drugs, and to include non-prescribed medications in the inquiry. For example, an antibiotic or a non-steroidal antiinflammatory drug (NSAID) started a week before onset of a maculopapular eruption is a more likely cause than a beta-blocker started 2 months

previously, partly because the former drugs are a more common cause of rash, and partly because the timing fits better with the pattern of eruption.

The diagnosis is often supported by the response to withdrawal of the suspect drug (Fig. 18.10), most eruptions improving over a few days or weeks (although some may initially worsen, usually for no more than a few days). Some patterns, such as quinine-induced photosensitivity, may take months to settle. For most drug reactions, there is no simple diagnostic test. Patch testing can be useful for identifying some drug reactions (such as to carbamazepine) but is considered unreliable for others (such as to local anesthetics) and is simply unhelpful in most instances. Prick tests and intradermal tests are not routinely helpful, and have a potential risk, but can be performed for penicilloyl residues if there are important reasons requiring use of a penicillin rather than of an alternative antibiotic. Lymphocyte transformation tests, basophil activation tests, and other laboratory tests are not routinely available. Rechallenge is generally not performed unless the drug is important to the patient (e.g. to treat a condition where there are few alternatives), and the expected reaction is not likely to be severe. Challenge testing can be a very time-consuming process but may be required occasionally (e.g. in some cases of local anesthetic reaction).

Assessment and treatment overview

The most common patterns of drug eruption will respond to drug withdrawal and administration of a topical corticosteroid and oral antihistamines as required on a symptomatic basis. Antihistamines are most useful for urticarial reactions, whereas short-term potent topical corticosteroids are generally the most effective way to treat maculopapular eruptions.

Some eruptions require other specific measures, for example anaphylaxis or severe urticaria (see Ch. 9), toxic epidermal necrolysis (treated along the lines used for thermal burns, with particular attention to fluid balance, secondary infection, and skin fragility), or erythroderma (which may be complicated by impaired temperature control, high-output cardiac failure, and malabsorption).

Desensitization may be used for some drug eruptions, for example urticarial reactions to sulfasalazine or penicillins. Desensitization to penicillin is not routine, and is generally performed only in situations where there is no easy alternative to treat a specific infection; the process requires careful intensive care unit monitoring for safety.

In many situations, it is important to consider whether an alternative drug can be substituted. For example, in an infection, an antibiotic can usually be chosen for which cross-reactions would be unlikely. In the case of NSAIDs, most selective cyclooxygenase (COX)-2 inhibitors have been shown to be safe in the vast majority of patients with urticarial or with pseudoallergic reactions to traditional NSAIDs.

Generally, when considering therapy, it is also important to consider severity issues. These include the following.

- Factors that suggest a significant systemic effect, such as fever, malaise, lymphadenopathy, eosinophilia, and transaminitis (some severe drug eruptions, often to agents such as anticonvulsants, may be termed hypersensitivity syndrome or fit the acronym DRESS: drug reaction with eosinophilia and systemic symptoms).
- Severity of cutaneous component—erythema of more than 60% of body surface area (BSA) or blistering of over 10% are generally considered significant (specific scoring systems may be applied to some eruption patterns, such as SCORTEN for toxic epidermal necrolysis).
- Subjective symptoms, such as severity of itch.
- Impact on future treatment—for example, urticarial eruptions will usually recur on further exposure, but the significance of this is greater in a patient planned to have further cycles of a chemotherapy drug than it is in a patient treated with a type of antibiotic for which there is a sensible alternative.

PATTERNS OF DRUG ERUPTION

Urticaria, angioedema, and anaphylaxis

Numerous drugs may cause acute urticaria or anaphylaxis (Table 18.2). In many cases, the eruption is IgE-mediated and lasts less than 24 h, usually occurring rapidly after the second exposure to the causative agent. It should, however, be stressed that anaphylaxis due to drugs is rare; a UK study of anaphylaxis identified less than one case per 10 000 person years, 10% needing urgent treatment, and only 30% of these were due to drugs.

The risk of severe urticarial or anaphylactic reactions is greatest with intravenous administration. Penicillins, NSAIDs, contrast media, and serum products or desensitizing agents are the most frequent cause of acute reactions. Vaccines may cause transient urticaria (Fig. 18.11). Reactions to anesthetics are difficult to interpret sometimes (see later discussion of local anesthetic reactions). Intravenous immunoglobulin and monoclonal antibodies are an increasingly common cause of immediate urticarial or angioedema reactions of relevance in dermatologic usage, but the cause is generally readily apparent.

Aspirin and angiotensin-converting enzyme (ACE) inhibitors are relatively common and underdiagnosed causes of intermittent urticaria or angioedema (Fig. 18.12); aspirin is often taken without medical prescription, and related salicylates are also present in numerous foods. NSAIDs may also trigger or aggravate chronic urticaria. Such reactions have non-immunologic ('pseudoallergic') mechanisms, for example due to overproduction of cysteinyl leukotrienes in NSAID-aggravated chronic

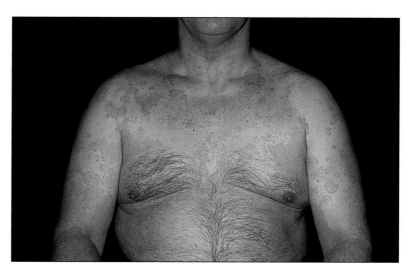

Figure 18.11 Rashes due to vaccines and related agents are often of urticarial pattern. In this case, the presumed cause was an influenza vaccination some days previously.

Category	Drugs
Antiinfective	Penicillins, cephalosporins, sulfonamides, aminoglycosides, vancomycin (rapid infusion), azole antifungals
Antirheumatics	Salicylates, non-steroidal antiinflammatory drugs, allopurinol
Investigative	Radiographic contrast media (iodine)
Cardiac	Angiotensin-converting enzyme inhibitors, streptokinase, simvastatin, hydrochlorothiazide
Gastroenterology	Sulfasalazine, proton pump inhibitors
Vaccines etc.	Animal sera, due to egg proteins, desensitizing
Anesthesia or emergency medicine	Anesthetic agents, muscle relaxants, dextrans, opiates
Other	Hydantoins, cytotoxics, oral hypoglycemics, amitriptyline, intravenous immunoglobulin, interleukins, and other monoclonal biologicals

Table 18.2   DRUG CAUSES OF URTICARIA, ANGIOEDEMA, AND ANAPHYLAXIS

urticaria. Angioedema due to ACE inhibitors occurs in an older population than does most idiopathic angioedema, although there may be a higher frequency of previous angioedema than in the average population, and onset may be delayed. As with NSAIDs, the mechanism is non-immunologic, in this case increased bradykinin activity due to reduced degradation. In these non-immunologic triggers of urticaria, the problem is likely to occur with other drugs of the same type.

Postoperative opiates are common non-immunologic causes of urticaria. Their ability to non-specifically cause mast cell degranulation is a particular concern in mastocytosis, discussed earlier. A reaction that appears to relate specifically to rapid infusion is the 'red man' syndrome due to vancomycin, which may be associated with severe hypotension.

Treatment of drug-induced urticaria or anaphylaxis is the same as for other triggers, such as foods, insect stings, or blood products, and is discussed in Chapter 9.

Exanthem or maculopapular pattern

This is the most common pattern of eruption (Table 18.3) and usually occurs within 2 weeks of exposure to the causative drug. It is important to recognize that the rash may therefore start or worsen after the causative drug has been discontinued, especially after short courses of antibiotics, which are the most frequent cause of this reaction pattern (Fig. 18.13). Maculopapular eruptions occur particularly with ampicillin derivatives

if used in the context of a viral infection (Figs 18.3 and 18.4). Cross-reactions (e.g. between penicillins and cephalosporins, or between the sulfa drugs including sulfonamides, sulfonylureas, and thiazides) are common with this pattern of eruption.

The skin involvement is usually generalized but often initially apparent on the trunk. Pressure areas under clothing, and flexures, are sometimes spared. Lips may be affected, facial swelling may be a feature, diffuse erythema of palms and soles may occur, and a purpuric component on the lower legs (Fig. 18.4) is common, especially if there is associated dependent edema.

Most such reactions settle within a week or so of withdrawal, but some may be complicated (e.g. the pityriasis rosea-like eruption due to captopril may become lichenoid in appearance and last for several weeks), and a few may progress to a more generalized form or may be associated with systemic hypersensitivity symptoms (see discussion in the section on anti-convulsants, the commonest cause of this progression). In uncomplicated cases, a topical steroid is generally much the most effective therapy; as symptoms in most eruptions of this type are self-limiting over days, a potent or moderately potent agent can be used safely.

A specific pattern of maculopapular eruption that is rare but distinctive is the 'baboon syndrome', in which a systemic contact dermatitis affects the buttocks and flexures (also termed an inverse pattern of exanthem, Fig. 18.7). Mercury is the best documented trigger, although other metals,

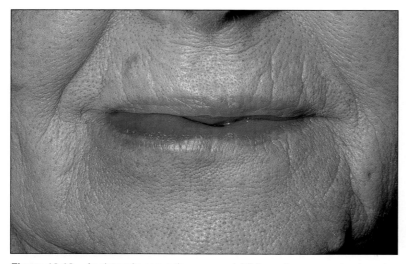

Figure 18.12 Angiotensin-converting enzyme inhibitors all cause angioedema in a small proportion of patients. This appears to be most common in older patients, often with mild preceding angioedema problems. This patient has swelling of the right side of the lower lip.

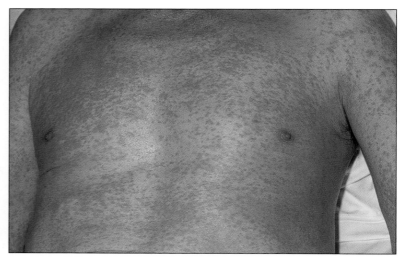

Figure 18.13 Antibiotics are the most common cause of maculopapular drug eruptions, usually with an interval of several days before the eruption develops. This rash was due to penicillin.

Table 18.3   COMMON CAUSES OF EXANTHEMATOUS OR MACULOPAPULAR (INCLUDING PITYRIASIS ROSEA–LIKE) DRUG ERUPTION[a]

Category	Drugs
Antimicrobials	Penicillins (especially ampicillin and derivatives), sulfonamides, isoniazid, amphotericin B, antiretroviral agents (especially nucleoside reverse transcriptase analogs and abacavir)
Anticonvulsants and psychiatry	Phenytoin, carbamazepine, barbiturates, phenothiazines, lithium
Antirheumatics	Non-steroidal antiinflammatory drugs, gold, allopurinol
Hypoglycemics	Sulfonylureas
Diuretics	Thiazides
Cardiology	Captopril, enalapril, beta-blockers, quinidine
Others	Carbimazole, imatinib, bismuth compounds, thalidomide

[a]Includes some drugs that are less commonly used but that commonly cause this pattern of eruption.

such as nickel, are also relevant; triggering by drugs may occur with antibiotics (especially ampicillin and derivatives), aminophylline, pseudoephedrine, heparin, and terbinafine.

Eczematous pattern

Other than predictable dry skin with eczematous change with oral retinoid drugs, eczematous drug eruptions are not very common. However, this pattern (Table 18.4) is a particular cause of diagnostic difficulty, as it may be gradual in onset and may be difficult to distinguish from endogenous eczema; for example, infliximab may cause a pattern that resembles atopic dermatitis, and interferon–alpha a rash similar to discoid eczema. Some of the systemic agents that cause an eczematous drug eruption are also known to cause eczematous reactions due to external contact (allergic contact dermatitis); in some cases where there is a history of preceding contact hypersensitivity to the same agent, the eruption will affect previous sites of external contact reactions. Penicillins and sulfonamides are of particular importance, as both were used topically for many years; older patients and some senior nursing staff who have handled topical penicillins or sulfonamides are at particular risk. Patch tests are positive in such individuals.

Erythroderma

Drug reactions account for about 5–15% of cases of erythroderma (Figs 18.14 and 18.15, Table 18.5). When it occurs, it has all the implications of erythroderma due to a primary skin disease (Ch. 7). It often overlaps with exfoliative patterns, as generalized peeling may occur in the resolution phase.

Erythema multiforme and toxic epidermal necrolysis

These patterns are considered together, because some patients may progress from erythema multiforme (EM) lesions to toxic epidermal necrolysis (TEN), although others are firmly at one end of the spectrum from the outset. The intermediate picture has given rise to terms such as acute disseminated epidermal necrolysis (ADEN), but such terms have

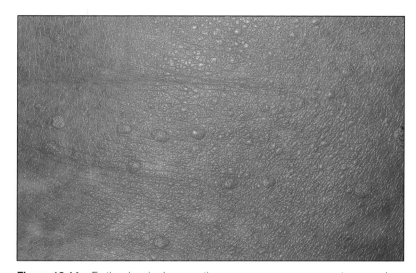

Figure 18.14 Erythrodermic drug reactions may cause severe symptoms, and may be difficult to distinguish from other causes of erythroderma. An underestimated feature of erythroderma that may cause diagnostic concern is the eruption of multiple tiny acanthomas resembling seborrheic keratoses. This case was due to phenytoin.

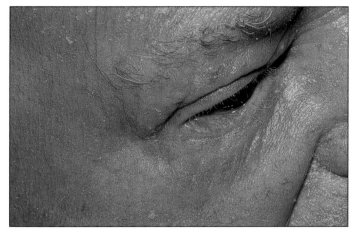

Figure 18.15 Ectropion is common in erythroderma, in this case due to a thiazide diuretic. It resolves as the skin settles but may need treatment with lubricant or antibiotic eye ointments.

Table 18.4   CAUSES OF ECZEMATOUS DRUG ERUPTION

Category	Drug(s)
Antibiotics	Penicillins, cephalosporins, sulfonamides
Diuretics	Thiazides
Antihypertensives	Methyldopa, beta-blockers
Hypoglycemics	Sulfonylureas
Anticonvulsants	Phenytoin, carbamazepine, lamotrigine
Psychiatry	Chlorpromazine
Other	Quinine, quinidine, gold, bleomycin, isotretinoin, statins (ichthyosis), infliximab, interferon-alpha

Table 18.5   CAUSES OF ERYTHRODERMIC DRUG REACTIONS

Category	Drug(s)
Anticonvulsants	Phenytoin, carbamazepine
Antiinflammatory	Gold, allopurinol, phenylbutazone and other pyrazolones, chloroquine, hydroxychloroquine, thalidomide
Psychiatry	Chlorpromazine, lithium
Antiinfective	Sulfonamides, nitrofurantoin, penicillins, antituberculous drugs, pristinamycin
Miscellaneous	Cimetidine, quinine, captopril

currently been discarded. Blistering may also occur in fixed drug eruptions, mimicking immunobullous disease, at pressure sites in drug-induced coma, in pseudoporphyria, and in eczematous drug reactions.

Erythema multiforme is most commonly due to herpes simplex infection (discussed in Ch. 11); drug-induced EM (Figs 18.16 and 18.17, Table 18.6) generally produces rather more variable and less well-defined 'target lesions'. In cases due to antibiotics, it is often difficult to confidently distinguish between EM due to the drug or due to the underlying infection. Mucous membrane involvement (Stevens–Johnson syndrome) may occur, but pure mucous membrane involvement is more likely to be due to mycoplasma infection than to drugs. The fixed lesions of EM should be distinguished from the much rarer, slowly migrating, annular erythema that may occur due to H_2 antagonists, penicillins, thiazides, chloroquine, and estrogens.

In TEN (Figs 18.18 and 18.19, Table 18.7), there is much more widespread superficial blistering, with mucous membrane involvement and significant malaise. The cause is usually a drug, but rare cases of adult staphylococcal scalded skin syndrome (SSSS) need to be excluded; in this condition, the blistering is subcorneal rather than a full-thickness epidermal cell death. Many patients have some areas of EM-like lesions (sometimes termed TEN with spots); these strongly suggest the diagnosis of TEN, as they are not a feature of SSSS. Other differential diagnoses include extensive drug-induced linear IgA disease (see later) and, if the condition occurs in the right hematologic context, graft-versus-host

Table 18.6 DRUG CAUSES OF ERYTHEMA MULTIFORME

Category	Drug(s)
Antimicrobials	Sulfonamides, penicillins, tetracyclines, thiabendazole, isoniazid, didanosine
Anticonvulsants	Phenytoin, carbamazepine, barbiturates
Analgesics and rheumatology	Aspirin, codeine, non-steroidal antiinflammatory drugs, leflunomide
Diuretics	Furosemide, thiazides
Others	Phenothiazines, quinine, sulfonylureas, progestogens, omeprazole

disease. The commonest causes are probably antibiotics, anticonvulsants, and allopurinol. Among the NSAIDs that may provoke TEN, there is some evidence that it may be commonest with oxicams; there are also several recent reports of TEN due to celecoxib.

For prognostic purposes and to allow comparison between different interventional studies, it is helpful to record the following.

- Whether there are classic EM lesions (and whether these are bullous), atypical target lesions, or erythematous or purpuric macules.
- Whether there is mucosal involvement (Stevens–Johnson syndrome).
- The extent of epidermal detachment expressed as a percentage of BSA, usually now divided as < 10%, 10–30%, or > 30% BSA.
- A severity scoring system such as SCORTEN, specifically generated for use in this disorder, is useful.
- The causative drug and the timing of its withdrawal.

Toxic epidermal necrolysis is a rare condition but can be fatal due to the problems of toxemia, electrolyte control, and secondary infection of denuded areas of skin. Intensive care similar to that for burns is required. The earlier a suspect drug is withdrawn, then the better the overall outcome, but this is also influenced by the half-life of the causative agent (there is higher mortality if drug persistence is longer). Treatment has been the subject of much argument, but demonstration of abnormality of Fas and its ligand has generated interest in approaches that influence this. In two of three recent studies, high-dose intravenous immunoglobulin was beneficial; there is also some support for use of ciclosporin.

Erythema nodosum

Most cases of erythema nodosum (mainly discussed in Ch. 22) are due to systemic diseases such as streptococcal infection, inflammatory bowel disease, or acute sarcoidosis, but it may also be caused by drugs such as penicillins, sulfonamides, dapsone, gold, codeine, NSAIDs, sulfonylureas, amiodarone, thiouracils, halogens, and oral contraceptives.

Lichenoid drug eruption

Lichenoid drug eruptions (Figs 18.20 and 18.21, Table 18.8) are often difficult to diagnose, for the following reasons.

- They may start weeks or months after a causative drug has been introduced.
- They may be preceded by pruritus without rash (e.g. due to mepacrine).
- They may evolve from other clinical patterns (e.g. captopril causing an initial pityriasis rosea-like pattern) or progress to erythroderma or exfoliative dermatitis.
- They often have mixed morphology, with eczematous areas, psoriasiform areas, or areas that resemble lupus erythematosus (see Ch. 13 for causes of drug-induced lupus erythematosus).
- They may be bullous (lichen planus pemphigoides pattern); see Table 18.15.
- They may affect relatively unusual sites for lichen planus, such as dorsal hands or feet (e.g. due to hydroxycarbamide [hydroxyurea]) or the scalp (in which case permanent alopecia may occur), or have other unusual localization (e.g. to Blaschko lines, provoked by ibuprofen, or

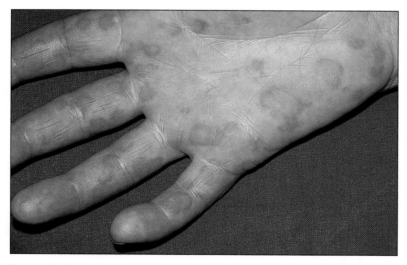

Figure 18.16 Erythema multiforme on the palm of the hand, due to sulfasalazine. Note the typical grayish center of the target lesions, due to epidermal necrosis.

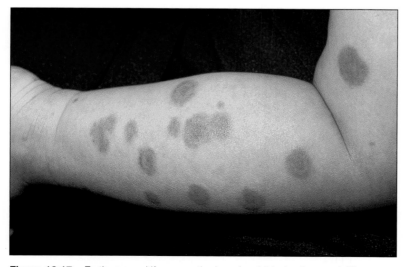

Figure 18.17 Erythema multiforme on the leg of a child, due to amoxicillin. Herpes simplex should always be excluded as a cause of this reaction pattern. Remember that the cause may be the underlying infection rather than the drug used to treat it.

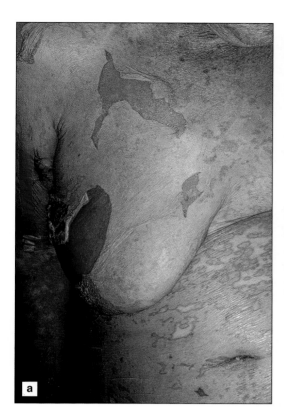
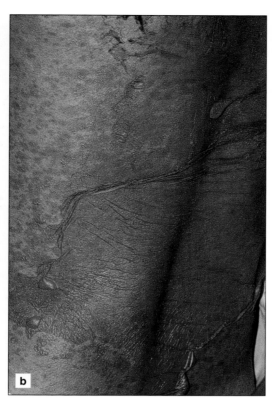

Figure 18.18 Examples of toxic epidermal necrolysis. In (**a**), the eruption was due to allopurinol, one of the more common causes of this reaction; no cause could be identified in (**b**). Note the semiconfluent, rather erythema multiforme–like, annular areas ('atypical target lesions') with central epidermal necrosis, most apparent in (a); these areas of necrosis should be counted as blisters when evaluating the extent of the eruption.

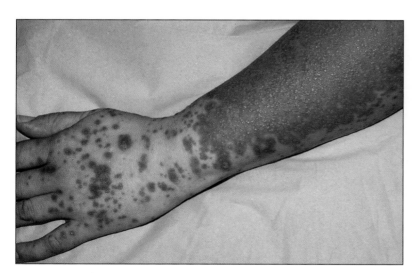

Figure 18.19 Atypical target lesions are shown in this patient with carbamazepine-induced erythema multiforme, in whom there were also areas of blistering.

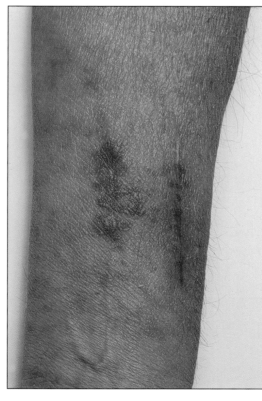

Figure 18.20 This eruption appears to be typical lichen planus in a scar, but was due to captopril. It started as a pityriasis rosea–like pattern on the trunk, with evolution to a more lichen planus–like morphology over 2 weeks, and resolved after withdrawal of the trigger.

localized to injection sites [hepatitis B vaccination, granulocyte-colony stimulating factor]).

- They may be photodistributed (particularly in the case of NSAIDs, thiazides, isoniazid, and pyrazinamide).
- They usually lack features such as Wickham's striae, although lichenoid pigmentation is usually present.
- They may mimic naturally occurring dermatoses, not just lichen planus but also eczemas, dermatomyositis, and others.
- They do not usually exhibit mucosal lesions (although some are purely oral in at least some patients, e.g. due to zidovudine).
- They resolve slowly.

Histologic examination of a skin biopsy may show typical lichen planus, but usually there is a more mixed cellular infiltrate with some prominence of eosinophils, and infiltrate around sweat glands.

External agents that cause a lichenoid reaction, and localized causes such as tattoo pigments, are discussed in Chapter 8.

Fixed drug eruption

Fixed drug eruption (FDE) is an uncommon and usually characteristic pattern of drug reaction (Figs 18.22–18.25, Table 18.9). The acute lesion is a well-demarcated erythematous plaque, sometimes with blistering (Fig. 18.22), and usually a few centimeters in diameter. Brown staining may be prominent as it resolves, particularly after repeated episodes, as the eruption recurs at the same site on reexposure. Lesions are usually solitary but may be multiple initially, or may increase in number with several episodes (Fig. 18.23). Distal limbs or the glans penis (Figs 18.24 and 18.25) are favored sites; the latter is particularly linked with FDE due to co-trimoxazole. FDE on the face or lip has been linked with naproxen as a

Table 18.7   SOME CAUSES OF TOXIC EPIDERMAL NECROLYSIS

Category	Drugs
Antibiotics	Penicillins, sulfonamides, tetracyclines, chloramphenicol, macrolides, nitrofurantoin, ciprofloxacin, metronidazole, vancomycin
Antiretrovirals	Nevirapine, foscarnet
Anticonvulsants and psychiatry	Phenytoin, carbamazepine, lamotrigine, barbiturates, valproate, fluoxetine, fluvoxamine
Rheumatologic and analgesics	Allopurinol, gold, non-steroidal antiinflammatory drugs and aspirin, celecoxib, colchicine, codeine, opiates, acetaminophen
Antimalarials	Sulfadoxine or pyrimethamine, mefloquine, hydroxychloroquine
Antidiabetic	Sulfonylureas
Cytotoxics	Cyclophosphamide, methotrexate, cytosine arabinoside, docetaxel, gemcitabine, Adriamycin (doxorubicin), mithramycin, amifostine, interleukin-2
Radiology	Iohexidol, iopamidol
Cardiology	Quinidine, captopril
Others	Vaccines (various), thalidomide

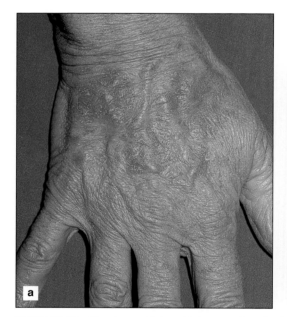

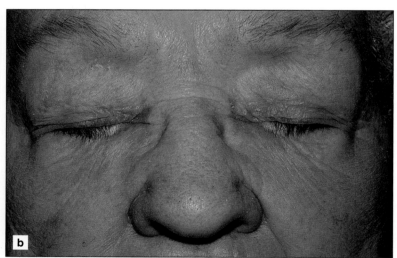

Figure 18.21   Spectrum of lichenoid drug eruption due to quinine (**a**) on the dorsum of the hand, and (**b**) mimicking dermatomyositis on the eyelids. Lichenoid eruptions often have the purple color of idiopathic lichen planus, but are usually broader and less discrete lesions, without the typical Wickham's striae of the idiopathic pattern (Ch. 8). (Panel b courtesy of Dr. L. Barco.)

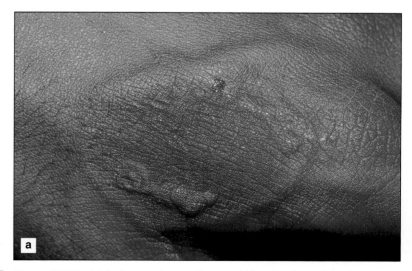

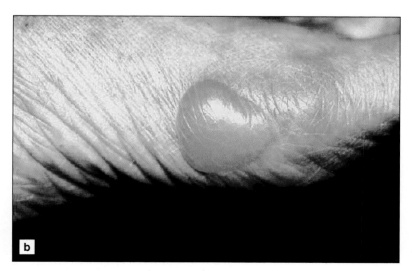

Figure 18.22   (**a**) A discrete plaque with central blistering due to fixed drug eruption (FDE). (**b**) In some cases, blistering may be the dominant feature of FDE, in this case due to ibuprofen. (Panel b courtesy of Dr. G. Dawn.)

Table 18.8   SYSTEMICALLY ADMINISTERED DRUGS THAT MAY CAUSE A LICHENOID REACTION

Category	Drugs
Cardiology	Beta-blockers, methyldopa[a], captopril and other angiotensin-converting enzyme inhibitors[a,b], nifedipine, quinidine[c], thiazides[c], furosemide[b,c], spironolactone, simvastatin, pravastatin, diazoxide[c], hydralazine, acetylsalicylic acid, clopidogrel
Antimicrobials	Isoniazid, p-aminosalicylic acid, ethambutol[c], isoniazid, tetracyclines[c], interferon or ribavirin, zidovudine[a], hepatitis B vaccine[a], dapsone, ketoconazole[a], terbinafine
Antimalarials	Mepacrine, chloroquine, hydroxychloroquine
Rheumatologic	Gold[a], penicillamine[a], non-steroidal antiinflammatory drugs[a], allopurinol[a], leflunomide and anti-tumor necrosis factor agents
Hematologic and cytotoxic	Hydroxycarbamide, bleomycin, 5-fluorouracil[c], imatinib[a], granulocyte-colony stimulating factor (localized to injection site)
Anticonvulsants	Carbamazepine[c], phenytoin, valproate
Psychiatry	Phenothiazines, especially chlorpromazine[c]; chloral hydrate; lithium carbonate
Gastroenterology	Ursodeoxycholic acid, histamine H_2 antagonists, proton pump inhibitors
Heavy metals	Bismuth, mercury, arsenicals
Others	Sulfonylureas[a], iodides, quinine[c], cyanamide (= carbimide)[a], cinnarizine[b], infliximab, thalidomide[a], isotretinoin, sildenafil

[a]May cause oral lichenoid eruption.
[b]May cause bullous lichenoid reaction or lichen planus pemphigoides.
[c]May be photodistributed.

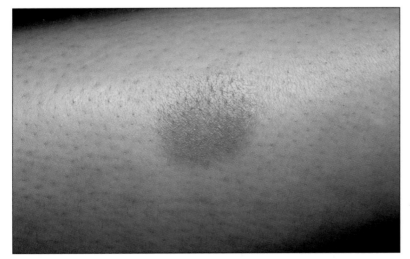

Figure 18.23   Residual pigmentation is common in fixed drug eruption, especially after multiple episodes; in this patient, the cause was mefenamic acid taken for premenstrual symptoms.

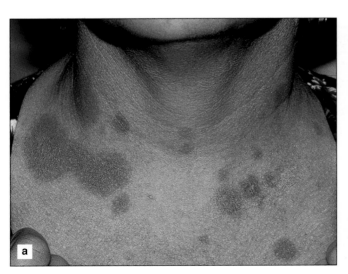

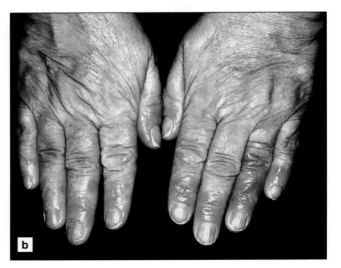

Figure 18.24   Multiple lesions of fixed drug eruption are less common than a solitary lesion, and may cause greater diagnostic problems. The typical discoid morphology is apparent in (**a**); the acral pattern in (**b**), due to a sulfonamide, is more unusual. (Panel b courtesy of Dr. G. Dawn.)

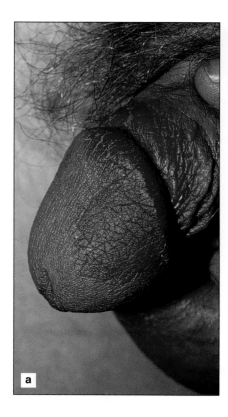

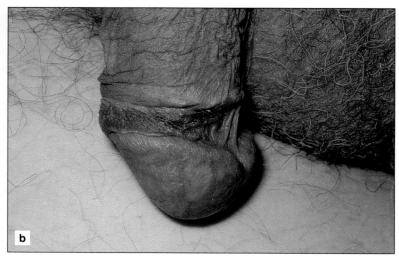

Figure 18.25 The glans penis is a disproportionately common site for fixed drug eruption (FDE) (**a**). Residual pigmentation (**b**) is a common feature of FDE, especially after repeated episodes and especially on the penis. This case was probably due to sulfamethoxazole some years previously.

Table 18.9 SOME CAUSES OF FIXED DRUG ERUPTION

Category	Drugs
Antimicrobials	Sulfonamides, trimethoprim, tetracyclines, metronidazole, quinolones, macrolides, rifampin, terbinafine, fluconazole, nystatin, saquinavir, aciclovir, interferon-alpha with ribavirin, influenza vaccine
Rheumatologic and analgesics	Non-steroidal antiinflammatory drugs including cyclooxygenase-2 agents and acetylsalicylic acid, acetaminophen, opiates, allopurinol
Anticonvulsants and psychiatry	Phenytoin, barbiturates, carbamazepine, lamotrigine, chloral hydrate, disulfiram, chlordiazepoxide, imipramine, oxazepam
Antiallergy preparations and steroids	Ephedrine, pseudoephedrine, atropine, diphenhydramine, cetirizine, hydroxyzine, loratadine, betahistine, triamcinolone
Gastroenterology	Cimetidine, omeprazole, sulfasalazine
Cytotoxics and immunosuppressives	Paclitaxel, hydroxycarbamide, interferon-alpha
Others	Phenolphthalein, quinine, quinidine, dapsone, radiocontrast media, lidocaine (lignocaine)

likely cause. HLA associations of FDE were discussed earlier in this chapter.

Rarer variants include non-pigmented FDE (typically a pattern seen with ephedrine or pseudoephedrine), 'wandering' FDE, periorbital FDE, bilateral symmetric FDE, urticarial or eczematous FDE, linear or extensive sheets of FDE, and mucous membrane FDE.

Some cases of clinically typical FDE may be caused by food additives and colorings (e.g. tartrazine), drinks (e.g. tonic water), or herbal preparations; many are due to non-prescribed medications such as acetaminophen or agents for upper respiratory tract infections. Drugs that may be used to treat skin conditions may be the cause, notably antihistamines (especially cetirizine and chemically related antihistamines). Intraarticular steroid injections have been reported as a cause, as has injected botulinum toxin and influenza vaccine, although most cases are due to orally administered agents. The cause may not therefore be immediately apparent even if FDE is correctly suspected. In some instances, FDE may occur due to cross-reacting drugs, especially between NSAIDs and between tetracyclines. Several drugs have been reported to cross-react with sulfonamides, causing FDE, including indapamide and rofecoxib. Some cases are due to

excipients rather than the active drug, and a type of 'compound' allergy may occur in which two drugs have to be present together to cause the reaction.

Patch tests to the suspect drug may be positive on the lesional skin (but usually not on unaffected skin) between episodes.

Cytotoxic drug reactions

Cytotoxic agents may cause a variety of skin and systemic reactions (Figs 18.26–18.30, Table 18.10). Some reactions are common to many of the drugs used and are not listed in the table. Most cause some degree of stomatitis and alopecia due to effects on rapidly dividing cells of the gastrointestinal tract and hair follicles, respectively. The alopecia (anagen effluvium) may be prevented by local cooling of the scalp during administration, but this may be uncomfortable and is usually reserved for drugs that exhibit this effect strongly, such as doxorubicin. Other non-specific effects include Beau lines, onycholysis, and multiple parallel transverse white bands in the nails, which are due to cycles of therapy (Fig. 18.28). Local extravasation and injection site reactions are a particular problem with drugs used in leukemia treatment. Urticarial or angio-

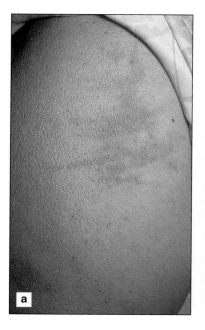

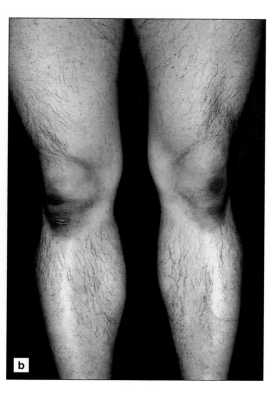

Figure 18.26 Pigmentation is a potential side effect of several chemotherapeutic drugs. (**a**) Pigmentation due to bleomycin often has a streaky pattern, termed a flagellate pattern of eruption. (**b**) A more unusual pattern of pigmentation, caused by systemic 5-fluorouracil. (Panel a courtesy of Michael O. Murphy, M.D., panel b courtesy of Dr. G. Dawn.)

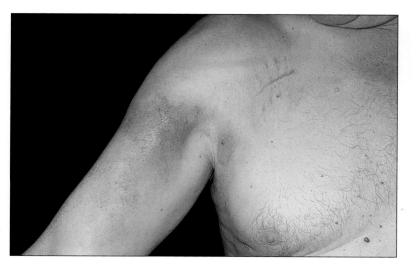

Figure 18.27 Local reaction due to chemotherapy extravasation from a subcutaneous subclavian line. This type of reaction is less common than it used to be, due to better methods of long-term venous access and specific extravasation regimens for many cytotoxic agents.

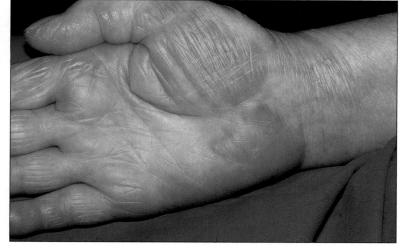

Figure 18.29 Neutrophilic eccrine hidradenitis (NEH). Acral erythema is a common effect of cytotoxic drugs and occasionally other drugs. In some cases, this is related to inflammatory changes affecting sweat ducts, known as NEH. This biopsy-proven case was due to an amoxicillin product.

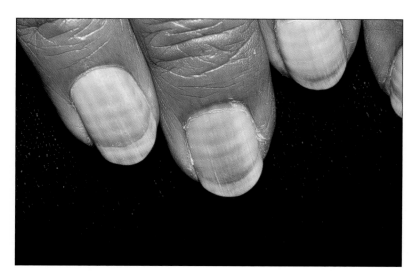

Figure 18.28 Multiple white bands in the nails, representing periods of growth arrest, in this case due to cycles of treatment with 5-fluorouracil.

edematous hypersensitivity reactions are a feature of some monoclonal biologicals, although they also occur with other drugs, such as docetaxel.

Pigmentation may affect the skin (a streaky pattern is typical of bleomycin especially, Fig. 18.26), nails, or oral mucosa. Radiation recall (inflammation in the skin over a radiotherapy field), and occasionally sunburn reactivation, may also be followed by hyperpigmentation. Thiotepa may cause pigmentation where the skin is occluded, possibly due to secretion in sweat.

Neutrophilic eccrine hidradenitis (NEH) is a relatively recently described reaction of papules and plaques that last for several days, affecting areas where sweating occurs, such as the hands. It is characterized by neutrophilic inflammation around the eccrine glands, with necrosis of the secretory epithelium. Chemotherapeutic agents, especially cytosine arabinoside, are most commonly implicated, but it can occur due to other drugs (Fig. 18.29). Eccrine squamous syringometaplasia is associated with high-dose chemotherapy (such as pre-marrow transplant) and presents as erythematous plaques in the axillae and groins, often with localized areas of painful palmoplantar erythema.

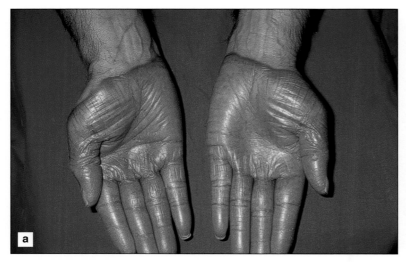

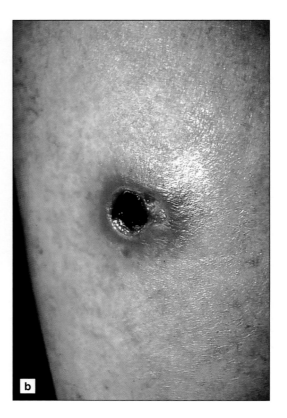

Figure 18.30 (**a**) Palmoplantar syndrome due to continuous infusion of 5-fluorouracil for bowel cancer. This reaction occurs in about 30% of patients, and has a typical sharp demarcation, as shown here. Associated nail changes are seen in some cases, but symptoms are relatively mild in most. (**b**) By contrast, ulceration due to 5-fluorouracil is rare. (Panel b courtesy of Dr. G. Dawn.)

Table 18.10 SOME CUTANEOUS SIDE EFFECTS OF CYTOTOXIC DRUGS

Side effect	Drug(s)
Urticaria	Asparaginase, cisplatin, melphalan (intravenous)
Radiation recall	Dactinomycin, doxorubicin, bleomycin, 5-fluorouracil
Pigmentation	Bleomycin (may be flagellate pattern), cyclophosphamide, busulfan, doxorubicin, 5-fluorouracil (may follow veins), hydroxyurea (nails)
Photosensitivity	Dacarbazine, vinblastine, mitomycin, 5-fluorouracil
Acral erythema	5-fluorouracil, cytosine arabinoside, doxorubicin
Neutrophilic eccrine hidradenitis	Cytosine arabinoside, bleomycin, docetaxel
Dermatomyositis-like (acral)	Hydroxyurea (long term)
Dermatitis	Mitomycin (intravesical)
Toxic epidermal necrolysis	See Table 18.7
Acute generalized eruptive pustulosis	Cytosine arabinoside
Scleroderma-like reaction	Paclitaxel

Palmar erythema

Palmar erythema is seen as part of several exanthematous drug eruptions. Palmar crease purpura is a feature of drug-induced vasculitis in some patients and may occur in TEN.

Isolated palmar erythema may occur due to several non-drug causes, such as in pregnancy, liver disease, and acutely in the purpuric gloves and stocking pattern of parvovirus B19 infection.

Erythromelalgia is a palmoplantar disorder consisting of erythema and burning pain, which may be relieved in some patients by immersing the affected sites in cold water or walking on a cold floor. It may be idiopathic, but may also be due to drugs; nifedipine and nicardipine have been particularly implicated. It may respond to aspirin and drug withdrawal, but can be very resistant to treatment.

Some cytotoxic agents commonly cause palmoplantar erythema. The most consistent is 5-fluorouracil given by continuous infusion for bowel carcinomas, about 30% of patients developing 'palmoplantar syndrome' with this regimen (Fig. 18.30). This reaction takes a few months to develop, may affect the face and nails as well as the palms and soles, and is relatively asymptomatic but can be reduced in degree by treatment with oral pyridoxine. A more acute palmoplantar erythema and desquamation may occur due to doxorubicin, daunorubicin, cytosine arabinoside, and others.

Anticonvulsant rashes and drug hypersensitivity syndrome

Anticonvulsant reactions (Figs 18.2, 18.31 and 18.32) are important as:
- they are common,
- they are often severe,
- internal organs are often affected, and
- cross-reactions are common.

The usual cutaneous reaction pattern to anticonvulsants is exanthematous or maculopapular, but may be urticarial, EM, TEN, FDE,

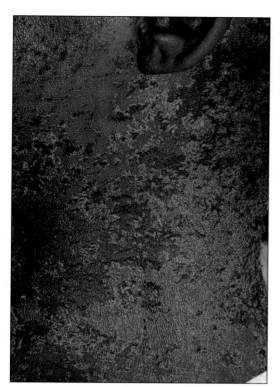

Figure 18.31 An eczematous pattern of drug eruption as part of the anticonvulsant hypersensitivity syndrome.

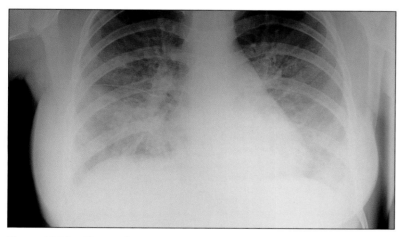

Figure 18.32 Chest radiograph of a patient with a severe carbamazepine reaction. She had extensive rash, lymphadenopathy, fever, hepatitis, and eosinophilia.

and others. Facial edema is common in the more severe cases. The anticonvulsant syndrome, which occurs in up to 1% of patients on aromatic anticonvulsants, especially phenytoin, consists of fever, headache, sore throat, arthralgia, hepatitis, pneumonitis (Fig. 18.32), nephritis, and lymphadenopathy. Laboratory features include leukocytosis with eosinophilia and atypical lymphocytes, presence of cold agglutinins, positive rheumatoid factor or antinuclear antibody, and increased polyclonal hypergammaglobulinemia. It may take several weeks to develop after the drug is started. In cases where carbamazepine is suspected to be the cause, patch testing is useful to confirm the diagnosis, but is retrospective. Less severe, usually morbilliform, skin reactions occur in a further 2% of patients but can be difficult to distinguish from the hypersensitivity syndrome, as rash and fever are usually the initial features of the more severe reactions. There is extensive cross-reaction between anticonvulsants due to common arene oxide metabolites.

Lamotrigine, a more recently introduced drug, has also been increasingly implicated as a cause of severe skin rash with fever, multiorgan dysfunction, and sometimes disseminated intravascular coagulation; this severe reaction is more frequent in children and may be more likely if valproate is given concurrently (as it increases plasma lamotrigine levels). However, valproate in isolation is a rare cause of significant rash and, as it has a different structure to the cross-reacting aromatic anticonvulsants, is the usual substitute in patients with severe drug reactions.

Severe reactions of this type with systemic features are also termed the drug hypersensitivity syndrome (DHS) or drug reaction with eosinophilia and systemic symptoms (DRESS). Anticonvulsants account for most cases, but this pattern of hypersensitivity may also occur with sulfonamides, allopurinol, gold, dapsone, minocycline, nitrofurantoin, terbinafine, abacavir, diltiazem, and many others less commonly.

A pseudolymphoma picture, with lymphadenopathy and variable skin plaques or nodules resembling B-cell lymphoma or mycosis fungoides, may occur with phenytoin. This is occasionally fatal due to agranulocytosis or neutropenia, and the incidence of true lymphoma is increased.

PRACTICE POINTS

Severe drug eruptions are important! Don't forget the following points.

- Anticonvulsants have about a 1% risk of severe rash with eosinophilia and systemic features such as fever, arthralgia, lymphadenopathy, hepatitis, pneumonitis, and nephritis, and many will cross-react.
- Allopurinol is one of the commoner causes of toxic epidermal necrolysis (TEN) and of erythrodermic drug eruptions.
- If they have not already been discontinued, likely culprit drugs should be stopped immediately if blisters or erosions appear during the course of a drug eruption: the blistering may be the start of TEN.
- Erythema affecting more than about 60% of the body surface area or evidence of systemic involvement is a feature suggesting a severe reaction.
- Extensive pustular drug eruptions are usually due to antibiotics and develop rapidly after exposure, usually within a couple of days.

Drug-induced pigmentation

Pigmentation due to postinflammatory pigmentary incontinence may be a feature of any lichenoid reaction, and is usual in FDE. There are many other patterns of drug-induced pigmentation (Table 18.11), involving a variety of mechanisms, the most frequent being:

- postinflammatory (most are due to this);
- stimulation of melanin synthesis, for example by psoralens (Ch. 17);
- chemical deposition, for example argyria and other heavy metals;
- mixed chemical deposition and increased melanin, for example minocycline (Figs 18.33–18.35, see also Fig. 4.3) and mepacrine (Fig. 18.36); and
- mixed drug and other chemicals, for example clofazimine with a ceroid–lipofuscin pigment in macrophages.

Some drugs seem to have an association with particular patterns or site combinations of pigmentation, which may strongly suggest a certain drug or group of agents as being responsible. Examples include the following.

- Minocycline—may affect scars (face, back, and other sites), diffuse facial, circumscribed areas on distal limbs, nails, and teeth.

Table 18.11   DRUGS THAT CAUSE PIGMENTATION

Category	Drug(s)
Cytotoxic	Bleomycin, cyclophosphamide, busulfan, Adriamycin (doxorubicin), others
Antimalarials	Mepacrine, chloroquine
Psychiatry	Chlorpromazine, imipramine
Anticonvulsants	Phenytoin
Cardiac	Amiodarone, methyldopa, beta-blockers
Hormonal	Adrenocorticotropic hormone, oral contraceptives
Metals	Gold, silver, bismuth, mercury, arsenic
Tetracyclines	Minocycline, tetracycline
Others	Psoralens, quinine, co-danthramer

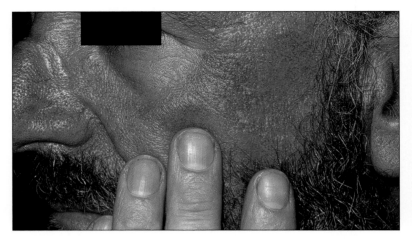

Figure 18.33 Pigmentation due to long-term administration of minocycline for rosacea. In this case, the pattern is a diffuse blue-gray pigmentation affecting the face and nail beds.

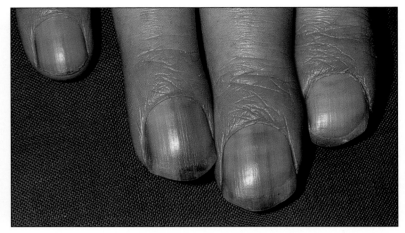

Figure 18.36 Pigmentation due to mepacrine commonly affects the palate, sclera, or nails, as shown here. The color is usually brownish or blue-gray, but skin pigmentation may be rather yellowish.

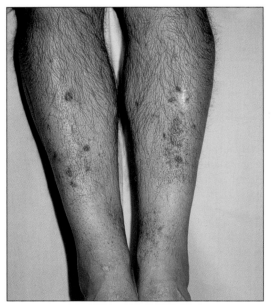

Figure 18.34 Pigmentation due to long-term administration of minocycline. In this instance, the pigment is localized to old scars on the lower legs. The same process may occur in facial acne scars. See also examples in Figure 4.3.

Table 18.12	SOME DRUGS THAT MAY CAUSE ALOPECIA
Category	**Drugs**
Chemotherapy and related drugs	Doxorubicin or daunorubicin, cyclophosphamide, azathioprine, methotrexate
Anticoagulants	Heparin or heparinoids, coumarins
Endocrinology	Thiouracils, carbimazole, bromocriptine
Neurology and psychiatry	Carbamazepine, valproate, levodopa, tricyclics, lithium, haloperidol
Rheumatology	Gold, allopurinol, ibuprofen
Cardiology	Captopril, propranolol, some lipid-lowering drugs
Others	Retinoids, colchicine, cimetidine, amphetamines

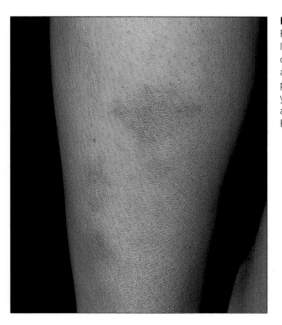

Figure 18.35 Pigmentation due to long-term administration of minocycline, showing a more bruise-like pattern on the legs in a younger patient. See also examples in Figure 4.3.

- Antimalarials—hard palate, nails, and ocular.
- Phenothiazine, anticonvulsants, amiodarone, and diltiazem—photoexposed.
- Co-danthramer—perianal and thighs (skin staining after excretion in the stools, Fig. 18.8).

Hair changes

Alopecia is frequently considered to be a side effect of drugs but in many instances is not well substantiated; drugs perhaps account for about 5% of cases of diffuse alopecia. Some potential causes are listed in Table 18.12. Mechanisms vary; in some cases, such as alopecia due to cytotoxic agents, the cause is well understood (see anagen effluvium, Ch. 28). Poisons such as thallium may do the same. Some drugs may cause other patterns of hair change, such as the generalized curliness or marginal 'acquired progressive kinking' that can occur in some patients taking systemic retinoids.

Hypertrichosis due to drugs is mainly due to a small number of agents, including corticosteroids, androgenic steroids, ciclosporin, diazoxide, and minoxidil.

Anticoagulant drug eruptions and vitamin K

Any anticoagulant may predispose to bruising (Fig. 18.37), which may be localized (e.g. to areas of heparin injection) or more widespread.

Heparin may also cause local allergic reactions (Fig. 18.38); some of these are due to preservatives such as chlorocresol in the vehicle, but others are true allergy to heparin, which causes local eczematous plaques at injection sites. Change to a heparin of different molecular weight usually

- Cytotoxics—patterns include pigmentation of nails (mainly bleomycin, cyclophosphamide, and doxorubicin), mucous membranes (busulfan and doxorubicin), a 'flagellate' pattern (bleomycin and busulfan), localization to striae (bleomycin), and a serpiginous pattern overlying veins (5-fluorouracil).

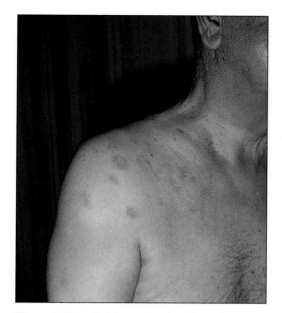

Figure 18.37 Bruising on the shoulder and upper trunk in a patient taking an excessive dose of warfarin (coumarin) anticoagulant.

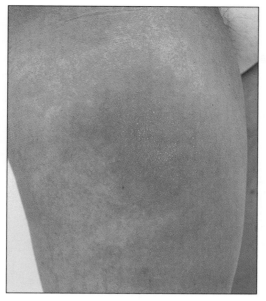

Figure 18.38 Local allergy to subcutaneous heparin injections, in this case in a pregnant patient with high risk of thromboembolism, caused multiple erythematous or eczematous plaques at the injection sites on the anterior thighs.

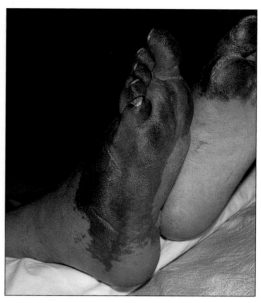

Figure 18.39 Coumarin necrosis affecting the feet, in a patient with paraneoplastic venous thrombosis who received anticoagulation with standard doses.

resolves the problem. Local heparin-induced necrosis at injection sites is very rare, and is due to a heparin-dependent platelet-activating IgG, which may also cause thrombocytopenia and paradoxical thrombosis.

Coumarins such as warfarin may rarely cause a severe reaction known as coumarin necrosis, in which erythematous and bruised areas progress to blistering and necrosis (Fig. 18.39). This usually starts on about the third day of anticoagulation, and is fairly symmetric over fatty areas or sometimes at the extremities. It is associated with thrombophilic states, usually heterozygous protein C deficiency. The condition occurs because warfarin depresses circulating levels of protein C (which has an anti-coagulant function) before it decreases levels of other (procoagulant) vitamin K-dependent clotting factors; once the additional anticoagulant effect of heparin is withdrawn, there may therefore be a period of hypercoagulability. This effect is most prominent in individuals who have low levels of protein C, protein S, or antithrombin III.

Vitamin K injections may cause prolonged local injection site macules and plaques, in a minority of cases progressing to localized scleroderma- or morphea-like changes (Texier syndrome).

Acneiform eruptions

Acneiform drug eruptions (Table 18.13) generally differ from ordinary acne by having relatively monomorphic papules and pustules, and no comedones. The commonest cause is corticosteroid therapy. However, some drugs such as lithium may aggravate ordinary acne, and some such as halides cause a more inflammatory pustular eruption in which there may also be plaques, nodules, and necrotic lesions; this may mimic pyoderma gangrenosum or Sweet disease (Ch. 14).

Pustular eruptions, acute generalized exanthematous pustulosis

Pustular eruptions distinct from acneiform drug eruptions are increasingly recognized, for example eosinophilic pustular folliculitis related to carbamazepine, a pustular psoriasiform eruption due to terbinafine, and provocation of true pustular psoriasis by bupropion.

A particularly acute and severe pustular pattern of drug eruption has been described as acute generalized exanthematous pustulosis (AGEP; Figs 18.40 and 18.41, Table 18.14). In this disorder, the eruption consists of small, superficial, semiconfluent, non-follicular pustules that may resemble acute pustular psoriasis; occasionally, purpuric lesions resembling atypical target lesions may be seen. Most cases are drug-induced; a

Table 18.13	**CAUSES OF ACNEIFORM DRUG ERUPTION**
Category	**Drug(s)**
Steroids	Anabolic or androgenic, glucocorticoids
Halogens	Iodides, bromides
Anticonvulsants	Phenytoin
Antituberculous	Ethambutol, isoniazid
Psychiatry	Lithium
Other	Danazol, quinidine, azathioprine

minority appear to follow viral infections (especially enteroviruses) or to occur in patients with autoimmune diseases (such as thyroid disease or ulcerative colitis). Overall, antibiotics account for about two-thirds of cases; the most common cause is penicillins (especially ampicillin and derivatives). The eruption is usually of rapid onset (typically within a day or two in antibiotic-triggered cases) with fever and malaise, and often involves flexures initially. Lymphocyte transformation tests, and sometimes patch tests to the suspect drug, may be positive. Primary skin infections, other neutrophilic dermatoses, pustular vasculitis (both Ch. 14), and generalized pustular psoriasis (Ch. 7) should be excluded.

Photosensitivity

This is discussed in more detail in Chapter 17. Many drugs can cause this pattern of reaction (Fig. 18.42).

Purpura, vasculitis, and serum sickness

Vasculitis and purpura are discussed in more detail in Chapter 14. Drugs that cause this reaction pattern include antibiotics (especially penicillins and sulfonamides), diuretics (especially thiazides and furosemide, Fig. 18.43), NSAIDs, hydantoins, thiouracils, systemic imidazole antifungals such as itraconazole, intravenous immunoglobulins, and anti-tumor necrosis factor agents. Provocation of pigmented purpuric dermatosis is discussed later.

Figure 18.40 Acute generalized exanthematous pustulosis, showing more confluent pustules.

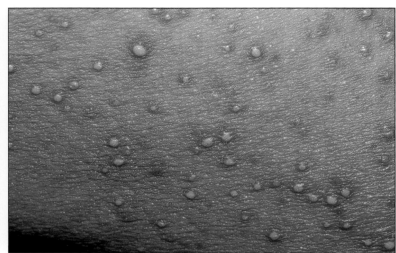

Figure 18.41 Acute generalized exanthematous pustulosis, showing grouped pustules.

Table 18.14 DRUG AND CHEMICAL CAUSES OF ACUTE GENERALIZED EXANTHEMATOUS PUSTULOSIS (AGEP)	
Category	**Drugs**
Antimicrobials	Penicillins (most cases), macrolides, vancomycin, sulfonamides (relatively uncommon), nystatin, fluconazole, terbinafine, others
Analgesics	Non-steroidal antiinflammatory drugs, celecoxib, acetaminophen
Neurology and antidepressant	Carbamazepine, clobazam, amoxapine
Cardiac and respiratory	Calcium channel blockers, quinidine, theophyllines, furosemide
Others	Mercury, cytosine arabinoside, mesalazine, hydroxychloroquine

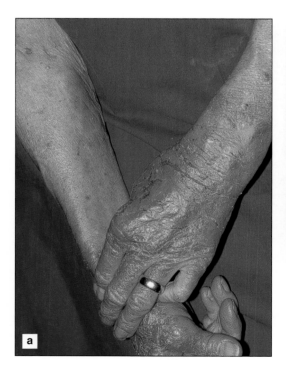

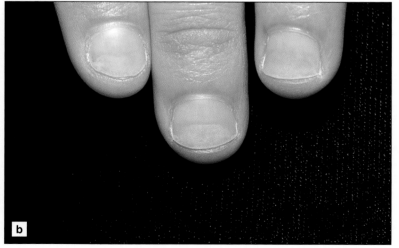

Figure 18.42 (**a**) Acute photosensitivity due to chlorpromazine. The diagnosis was confirmed by grossly abnormal phototest results. (**b**) Photoonycholysis is a less common phototoxic reaction; it was common with a non-steroidal antiinflammatory drug called benoxaprofen (withdrawn from sale for may years) and is currently seen most often due to tetracyclines, as in this case (see also Fig. 17.40).

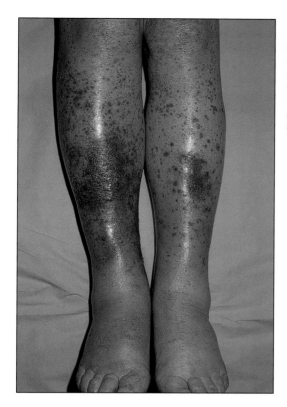

Figure 18.43 Vasculitis of 'palpable purpura' type (see Ch. 14), due to furosemide. Some cases of vasculitis due to furosemide present months or even years after the drug has been started.

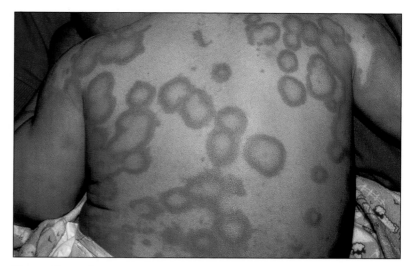

Figure 18.44 Serum sickness–like reaction, in this case due to amoxicillin. The acute onset in a child of inflammatory, red papulonodules that spread out into annular, urticarial plaques with dusky centers ('purple-colored urticaria') is characteristic. Note the coalescence of some lesions.

Serum sickness is a type III reaction with immune complex-mediated vascular damage. It presents as a vasculitis (palpable purpura, hemorrhagic blisters and ulcers, sometimes digital necrosis) with associated morbilliform and urticarial rash, arthralgia, fever, and malaise. Apart from true serum sickness due to serum products and vaccines, a serum sickness-like eruption may occur due to antibiotics (especially some cephalosporins, also ampicillin and derivatives, other β-lactam antibiotics, minocycline, and doxycycline), beta-blockers, bupropion, and streptokinase. Complement levels (C3 and C4) are reduced in true serum sickness but not in these drug-induced eruptions.

Serum sickness–like reaction
Serum sickness-like reaction is a recognizable reaction to a drug. It has occurred most frequently following cefaclor, but may occur with other cephalosporins, penicillins, or other drugs. Prior treatment with the drug is not necessary.

The acute onset in a child of inflammatory, red papulonodules that spread out into annular, urticarial plaques with dusky centers is characteristic (it has been termed purple-colored urticaria; Fig. 18.44). The onset is usually 7–10 days after the causative drug was begun. There are no true target lesions as with EM, and the lesions may expand but do not have the day-to-day fluctuation seen in urticaria. The child often has joint pains and fever. Lymphadenopathy and renal involvement usually do not occur, in contrast to true serum sickness. The causative medication should be stopped. Prednisone (e.g. 2 mg/kg per day) can be dramatically helpful, if needed.

Bullous eruptions
Drug-induced blisters (Table 18.15) may occur in several ways.
- As part of a drug eruption with a specific recognizable morphology— for example, in EM or TEN, FDE, or photosensitivity (all discussed earlier).
- Provoking or closely mimicking an immunobullous eruption or a metabolic cause of blistering (Table 18.16).
- Causing less specific patterns of bullous lesions.

Drug-induced porphyria and pseudoporphyria (Fig. 18.45) are described in Chapter 17. Blistering at pressure areas due to barbiturate-induced coma is now uncommon.

Drug eruptions that resemble immunobullous disorders are increasingly recognized (Table 18.16). Some of these occur only after months or years of treatment (e.g. penicillamine-induced pemphigus, Figs 18.46 and 18.47), but others may be relatively acute (e.g. vancomycin-induced linear IgA disease, Fig. 18.48). Drug-induced pemphigus is generally of foliaceous or erythematosus type. Several cases of drug-induced linear IgA disease have been reported in which the morphology resembled TEN.

Injection site reactions
In addition to simple effects of tissue damage, such as bruising or transient tenderness, and reactions to vitamin K discussed earlier, a number of local reactions may occur related to injections, summarized in Table 18.17 (Fig. 18.49). Generalized rash may also be triggered, such as urticaria due to the hepatitis B vaccine (urticarial rash is a feature of early hepatitis B infection in some cases); there are even occasional reports of TEN temporally related to vaccine administration. Occasionally, a viral exanthem that would normally be expected to be generalized will occur locally around a recent vaccination site.

Local anesthetic reactions
Local anesthetics may cause dose-related systemic toxicity due to either lidocaine (lignocaine; tinnitus, numb lips, metallic taste, nausea, diplopia, nystagmus, tremor, and convulsions) or adrenaline (epinephrine; local vasoconstriction, tachycardia, dysrhythmias, and tremor). These are most likely in children, the elderly, and those with existing heart, liver, or renal disease.

Idiosyncratic reactions to local anesthetic agents are unpredictable and less easy to interpret. Allergy to topical esters such as benzocaine is not uncommon, but reactions to amides such as lidocaine are very rare. The vast majority of such events after skin or dental surgery are simple fainting episodes, which are unrelated to the anesthetic agent. Collapse that is not associated with injection site urticaria, facial angioedema, or respiratory symptoms, and especially if occurring after an uneventful procedure, is unlikely to be due to local anesthetic allergy. Urticaria confined to a surgical area or around the mouth may alternatively be due to other allergies, such as to latex gloves. Palpitations and sweating may be due to inadvertent injection of adrenaline (epinephrine) into a vessel.

In a case where allergy to lidocaine appears unlikely but a degree of caution is required, prilocaine can be used (with octapressin as a vasoconstrictor if necessary). Lidocaine cross-reacts with dibucaine (cinchocaine) and mepivacaine, but reactions to prilocaine are extremely rare. In patients with a strong suspicion of lidocaine allergy, it is possible to perform testing, but this is time-consuming and requires adequate resuscitation facilities. The usual sequence is patch testing to 20% lidocaine, followed by prick testing, intradermal testing, and a gradually increasing sequence of challenge doses, but results are often not reliable; for example, patients may have a positive skin test to an agent that has been used clinically without any problem, or vice versa.

Table 18.15   SOME CAUSES OF DRUG-INDUCED BLISTERING

Category	Drugs
Antibiotics	Tetracyclines, sulfonamides, rifampin, vancomycin, nalidixic acid
Antiinflammatory	Non-steroidal antiinflammatory drugs, thalidomide, dapsone, gold, chloroquine, colchicine
Neurologic	Barbiturates, chloral hydrate, phenytoin
Cytotoxics and oncology	Vinblastine, 5-fluorouracil, interleukin-2
Cardiac	Thiazides, furosemide, quinidine, captopril
Other	Insulin, sulfonylureas, phenolphthalein, quinine, epsilon-aminocaproic acid

Table 18.16   SOME DRUGS THAT MAY PROVOKE ERUPTIONS OF IMMUNOBULLOUS OR METABOLIC PATTERN

Clinical disease pattern	Example(s) of provocative drugs
Pemphigus	Thiol drugs (penicillamine, captopril, gold sodium thiomalate), piroxicam, rifampin, levodopa, penicillin, propranolol, phenobarbital
Pemphigoid	Psoralens, furosemide, clonidine, ibuprofen, sulfa drugs, ciprofloxacin, penicillins, chloroquine, captopril, enalapril
Cicatricial pemphigoid	Penicillamine
Lichen planus pemphigoides	Captopril, ramipril, cinnarizine, furosemide, simvastatin
Linear IgA disease	Vancomycin (most), co-trimoxazole, phenytoin, carbamazepine, furosemide, somatostatin, some non-steroidal antiinflammatory drugs, amiodarone, captopril, ciclosporin, atorvastatin, vigabactrin, lithium carbonate, acetaminophen, interleukin-2
Pseudoporphyria (see also Ch. 17)	Furosemide, naproxen, nalidixic acid, simvastatin

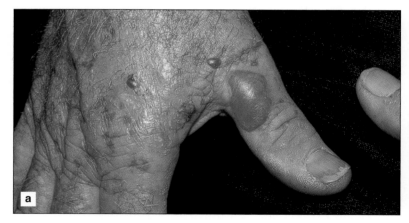
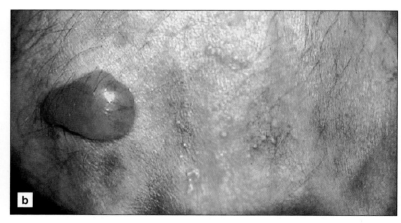

Figure 18.45   Pseudoporphyria due to (**a**) tetracycline and (**b**) naproxen. (Panel b courtesy of Dr. G. Dawn.)

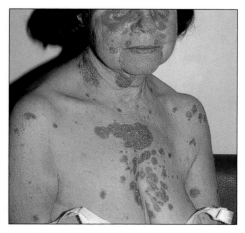

Figure 18.46   Penicillamine-induced pemphigus, of pemphigus foliaceus type (see also Ch. 16) with lesions predominantly on the face and upper trunk. This can be a prolonged and potentially serious eruption, which presents in a delayed manner.

PRACTICE POINTS

In considering local anesthetic reactions, the following points should be remembered.

- True allergic reactions to injected local anesthetic agents are very rare.
- Collapse that is not associated with injection site urticaria, facial angioedema, or respiratory symptoms, and especially if occurring after an uneventful procedure, is unlikely to be due to local anesthetic allergy.
- Urticaria confined to a surgical area or around the mouth may be due to other allergies, such as to latex gloves.
- If there is concern about allergy to lidocaine (lignocaine) but the likelihood is low, prilocaine can usually be substituted.
- Proving local anesthetic allergy is time-consuming and may not be reliable.

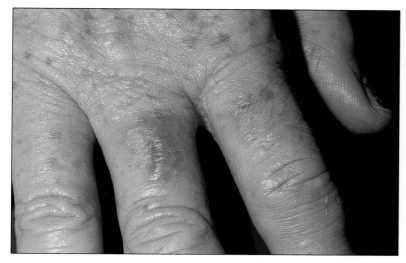

Figure 18.47 Penicillamine-induced pemphigus affecting the hand. Intact blisters are relatively uncommon in pemphigus, and tend to rupture to produce erosions and crusting.

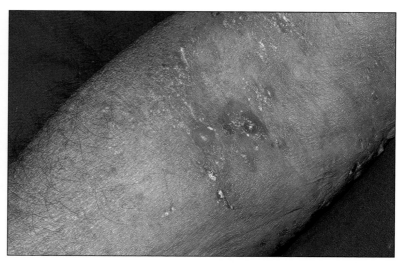

Figure 18.48 Vancomycin-induced linear IgA disease in a patient treated with intravenous vancomycin for an infected hip replacement wound. There was no recurrence of blistering during the following 2 years, when he was seen about an unrelated skin lesion.

Table 18.17   INJECTION SITE REACTIONS

Drug(s)	Reaction
Vaccines	Local erythema, exanthem; granulomas (due to aluminum or bacillus Calmette–Guérin [BCG] vaccine); allergic reaction (to preservatives such as thiomersal); localization of viral exanthema
Insulin	Lipoatrophy, lipohypertrophy (see Ch. 22)
Corticosteroids	Atrophy, depigmentation
Hematologic drugs	Heparin: bruising, allergy, necrosis; vitamin K morphea-like lesions (Texier syndrome); cytotoxic extravasation reactions; granulocyte-colony stimulating factor: localized lichenoid reaction
Others	Apomorphine nodules; pentazocine panniculitis, vasculitis due to interferon-alpha
Non-specific	Bruising, transient tenderness; thrombophlebitis, ulceration, or abscesses (especially narcotics); hypertrichosis

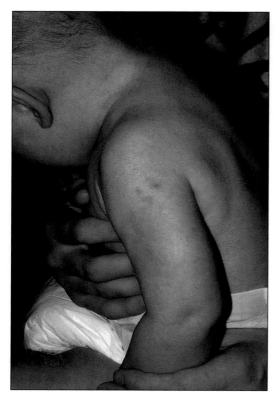

Figure 18.49
Vaccination site granuloma due to aluminum in the vaccine; these lesions may persist for years as subcutaneous nodules.

Other patterns of eruption

A few other patterns of eruption warrant specific mention.

- The baboon syndrome has been discussed earlier as a form of systemic contact dermatitis that presents as a flexural and buttock exanthema. However, multiple lesions of FDE with a similar distribution have been reported.
- A papular eruption with methotrexate appears to be limited to patients with an underlying collagen vascular disorder; the papules occur mainly on the proximal limbs soon after starting methotrexate.
- A dermatomyositis-like, or acral lichenoid, eruption may occur with hydroxycarbamide (Fig. 18.50) and occasionally with simvastatin.
- Hydroxycarbamide may also cause chronic leg ulceration resembling venous disease.
- Iododerma and bromoderma are rare reactions to iodine and bromine, respectively; iododerma is more common, as iodine is used therapeutically (in thyroid disease, radiocontrast media, and some inflammatory dermatoses), but these chemicals are also in some foods and drinks that may occasionally be consumed to excess. Lesions are inflammatory nodules with blistering, postulation, or necrosis, clinically resembling pyoderma gangrenosum.
- A 'burning erythema' may occur with some monoclonal biologicals, such as interleukin-2 (which may also cause skin necrosis).
- A scleroderma-like pattern may occur with paclitaxel.
- Edema is a common side effect of imatinib (also known as STI 571); over 60% get this, together with pruritus in 40% and various

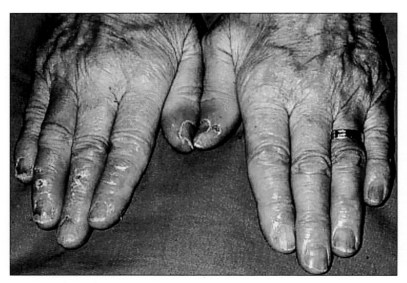

Figure 18.50 Hydroxycarbamide (hydroxyurea) may cause an acral lichenoid or dermatomyositis-like rash; acral or leg ulceration may also occur. Such problems may be missed, as they can occur after therapy has been used for several years. (Courtesy of Dr. G. Dawn.)

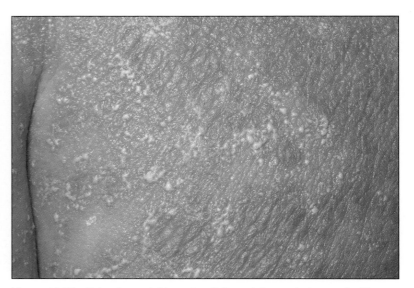

Figure 18.51 Extensive unstable and partially pustular psoriasis provoked by bupropion for smoking cessation in a patient with previously stable plaque psoriasis. (From Cox NH, et al. Br J Dermatol 2002; 146: 1061–3.)

morphologies of rash (mainly exanthematous, exfoliative dermatitis, and lichenoid eruption) in two-thirds.

- Cheilitis is an inevitable dose-related side effect of systemic retinoids; it may also occur with indinavir. Circumoral paresthesia commonly occurs with ritonavir.
- Progesterone and estrogen dermatitis may be eczematous, urticarial, or EM-like; see Chapter 12.

Provocation or exacerbation of preexisting skin disease

A number of drugs may occasionally provoke an apparently idiopathic dermatosis, or may aggravate an existing dermatosis; some of these are listed here (see also the earlier text on bullous drug eruptions).

Psoriasis

Drugs that may worsen psoriasis include the following.

- Lithium. Management of psoriasis in patients on this drug may be very difficult, particularly as lithium has so many potential drug interactions and is often used where other psychiatric medications have failed. The effect is probably on neutrophil function, as lithium-induced psoriasis is often of pustular type. Potassium iodide may worsen psoriasis by a similar mechanism.
- NSAIDs. These interfere with cyclooxygenase and lipoxygenase enzymes in the prostaglandin synthesis pathway, and may cause an increase in proinflammatory leukotrienes such as leukotriene B4. Fortunately, this potential adverse effect is rarely clinically apparent, as a significant number of patients with psoriasis have arthropathy, which may require this type of treatment. NSAIDs are also potential causes of photosensitivity and may occasionally interfere with PUVA photochemotherapy.
- Beta-blockers. Aggravation of psoriasis due to beta-blockers is recorded; studies vary in determining the strength of the association, but worsening in up to 75% has been recorded. The significance of this in a variable disorder is uncertain; marked deterioration is uncommon.
- Bupropion. The mechanism for worsening psoriasis is unknown, but deterioration may be severe; generalized pustular or erythrodermic psoriasis has been reported, usually a few weeks after starting this medication for smoking cessation (Fig. 18.51).
- Terbinafine may apparently provoke psoriasis de novo or may aggravate existing psoriasis.
- Gemfibrozil has been reported to aggravate psoriasis.
- Abrupt withdrawal of corticosteroids may cause a rebound flare of psoriasis; at worst, pustular psoriasis may be provoked. Corticosteroids should therefore be used with caution in patients with severe rashes or erythroderma that may actually be due to psoriasis.

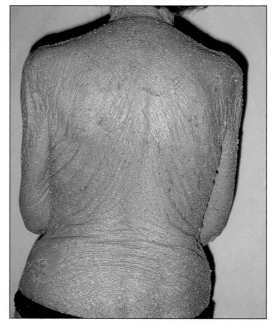

Figure 18.52 An extensive exfoliative psoriasis pattern in a patient taking captopril.

Other drugs that may cause a psoriasiform pattern of drug eruption include captopril (Fig. 18.52), methyldopa, imatinib, and interferons.

Lupus erythematosus

Drug-induced lupus, with a list of causes, is discussed in Chapter 13. Thiazides may cause a lupus-like rash.

Porphyria cutanea tarda

A huge number of drugs may provoke the neurologic symptoms of acute intermittent porphyria or variegate porphyria, but drug induction or aggravation of porphyria cutanea tarda (PCT) is much less convincing. Alcohol is the most important trigger; of physician-prescribed medications, estrogens for prostatic neoplasia are an important trigger. Chloroquine and hydroxychloroquine can be used to treat PCT in low dose, but at higher doses may provoke symptoms. This is discussed in more detail in Chapter 17.

Dermatitis herpetiformis

Drug-induced aggravation of dermatitis herpetiformis (DH) is rare. Topical nicotinamide provokes lesions, but the potentially more severe problem is more generalized triggering of DH by iodides in radiocontrast media or in thyroid treatment (Lugol's iodine). The mechanism is probably by increasing activity of neutrophil enzymes such as myeloperoxidase.

Urticaria

The role of non-immunologic mechanisms of drug-triggering of urticaria and angioedema is discussed in the section on urticarial drug eruptions.

Rosacea

Any vasodilator may potentially aggravate the erythematous component of rosacea. Some, such as nifedipine, may cause development of telangiectasia in a photodistributed pattern. The drug trigger frequently noticed by patients is alcohol.

Sweet syndrome

Several drugs have been implicated as triggers of Sweet syndrome (acute febrile neutrophilic dermatosis; see also Ch. 14). Most implicate either all-*trans*-retinoic acid or granulocyte colony-stimulating factor (both agents used in hematology that induce an increase in neutrophil count) or minocycline. Other reported drug triggers include other tetracyclines, hydralazine, trimethoprim–sulfamethoxazole, nitrofurantoin, celecoxib, furosemide, lithium, isotretinoin, clonazepam, diazepam, oral contraceptives, cytosine arabinoside, and bacillus Calmette-Guérin (BCG) vaccination.

Others

- A mycosis fungoides-like rash has been reported with phenytoin, carbamazepine, and fluoxetine, and it has been suggested that the last may worsen preexisting mycosis fungoides. A pityriasis lichenoides-like eruption may also occur due to drugs (Fig. 18.53).
- Pigmented purpuric dermatoses (PPD) may occasionally be provoked by drugs, including various cardiac agents (beta-blockers, calcium channel blockers, ACE inhibitors, furosemide, and nitrites), some antidepressants, chlordiazepoxide, some antihistamines, glipizide, acetaminophen, interferon–alpha, and infliximab (the last provoking the 'itching purpura' or Doucas and Kapetenakis pattern of PPD).
- Livedo reticularis, a network-like vascular patterning, occurs in a variety of vascular occlusion disorders and in vasculitides such as polyarteritis nodosa (all discussed in Ch. 14). However, it may also occur due to drugs such as amantadine or ergotamine, as well as being associated with microangiopathy related to heparin and others. Localized triggering of livedo has been reported after injection of bismuth, cocaine, glucocorticoids, NSAIDs, depot penicillins, and copolymer.
- Inflammation of actinic keratosis may occur with systemic 5-fluorouracil (as it does with the topical formulation).
- Penicillamine may cause elastosis perforans serpiginosa, as well as various immunobullous disorders (Table 18.15).

Cross-reactions

Some groups of drugs exhibit important cross-reactions; a previous severe reaction with a chemically related drug is thus a reason to avoid unnecessary exposure. Some examples are given here.

Antibiotics

There are frequently cross-reactions between penicillins, and about 10% cross-reactivity between penicillins and cephalosporins. Using drug-

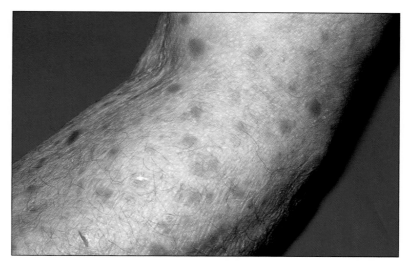

Figure 18.53 A pityriasis lichenoides–like eruption due to diclofenac.

specific T-cell clones from patients with ciprofloxacin-triggered exanthema, half demonstrated cross-reactivity with other quinolones. Cross-reactions between aminoglycosides are also very frequent, but of greater dermatologic importance during topical use.

Cross-reactions between pristinamycin and other synergistins are particularly common, and have been proved by skin testing.

Sulfa drugs

Sulfonamide antibiotics, sulfonylurea drugs for diabetes, and thiazide diuretics all share a similar structure. A similar spectrum of reactions is therefore seen for each of these groups; for example, they are all reasonably common causes of drug-induced photosensitivity reactions.

Anticonvulsants

The cross-reactions between aromatic anticonvulsants, due to arene metabolites that they have in common, are discussed earlier.

Local anesthetics

Cross-reactions between these agents are discussed earlier. Additionally, the *para*-amino agents may cross-react with topical agents (discussed later).

Cross-reactions of systemic drugs with topical allergens

Medications such as antibiotics may cause a rash when taken orally, and also cause contact sensitivity by external application or inadvertent contact (e.g. penicillins, especially in older patients who have been treated with topical penicillin or nurses who have handled such agents).

Antabuse, for alcohol abstinence, is a thiuram chemical and may cause severe reactions in patients who are allergic to thiurams by contact sensitivity (used in rubber manufacture); flushing is part of the reaction (anticipated rather than idiosyncratic).

Aminophylline (for asthma) is chemically related to ethylene diamine (a stabilizer in some creams) and may cross-react.

The *para*-amino types of local anesthetic may cross-react with topical agents containing a similar structure, such as hair dyes.

FURTHER READING

Bachot N, Roujeau J-C. Differential diagnosis of severe drug eruptions. Am J Clin Dermatol 2003; 4: 561–72

Bigby M, Jick S, Jick H et al. Drug-induced cutaneous reactions: a report from the Boston collaborative drug surveillance program on 15,438 consecutive inpatients, 1975 to 1982. JAMA 1986; 256: 3358–63

Bork K. Cutaneous Side-effects of Drugs. Philadelphia: Saunders, 1988

Breathnach SM, Hintner H. Adverse Drug Reactions and the Skin. Oxford: Blackwell Scientific Publications, 1992

Dereure O et al. Drug-induced skin pigmentation. Epidemiology, diagnosis and treatment. Am J Clin Dermatol 2001; 2: 253–62

Halevy S, Shai A. Lichenoid drug eruptions. J Am Acad Dermatol 1993; 29: 249–55

Mahboob A, Haroon TS. Drugs causing fixed eruptions: a study of 450 cases. Int J Dermatol 1998; 37: 833–8

Roujeau J-C, Stern RS. Severe adverse cutaneous reactions to drugs. N Engl J Med 1994; 331: 1272–85

Roujeau J-C et al. Acute generalized exanthematous pustulosis. Analysis of 63 cases. Arch Dermatol 1991; 127: 1333–8

Susser WS et al. Mucocutaneous reactions to chemotherapy. J Am Acad Dermatol 1999; 40: 376–98

Wolff K, Tappenheimer G. Treatment of toxic epidermal necrolysis: the uncertainty persists but the fog is dispersing. Arch Dermatol 2001; 139: 85–6

Wolverton SE. Update on cutaneous drug eruptions. Adv Dermatol 1997; 13: 65–83

INTRODUCTION

The area of pediatric dermatology is a specialty of its own. It combines aspects of neonatology, genetics, and pediatrics, and is much more than just 'adult dermatology in little people'. This chapter begins with congenital lesions or birthmarks. It then considers conditions common in the infant, including diaper dermatitis. The last part of the chapter considers inherited conditions, also known as genodermatoses. Subsections include ichthyoses and palmoplantar keratodermas (see Ch. 7).

CONGENITAL LESIONS

Common skin conditions in the newborn

A variety of skin conditions are common incidental findings in the newborn. In general, no treatment is needed (Figs 19.1–19.8).

Congenital and early-onset vascular anomalies

Congenital vascular anomalies are divided into two broad categories.

- Hemangiomas—proliferative lesions that grow and ultimately may involve.

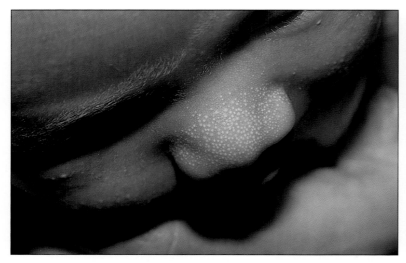

Figure 19.1 Sebaceous hyperplasia. The sebaceous glands of the newborn may be temporarily enlarged at birth secondary to stimulation by maternal hormones. Note the pinpoint yellow papules on this infant's nose.

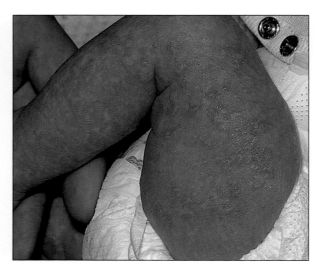

Figure 19.4 Erythema toxicum. Erythematous macules (1–3 cm in diameter) with a central papulopustule in a newborn is characteristic of this benign and transient condition.

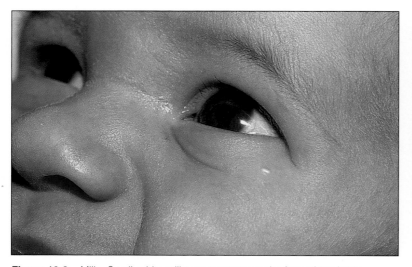

Figure 19.2 Milia. Small, white milia are common on the face of newborns. Spontaneous resolution is expected.

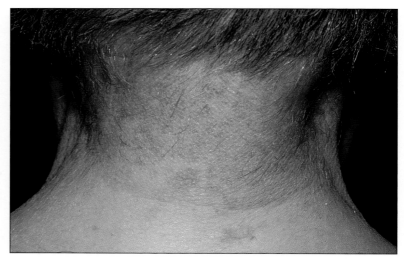

Figure 19.5 Erythema nuchae. A congenital vascular patch on the nape occurs very commonly and may persist throughout life.

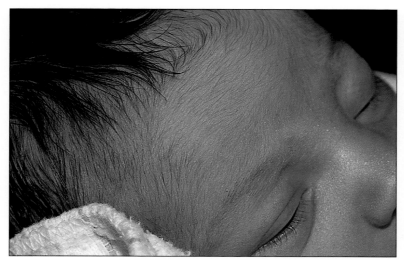

Figure 19.3 Lanugo hair. The presence of increased hair in an infant, as shown here on the forehead, is common and temporary.

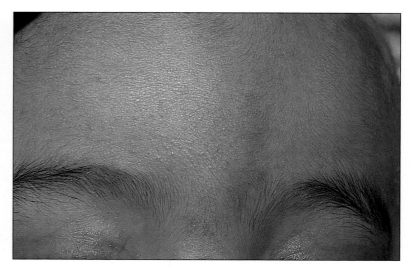

Figure 19.6 Salmon patch. A vascular blanching red patch or streak across the forehead or glabella occurs in many newborn infants. It usually fades, in contrast to port wine stains or vascular patches on the nape, which persist.

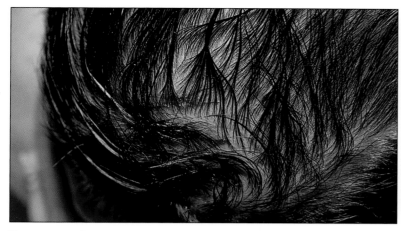

Figure 19.7 Scalp: electrode laceration. Superficial lacerations may be seen in the newborn, caused by the scalp fetal monitor. Herpes simplex infection has also been associated. Rarely, scalp abscesses may occur.

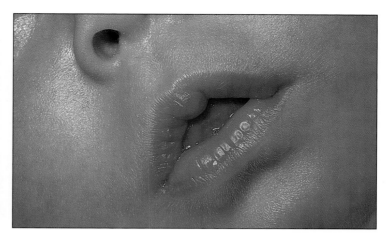

Figure 19.8 Sucking pad.

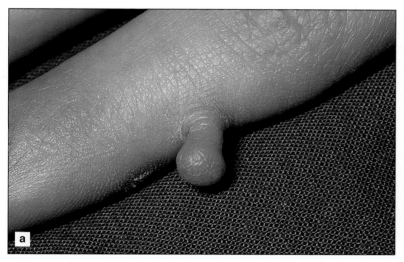

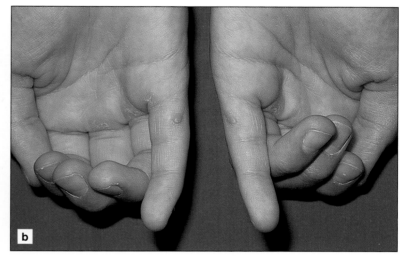

Figure 19.9 Supernumerary digit: (**a**) a solitary lesion; (**b**) bilateral lesions in a typical location.

- Vascular malformations—generally static lesions, although they may grow as the patient grows.

These conditions and their classification are discussed in Chapter 15.

Common infantile lesions such as nevus flammeus, 'stork bite', and 'salmon' patch are excluded from modern classifications of vascular anomalies. They occur mainly on the nape of the neck and forehead, and are viewed as dermal vascular ectasias that will fade. However:

- facial lesions may be in the differential diagnosis of early lesions of port wine stain, and
- nape of neck lesions may persist and become apparent again as hair thins in older patients.

Supernumerary digit

A supernumerary digit is congenital and usually located at the ulnar side of the base of the fifth finger. It may range in size from a small papule to a large (sixth) digit (Fig. 19.9). Surgery is appropriate if needed.

Accessory tragus

A congenital, firm papule or multilobular nodule occurring in the preauricular area is characteristic (Fig. 19.10). The lesion may consist of skin only, or skin and cartilage. It presumably developed from the auricular hillocks of the first branchial arch. These lesions may occasionally be bilateral or familial, or occur in association with other facial abnormalities. Congenital ear defects may be associated with kidney abnormalities, as both are formed at the same embryologic stage.

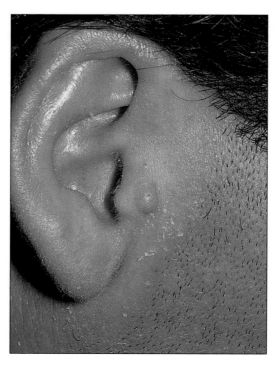

Figure 19.10 Accessory tragus. This congenital lesion is thought to represent a remnant of the first branchial arch.

The preauricular tag may be simply excised. However, if there is any question of a sinus or deep extension, excision should be done by a pediatric otolaryngologist.

Congenital preauricular sinus

A preauricular pinpoint opening (Fig. 19.11) may indicate an underlying sinus or fistula. Acute swelling and pain indicate a bacterial infection. This sinus may be familial (autosomal dominant). A sinus is much more common than a fistula and usually ends blindly, joining with the periosteum of the auditory canal. Rarely, there is an auricular fistula that connects with the tympanic or intratonsillar cleft. There are rare associations, most commonly with deafness and branchio–oto–renal (BOR) syndrome. If other anomalies are present, auditory and renal testing should be considered. An oral antibiotic should be given for any infection. A pediatric otolaryngologist may perform a surgical excision on the uninfected sinus.

Accessory nipple

Also known as polythelia, this lesion appears as a small, brown papule that may resemble a nipple, along the milk line that stretches from the axilla through the normal nipple to the groin. Only if there is breast tissue can conditions such as fibrocystic disease, abscess, or cancer develop. An association with urinary tract abnormalities has been reported. In one study, kidney and urinary tract malformations (e.g. adult polycystic kidney disease, unilateral renal agenesis, cystic renal dysplasia, familial renal cysts,

and congenital stenosis of the pyeloureteral joint) occurred in 7.5% of patients with polythelia versus 0.7% of controls. If an analysis of the urinary system is indicated, an ultrasound examination may be done.

One, two, or more lesions may occur. If two occur, they often appear on opposite sides at the same level (Fig. 19.12). There is an equal sex and side incidence. No treatment is needed. Simple excision may be done.

Wattle

Also known as cutaneous cervical tag, the wattle presents as a pedunculated, flesh-colored tag on the neck (Fig. 19.13). Onset is usually by 3 years of age. A branchial sinus may be associated. The wattle probably represents either ectopic auricular cartilage or a remnant of the branchial arch system. Simple excision may be done if no sinus or fistula is associated.

Absent fingerprints

Rarely, a person may be born without fingerprints (Fig. 19.14).

Midline sacral lesions
Clinical

Lipomas, sinus tract, pigmented lesions, tufts of hair (e.g. fawn tail nevus), and vascular patches are some of the congenital, sacral, cutaneous abnormalities that may be associated with an underlying spinal malformation (Fig. 19.15), also known as spinal dysraphism. Potential associations include tethered cord, spina bifida, and vertebral anomalies. In one study,

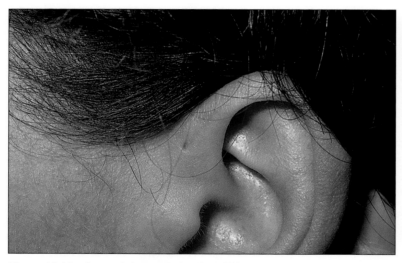

Figure 19.11 Congenital preauricular sinus. This preauricular hole most often ends blindly. The main risk it poses is secondary infection.

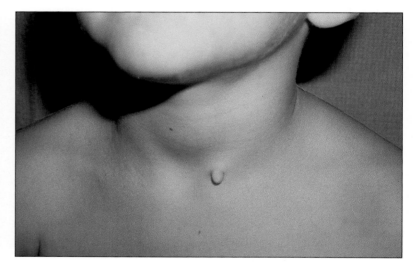

Figure 19.13 Wattle. (Courtesy of Tanya Forman, M.D.)

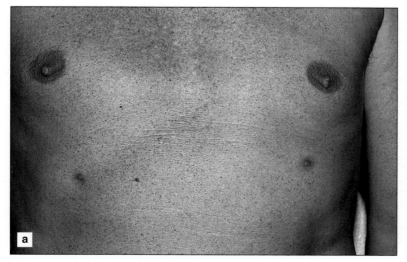

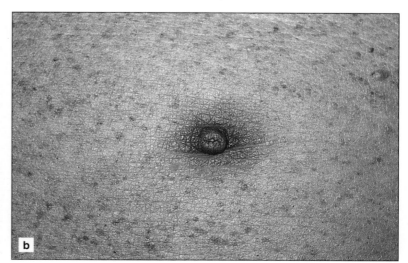

Figure 19.12 Accessory nipple. (**a**) Also known as polythelia, this lesion appears as a small, brown papule that may resemble a nipple. One, two (as shown), or more may occur. If two occur, they often appear on opposite sides at the same level. (**b**) Close-up view.

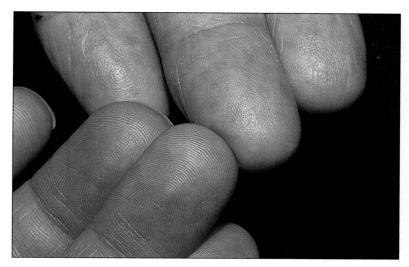

Figure 19.14 Absent fingerprints. This patient was on record with the FBI for being born without fingerprints (or so he said!).

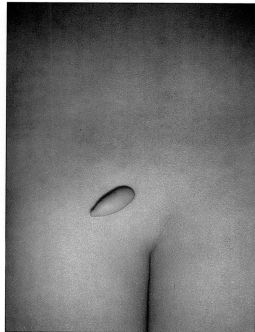

Figure 19.16 Embryonic tail. (Courtesy of Mary M. Dobry, M.D.)

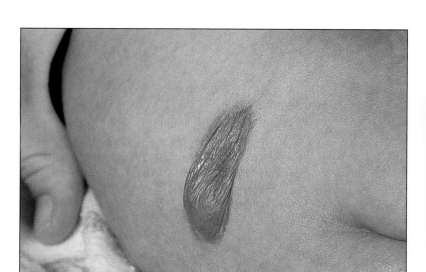

Figure 19.15 Meningomyelocele. (Courtesy of O. Dale Collins III, M.D., Ph.D.)

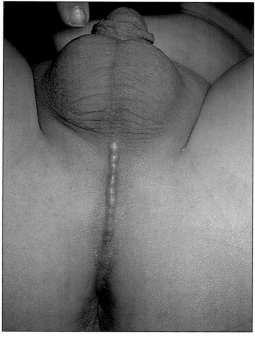

Figure 19.17 Multiple congenital milia or small epidermoid cysts along the raphe. (Courtesy of O. Dale Collins III, M.D., Ph.D.)

dimples or pits (defined as a depression whose base could not be visualized with or without traction) alone were not associated with an underlying abnormality. It appears that the presence of two or more lesions makes finding an underlying abnormality more likely.

If occult spinal dysraphism is suspected, magnetic resonance imaging (MRI) is the imaging method of choice. Plain radiographs may be negative. If a dermal sinus tract is not suspected, MRI may be delayed until 4 months of age to allow for better imaging. Until approximately 6 months of age, when the posterior vertebral elements ossify, ultrasound is an excellent screening tool. If plain radiographs and spinal ultrasound are unremarkable in an infant with a suspicious cutaneous sacral lesion who is otherwise normal, MRI may not be necessary.

Biopsy or surgical removal of a cutaneous midline lesion should not be attempted before a non-invasive work-up has been done.

Embryonic tail

A congenital, pedunculated, tail-like lesion attached to the sacrum is characteristic of a 'human tail' (Fig. 19.16). It may contain adipose, collagen, skeletal muscle fibers, blood vessels, and nerves, but it does not contain bone, cartilage, or spinal cord elements. Some reports have documented movement and contraction. Associated abnormalities are common, including spina bifida, meningocele, cleft palate, and skeletal defects.

After careful physical examination and radiographic imaging of the area, surgery may be done.

Median raphe cyst

There is a barely raised line or fold, termed the raphe, that runs along the midline from the urethra, along the penis, scrotum, and perineum to the anus, in a male. Congenital cysts that are found along this line are called median raphe cysts. These cysts are thought to arise as a fusion defect or entrapment phenomenon occurring during the embryonic development of the raphe. An asymptomatic (unless infected) cyst, which may form along the raphe from the glans to the anus, is characteristic. It may present with acute inflammation and enlargement at puberty or soon after due to infection with staphylococcus, *Neisseria gonorrhoeae*, or simple trauma from intercourse. Culture for gonorrhea should be done. Inquiry about penile discharge or other signs of sexually transmitted disease is appropriate. Multiple congenital milia along the median raphe have been reported (Fig. 19.17).

Simple surgical excision may be performed. Observation alone may be appropriate, with intervention anticipated if symptoms arise.

Nasal glioma

Etiology and pathogenesis

The nasal glioma (also known as nasal glial heterotopia) falls under the category of heterotopic brain tissue (Fig. 19.18). There is no connection with the central nervous system, in contrast to an encephalocele or meningocele, and thus nasal gliomas do not change size or shape as a result of crying or straining, nor do they distend with jugular vein compression (Furstenberg sign).

Clinical

A congenital, firm, non-transilluminating, blue or red nodule just lateral to the nasal root (extranasal glioma) is characteristic. It may also protrude from the nasal cavity (intranasal glioma) or be mixed. Some degree of nasal obstruction may occur.

Differential diagnosis

This includes other congenital nodules of the face, notably the following.
- Dermoid cyst—most common on the lateral eyebrow or temple.
- Hemangioma—usually red, softer, and more compressible.
- Tumors—for example rhabdomyoma (all rare, expand in size).

Treatment

Preoperative imaging and surgical excision by a neurosurgical specialist is recommended. Surgery should be performed in childhood to prevent the deforming effects on developing facial bones.

Dermoid cyst

Etiology and pathogenesis

The dermoid cyst is present at birth and is composed of epithelium and appendageal elements; it may contain bones, hair, or teeth.

Clinical

A round, subcutaneous, asymptomatic congenital nodule at the tail of the eyebrow (Fig. 19.19), periorbitally, or on the nose or scalp is characteristic. In a recent retrospective review of orbitofacial dermoids, those of the brow–frontotemporal region were the most common. In none of the 54 was there a bony attachment or transcranial communication. The second most common location was in the orbit. In this group of 21 orbital dermoids, none had an intracranial connection. However, of nine naso-glabellar dermoids included in the analysis, several showed an intracranial connection.

Preoperative MRI is recommended, although the yield for brow–frontotemporal lesions is low. An ophthalmologist should be consulted for orbital lesions.

Differential diagnosis

Lesions discussed in the differential diagnosis of nasal glioma should be considered.

Patients with a dermoid cyst may be referred at an older age with a diagnosis of epidermoid cyst, but the site, congenital nature, and lack of punctum should rapidly distinguish the two.

Treatment

Dermoids may be removed surgically. For isolated dermoids in the brow–frontotemporal region, simple excision may be done, although incision through the frontalis muscle is needed. After removal of lesions of the orbit, volume replacement may be needed for the larger lesions. Finally, those in the nasoglabellar region may show transcranial extension, and craniotomy may be needed.

Median nasal dermoid fistula

The median nasal dermoid fistula is a dermoid cyst with a connection to the surface. A midline pit or fistula, often with hairs emanating from it, on the dorsum of the nose is characteristic (Fig. 19.20). Sebaceous material may emanate spontaneously or on compression. The fistula communicates with a dermoid cyst, which usually occurs posterior to the nasal bones but may also occur in the nasal septum, ethmoid, or sphenoid bones, or attached to the dura. A firm, painless swelling may be noted anywhere from the glabella to the tip of the nose. Intermittent drainage, abscess formation, meningitis, or osteomyelitis may occur.

Surgical excision is recommended by a trained specialist able to remove the entire lesion.

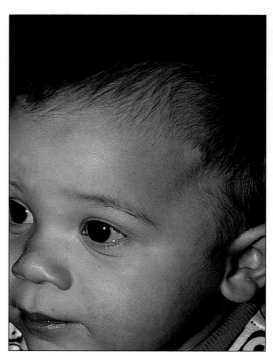

Figure 19.19 Dermoid cyst. This round, subcutaneous, asymptomatic, congenital nodule at the tail of the eyebrow was presumed to be a dermoid cyst.

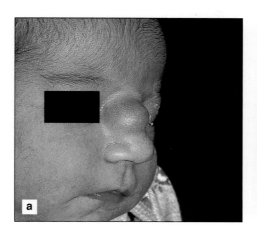

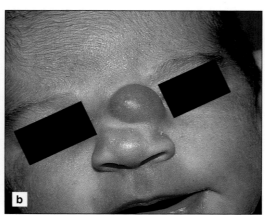

Figure 19.18 (**a,b**) Nasal glioma. The nasal glioma represents a congenital deposit of brain tissue. There is no connection with the central nervous system, in contrast to an encephalocele or meningocele.